Total Iron-Binding Capacity (TIBC):
300–360 μg/dl of serum
<300 μg/dl of elderly serum

Transferrin Saturation:
20–55% in serum

Erythropoietin (EPO):
5–36 mU/ml of serum

Glucose-6-Phosphate Dehydrogenase (G-6-PD):
10–14 U/g of hemoglobin

Erythrocyte Folate:
166–640 μg/l of whole blood

Vitamin B$_{12}$:
200–835 pg/ml of serum
1300 pg/ml of newborn serum
<200 pg/ml of elderly serum

Folate:
3–20 ng/ml of serum

Lead:
25 μg/dl of serum
>100 μg/dl of serum is toxic

Free Erythrocyte Protoporphyrin:
<35 mg/dl of whole blood
1.3–7 mg/dl in a 24-hr urine

Red Blood Cell Survival:
25–35 days (½ radioactivity gone)

Red Blood Cell Mass:
>0.36 ml/kg of male whole blood
>0.32 ml/kg of female whole blood

Plasma Volume:
44 mg/kg in average men; 43 mg/kg in average women
29 mg/kg in short, fat men; 27 mg/kg in short, fat women
46 ml/kg in tall, thin men; 41 mg/kg in tall, thin women

Thrombocyte Count (Platelet Count):
150–450 $\times$ 10^9/l
Average 8–20/100 $\times$ microscopic oil field
2–4 μ diameter

Thrombocyte Indices:
 Mean Platelet Volume (MPV):
 3–15 femtoliters (fl)
 Platelet Distribution Width (PDW):
 <20%

Capillary Fragility:
0–5 petechia as a result of the tourniquet test

Bleeding Time Test:
<10 minutes for bleeding to stop (varies by method)

Activated Partial Thromboplastin Time (APTT):
<35 seconds

Prothrombin Time (PT):
11–13 seconds
INR 2.0

Thrombin Time (TT):
17–25 seconds

Fibrinogen Level:
200–400 mg/dl

Fibrin Degradation Products (FDP):
(Fibrin Split Products [FSP])
<2 μg/dl providing a negative result

pH:
7.2–7.6 units, ideal 7.4 units in whole blood

Partial Pressure of Carbon Dioxide (Pco_2):
40 mmHg in arterial whole blood

BODY FLUID VALUES
Cerebrospinal Fluid (CSF):
0–5 mononuclear cells/μl for adults
0–10 mononuclear cells/μl for children

Serous Fluids:
<1000 white blood cells/μl of fluid
<10,000 red blood cells/μl of fluid

Exudates: Pleural Fluid, Pericardial Fluid, Peritoneal (Ascites) Fluid
Specific gravity >1.015
Total protein >3 g/dl
Leukocyte count is >1 $\times$ 10^9/l, > neutrophils
Erythrocyte count is >100 $\times$ 10^9/l

Transudates:
Specific gravity is <1.015
Total protein is <3 g/dl
Leukocyte count is <100 $\times$ 10^9/l, > mononuclear cells

Sperm Count:
20–250 $\times$ 10^6 sperm/ml of specimen

Synovial Fluid:
<2000 erythrocytes/μl of fluid
<200 leukocytes/μl:
 60% monocytes and macrophages
 30% lymphocytes
 10% neutrophils
⅓ total protein of the plasma value
fasting glucose within 10 mg/dl of plasma value

TEMPERATURES RELEVANT TO LIFE AND RESEARCH

Inactivation and Denaturization of Proteins, such as Complement and Coagulation Factors:
56° C for 30 minutes

Room Temperature:
25° C (Celsius)

Body Temperature:
37° C

Refrigerator Temperature:
4° C

Freezer Temperature:
−20° C

Deep Freeze Temperature:
−70° C

Dry Ice:
−100° C

Liquid Nitrogen Temperature:
−196° C (boiling point of this gas condensed to a liquid)

Fundamentals of
Clinical Hematology

Fundamentals of
Clinical
Hematology

Marcella Liffick Stevens, MA, MS, CLS(NCA), MT(ASCP)
Assistant Professor of Life Sciences
Clinical Laboratory Science Program Coordinator
Indiana State University
Terre Haute, Indiana

W.B. SAUNDERS COMPANY
A Division of Harcourt Brace & Company
Philadelphia London Toronto Montreal Sydney Tokyo

W.B. SAUNDERS COMPANY
A Division of Harcourt Brace & Company

The Curtis Center
Independence Square West
Philadelphia, Pennsylvania 19106

Library of Congress Cataloging-in-Publication Data

Fundamentals of clinical hematology / Marcella Liffick Stevens.—1st ed.

   p. cm.

   ISBN 0-7216-4177-6

   1. Hematology. 2. Blood—Diseases.
   [DNLM: 1. Blood Cells. 2. Hemostasis. 3. Hematopoiesis.
   4. Hematologic Diseases. 5. Body Fluids. WH 140 S485f 1997]

RB145.F862 1997
616.1'5—dc20

DNLM/DLC   96-16711

Fundamentals of Clinical Hematology   ISBN 0-7216-4177-6

Printed in the United States of America.

Last digit is the print number: 9   8   7   6   5   4   3   2   1

*This book is dedicated to
the laboratory practitioners who keep the faith.*

*The profession of clinical laboratory science
is crucial to the quality of health care but is yet
unknown to the people for whom we toil.*

In memory of

Becky (Elizabeth Ann) Burget
August 5, 1944–July 7, 1965

*who died of leukemia in 1965. She was my sister's best friend,
someone I admired and loved. On the day of her death I decided,
at age 13, to do something that would help people with leukemia;
thus, I became a clinical laboratory scientist/hematologist.*

Reviewers

Special thanks go to the following people who graciously reviewed various elements of this book.

Lorri Huffard, MS, MT(ASCP), SBB
Wytheville Community College
Wytheville, Virginia

Cynthia Martine, MT(ASCP), MEd
University of Texas Medical Branch at Galveston–School of Allied Health Sciences
Galveston, Texas

Joseph K. Semak, EdD, MT(ASCP)
Cleveland State Community College
Cleveland, Texas

Thomas B. Wiggers, BS, MS
University of Mississippi Medical Center
Jackson, Mississippi

Katherine Nisi Zell, MT(ASCP), SH, MEd, EdS
Brunswick College
Brunswick, Georgia

Preface

I have written this book, *Fundamentals of Clinical Hematology,* after working in hospital laboratories and after 20 years of teaching clinical laboratory science at both the 2-year level and the 4-year level. Over the years I have seen students become more and more harassed by life. The philosophy that I try to incorporate into my life and into this book is to keep life in perspective and to "enjoy" hematology instead of just struggling to learn the subject.

In order to facilitate the learning of a maximum amount of information in the minimum amount of time and effort, I have included as many learning features as I considered appropriate and possible. My goal was to produce a "student friendly" textbook that facilitates learning. The chapter outlines list the contents of the chapters, and the objectives state the learning outcomes or goals. "Do It Now" exercises are inserted periodically throughout the book. These exercises are used to encourage thought and application of the previously presented information. "Fast Facts" are included in every chapter (except Chapter 16) in an attempt to summarize the basic information. Special statements of significance are separated from the text by blue lines for emphasis. The primary information in each paragraph is printed in bold face to allow meaningful use of the text when there is little time to read an entire paragraph or chapter. Study questions conclude each chapter to provide a review and self-assessment tool. The comprehensive glossary, a shortcut to knowledge, contains more than just a brief definition in an effort to keep a unified understanding of each word or term. The bibliography is provided to offer additional reading to supplement the material in the book.

A central theme throughout the book is integration, collaboration, balance, and wholeness. Hematology is not isolated or independent of the other laboratory areas, likewise, the blood does not exist independent of the other parts of the patient's body. If the study of hematology (and of life in general) is approached with an attitude of adventure and challenge, with the student asking "What is it I need to know, and how does this relate to life?", this experience will be successful and rewarding—so please ENJOY!!!

Acknowledgments

No book is written alone. I would like to acknowledge and thank the following people:

My husband, **Randy Stevens, M.D.,** for showing me throughout our 22-year journey that I can make a difference and have a lot to offer others.

My daughter, **Ann Marie,** a beautiful person who is a constant source of encouragement for me to follow my heart and soul.

My son, **Chad,** whose awesome hugs, wit, and creativity have kept me balanced.

The rest of my family including my parents **Margaret and Warren Liffick,** my brother **Michael,** and especially my sisters **Mary Lou Eastep** and **Margaret Ann Reed** (deceased), for their unconditional love and support.

Randy's parents, **Dorothy and Jim Stevens,** who always step in when we need them.

Patricia Canfield, M.D., for providing her slide collection, professional advice, and personal support.

Hal Broxmeyer, PhD., for the excitement of hematopoietic research and taking the time to encourage me.

Sharon Bastian, who provided endless work and support without a complaint.

Ann Farese, a colleague and good friend who has demonstrated the application of CLS skills in hematopoietic research and given me a different perspective on life.

Tony Brentlinger, for helping me with the photography and also for keeping my spirit soaring.

Bunny Rodak, for having faith in me as a colleague and an author and encouraging me, by example, to keep my faith.

Linda Kasper, who never ceases to amaze me with her calm, quiet, caring persona, which provides needed wisdom and spurs others to pursue life.

Kathy Waller, PhD., my professional mentor and good friend, who has had a positive impact on my personal life and has cultivated my professional enthusiasm.

David Prentice, PhD., and **Jim Hughes, PhD.,** for providing computer consultation and for keeping me in touch with reality.

Cheryl Selvage, for reviewing my work from her knowledge and her heart.

Peter Doung, Ph.D., Eric Chaney, and the **Terre Haute Center for Medical Education,** for the use of their microscopy equipment, facilities, and expertise.

Roland Kohr, M.D., for providing microscope slides and review comments.

Union Hospital and **Terre Haute Medical Laboratory** for allowing photographs of the hospital and the laboratory to help tie it all together.

Selma Kaszczuk, who excited me about the possibility of sharing my knowledge through publishing.

Helaine Barron, for keeping me on track and teaching me what publishing is all about.

J. Bruce Francis, Ph.D., and **The Graduate School of America,** who presented new thoughts and opened new doors for me.

Melody Drake Spicklemire, M.D., who listened to me struggle through this, a month at a time.

Sherry Mangin and **Karla Zody, M.D.,** for insisting that I escape from the computer to meet with Lavinia.

Karen Childress, whose friendship, strength, and accomplishments are an inspiration to me.

My many friends and relatives not mentioned, who share their energy to encourage me and excite me regarding life and my profession—you know who you are!!!!

Brief Contents

STUDENT LEARNING GUIDE xxi

PART I: **INTRODUCTION TO FUNDAMENTAL CLINICAL HEMATOLOGY**

CHAPTER 1   **Basic Principles of Clinical Hematology** 5

CHAPTER 2   **Hematopoiesis** 35

PART II: **LEUKOCYTES**

CHAPTER 3   **Granulocytic Blood Cells** 53

CHAPTER 4   **Monocyte/Macrophage Blood Cells** 75

CHAPTER 5   **Lymphocytes and Plasma Cells** 87

CHAPTER 6   **Leukocyte Testing** 109

PART III: **ERYTHROCYTES**

CHAPTER 7   **Erythrocytic Blood Cells** 141

CHAPTER 8   **Hemoglobin** 159

CHAPTER 9   **Normal Responses and Diseases of Erythrocytes** 173

CHAPTER 10   **Erythrocyte Testing** 199

PART IV: **HEMOSTASIS**

CHAPTER 11   **Thrombocytes (Platelets) and Vasculature (Blood Vessels)** 229

CHAPTER 12   **Blood Coagulation and Fibrinolysis** 245

CHAPTER 13   **Hemostasis Testing** 259

xiii

PART V: BODY FLUIDS

CHAPTER 14   **Body Fluid Analysis**...283

CHAPTER 15   **Body Fluid Testing**..299

PART VI: CLINICAL LABORATORY PRACTICE

CHAPTER 16   **Correlation, Validation, Verification, and Considerations**..315

BIBLIOGRAPHY 321

COMPREHENSIVE GLOSSARY: A SHORT CUT TO KNOWLEDGE! 323

INDEX..369

Contents

STUDENT LEARNING GUIDE............................ xxi

PART I: **INTRODUCTION TO FUNDAMENTAL CLINICAL HEMATOLOGY**

CHAPTER 1   **Basic Principles of Clinical Hematology**.............. 5

Composition of Blood, 6
Terminology, Measurement, and Mathematics, 7
    Terminology, 7
    Measurement and Mathematics, 8
Basic Physiologic Concepts of Hematology, 15
    Homeostasis, 15
Phlebotomy, 17
    Preparation of the Patient, 17
    Equipment, 18
    Notes, 20
Microscopy, 23
    Peripheral Blood Smear Preparation, 24
    Hematology Stains, 26
    The Microscope, 27
    Microscope Components and Their Functions, 27
    Care and the Use of the Microscope, 28
    Calculation of Magnification, 29
Safety, 29
Quality Assurance, 30
The Practice of Clinical Laboratory Science, 31
Study Questions, 32

CHAPTER 2   **Hematopoiesis** 35

Fetal Hematopoiesis, 36
Pediatric and Adult Hematopoiesis, 36
    Bone Marrow, 36
    Whole Blood, 39
Blood Cell Proliferation and Differentiation, 39
    Scheme of Hematopoiesis, 39
    Cell Adhesion Molecules, 39
    Specific Growth of Factors and Differentiation of Cells, 39
Cellular Identification and Evaluation, 43
Bone Marrow, 44
Basic Cell Structure and Maturation Characteristics, 44
Study Questions, 47

PART II: LEUKOCYTES

CHAPTER 3   **Granulocytic Blood Cells** 53

Origin, Maturation, and Morphology of Granulocytes,   54
Neutrophils, 58
Eosinophils, 58
Basophils, 59
Physiology and Function of Granulocytes, 60
Normal Response and Diseases of Granulocytes, 62
Increased Neutrophil Count (Neutrophilia), 62
Decreased Neutrophil Count (Neutropenia), 68
Abnormal Neutrophil Function, 69
Anomalies, 70
Lupus Erythematosus Cell, 70
Increased Eosinophils (Eosinophilia), 71
Decreased Eosinophils (Eosinopenia), 72
Increased Basophils, 72
Study Questions, 73

CHAPTER 4   **Monocyte/Macrophage Blood Cells** 75
Origin, Maturation, and Morphology of Monocytes/Macrophages, 76
Physiology and Function of Monocytes/Macrophages, 77
Normal Response and Diseases of Monocytes/Macrophages, 80
Increased Monocytes (Monocytosis), 80
Decreased Monocytes (Monocytopenia), 82
Study Questions, 85

CHAPTER 5   **Lymphocytes and Plasma Cells** 87
Origin, Maturation, and Morphology of Lymphocytes and Plasma Cells, 88
Physiology and Function of Lymphocytes and Plasma Cells, 90
T Lymphocytes, 90
B Lymphocytes and Plasma Cells, 94
K Lymphocytes and NK Lymphocytes, 96
Normal Response and Diseases of Lymphocytes and Plasma Cells, 96
Increased Lymphocytes (Lymphocytosis), 97
Decreased Lymphocytes (Lymphocytopenia), 104
Malignant Lymphomas, 104
Study Questions, 107

CHAPTER 6   **Leukocyte Testing** 109
Leukocyte Counts, 110
Automated Complete Blood Count (CBC), 110
Manual Leukocyte Count, 114

Microscopic Leukocyte Evaluations, 119
   Leukocyte Differential and Peripheral Blood Smear
     Evaluation Procedure, 119
   Cytochemical Stains, 122
   Leukocyte (Neutrophil) Alkaline Phosphatase (LAP/NAP)
     Score, 123
   Arneth Count for Neutrophil Segmentation, 123
   Buffy Coat Preparation for Leukocyte Evaluation, 124
Special Leukocyte Tests, 124
White Blood Cell Function Tests, 125
Related Methodologies for Protein and Vitamin Identifica:
tion and Quantitation, 127
Study Questions, 136

PART III: **ERYTHROCYTES**

CHAPTER 7   **Erythrocytic Blood Cells** 141
Origin, Maturation, and Morphology of Erythrocytes, 142
Metabolism, Physiology, and Function of Erythrocytes, 150
Study Questions, 156

CHAPTER 8   **Hemoglobin** 159
Hemoglobin Structure, Synthesis, and Breakdown, 160
Hemoglobin Iron Kinetics, 163
Classification and Function of Hemoglobin, 165
Study Questions, 170

CHAPTER 9   **Normal Responses and Diseases of**
                  Erythrocytes 173
Physiologic Decreases in Erythrocyte Count, 174
Abnormal Decreases in Erythrocyte Count or Hemoglobin
(Anemia), 178
Physiologic Increases in Erythrocyte Count, 191
Abnormal Increases in Erythrocyte Count (Polycythemia
and Erythroleukemia), 194
Study Questions, 196

CHAPTER 10   **Erythrocyte Testing** 199
Complete Blood Count, 200
Hemoglobin and Hematocrit, 206
Microscopic Evaluation of Erythrocytes, 206
Special Erythrocyte Tests, 213
Study Questions, 223

PART IV: HEMOSTASIS

CHAPTER 11   **Thrombocytes (Platelets) and Vasculature (Blood Vessels)** 229
Origin, Maturation, and Morphology of Thrombocytes, 230
Physiology and Function of Thrombocytes and Vasculature, 233
Normal Responses and Diseases of Thrombocytes and Vasculature, 235
Study Questions, 242

CHAPTER 12   **Blood Coagulation and Fibrinolysis** 245
Coagulation and Fibrinolytic Proteins and Pathways, 246
Appropriate Coagulation and Fibrinolysis, 249
Inappropriate Coagulation and Fibrinolysis, 251
Study Questions, 255

CHAPTER 13   **Hemostasis Testing** 259
Vascular Testing and Evaluation, 260
Thrombocyte Testing and Evaluation, 261
Coagulation Testing and Evaluation, 268
Fibrinolysis Testing and Evaluation, 273
Study Questions, 276

PART V: BODY FLUIDS

CHAPTER 14   **Body Fluid Analysis** 283
Cerebrospinal Fluid, 284
Synovial Fluid (Joint), 288
Serous Fluids, 291
Urine Analysis and Miscellaneous Body Fluids, 294
Study Questions, 296

CHAPTER 15   **Body Fluid Testing** 299
Physical Characteristics of the Body Fluid, 300
Body Fluid Cell Counts, 301
Microscopic and Cytologic Evaluation of Body Fluids, 303
Chemical Analysis of Body Fluids, 306
Microbiologic and Immunologic Tests of Body Fluids, 307
Study Questions, 310

PART VI: CLINICAL LABORATORY PRACTICE

CHAPTER 16   **Correlation, Validation, Verification, and Considerations** 315

Correlation of Clinical Laboratory Results, 316
Validation of Fact Versus Fiction, 316
Documentation, Verification, and Dissemination, 318
Important Considerations of Clinical Hematology and
Clinical Laboratory Practice, 319
Study Questions, 320

BIBLIOGRAPHY 321

COMPREHENSIVE GLOSSARY: A SHORTCUT TO KNOWLEDGE! 323

INDEX 369

STUDENT LEARNING GUIDE

Dear Student:

My goal is to produce a "student friendly" textbook that makes learning as painless as possible. I have included as many learning features as I felt appropriate and possible and that I could talk the editors into including, so take advantage of these learning tools. This textbook can be your "personal hematology trainer," analogous to a fitness trainer, if you follow the suggestions and use the learning tools. These learning tools include: basic information in each paragraph written in **boldface** for your convenience; **"Do It Now"** exercises providing suggestions for discussion and application of the information; **"Fast Facts"** sheets summarizing the information; **"Study Questions"** for review and self-assessment of the information learned; **"Critical Thoughts"** emphasized by blue line separations; a **"Comprehensive Glossary"** to help clarify information; and repetition of information and figures throughout the book to facilitate learning and retention of information. As a personal hematology trainer, this textbook suggests how to make learning interesting to help you get in shape academically in order to reach your professional goals, in addition to any physical fitness goals.

If the study of hematology (and life in general) is approached with an attitude of adventure and challenge, with the student asking "What is it I need to know, and how does this relate to life?", it will be a successful and rewarding experience—so please ENJOY!!!

CONCEPT MAPPING

One learning tool not mentioned in the text but that can be applied throughout the entire text is **concept mapping.** Learning is boring and difficult if the information involves mere facts to memorize or concepts that do not seem relevant. Through concept mapping, the information in this book (and lifelong learning) is made meaningful by integrating the various topics, through concept mapping, collaborating with other individuals (e.g., students, faculty, friends), and balancing your life to achieve wholeness.

Concept mapping is a way of making links between the relevant useful knowledge that you already have and new knowledge being presented in this book. The **process of creating** the concept map is the learning experience—**not the finished map.** Your concept maps will change over time as you learn more and relate the new information to your previous knowledge, which is constantly growing and changing. Concept mapping is like brainstorming in which a topic (concept) is chosen and then you link it with all the relating topics (concepts) that you can think of and already know. This may help you to make connections that will keep the concepts and learning in perspective.

Also take advantage of the following features of this textbook that were written to be "student centered."

● OBJECTIVES are for use as study questions. If you can look at the objectives in the front of each chapter as questions to be answered, you will have studied the right material.

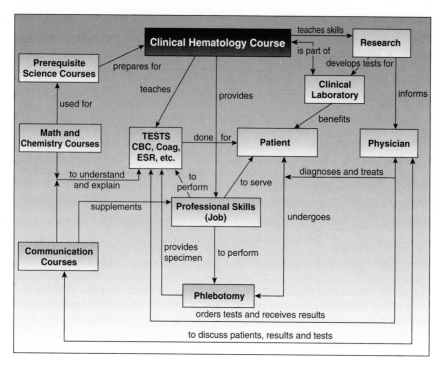

Using hematology as the starting point concept, here is an example of a concept map.

● BOLDFACE WORDS are designed to highlight the basic concept of each paragraph. Students highlight textbooks to emphasize the basic concepts and provide a method for rapid reading and review. This is already done for the student. If time does not allow the student to read every word of a paragraph, reading the boldface words provides quick information.

● SPECIAL EMPHASIS REMARKS are separated from the body of the text by blue lines to denote that this information is a "must learn" concept.

● DO IT NOW EXERCISES are suggestions for activity associated with the presented material to encourage student interaction and thinking about the information in other ways.

● FAST FACT SHEETS are dispersed throughout to serve as a summary of facts, figures, and associations described and discussed in each chapter.

● STUDY QUESTIONS provide samples for the students to demonstrate their knowledge and get some insight into future examination performance.

● TABLES AND FIGURES dispersed throughout the book depict visually what is presented in the text.

● COMPREHENSIVE GLOSSARY, a shortcut to knowledge, will serve as a quick reference. The glossary includes phrases as well as words, explanations, examples, and chapter references, all of which add to the usefulness.

● BIBLIOGRAPHY lists sources used in preparing this book for the student's further reading in areas of interest.

Good luck on this academic adventure.

Sincerely,

MARCELLA LIFFICK STEVENS

Introduction to Fundamental Clinical Hematology

In this part, the basic principles and foundations of the discipline of hematology are presented. To facilitate understanding of the material, there are objectives, key terms, and concepts presented in bold print; "Fast Fact" sheets are available to summarize and emphasize key information; "Do It Now" exercises are located after each section to apply what was presented; and study questions are included at the end of each chapter.

Hematology literally means the **study of blood.** The discipline of hematology is limited to the study of the formed elements (red blood cells, white blood cells, and platelets) and hemostasis (blood vessels and blood coagulation). The hematologist examines the **quantity (too many or too few)** of the blood components as well as the **quality (morphology and function)** of these components. In order to study the various aspects of blood, an understanding of the terminology, units of measurement, and basic physiologic concepts must be mastered. The information in this chapter will provide the foundation to an understanding of hematology.

CHAPTER 1

OUTLINE

Composition of Blood

Terminology, Measurement, and Mathematics
Terminology
Measurement and Mathematics

Basic Physiologic Concepts of Hematology
Homeostasis

Phlebotomy
Preparation of the Patient
Equipment
Notes

Microscopy
Peripheral Blood Smear Preparation
Hematology Stains
The Microscope
Microscope Components and Their Functions
Care and the Use of the Microscope
Calculation of Magnification

Safety

Quality Assurance

The Practice of Clinical Laboratory Science

Study Questions

Basic Principles of Clinical Hematology

OBJECTIVES

Upon completion of this chapter the student should be able to:

1. Identify or define the meaning of commonly used prefixes, suffixes, and stems in hematology vocabulary.

2. Write the various measurements used in hematology in both the conventional and standard international (SI) units.

3. Demonstrate application of the calculations used in hematology in various laboratory situations.

4. Apply basic physiologic concepts to clinical hematology practice.

5. Demonstrate knowledge of phlebotomy equipment and techniques.

6. Prepare acceptable stained peripheral blood smears and explain the parameters that determine the characteristics of the smear.

7. Demonstrate the proper use of a binocular light microscope.

8. Describe, define, and demonstrate the proper safety requirements in the laboratory, including Occupational Safety and Health Administration (OSHA), universal precautions (UP), personal protective equipment (PPE), material safety data sheets (MSDS), body substance isolation (BSI), isolation signs, safety equipment, and hazardous warning signs.

9. Explain quality assurance (QA) in terms of quality control (QC), Clinical Laboratory Improvement Act (CLIA), total quality management (TQM), and continuous quality improvement (CQI).

COMPOSITION OF BLOOD

Whole blood as it exists in the body consists of **erythrocytes** (i.e., red blood cells), **leukocytes** (i.e., white blood cells), **thrombocytes** (i.e., platelets), and **plasma** (i.e., fluid). When whole blood is taken from the body, prevented from clotting, and allowed to settle or to be centrifuged, the components settle out by density (Fig. 1–1). The erythrocytes are very heavy, primarily due to the oxygen-carrying protein, hemoglobin, and settle to the bottom of the tube. Erythrocytes make up approximately 45% of whole blood. The leukocytes settle out next, followed by the thrombocytes. The layer of leukocytes and thrombocytes together is called the **buffy coat,** and this layer makes up approximately 1% of whole blood. The plasma volume is approximately 54% of whole blood. **Plasma** consists of 90% water and 10% dissolved substances (solutes) such as proteins, nutrients, metabolites, various ions, and electrolytes necessary for body function. The various **solutes** in plasma, especially **fibrinogen protein,** result in a **slightly cloudy,** pale straw-yellow

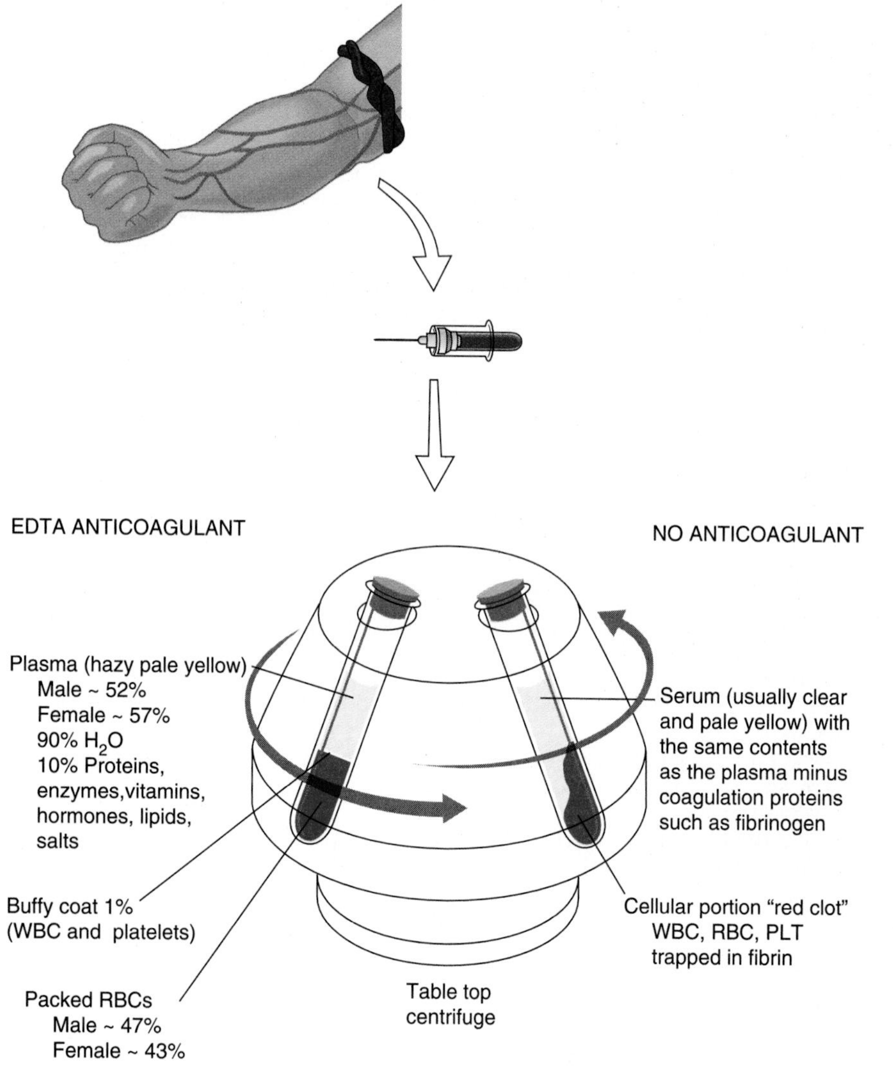

FIGURE 1–1
Blood from the circulatory system can be coagulated or anticoagulated and separated by centrifugation or sedimentation into the component parts. (EDTA = ethylenediaminetetraacetic acid; PLT = platelet; RBC = red blood cell; WBC = white blood cell.)

EDTA ANTICOAGULANT

NO ANTICOAGULANT

Plasma (hazy pale yellow)
Male ~ 52%
Female ~ 57%
90% H$_2$O
10% Proteins, enzymes,vitamins, hormones, lipids, salts

Serum (usually clear and pale yellow) with the same contents as the plasma minus coagulation proteins such as fibrinogen

Buffy coat 1% (WBC and platelets)

Cellular portion "red clot" WBC, RBC, PLT trapped in fibrin

Packed RBCs
Male ~ 47%
Female ~ 43%

Table top centrifuge

color. If **blood is allowed to clot,** it is no longer whole blood and the erythrocytes, leukocytes, and thrombocytes (formed elements) become trapped in strands of fibrin (converted fibrinogen) protein, which hold the clot together. The fluid expressed after centrifugation is **serum** instead of plasma, which is the fluid portion of whole blood. Due to the **lack of coagulation proteins, such as fibrinogen,** which are consumed in the blood clot, serum is a **clear,** straw-yellow color. This characteristic of serum, containing less protein, renders **serum the specimen of choice for most chemical laboratory analysis.**

Many factors may affect or alter the composition of blood. The **fluid portion** (plasma or serum) is a **balance of the nutrients, proteins, ions, salts, waste products, and water.** The percentage of **erythrocytes** is a result of their **production versus destruction** (i.e., death). The percentage of **buffy coat** is related directly to the **number of leukocytes** and to a lesser extent to the **number of thrombocytes.** The numbers of these components reflect their production or destruction.

Do It Now | Composition of Blood Exercises

1. Ask the instructor for a variety of blood specimens with a range of volumes of erythrocytes, plasma colors and consistencies, and buffy coat volumes (leukocyte counts).
2. Describe these specimens using the following criteria: Collection container and contents consisting of tube stopper color and additive; specimen obtained, which may be whole blood with plasma and cells or clotted blood with serum; characteristics of serum or plasma, which may be light or dark, clear, cloudy, or milky and straw, yellow, red, white, or other colors; proportion of components (e.g., percentages of fluid, erythrocytes, and buffy coat [leukocytes]), volume of blood.
3. Correlate the descriptions of each of these components for each of the specimens provided with a possible reason.

TERMINOLOGY, MEASUREMENT, AND MATHEMATICS

Terminology

Many of the hematology terms are proper names and must be learned as such. Many of the terms and concepts, however, are derived from Latin or Greek, and a basic knowledge of a variety of stems, prefixes, and suffixes will facilitate the understanding of most of the vocabulary encountered in hematology and clinical laboratory medicine. In order to avoid constant turning to the glossary or dictionary when beginning the study of hematology, the following prefixes, stems, suffixes, and terms associated with hematology, and essential to the study of blood, are listed in the following charts. These charts are only a sample of the most common vocabulary of hematology. A medical dictionary is recommended for clinical laboratory practice.

SOME STEMS, PREFIXES, AND SUFFIXES USED IN MEDICAL TERMINOLOGY

a = without
blast = young, nucleated
cyte = cell
chromatic, chromic = color
dys = abnormal
emia = blood
ferro = iron
hyper = more, increased
hypo = less, decreased
iso = equal to, same as
lympho = of the lymph
macro = large
mega = large
micro = small
myelo = marrow
normo = normal
oid = like
osis = increase
penia = decrease
plasia = formation
poiesis = cell production
poly = many
pro = before, previous
sidero, side = side
uria = urine

Benign = not life threatening
Colony-stimulating factor (-CSF) = a growth factor for a cell line, such as granulocytes (G-CSF)
Colony-forming unit (CFU) = the parent cell of a cell line
Cerebrospinal fluid (CSF) = fluid from the spinal column that is sterile and cell free
Cytokines = proteins secreted by cells that regulate other cells (there are specific cytokines: lymphokines and monokines)
Erythrocyte = red blood cell
Erythropoietin (EPO) = a hormone produced in the kidney in response to low O_2 which stimulates erythrocyte production by the bone marrow
Etiology = study of the cause of disease
Hematoma = a blood tumor, collection of blood clotted beneath the skin
Hypoxia = decreased oxygen
Interleukin = protein produced by one leukocyte, which acts on other leukocytes
Leukocyte = white blood cell
Malignant = life threatening
Necrotic = dead, no longer living
Neoplasm = new growth, of different cells
Phlebotomy = removing blood from a vein
Plasma = liquid portion of whole blood, cloudy
Palpate = feel by touch
Serum = liquid portion of clotted blood, clear
Thrombocyte = platelet (clot-forming cell fragment)

Do It Now Terminology Exercise

1. Make up your own terminology by matching stems, prefixes, and suffixes from the aforementioned terms. Present the new words to a classmate to define verbally.
2. List all the words you can think of that include the prefix "hyper" or "mega." Ask a classmate to do the same. Compare lists. Repeat this exercise with any part of a word.

Measurement and Mathematics

Mathematics of measurement is a constant aspect of hematology, as well as analysis of urine and other body fluids, and the microbiology area of the clinical laboratory. Very few concepts are unique to one area of the laboratory. This is why an understanding of the concepts and the application of laboratory mathe-matics is crucial in order to apply knowledge from one area of the laboratory to another successfully.

Size and Shape

The **size** and **shape** of a cell, a microorganism, or any biologic particle are important concepts associated with cell, microorganism, and particle **identification** and **evaluation.** In order to determine the size of a cell when looking through the microscope, the microscopic field or the size of surrounding elements must be known in order to assess an abnormal size and shape. The thrombocytes, the smallest of the formed elements, can be compared with erythrocytes in order to determine increased size. The erythrocytes can be compared with a small lymphocyte to determine increased or decreased size. The leukocytes can be compared with the erythrocytes in order to determine size. Cell size is expressed in micrometers (μm).

FORMED ELEMENT SIZES ARE:

Thrombocytes = 2–4 μm
Erythrocytes = 6–8 μm
Lymphocytes = 8–10 μm
Basophils = 8–10 μm
Neutrophils = 10–12 μm
Eosinophils = 10–15 μm
Monocytes = 10–15 μm

The aforementioned cell **sizes** are relevant for **microscopic evaluation** and morphologic point of reference. The cell **volume,** the variation in cell size, and sometimes the weight of the cell contents are also important in describing and learning about the **physical characteristics** of the formed elements of the blood.

Some diseases and disorders result in a change in cell size, or contents, and this can be calculated manually or by using the testing instrument and reported as an index of cell characteristics. The volume of the formed elements is expressed in femtoliters (fl), cubic micrometers (μm^3), or cubic millimeters (mm^3). The number of cells of an abnormal size or the number of specific cells present is expressed as a percentage (%) of the cells involved. The weight of the contents of the cell is expressed in picograms (pg) or as a percentage (%). Erythrocytes and thrombocytes are evaluated **microscopically** by **size** and through cell counting **instrumentation** by **size and volume,** as provided by the erythrocyte indices and thrombocyte index in the following chart.

RED CELL INDICES AND PLATELET INDEX

Erythrocyte indices:

Mean corpuscular volume **(MCV)** = 80–95 fl
Mean corpuscular hemoglobin **(MCH)** = 26–34 pg
Mean corpuscular hemoglobin concentration
   (MCHC) = 32–36%
Red blood cell distribution width
   (RDW) = 11.5–14.5%

Thrombocyte index:

Mean platelet volume **(MPV)** = 7.0–10.0 fl

Comparison of the **observed microscopic** morphology with the **indices** allows a more **accurate interpretation** of the blood picture. The calculations and additional application of these measurements are presented in this chapter and in Chapters 10 and 13. The purpose here is to introduce the importance of knowing the size and volume of the particles or cells of interest and learning to compare various pieces of laboratory information in order to obtain the most accurate interpretation to present to the physician.

Measurements, such as the hemoglobin concentration, are addressed in the specific chapter covering the theory and methodology of each specific test. Values are presented in both conventional and standard international (SI) units. A list of clinical hematology reference values in both conventional and SI units is printed inside the textbook cover.

In any area of the clinical laboratory, there will be the requirement for calculations and proper recording and interpretation of numerical data. Many of the hematology calculations are universal, that is, they will also be required for the clinical chemistry laboratory, the immunohematology (blood bank) laboratory, the clinical microbiology, clinical immunology,

and special clinical laboratory areas. For this reason, the knowledge of the use of the calculation is much more important than is the calculation itself.

Many textbooks provide the formulas, but the appropriate use, application, and interpretation of the data require a knowledgeable laboratory practitioner. Don't just memorize!

Manual Cell Counts

The important aspect of reporting cell counts, or any value in the clinical laboratory, is the **consistency and relevance to reference values.** Every laboratory performs cell counts on a different instrument and has its own procedure and protocol that will determine the reference values, abnormal indicators, and interpretation of the information generated. The physician, nurse, or other health practitioner receiving the reported values must be able to determine immediately the relationship of the reported value and the reference value. If these values are not presented in the same units or same exponents, they become confusing and meaningless for patient care. The various options for reporting values presented here can be utilized equally well. The individual institution must decide which one will be used and conform all reports to this method of presentation.

VALUES

**Thrombocyte and Leukocyte Counts
Are Reported As:**

The number of cells counted $\times 10^3/mm^3$
The number of cells counted $\times 10^3/\mu l$
The number of cells counted $\times 10^9/l$

Erythrocyte Counts Are Reported As:

The number of cells counted $\times 10^6/mm^3$
The number of cells counted $\times 10^6/\mu l$
The number of cells counted $\times 10^{12}/l$

An example of the application of a calculation is when cells are counted manually using a hemocytometer and microscope. This procedure and a picture of a hemocytometer are shown in Chapter 6. Manual cell counts using a hemocytometer utilize the following formula to determine cell number:

$$\frac{\text{Number of cells counted}^a}{\text{Number of large (1-mm) squares}^b}$$
$$\times \text{ depth}^c \text{ factor (10)} \times \text{ dilution}^d \text{ factor}$$
$$= \text{cells} \times 10^?/\text{mm}^3 \times 10^?/\text{l (or } /\mu\text{l)}$$

If a blood specimen was diluted $1:20^d$ and 200^a cells were counted in four large squares,[b] the calculation is as follows:

$$\frac{200^a}{4^b} \times 10^c \times 20^d = 10,000 = 10.0 \times 10^3/\text{mm}^3$$
$$\text{or } 10.0 \times 10^3/\mu\text{l or } 10.0 \times 10^9/\text{l}$$

Relative and Absolute Cell Counts

A relative versus an absolute cell count refers to the relationship of the component of interest to other blood components within the peripheral blood. Examples are: A **relative** lymphocytosis is an **increase in the percentage** of lymphocytes (60% instead of the usual 30%) in relation to the other cells seen in the peripheral blood with the **total cell count** remaining in the **normal** reference range. An **absolute** lymphocytosis would be seen when the total **cell count** is **increased** along with a **percentage increase** in lymphocytes. The absolute cell count is indicative of a true increase of a specific cell and is very important information to assist the physician in making a diagnosis.

The percentage of lymphocytes in the peripheral blood times the total leukocyte count is equal to the absolute lymphocyte count or:

% Lymphocytes × total leukocyte count
= absolute lymphocyte count

A **relative polycythemia** (proportional increase in erythrocyte mass) is observed when

---

[a] Any particle can be enumerated by this method. See Chapter 6 for specific details of how to count using the hemocytometer.

[b] Any area of the hemocytometer can be used for a count. The major factors determining which area is used are the need for **precision** (ability to duplicate) and **accuracy** (closeness to the true value) in the result. Precision and accuracy are dependent on a **random distribution.** If the count is very low as seen in body fluid counts, all nine squares may be counted. If the count is in the leukocyte range, the four large corner squares are counted. Thrombocytes have the next highest value, and one large square will provide an adequate sample for a count. When the count is high, such as is seen with erythrocytes and sperm counts, only one twenty fifth of one large square is counted.

[c] The hemocytometer is divided into 1-mm squares but is only 0.1-mm deep. In order to report cubic millimeters (mm³), the number of particles counted must be multiplied by 10 to achieve the same number present if the chamber were 1-mm deep instead of 0.1-mm deep.

[d] The dilution factor is determined by the procedure used. See Chapter 6 for specific details of diluting manual cell counts.

[?] The power of 10 appropriate to report an acceptable result for the cells or particles counted.

FAST FACTS

Basic Principles of Clinical Hematology

The composition of whole blood is 55% fluid (plasma), 1% leukocytes and thrombocytes (buffy coat), and 44% erythrocytes.

The composition of clotted blood is 55% fluid (serum), 45% clot containing erythrocytes, leukocytes, thrombocytes, and fibrin protein strands holding it together.

The size of platelets is 2 to 4μm, erythrocytes 6 to 8μm, and leukocytes 8 to 20μm, judged relative to a known structure in a microscopic field.

The shape of platelets (disk-shaped), erythrocytes (biconcave), and leukocytes (round).

Do It Now Measurement and Mathematics

1. The size and shape of a cell can be described using the *diameter, width,* and *volume.* List the units that can be used for each of these measurements.
2. A specimen of cerebrospinal fluid (CSF) is received in the laboratory. A manual hemocytometer count is done. There are 44 cells counted in four large (1 mm²) squares and the CSF fluid is diluted 1:10. What is the total leukocyte count in liters?

Do It Now Relative Versus Absolute Interpretation of Data

1. A patient sample had a leukocyte count of $8.0 \times 10^3/l$ (reference $5-10.0 \times 10^3/l$). The peripheral blood smear differential demonstrated 73% (reference 30–60%) lymphocytes and 26% neutrophils (reference = 40–70%). Is this a relative or absolute lymphocytosis?
2. A 4-year-old boy was admitted to the hospital with severe vomiting and diarrhea. The child's hematocrit (Hct) was 73%. One hour after the intravenous saline was administered, the Hct returned to normal (36%). Is this a relative polycythemia or an absolute polycythemia? Why?

the amount of fluid (plasma) portion of the blood is decreased. When testing is done, it appears as if the number of erythrocytes is increased, when in fact this is the same number of erythrocytes appearing increased due to the decrease in the fluid component. An **absolute polycythemia** occurs when the number of erythrocytes is actually increased (Fig. 1–2).

Hemoglobin Determinations

Hemoglobin determinations are discussed in Chapter 8 and presented in more detail in Chapter 10. This presentation relates only to the mathematics and reporting consistency involved in hemoglobin data. Hemoglobin values are reported as grams per deciliter (g/dl), such as 12.0 g/dl. The hemoglobin concentration is calculated by most automated instruments and is presented with one place to the right of the decimal. The **consistency of values** is important to **decrease clerical error and misinterpretation of results** by the clinician. The laboratory values and reference values should be reported in the same decimals, units, and format.

If a manual procedure is used, the hemoglobin concentration can be determined by using a standard line or a K value. Hemoglobin is measured by changing the hemoglobin to a colored substance that directly relates the con-

centration to the light absorbance (ABS) at a specific wavelength. The law forming the mathematical basis for colorimetric procedures, such as determination of hemoglobin concentration, is called **Beer's law.** This law states that a **relationship** can be made between the **light ABS of a colored solution** and the **concentration** of the colored substance. A standard line is made by using a known standard, in the procedure, diluted to various dilutions and making a graph by plotting ABS on the horizontal axis and hemoglobin concentration on the vertical axis. The unknown specimen ABS can then be read off of the standard line (Fig. 1–3). The use of a standard line is not limited to hemoglobin determinations. Many chemistry tests are also colorimetric procedures. Most procedures can produce a standard line from the known standards, and the unknowns can be determined from this line. Instruments utilized in the laboratories will perform the calculations and provide an acceptable result.

Another method to determine the hemoglobin (or any spectrophotometric color determi-

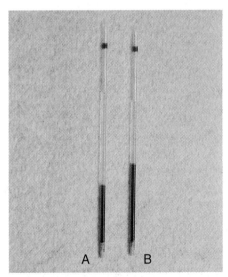

FIGURE 1–2
Microhematocrit tubes demonstrating a difference in packed red blood cell volume. Centrifuged blood allows the comparison of cells to plasma for evaluation of packed cell volume and hematocrit for diagnosis of anemia or polycythemia. *A,* Normal to slightly increased proportion of whole blood fluid (plasma, 52 to 57%) and red blood cells (43 to 47%). *B,* Decreased proportion of fluid and increased proportion of red blood cells.

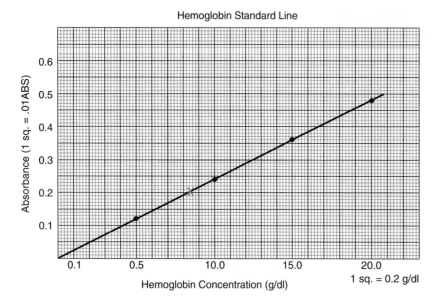

Unknown patient specimen ABS = 0.2
X reading from Hemoglobin Standard Line = 8.4 g/dl

FIGURE 1–3
The hemoglobin standard line produced from dilutions of a standard (known) solution in the test system used for the unknown specimen and plotted concentration versus light absorbance (ABS).

nation) concentration is to calculate a standard K value. A known standard is read, and the concentration is divided by the ABS, which gives the K value.

$$\frac{\text{Standard concentration}}{\text{ABS}} = \text{K value}$$

The unknown hemoglobin concentration is then determined by taking the ABS of the unknown multiplied by the K value.

ABS of an unknown test specimen
$\times$ K value = hemoglobin in g/dl

Hematocrit Determinations

Hematocrit determinations provide information relative to the percentage of erythrocytes in whole blood. Hematocrit determinations are reported as a whole number percentage (%) or a decimal in liters/liter (l/l), such as 36% or 0.36 l/l.

Erythrocyte and Thrombocyte Indices

Calculations on erythrocyte indices are presented in Chapter 10, and thrombocyte index calculations are presented in Chapter 13. The purpose of discussing indices here is to relate the reporting of indices to other laboratory-generated results. It is important to understand the various units of measurement and how they are reported in an acceptable manner. Therefore, this section is about how to report results rather than how to perform the test described. **Indices** are calculations that depict the expected cellular morphology, which is important in diagnosis and treatment. These values **should correlate with the histograms and cell morphology** to indicate the cell sizes, shapes, and content, in order to facilitate the accurate assessment of the cells. This mathematical correlation with the cell morphology is used to ensure accuracy of results and to provide additional information to the health care provider. The following chart contains terminology and units used for reporting the indices.

TERMINOLOGY AND UNITS USED FOR REPORTING INDICES

Mean corpuscular volume **MCV** in femtoliters (volume)

Mean corpuscular hemoglobin **MCH** in picograms (weight)

Mean corpuscular hemoglobin concentration **MCHC** in percentage (weight per cell)

Red cell distribution width **RDW** in percentage

Mean platelet volume **MPV** in femtoliters

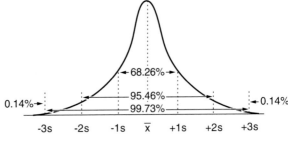

Gaussian Probability Curve

FIGURE 1–4

Chart of a normal gaussian curve. In the population, 95% falls within +1 standard deviation, and 99% falls within 2 standard deviations.

Quality Control Calculations

Quality control (QC) calculations are done to determine if: (1) the values generated from **known testing control** material fall **within acceptable limits,** and (2) the random **patient values are** as **accurate** as possible. The quality control calculations are used to assess the variation in values and the distribution of values within a laboratory. A **Levey-Jennings QC graph** (see Fig. 1–5) is used to plot laboratory QC results. The numerical result is plotted on the vertical axis, and the time is plotted on the horizontal axis. Within the chart, the solid center line represents the mean value, and the broken lines represent the control limits (range of acceptable values). The control limits are set at ±2 or 3* **standard deviations** (SD) from the mean. Of the population, 95% will fall within ±2 SD* and 99% within 3 SD in a normal **gaussian distribution** (Fig. 1–4). Plotting values on a regular basis will detect changes and out-of-control results as shown in Fig. 1–5. Graph A demonstrates random normal values with one error, outside of −2 SD, that may be caused by a practitioner's erratic pipetting or other causes. Graphs B and C demonstrate systematic errors due to a change in the reagent, instrumentation, and so forth.

The **Westgard multirule technique** can be used to interpret control charts and to detect error. The rules are as follows:

1. Reject when one observation falls outside of ±3 SD.

2. Reject when two consecutive observations fall outside of ±2 SD.

3. Reject when one control observation in a run is greater than +2 SD and another is less than −2 SD.

4. Reject when four consecutive control observations are greater than the mean +1 SD or are less than the mean −1 SD.

5. Reject when 10 consecutive control observations are on one side of the mean.

The most common of these QC calculations are:

> x = observed value
> Σ = sum of
> n = number of determinations

The **mean** ($\bar{x}$) is the average value.

$$\bar{x} = \frac{\text{Sum of all the determinations}}{\text{Number of determinations}}$$

The mean, or average value within a population, is required to determine each laboratory's own reference ranges as well as to calculate the additional quality assurance values. The average value for a test at one hospital or clinic may differ from another hospital or clinic. The **values generated by one clinical laboratory facility are only relevant to the population serviced by that specific facility.** Numbers mean nothing if there is no relevant point of reference.

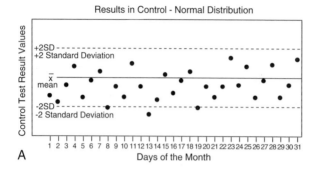

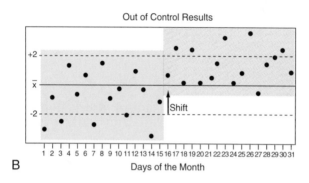

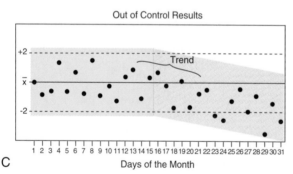

FIGURE 1–5

Levey-Jennings quality control charts demonstrating an abnormal distribution of results. *A*, Results are randomly distributed around the mean (average) value. *B*, Sudden change (shift) in testing. Results are all higher than normal. Must be investigated and corrected. *C*, Gradual change in test results. Values become lower than normal.

The **variance** (s^2) is the sum of squared deviations around the mean, divided by n − 1.

$$s^2 = \frac{**(\overline{x} - x)^2}{n - 1}$$

The **SD** is the square root of the variance.

$$SD = \sqrt{s^2} \text{ or } \sqrt{\frac{**(\overline{x} - x)^2}{n - 1}}$$

The **coefficient of variation** (CV) is relative (to the mean) SD.

$$CV = \frac{SD}{\overline{x}}$$

These calculations allow the laboratory to record, on a graph, values pertinent to precise and accurate test results. If the values are rising, falling, or erratic, steps can be taken to correct the problem with the procedure, reagents, instruments, or with the individual performing the test before the patient's results become erroneous.

Much of the **quality assurance** (QA) checks and balances are included in the computerized instrumentation. The **delta check** is an example of QA through correlation of more than one test result. If a count in the morning is 4000/mm³ and the count is 12,000/mm³ (>10% change) on an additional specimen drawn from the same individual, a delta check would be noted. The laboratory practitioner would address the delta check by repeating the test and by investigating any changes in the patient in order to resolve the discrepancy and to ensure accurate results. The most common cause of laboratory error is **clerical error,** due to the release of erroneous values or transcription or lack of correlation, **even when a test has been performed correctly.**

Do It Now Quality Control

1. Ask the instructor for a set of laboratory results for a specific test. Use these results to determine the mean, variance, SD, and CV.
2. Prepare a Levey-Jennings QC graph using the data from number 1. Analyze the data, and give an assessment.

BASIC PHYSIOLOGIC CONCEPTS OF HEMATOLOGY

Hematology involves determination of the number of formed elements, the correct morphology and function of the formed elements, the amount of coagulation proteins, and the correct function of coagulation proteins. All testing is done to determine the status within the patient's body, which is termed in vivo. Hematologic disease in vivo is caused by:

1. Not enough of a formed element or coagulation protein.
2. Too much of a formed element.
3. Adequate amount of the formed element or coagulation protein with abnormal function.

The laboratory must guard against changes that take place once the patient's specimen is taken from the body and placed in a glass or plastic container. The specimen in a container outside of a body is termed in vitro. In order to be relevant to the health of the individual or the disease process, the **laboratory values must reflect the in vivo values, not the in vitro changes** that have no bearing on the state of the individual specimen being tested.

Homeostasis

Homeostasis is the tendency of an organism such as the human body to move toward **stability** in the normal physiologic sense. This is done by maintaining the structures, the temperatures, and all the elements within the body to achieve a healthy balance. All aspects of clinical laboratory science involve evaluating and measuring this balance.

When a test is done in the laboratory, in vitro, it must be ascertained that the analytical results represent the body specimen values as they existed, in vivo, prior to collection. In order to ensure accurate results, blood and body fluids containing cellular elements require the following to truly reflect how they exist in the body:

1. **Osmotic concentration.** The cellular osmotic environment must remain isotonic, that is, maintain the same fluid or solute concentration as the body's environment. The normal concentration of fluids and cells within the body is equivalent to a 0.85% NaCl solution. Any diluent used to suspend cells must be isotonic. Some blood collection tubes contain salts or liquids that prevent the blood from clotting. The volume of additive, in the blood collection tube, is relative to a full tube of blood. If less than a full tube is drawn, the osmotic concentration may vary and the formed elements may be altered. If the cells are placed in a diluent that is **hypotonic** (i.e., containing more water and less solutes), water will pass into the cell and try to equalize or dilute the concentration within the cell to equal the exterior environment. This will cause the cell to become **swollen** (spherocytic) and burst. If the cells are exposed to **hypertonic** solutions (i.e., containing less water), they will lose water through the membrane into the diluent, resulting in a shriveling effect called **crenation**. Crenated and swollen cells are measured differently and behave differently in laboratory testing, generating erroneous results (Fig. 1–6).

2. **pH.** The pH of blood is determined by many factors, including respiration and metabolism. If an individual is not breathing properly, if the lungs are not functioning properly, if kidney problems exist, or if the individual's body is not metabolizing glucose properly, the blood pH may be altered. A normal blood pH for venous blood is 7.36 to 7.41 and 7.38 to 7.44 for arterial blood.

3. **Temperature.** Body temperature of **37° C** is the temperature at which metabolism is quite rapid to meet the needs and demands of the body. When blood is drawn from the body, the metabolism of the cells will continue in the test tube. If the specimen is not tested in a relatively short period of time, it should be refrigerated. The lower temperature (4° C) will slow down the metabolism and component degradation, which will keep the blood as close to the in vivo state as possible. A few special tests require the blood to be placed on ice immediately or to be kept warm (37° C) until testing. Most test protocols specify **room temperature (25° C) for testing.**

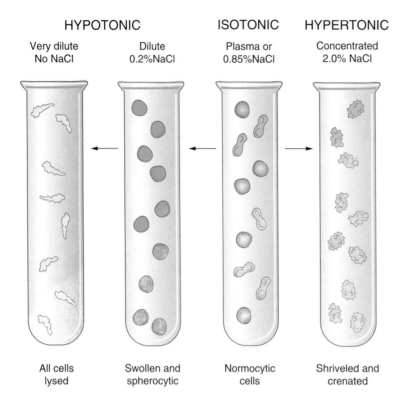

| HYPOTONIC | | ISOTONIC | HYPERTONIC |

| Very dilute No NaCl | Dilute 0.2%NaCl | Plasma or 0.85%NaCl | Concentrated 2.0% NaCl |

| All cells lysed | Swollen and spherocytic | Normocytic cells | Shriveled and crenated |

FIGURE 1-6
The effects of the osmotic microenvironment on cell morphology. Cells in a hypotonic diluent will become spherocytic and lyse; isotonic diluent will not be altered; hypertonic diluent will crenate (make scalloped or notched) and shrivel the cells.

If the test is done at an inappropriate temperature, the results will not be accurate. If blood is heated above 56° C, the cells will lyse and be destroyed. If blood is subjected to temperatures lower than 4° C, freezing and lysing of the cells may occur.

4. **Nutrients.** Blood cells require nutrients to remain viable until testing. Most routine testing is done within a few hours of blood collection. There are **enough nutrients** in the blood to sustain the blood for the routine testing time period, which is less than **4 hours.** After this time, the blood may remain viable, but changes will begin to take place. Testing over a prolonged period of time, or storage of units of blood for up to 35 days for transfusion, requires added nutrients to keep the cells viable. Glucose metabolism is a major source of energy. Glucose levels are measured as part of a routine chemistry profile. Accurate glucose levels depend on the diet prior to blood collection and the time in which the fluid portion of the blood remains in contact with the cells after blood collection. The cells will continue to metabolize the glucose, at the rate of 5% per hour, resulting in a lower glu-

cose value than is present in vivo. Heparin fluoride can be added to inhibit glycolysis. If bacteria are present in the specimen, they will utilize glucose also. The use of heparin fluoride will not affect bacterial glucose metabolism.

5. **Vitamins and Minerals.** Vitamins are required for normal body function; however, a few vitamins are more significant in relation to hematology. **Vitamin B$_{12}$** is necessary for normal **synthesis of deoxyribonucleic acid (DNA).** Abnormal DNA synthesis is observed in hematology by the appearance of large abnormal (megaloblastic) erythrocytes in the bone marrow and peripheral blood. The anemia associated with this deficiency is called pernicious anemia or vitamin B$_{12}$ deficiency anemia. **Vitamin C** is required **for normal blood vessel (vascular) integrity.** If an individual is deficient in vitamin C, small hemorrhagic spots (petechiae) will be seen as the blood vessels leak small amounts of blood under the skin. **Vitamin K** is essential for the production of **functional coagulation factors** in the liver. If an individual is vitamin K deficient or is taking warfarin sodium (Couma-

Do It Now Homeostasis

1. Prepare NaCl dilutions of 0%, 0.2%, 0.6%, 0.8%, 1.2%, and 2%. Prepare a 3% saline cell suspension from fresh whole blood. Place two drops of each NaCl solution on a slide, and add one drop of a 3% solution of erythrocytes. Cover with a glass coverslip, and let it stand in a moist chamber (Petri dish) for 5 minutes. Examine the slide under a microscope for changes in erythrocyte morphology.

din) (oral anticoagulant) or one of its derivatives, a lower level of coagulation factors will be produced and, therefore, less clotting will take place. A variety of minerals is necessary **for normal body function.** The most commonly known of these minerals are calcium **(Ca^{2+})** and iron **(Fe^{2+}).** Others include magnesium **(Mg^{2+}),** zinc **(Zn^{2+}),** and **iodine.** Calcium is a component of blood coagulation (clotting) as well as many other systems within the body. Several of the anticoagulants (ethylenediaminetetraacetic acid [EDTA], sodium citrate, sodium oxalate, and sodium fluoride) keep the blood from clotting by binding the calcium ions in the blood. Iron is necessary for erythrocyte formation. Lack of iron results in anemia. Overdoses of minerals may occur, due to storage in various organs of the body, and may be toxic. Tests to measure vitamin and mineral levels are performed in the clinical chemistry section of the laboratory.

PHLEBOTOMY

Phlebotomy literally means the cutting or wounding of a vein with a sharp instrument. In practice, phlebotomy is the entry of a vein with a needle to **obtain blood.** The art of phlebotomy requires specific knowledge of the blood vessel anatomy, equipment used, specific test requirements, proper patient identification, and personal relations including communication and ethics. The phlebotomist is the laboratory's major contact with the public by way of the patients, who are the clients and who require accurate, ethical, and personal treatment. The accuracy of the specimen drawn is critical. **If the correct specimen is not drawn on the correct individual, the laboratory results are meaningless.**

Preparation of the Patient

Approaching the patient is an important part of phlebotomy. The appropriate protocol involves a smile, a personal introduction, an explanation of the procedure to be done (in brief nontechnical terms), and any comforting or neutral conversation that you are comfortable carrying on while preparing for the procedure. Do not ask the individual how he or she is doing. This question will bring attention to his or her discomfort and involves confidential information. It may also take a while for the patient to explain how he or she is feeling. It is not appropriate to indicate the specific test associated with the specimen drawn. If this information is requested, please refer the patient to his or her physician.

Identifying the Patient

Proper identification of the patient is the most essential component of phlebotomy. The best identification is the **permanently attached arm band** on the hospital inpatient. This must **match the test request information exactly.** If one letter or number is different, a nurse or someone present should identify the patient and initial the request slip verifying this information. Never depend on the name above the bed or the patient's personal response. Patients are often sleepy or incoherent due to medication or illness and will respond inappropriately.

In outpatient, nursing home, or home health care settings, ask individuals to say and spell their name. If the individual is unable to do this, verify the identifying information with a health care worker or relative, being certain to note who identified the person.

Once the blood is drawn, the tubes must be properly labeled. The specimen identification and the request information must match identically, including the date, the time (military or A.M./P.M.), and the phlebotomist's initials.

Venipuncture Sites

The anatomic sites for routine venipuncture are the veins of the forearm as shown in Figures 1–7 and 1–8. The center vein (medial cephalic) of the nondominant arm is the best choice, if this vein is palpable. The center vein is anchored by joining veins on either side and by using the nondominant arm, the chance of use of the phlebotomized arm is decreased, resulting in less chance of a hematoma developing from bleeding. The vein chosen must be palpable (felt by touching). **Palpating a vein provides a wealth of necessary information.** The size, depth, direction, mobility, and wall thickness of the vein can all be estimated by accurate palpation. Vein palpation should be done using the forefinger of the opposite hand used for phlebotomy. Never use the thumb.

Equipment

Gloves

Gloves should be worn and either washed or discarded after each patient is drawn. Gloves are necessary to **protect against transfer of infection** from one patient to another as

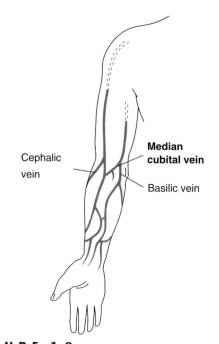

FIGURE 1–8

The median cubital vein is the best choice, followed by the cephalic vein and the basilic vein, which runs close to an artery.

well as to protect the phlebotomist from patient infections. There are many different types of gloves, the most common of which is latex. There are alternatives such as glove liners, protective hand creams, and alternative glove material.

Cleansing the Site

For routine phlebotomy, **70% isopropyl alcohol** is the cleanser of choice. Clean the area by wiping with alcohol in concentric circles from the inside out. Tests requiring alternative methods of cleansing are: blood cultures, which require a specific sterile Betadine technique, and blood alcohol tests, which require cleansing with an alcohol-free antiseptic. A few moments to allow the alcohol to dry will decrease the patient's sensitivity to entry of the needle.

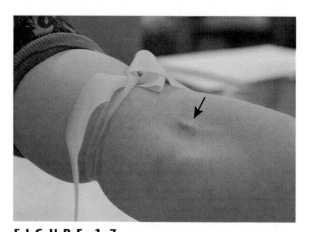

FIGURE 1–7

A forearm with prominent vein (*arrow*) due to pressure exerted by the application of a tourniquet.

Once the site has been cleaned, do not touch the clean site before venipuncture.

If additional palpation is required, cleanse the index finger with the same cleanser used on the vein and locate the vein. Enter the vein near the palpation point. This action eliminates any uncertainty of vein location, direction, or depth to ensure an accurate and successful venipuncture. A dry cotton swab or gauze must be available to place over the venipuncture site upon exiting the vein. If necessary, a Band-Aid can be applied.

Tourniquets

Tourniquets are used to give the veins prominence, which facilitates locating and entering the vein. A tourniquet must be applied to the arm approximately 2 inches above the elbow and should not be left on for more than 1 minute. Several types of tourniquets are available, two of which are shown in Figure 1–9. The Velcro tourniquet (A) is easily applied and removed; however, there is a specific range of arm sizes that will be suitable for this tourniquet. If the arm is too large or too small, an appropriate amount of pressure will not be applied. A second type of tourniquet is the latex band (B) or tube. This type is the most commonly used due to cost and versatility. The latex tourniquet is tied around the arm in such a way that it will not interfere with the phlebotomy and can be easily removed with one hand. Note that in Figure 1–7, the ends of the latex tourniquet have been pulled across the forearm and the bottom end is brought over the top end and tucked under to

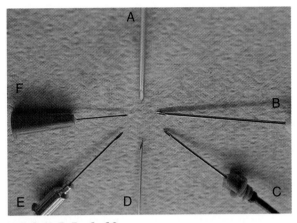

FIGURE 1–10
Various gauges and lengths of phlebotomy needles. Large gauge, A, to small gauge, F. Long (1½") needles, A and D. Shorter needles, C and E (1") and F (½").

secure. This allows the end which is tucked under to be pulled easily upward to remove the tourniquet.

A tourniquet should not be left on for more than 1 minute.

If left on the arm for more than 1 minute, **test values may be altered** due to the concentration of blood at the venipuncture site. The medial cephalic or medial cubital vein is the best choice for venipuncture. This vein is well anchored due to the location between the cephalic and basilic veins, which are the next best site choices. The basilic vein is the third choice because of the proximity to an artery.

Needles

Needles of a **20 or 21 gauge** (Fig. 1–10, B through F) are appropriate for routine phlebotomy. The larger the gauge, the smaller will be the diameter of the needle. If a larger-gauge needle is used, there is a risk of hemolyzing the erythrocytes as they are forced through such a small bore. Using a smaller-gauge needle may limit the choice to veins with a greater diameter than the needle. There are also various lengths of needles, selected by personal preference. The needle should be used with the slanted side (bevel) up (see Fig. 1–

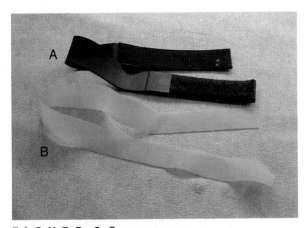

FIGURE 1–9
Velcro (A) and latex band (B) tourniquets.

10) and discarded immediately after the procedure into an appropriate sharps container.

Never re-cap the needle or lay it down.

Needle Holders

Needle holders are required for routine venipuncture with the vacuum tube technique. This technique requires that the needle be attached to a plastic needle holder (sometimes called a jacket) in which the tubes are inserted. The needle holders have various sizes and require a needle with the same method of attachment. As seen in Figure 1–11 (A–C), the needle holder **may require a threaded needle** (A) or a **bayonet-style needle** (B) that inserts and locks with a half-turn. Some needle holders are disposable and are available with protectors that cover the needle upon exit from the vein.

Vacuum Tubes

Vacuum tubes of various sizes and contents are available. Various phlebotomy tubes and their uses are shown in Table 1–1. The most commonly used blood collection vacuum tubes are shown in Figure 1–12. The specific **tube,** the **amount of blood** collected, the treatment of the blood in transit from the pa-

TABLE 1–1 PHLEBOTOMY TUBES

Tube Stopper Color	Contents	Use
Red	Nothing (silicon coated for uniform clotting)	Chemistry, blood bank
Pink	Clot accelerator	Blood bank, chemistry
Lavender	Ethylenediaminetetraacetic acid (EDTA)	Hematology, chemistry
Blue	Sodium citrate (9:1, blood:anticoagulant, must be full)	Coagulation tests
Green	Sodium heparin	Special tests: ammonia, lupus erythematosus preparation
Gray	Sodium fluoride	Glucose testing, inhibits utilization of glucose by cells
Light blue	Thrombin and soy bean trypsin	Fibrin degradation products test

Various special tubes are available for blood cultures, mineral-free testing, and other unusual tests.

tient to the laboratory (**well mixed** and maintained at the **proper temperature**), and the **identification** of the blood tube are all essential to obtain accurate test results.

If your specimen is not correct, none of the subsequent testing is meaningful.

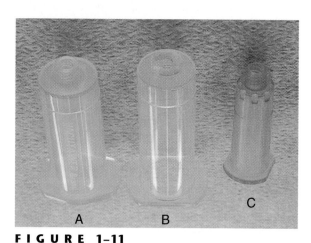

FIGURE 1–11
Various sizes of needle holders. Adult holders, *A* and *B.* Pediatric holder, *C.*

Notes

Upon completion of the phlebotomy, **apply pressure to the venipuncture site** by pressing on the cotton swab. **Invert anticoagulated tubes** several times in order to ensure adequate mixing. **Label all tubes** appropriately; check the venipuncture site; and determine if a Band-Aid is necessary or appropriate. Thank the patient and leave.

The **physical environment** should be returned to the way it was upon the phlebото-

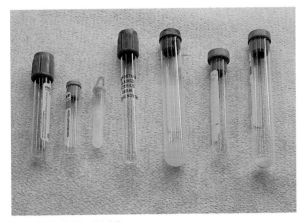

FIGURE 1–12
Vacuum blood collection tubes. The color of the stopper indicates additives or tube use listed in Table 1–1.

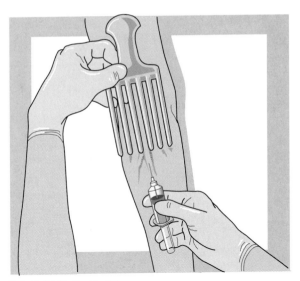

FIGURE 1–13
Hair pic method to immobilize veins. (From Bischof RD: Letter in "practical pointers." Consultant 32[4]:42, 1992.)

mist's entry into the room. All items brought into the patient's room should be taken out when the phlebotomist leaves. Never discard any items into the patient's waste containers. If it was necessary to move the patient's table or lower the side of the bed, these **items should be placed back in their original position before leaving.**

Confidentiality is an integral part of phlebotomy and laboratory medicine. Patients should be approached in a very friendly manner, and confidentiality is essential. The phlebotomist does not have the right to provide any medical information to the patient; he or she should be referred to the physician for explanations.

Never discuss a patient with anyone by name or other identifying information.

Often in **elderly patients** the veins are lying near the surface and are not well anchored. This makes entering the vein difficult due to the movement of the vein away from the needle point. This moving vein can be **anchored** by placing the **thumb below** the venipuncture site to hold the vein tight against the arm. The problem with this technique is the flattening of the vein, which increases the chances of complete puncture through both sides of the vein, resulting in excess bleeding. An alternative technique to

stabilize the vein requires the **prongs of a pic** placed on each side of the vein; this will keep the vein from moving while not affecting the round structure of the vein (Fig. 1–13). A phlebotomist should not attempt blood collection on the same individual more than twice during any one venipuncture event. A **syringe** or **winged needle apparatus** (Fig.

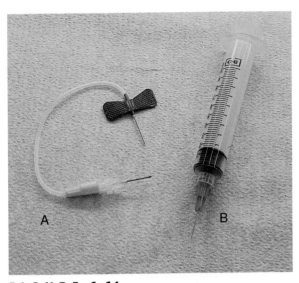

FIGURE 1–14
Winged needle apparatus (*A*) for use with vacuum blood drawing tubes and a syringe (*B*), both of which are used for difficult venipuncture.

TABLE 1–2   ADVANTAGES AND DISADVANTAGES OF THE ALTERNATIVE PHLEBOTOMY DEVICES

Syringe

Advantages:

1. *Controls the amount of vacuum* that is placed on the vein.
2. Basically the *same technique* as a vacuum tube procedure.
3. Ability to *distribute* the *blood between several tubes.*

   The routine vacuum tube systems contain a strong vacuum that may collapse the vein. The vacuum tube system draws blood into each tube until it is full; therefore, if you have a problem and only a portion of the required amount of blood is obtained, the entire volume of blood may be pulled into a single tube that may be inappropriate for the additional necessary testing. If blood drawn with a syringe must be distributed into vacuum tubes, the needle must be taken from the syringe and the appropriate vacuum tubes must be opened to allow the free flow of blood from the syringe into the tube. Entering the syringe needle into the closed vacuum tube will exert a great force of vacuum to draw the blood through the small needle, possibly damaging the erythrocytes. This may result in the need to re-draw blood from this patient, who was difficult to draw blood from initially.

Disadvantages:

1. More *expensive* than vacuum tube needles.
2. The amount of *blood drawn is limited* to the size of the syringe.
3. There is no anticoagulant in the syringe, therefore, a slow draw may result in *clotting* before transfer to an anticoagulated tube.

Winged Needle Apparatus

Advantages:

1. *Easy entry* into the vein.
2. Can be taped to the patient's arm to *avoid movement* and loss of blood flow.
3. Ability to draw blood *directly into vacuum tubes.*

Disadvantages:

1. *More expensive* than a syringe or vacuum tube needle.
2. The technique is not similar to that for using a vacuum tube or syringe and may seem *awkward.*

1–14) may facilitate blood collection if the patient has fragile surface veins, the patient is a child or is an adult with small veins, or an alternate site of venipuncture such as the hand or ankle must be used. Advantages and disadvantages of alternative phlebotomy devices are presented in Table 1–2.

Blood collection from newborns and infants requires a special technique. Lancets (Fig. 1–15) are used to access a blood supply in the foot of the newborn (Fig. 1–16) or the finger of an infant, child, or adult (Fig. 1–17). When performing a finger stick procedure, one of the center fingers that is used less should be chosen for the puncture to avoid constant irritation of the entry site. In order to obtain maximum flow of blood, a finger stick should be made across the fingerprint grain.

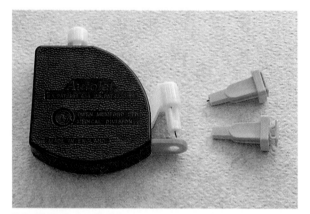

F I G U R E 1–15
Various lancet devices used for capillary blood collection.

Do It Now Phlebotomy

1. Ask one of your classmates to play the "patient." Perform a simulated phlebotomy, going through all the steps beginning with the introduction to and identification of the patient up to leaving the patient (without uncovering the needle and drawing blood). The "patient" should play the role and should not assume knowledge of any part of the process. This person should, however, be taking mental notes and critique your procedure upon completion. Switch places and repeat the scenario.

Another special procedure is the template **bleeding time test.** This procedure requires a special device that extends two lancets simultaneously into the forearm of a patient wearing a blood pressure cuff that is inflated

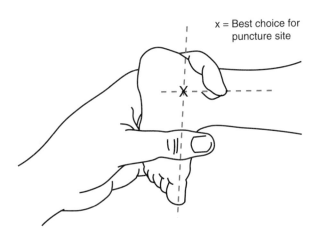

x = Best choice for puncture site

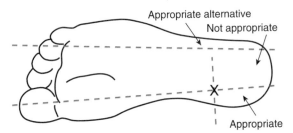

Appropriate alternative

Not appropriate

Appropriate

FIGURE 1-16
The richest capillary blood supply in the newborn foot is obtained from the point of intersection of a line from the big toe to the heel and a line from the ankle bone down to the bottom of the foot.

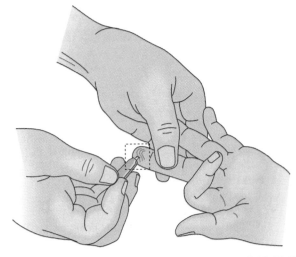

Finger Puncture Technique

- Choose the least used finger
- Cleanse the site
- Puncture across the grain of the skin

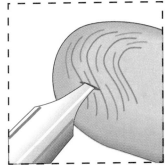

FIGURE 1-17
Appropriate skin puncture technique for an infant or an adult. The best blood flow requires a fast forceful incision that is *across the grain* of the fingerprint.

to 40 mm Hg. Once the incisions are made and the blood begins to flow, a stopwatch is started and the drops of blood are removed with filter paper. This procedure is provided in detail in Chapter 13.

MICROSCOPY

In order to evaluate or observe a specimen under the microscope, specific preparation is required. The correct size or number of objects must be considered. Objects that are too numerous, too few, too large, or too small are not suitable. Color enhancement through staining may also be required or helpful. The specimen preparation is a written procedure in

FAST FACTS

Phlebotomy

1. **Introduce yourself** and **identify the patient.** This is the most important step in specimen collection.
2. **Prepare the equipment.** Equipment consists of the needle, needle holder, tubes, alcohol swab, dry swab, and Band-Aid.
3. **Wash hands and wear gloves.** Wash hands and change gloves between each patient.
4. **Prepare the patient.** Situate the patient comfortably for both of you, and then explain the procedure.
5. **Apply a tourniquet.** Apply a tourniquet moderately tightly. *Do not* leave it on for more than 1 minute.
6. **Choose a vein.** The center vein is usually the best choice due to its size and stability.
7. **Cleanse the vein and enter.** Cleanse the area in concentric circles with 70% isopropyl alcohol.
8. **Obtain the required blood.** Anchor the needle and holder against the arm to maintain flow.
9. **Exit the vein and apply pressure.** Apply pressure to avoid bruising. Do not bend the arm.
10. **Discard the needle.** Discard the needle immediately in an appropriate sharps container.
11. **Invert the whole blood tubes** (anticoagulated). Invert six to eight times to avoid clotting.
12. **Label the specimen.** Before leaving the patient's bedside, ensure that all identification is correct.
13. **Check the patient** and **apply a Band-Aid if necessary.** Check to see if bleeding persists.
14. **Smile** and **bid farewell.** Be courteous, because this is part of public relations.

the laboratory manual. In hematology, the most common specimen is the prepared blood smear.

Peripheral Blood Smear Preparation

The best peripheral blood smear to reflect the in vivo condition of the patient is prepared at the bedside from blood, which remains in the needle after phlebotomy and does not come in contact with the anticoagulant or other additives. This technique, however, is not encouraged due to additional contaminated needle manipulation, which increases the risk of a needle stick. Peripheral blood smears are made from the anticoagulated specimen upon return to the laboratory. Several automated slide makers are available and have the advantage of making consistently reproducible slides. The manual method of slide preparation must continue to be available for instances in which the automated slide maker cannot be

used. The following techniques can be used to prepare an adequate blood smear.

Technique 1

Arrange several clean glass slides on a table. Place a drop of blood one quarter of the way from one end of the glass slide. Using another slide in a vertical (in approximately 15-degree angle) position, **back into the drop of blood,** allow the blood to spread evenly, and push the top slide **forward in a rapid even movement** to the end of the bottom slide. A smooth, fast motion is necessary for an adequate smear. The smear should stop approximately three quarters of the way from the point of application, ending in a macroscopically smooth feather edge of blood. Just inside this feathered edge of blood will be the monolayer of cells required for an accurate peripheral blood smear evaluation. If the smear is **too long, increase the angle** of the spreader slide or use less blood. If the smear is

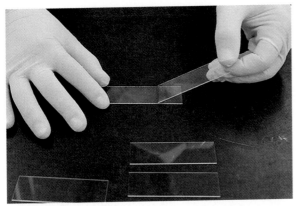

F I G U R E   1–18
Blood smear preparation technique 1. Place a drop of blood one quarter from the end and back the spreader slide into the drop.

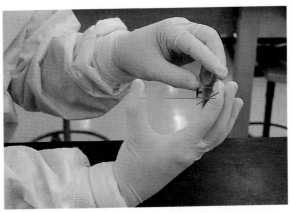

F I G U R E   1–20
Blood smear preparation technique 2. Place a drop of blood one quarter of the way from one end and back the slide into the drop.

too short, decrease the angle of the spreader slide or use more blood (Figs. 1–18 and 1–19).

Technique 2

Hold a clean glass slide with the thumb and forefinger of one hand, with the thumb facing toward you. Place a drop of blood one quarter of the way from the far end of the slide. Using a second glass slide, held horizontally (at ap-

proximately a 15-degree angle) with the thumb and forefinger of the other hand, **back into the drop of blood,** allow the blood to spread evenly, and **pull the spreader slide all the way toward you** (Figs. 1–20 and 1–21). A smooth, fast motion is necessary for an adequate smear. The smear should end approximately three quarters of the way from the point of application in a smooth, feathered edge of blood. If the smear is **too long, increase the angle of the spreader slide**

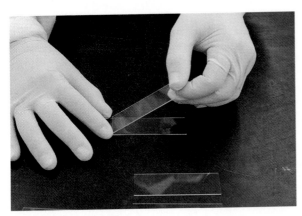

F I G U R E   1–19
Blood smear techique 1. Pushing the blood forward in a smooth, fast motion is necessary for an adequate smear.

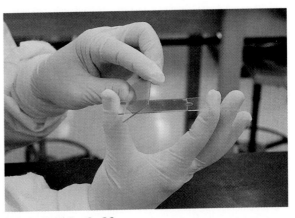

F I G U R E   1–21
Blood smear technique 2. Pulling the blood toward you in a smooth, fast motion is necessary for an adequate smear.

or use less blood. If the smear is **too short, decrease the angle** of the spreader slide or use more blood.

Hematology Stains

The **routine peripheral blood smear** is stained with a **polychrome (Romanowsky) stain,** such as **Wright-Giemsa** (Fig. 1–22). These stains require the cells to be fixed with methanol prior to immersion in the various stain components. Due to the fixation of the cells prior to staining, these are known as **nonvital stains.** The fixed cells in the blood smear are exposed to an orange **eosin (acid) dye,** which stains the *basic* components of the cell, such as the granules of the eosinophil and the hemoglobin of the red blood cell. After the eosin stain, the slide is exposed to a **methylene blue (basic) dye,** which stains the *acid* components of the cells such as the DNA and RNA. The pH of the stain must be 6.4 to 6.7 in order for the stain to appear accurately in the cell organelles. Another example of a nonvital stain utilized in hematology is the stain for siderotic (iron) granules called Prussian blue stain. Cytochemical stains are also used to demonstrate a specific component of a cell for identification purposes.

In addition to the polychrome Romanowsky type of blood smear stains, various **monochrome stains** are available to facilitate identification of specific cellular inclusions or contents. Some are applied to prepared peripheral blood and bone marrow smears, whereas oth-

ers are added to the blood while it is still viable. After the cells are stained, a slide is prepared. These stains are called **vital stains.** See Table 1–3 for examples of monochrome vital and nonvital stains.

Hematology Stains

1. A **hematology polychrome stain (Romanowsky stain)** is a slide stain of more than one color.
   a. **Methylene blue** is basic and stains *acid* components of cells, DNA, and RNA.
   b. **Eosin** is acid and stains *basic* components of the cells and some cytoplasmic organelles.
   Wright's, Giemsa, and **Wright-Giemsa** are the most common hematology polychrome stains.
2. A **hematology monochrome stain** is one color *specific* for one component of the cell.
   a. **Prussian blue** is an iron stain for prepared slides.
   b. A **vital stain** is added to viable cells before making a slide.
   Reticulocyte and **Heinz body stains** are vital monochrome stains.

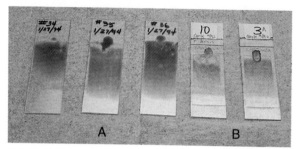

FIGURE 1–22
A, Unstained blood smears. *B,* Polychrome stained blood smears.

TABLE 1–3   HEMATOLOGY STAINS

Nonvital Polychrome Stain	Contents	Purpose of Stain
Romanowsky type; Wright, Giemsa, and Wright-Giemsa*	Methylene blue and eosin	Stain most cellular components
Vital Monochrome Stain	**Contents**	**Purpose of Stain**
Reticulocyte stain	Buffered methylene blue	Precipitates the RNA reticulum found in young erythrocytes
Heinz body stain	Brilliant cresyl green	Demonstrates denatured hemoglobin associated with G-6-PD deficiency
Nonvital Monochrome Stain	**Contents**	**Purpose of Stain**
Prussian blue stain	Potassium ferrocyanide Concentrated HCl Safranin counterstain	Demonstrates iron (Fe, hemosiderin) in peripheral erythrocytes, bone marrow histiocytes, and urine epithelial cells

* These stains vary in procedure, buffer, and dye concentration. G-6-PD = glucose-6-phosphate dehydrogenase; HCl = hydrochloric acid; RNA = ribonucleic acid.

The Microscope

Proper use and care of the microscope is an important aspect of the practice of hematology. Most hematology instrumentation is used to perform automated evaluations of the cells, including differentials; however, there is no substitution for microscopic evaluation of abnormal blood smears and random examination of normal smears to ensure instrument accuracy.

The light microscope is most commonly used in the hematology laboratory. The light microscope components are shown in Figure 1–23. In order to properly use the microscope, an **understanding of the function, use, and care** of each part of the microscope is essential.

Microscope Components and Their Functions

1. **Oculars**—lenses that adjust to the width of your eyes to allow the individual to see a full field of vision with both eyes open. The object viewed is **magnified 10×** by these lenses.

2. **Revolving nosepiece**—rotation of the objective lenses is done by rotating the nose-

piece until the desired lens is securely in place.

3. **Objective lenses**—these lenses range from a very low-power **scanning objective** to the oil immersion lens. The shorter scanning objective **(4 to 5×)** is used for large, gross specimens; the longer **low-power objective (10 to 15×)** is used for thinner and smaller specimens (e.g., peripheral blood smears) and for a clearer image of the gross specimen. Both the scanning objective and

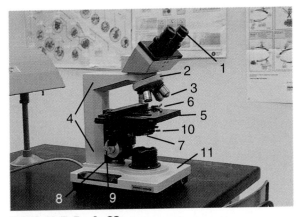

F I G U R E   1–23
The compound binocular light microscope. (1) Ocular, (2) revolving nosepiece, (3) objective lenses, (4) body tube, arm or neck, (5) stage, (6) glide stage, (7) substage condenser, (8) coarse adjustment, (9) fine adjustment, (10) iris diaphragm, (11) base.

low-power objective can be focused with the coarse adjustment control. The **high dry objective (40 to 45×)** is a little longer and is brought into **focus only with the fine adjustment** control. If the coarse adjustment is used, the objective may be driven through the specimen, thus damaging the objective lens and destroying the specimen. The **oil immersion objective (50 or 100×)** requires a **drop of oil** on the specimen to alter the light rays passing through the specimen to obtain better resolution for very small objects. **Only the fine adjustment control** can be used at this magnification.

4. **Body tube, arm,** or **neck**—a support for the head of the microscope. It is used to hold onto when transporting the microscope. The microscope should **never be carried by the neck alone!** Another hand should be placed underneath the base of the microscope.

5. **Stage**—a **stationary platform** on which the specimen is placed.

6. **Glide stage**—a mechanism used to secure and move the specimen on the stage.

7. **Substage condenser**—a lens that condenses the light from the bulb to pass through the hole in the stage and concentrate on the specimen. The angle and width of the light rays can be adjusted to best view each specimen by **raising or lowering the condenser** with the condenser knob. The adjustment of the condenser increases or decreases the contrast of the specimen.

8. **Coarse adjustment**—large movements of the stage are necessary on **lower-power objectives** (scan/4× and low/10×) to bring the specimen into focus. Always **observe from the side,** not through the oculars, when moving the stage and objectives toward one another with the coarse adjustment. Once the specimen and objectives are as close as they can be without touching, look **through the oculars** and move the specimen and the objectives **away from one another,** slowly, until the specimen comes into focus. The coarse adjustment is used only with the scanning objective and low-power objective.

Never use the coarse adjustment beyond the low/10× objective.

9. **Fine adjustment**—small, fine movements of the stage or objectives are necessary to bring the specimen into clear focus. The fine adjustment control should be adjusted to the mid-range of movement before focusing with the coarse adjustment. This allows a full range of use once the specimen is in focus on **high power (40×)** or **oil immersion (100×).**

10. **Iris diaphragm**—a mechanism to close off the amount of light passing through the stage and also the specimen. This may decrease the field of view.

11. **Base**—supports the microscope and contains the light source.

Care and Use of the Microscope

Care must be taken when transporting a microscope from the storage area to the work area to place one hand securely around the neck and another hand under the base. The microscope should be stored with the light off, the lenses clean, and the shortest objective in place on the revolving nosepiece. To properly use a binocular parfocal light microscope, the following procedure should be employed:

a. Place the specimen securely in the glide stage.

b. Turn on the light.

c. Adjust the oculars to fit your eye span to allow one clear field of vision. Note: do not allow eyelashes to touch the oculars. This may result in scratches on the lens.

d. Adjust the **fine focus control to mid-range.**

e. With the **10×-objective** in place, **observe from the side** as you bring the stage and low-power (or scan) objectives together, being careful not to touch the objective to the specimen. Note: 4×/scanning objective is used for large gross specimens only.

The 10× objective is observed from the side when moving toward the specimen.

---

f. Look through the oculars and slowly **move the stage** or objective **away** from one another until the specimen comes into focus.

Note: if the specimen is unstained, the substage condenser must be lowered to increase the contrast of the specimen structure. If the light is too great with the condenser up, no cells will be visible.

g. Adjust the substage **condenser** to provide optimum light to clearly see the specimen. An unstained specimen will usually require the condenser to be in a lower position that provides a greater contrast due to the angle of the light.

h. Move to the **high-power** objective (40×), and focus only with the **fine adjustment** control. The condenser may need to be adjusted at each level of magnification.

i. Rotate the nosepiece between the **high power** and the oil immersion objective, place a large drop of oil on the specimen directly over the opening in the stage, and turn the oil objective into the **drop of oil.** Focus only with the **fine adjustment.** Oil immersion requires that the condenser be in the uppermost position to allow maximum light to pass through the specimen in a small area.

j. View the specimen, making any **quantitative** or **qualitative evaluations** necessary.

k. Upon completion of the microscopic evaluation, **turn off the light,** immediately **turn** the nosepiece **to the shortest objective** (scan/5×), move the objectives and stage apart with the coarse adjustment control, remove the specimen, and clean all lenses of the microscope with **lens paper only** (any other material will scratch the lenses). **Cover** the microscope and **store** it in a safe place.

Calculation of Magnification

In order to determine total magnification, the magnification of the oculars (10×) must be multiplied by the objective magnification (10×, 40×, or 100×). If a specimen is evaluated using the high-power objective (40×), the specimen magnification is: 10× (oculars) × 40× (objective) = 400× total magnification. Some microscopes have the capability of adding additional lenses throughout the microscope to increase magnification.

Various specimens and procedures require a variety of microscopic techniques. Some additional types of microscopes and their uses are listed in Table 1–4.

TABLE 1–4 TYPES OF MICROSCOPES

Microscope	Use
Light microscope	Unstained and stained blood and bone marrow smears and cell counting
Phase contrast	Unstained specimen, such as urine sediments and platelet counts
Polarized	Urine sediments to visualize the crystal characteristics
Fluorescent	Fluorescent marker studies and fluorescent antibody tests
Transmission electron	Magnifies >100,000× to see organelles, viruses, and so forth, within a cell
Scanning electron	Magnifies >1000× to see the surface of cells, viruses, and so forth

There are other microscopes, such as the inverted and tunneling microscopes, which are not used in most clinical laboratories and, therefore, are not addressed.

SAFETY

The foremost safety issue of importance in the clinical laboratory is exposure to contagious diseases such as hepatitis and acquired immunodeficiency virus (AIDS). These diseases are spread by **bloodborne pathogens** that pose a high risk for the laboratory practitioner. The realization that apparently healthy individuals as well as patients with totally unrelated diag-

Do It Now Microscopy

1. Place a peripheral blood smear specimen on the microscope for evaluation. Beginning with the 10× objective, slowly move the condenser all the way up and all the way down to experience the change in visibility of the specimen in the various light contrast levels. Repeat this with the 4× and then the 100× oil immersion objective. What is the total magnification of the specimen under the 100× objective?
2. Calculate the total magnification for each objective on the microscope, which will be utilized in the classroom. Check your calculations with an instructor.

noses may be actively infected with hepatitis or with AIDS, as well as other organisms, has influenced safety practices. Today all laboratories must observe **universal precautions (UP),** which require that all blood and body fluid specimens be treated as if they were contaminated. UP specify the use of gloves, disposable or on-site laundered laboratory coats, appropriate containers for sharps, biohazard bags, goggles, face guards, fresh (less than 1 week old) 10% bleach on the hand for spills, and **no mouth or mucous membrane contact.** The safety attire worn is referred to as **personal protective equipment (PPE).** The practice of **body substance isolation (BSI)** is a more comprehensive approach that requires protective measures against all body specimens and exposure, not just to fluids. Following a protocol for personal protection is important to safety in the clinical laboratory and throughout any health care facility.

Each laboratory, although following the same basic safety mandates, will have their own protocol or system established to meet the safety requirements and needs. Each individual must demonstrate knowledge and familiarity with the safety environment with which he or she works.

Never touch objects from the laboratory or your hands to any mucous membranes, such as the mouth and eyes. If you must rub an eye or remove something from the mouth, remove gloves and wash hands first or use a sterile gauze. Never pipette by mouth!

Safety issues of concern in any work environment are mandated by the Occupational Safety Health Act of 1970, which established the **Occupational Safety and Health Administration (OSHA).** OSHA specifically requires safety devices, exits, and so forth. Each laboratory is also required to have comprehensive **Safety Manual and Material Safety Data Sheet (MSDS)** available for each chemical used in the laboratory. The MSDS provides instructions on storage, use, and emergency procedures.

Safety equipment and warning signs are essential in any work environment. Each student must be familiar with the **safety equip-**

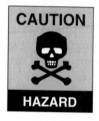 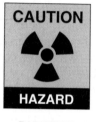 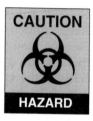

CHEMICAL RADIATION BIOLOGICAL

F I G U R E   1–24
These hazardous warning signs must be visibly posted in all areas associated with danger.

ment, warning signs (Fig. 1–24), and **safety manual.** Recognition and response to patient isolation precaution signs and procedures are also essential. If UP, protection against bloodborne pathogens, is the observed method of protection, isolation is needed for category or disease-specific infectious agents that are not bloodborne. Body substance isolation applies to all blood and body substances and eliminates isolation protocols, except for airborne diseases such as chickenpox, influenza, and tuberculosis. Each inpatient institution is required by the **Joint Commission for Accreditation of Healthcare Organization (JCAHO)** to establish an infection control committee and assign an individual as the epidemiologist or infection control practitioner (ICP). This individual is responsible for documenting and monitoring the infections, preventing new infections, and establishing appropriate infection control guidelines.

QUALITY ASSURANCE

QA is an all-encompassing term that is used to address the **accuracy, precision,** and **correlation of laboratory testing** as well

---

Do It Now Safety

1. Create an MSDS for something you work with on a daily basis.
2. Make flash cards with the safety abbreviations, precautions, and signs on one side and an explanation on the other side.

as the overall application of **quality to the personnel, environment, equipment, supplies, procedures, data presentation and interpretation, and personal relations.** QA is addressed and administered by the entire laboratory from the bench technician to the laboratory manager. The constant monitoring of quality is termed **continuous quality improvement (CQI)** and is practiced in most clinical laboratories. QA may be accomplished through **total quality management (TQM)** and involves all of the concepts listed above, including **QC,** which refers to a variety of controls and standards (known specimen results) within each system to ensure accuracy.

QA begins with patient or specimen identification. The most common cause of laboratory error is clerical error. The wrong specimen is drawn on the wrong patient, the specimen is labeled wrong, or the wrong values are recorded on the wrong patient. **If the specimen is incorrect, the identification is inaccurate, or the data are recorded in error, the test results are useless and may even hurt the patient.** Nurses and other health care professionals are now collecting many of the specimens, and the quality of these specimens may be unknown to the laboratory practitioner. The laboratory must examine the specimen and correlate results in order to, if possible, detect an inadequate specimen.

> It doesn't matter how well you perform a test—if the specimen or identification is incorrect, the test result is meaningless or even harmful.

Clinical laboratories are required to monitor the accuracy of their data by utilizing standards and controls on a regular basis and by undergoing competency testing periodically as part of their quality control. **Standards are specimens purchased with a known value,** such as a hemoglobin standard, to monitor the procedure and provide a comparison for unknown results. When this standard is measured in your test system, the value obtained must agree with the manufacturer's stated value to **ensure accuracy** of the pa-

tient's unknown results. Standards are also used to calibrate instrumentation and, in this setting, are referred to as calibrators. **Controls are prepared within the testing institution,** such as storing several cell count specimens at 4° C for 24 hours and performing the tests that were performed the day before. The same values should be obtained in order to support the continued accuracy of the test system. If the standard or control values are not accurate, corrective measures must be taken. Each laboratory will have a written protocol for solving problems such as this one.

> Every test performed in the clinical laboratory must have standards or control values to validate the unknown patient results.

Outside agencies may offer **proficiency testing (PT)** by providing a specimen with known values to be analyzed in your laboratory. Some agencies providing PT are state boards of health. This testing is required by the **Clinical Laboratory Improvement Act (CLIA)** and the **College of American Pathologists (CAP).**

Calculations used to determine the status of the quality control are the mean ($\bar{x}$), variance (s^2), standard deviation (SD), and coefficient of variation (CV). These are explained in the mathematics section of this chapter and are taught with more emphasis in clinical chemistry. These quality control values are recorded and often displayed as an ongoing wall chart. By displaying the daily values obtained over a period of time, any abnormal tendency may be detected. Accrediting agencies examine this recorded information and utilize this in the decision-making process to grant accreditation to an institution.

> The most common cause of laboratory error is clerical error, from the release of erroneous values, due to transcription error or lack of correlation of results. This clerical error results in ineffective health care even when a test has been performed correctly.

THE PRACTICE OF CLINICAL LABORATORY SCIENCE

The practice of clinical laboratory science requires the mastery of a specific body of knowledge, ability to perform specific skills, a knowledge of QA, a strong sense of teamwork, and good communication skills. The various disciplines of hematology, chemistry, microbiology, body fluids, and immunology, although unique, are integrated and must be seen as overlapping areas. In recent years the laboratory practice has been subject to tests moving out of the laboratory to alternative sites, **"managed care"** dictated by third party payers, which requires streamlining, collaboration, and cooperation of a variety of health care providers to deliver quality care in an efficient and least costly manner.

> The clinical laboratory scientist or clinical laboratory technician is no longer an isolated practitioner.

Today more and more testing is being done at the patient's bedside, in doctor's offices, or in the patient's home. This is called **"point of care" testing (POCT).** The laboratory practitioner must be prepared to work and communicate with individuals outside of the laboratory environment. This requires an adequate vocabulary, knowledge, and communication skills as well as the highest quality of clinical laboratory practice.

STUDY QUESTIONS

Choose the best answer:

1. A microcytic hypochromic erythrocyte would be:
   A. Small with less color
   B. Large with more color
   C. Small with more color
   D. Large with less color

2. Anemia due to aplasia would be:
   A. Due to overproduction
   B. Small erythrocytes due to lack of iron
   C. Lack of formation
   D. Due to loss of blood

3. After preparing a peripheral blood smear, fixing with methanol, and staining with Wright-Giemsa stain, the cells appear blue. What is the problem?
   A. Inappropriate fixation of the smear
   B. pH too basic
   C. pH too acidic
   D. Staining for too long a time in eosin stain

4. A clinical laboratory practitioner was preparing to wash some erythrocytes in a test tube. The plastic wash bottles in the laboratory usually contain 0.85% saline. The new laboratory assistant switched one of the saline bottles with a bottle of distilled water. The clinical laboratory practitioner didn't look at the label on the bottle and began washing the cells. What do you think happened?
   A. Nothing, the 0.85% NaCl solution (isotonic saline) is suspended in water anyway.
   B. Water is a hypotonic solution; the cells will become spherocytic and lyse.
   C. Water is a hypertonic solution and the cells will lose water and crenate (become scalloped and notched) and shrivel.

5. The blood collector (phlebotomist) had trouble getting a blood specimen, and the tube with the powdered form of the anticoagulant was only one-third full. This resulted in the anticoagulant dissolving in only one third of the amount of fluid portion of the blood as intended. This would affect the cells:
   A. By resulting in a hypertonic environment in which the osmotic pressure would force water from the cells and they would crenate.

   B. By resulting in a hypotonic environment in which the osmotic concentration would force the water into the cells rendering them spherocytic.

   C. Nothing would happen to the cells. The anticoagulant would have no effect on osmotic concentration of the blood.

Match the Following Situations with the Appropriate Use of the Microscope:

6. Unstained specimen

7. Stained specimen on 100× oil immersion

8. Large (gross) specimen, such as a worm

A. Increased light, raise condenser

B. Use the 4× (scan) objective

C. Decrease light, lower condenser

Choose the Best Answer:

9. A specimen is examined on a 15× objective with a 10× ocular. An additional 1.25× lens is in a camera that is used to photograph the specimen. When the picture is taken, what will be the total magnification of the photographed specimen?
   A. 150×

   B. 151.25×

   C. 187.5×

   D. 175×

Match the Following, Each Answer Is Used Only Once:

10. The organization that mandates and enforces a safe employment environment is

    _____.

11. One approach to guard against exposure to bloodborne pathogens is to treat specified body fluids (e.g., blood) as contaminated by following _____

    _____

12. One approach to protect oneself from bloodborne pathogens is to isolate oneself from all body specimens or substances, not just the fluids, which is the practice of _____
    A. BSI

    B. UP

    C. OSHA

    D. Organization of Safety and Health Advisory

13. Contrast and compare QA and QC. Be sure to address the method of administration and specific components of each.

    _____

    _____

    _____

    _____

O U T L I N E

Fetal Hematopoiesis

Pediatric and Adult Hematopoiesis
Bone Marrow
Whole Blood

Blood Cell Proliferation and Differentiation
Scheme of Hematopoiesis
Cell Adhesion Molecules
Specific Growth of Factors and Differentiation of Cells

Cellular Identification and Evaluation

Bone Marrow

Basic Cell Structure and Maturation Characteristics

Study Questions

Hematopoiesis

O B J E C T I V E S

Upon completion of this chapter the student should be able to:

1. Define hematopoiesis and terms associated with blood cell production.

2. Draw and label a diagram or explain the current concept of fetal hematopoiesis.

3. Compare and contrast pediatric and adult hematopoiesis with fetal hematopoiesis.

4. List and discuss the early hematopoietic cells and their regulators.

5. Compare and contrast proliferation and differentiation in terms of the cells involved and the changes that take place.

6. Demonstrate an understanding of the role of the bone marrow in hematopoiesis by determining the bone marrow involvement when given a hematopoietic situation (e.g., percentage of red bone marrow at age 70, changes in hematopoiesis due to a cancer infiltrating the bone marrow).

7. List the basic characteristics of cell maturation and, when given cell characteristics, determine the stage of maturation.

Hematopoiesis is the production of blood. Hematopoiesis results from a unique interaction of the pluripotent stem cells of the body, the microenvironment (stromal cells include fibroblasts, macrophages, endothelial cells, adipocytes/fat cells) in which hematopoiesis is taking place, and the growth factor or regulatory proteins (Fig. 2–1). These components of hematopoiesis work in a unique balance to produce normal healthy blood. This process takes place initially in the embryonic **yolk sac,** followed by the fetal **liver** and spleen, and hematopoiesis finally establishes within the **bone marrow,** where it continues to produce blood throughout life (Fig. 2–2). During a bone marrow transplant, the donor cells are administered to the patient through the peripheral blood. The hematopoietic stem cells migrate to the bone marrow, called homing, and locate in the microenvironment for proper development. If hematopoietic stem cells are transplanted into another area of the body, they will not develop due to a lack of the appropriate environmental influences. This explains why any alteration in this microenvironment due to genetic bone marrow cell abnormalities, radiation, toxic chemicals, or infiltration of the bone marrow with malignant cells will significantly affect hematopoiesis.

FETAL HEMATOPOIESIS

The yolk sac, located outside of the early developing embryo, is the first hematopoietic organ. This is described as **extramedullary hematopoiesis.** This refers to blood cell production outside of the bone marrow. Within the mesenchyme (cells of the mesodermic developmental layer) of the embryonic yolk sac the first primitive erythroblast, also called **hemocytoblast,** blood cells are produced. These primitive cells remain nucleated and exist intravascularly in **blood islands.**

The liver begins producing more definitive erythroblasts at approximately 6 weeks as the yolk sac decreases cell production. From 6 to 28 weeks of gestation the liver produces erythroblasts (nucleated erythrocytes), followed by granulocytes (leukocytes), and finally megakaryocytes (thrombocyte precursors). The erythro-

blast produced in the liver is capable of becoming anucleate, which allows more oxygen-carrying capacity and flexibility. The spleen also minimally contributes to hematopoiesis during this period of time. The liver continues to be the major (extramedullary) hematopoietic organ until about 7 months. As the liver hematopoiesis diminishes, the bone marrow hematopoiesis increases with a minor contribution from the lymph nodes.

At birth, the liver ceases to produce blood cells and **90%** of the bones of the body demonstrate **red marrow,** which indicates active production of blood cells. Over time, the demand for hematopoiesis is less and the bone marrow of the long bones becomes white marrow. **White marrow** is primarily adipose or fat tissue, which, under stress, is able to engage in hematopoiesis.

PEDIATRIC AND ADULT HEMATOPOIESIS

Bone Marrow

The bone marrow, as well as other organs, of the **newborn** is still developing and therefore **nucleated red blood cells (NRBC),** an **increased** amount of **lymphocytes,** and a **higher level of hemoglobin** may be seen. The **bilirubin level may** also **be slightly elevated** due to the inability of underdeveloped enzymes of the liver to break down the normal products of erythrocyte destruction. An increase in bilirubin may be indicated by a yellow (jaundiced) skin and membrane color. The enzymes that degrade bilirubin in the liver are not yet developed, and the infants are placed under a light source in the nursery that will break down the light-sensitive bilirubin without enzymes. The tests for bilirubin level and the liver enzyme levels used to investigate these alterations are performed in chemistry using fresh clear serum as the specimen. The infant hematopoiesis occurs in 80 to 90% of the bone marrow. The blood picture gradually moves toward the adult reference range. Figure 2–2 shows fetal hematopoiesis, including the hemoglobin changes within the

BONE MARROW MICROENVIRONMENT

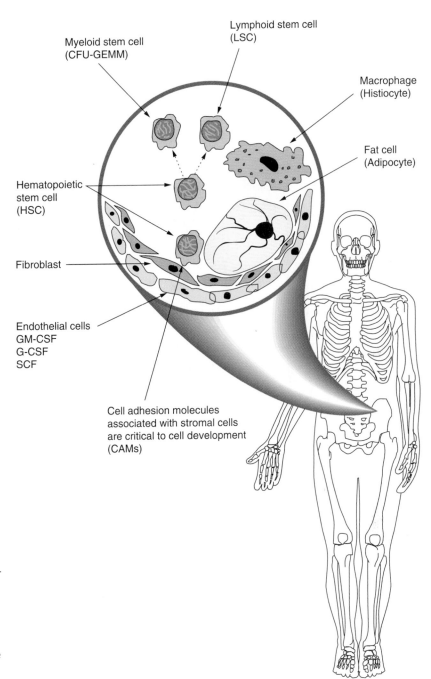

FIGURE 2–1

Bone marrow hematopoiesis. Adhesion to stromal cells (endothelial, fibroblast, adipose, and macrophage) and cytokines (proteins) produced by the stromal cells and accessory cells (macrophages, T lymphocytes) are essential for normal bone marrow cell development and maturation. (CFU-GEMM = colony forming unit: granulocyte, erythrocyte, monocyte, megakaryocyte; G-CSF = granulocyte colony stimulating factor; GM-CSF = granulocyte and monocyte CSF; SCF = stem cell factor.)

erythrocyte, which take place throughout hematopoiesis. This is covered in Chapter 8 within the hemoglobin presentation.

By age 20, approximately 60% of the bone marrow is actively producing cells as **red marrow.** The red marrow of the adult exists primarily in the large flat bones of the body. The site most often aspirated for bone marrow

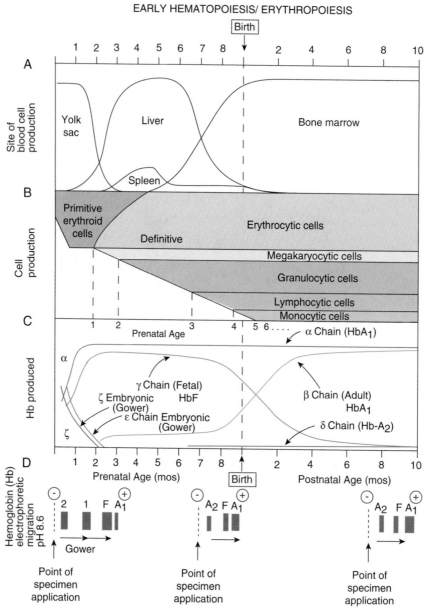

EARLY HEMATOPOIESIS/ ERYTHROPOIESIS

FIGURE 2-2

Fetal hematopoiesis. Beginning with yolk sac production, progressing to the liver as the primary fetal blood cell–producing organ, and converting to primarily bone marrow production by birth. The spleen and lymph nodes contribute minimally. (*A*) Leukocytes and hemoglobin are produced throughout fetal blood cell development. (*B* and *C*) Various hemoglobins are identified by their migration pattern on electrophoresis (*D*).

is the anterior or posterior iliac crest. If this area has been radiated or is not suitable for aspiration for any reason, the sternum is the alternative site for bone marrow aspiration. As age increases, the red marrow continues to be replaced by white (fatty) marrow. By **age 65, approximately only 40%** of the bone mar-row is still **actively producing blood cells.** There is evidence that the elderly have a re-duced response to the red blood cell growth hormone, resulting in a chronic normocytic anemia. An attempt is being made in research to determine if the elderly population have a consistently different reference range than do the pediatric and adult population. Newborns and children have demonstrated some variation in their reference range for laboratory tests. These **age-related reference values** are addressed in subsequent chapters.

Whole Blood

The average **adult body** contains approximately **6 liters (4 quarts)** of **blood.** This life-giving fluid is made up of approximately **45% formed elements** (erythrocytes, leukocytes, and thrombocytes) and **55% plasma.** The plasma consists of 90% water and 10% of various proteins, vitamins, nutrients, ions, and solutes. These proteins, vitamins, nutrients, ions, and other solutes are necessary for life or are the breakdown products of body processes that will be excreted through the renal system or gastrointestinal tract. The majority of the proteins present in plasma include albumin (a transport and osmotic-regulating protein), fibrinogen (a coagulation protein), and antibodies/immunoglobulins (part of the body's defense mechanism against disease). Other proteins include enzymes, hormones, growth factors, and coagulation factors, which are necessary to clot the blood when bleeding occurs. The bone marrow is constantly engaged in cell production to meet the body's needs as leukocytes are destroyed while fighting disease or die due to age, erythrocyte destruction or normal cell death occurs, and platelet utilization in coagulation or age-related death takes place.

BLOOD CELL PROLIFERATION AND DIFFERENTIATION

Scheme of Hematopoiesis

The scheme of hematopoiesis demonstrating the various cells and their major regulatory proteins is presented in Figure 2–3. The initial cell of blood origin is called the **pluripotent stem cell (PSC).** This cell makes up a significant percentage (approximately 10%) of the umbilical cord blood cells of a newborn and

less than 1% of the blood cells of an adult. This is the parent cell to a variety of cells within the body. Due to the enriched population of these PSCs, the cord blood is under investigation as an excellent source of cells for bone marrow transplantation. The **direction of development** and **differentiation** is determined by the protein factors that interact with the PSC. These factors can be stimulatory or inhibitory, and the cellular response to these factors depends on the presence of functional proteins and receptors on the cell that will allow the factor to bind to the cell and induce a reaction. One observation to explain hematopoietic regulation is the competition of protein regulatory factors (cytokines) for the stem cell receptors. The cytokine in highest concentration would bind an increased number of receptors and influence the direction of lineage-specific differentiation.

Cell Adhesion Molecules

Cell adhesion molecules (CAMs) located on various cells throughout the body influence and guide cells through development and function. Examples of these molecules are found in the bone marrow associated with the fibroblasts and endothelial cells and in the vasculature endothelial cells associated with lymphocyte movement out of the blood vessels.

Specific Growth of Factors and Differentiation of Cells

Specific **growth factors** such as stem cell factor (**SCF,** also known as *kit* ligand and the

Hematopoietic Chart of Cell Differentiation.

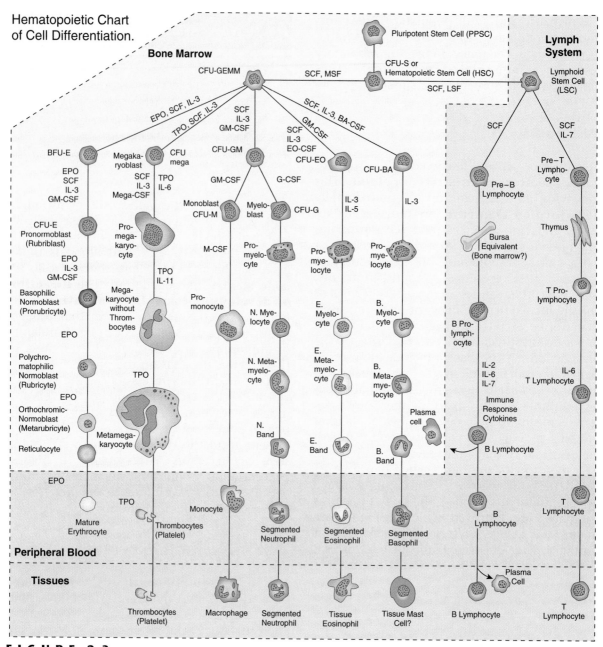

FIGURE 2–3

Scheme of hematopoiesis with regulators. All blood cells originate from the pluripotent stem cell (PPSC). The amount of proliferation and direction of differentiation is determined by cell-to-cell contact in the bone marrow microenvironment and the protein regulators (cytokines) produced in response to the body's needs.

Steel factor), interleukin-1 **(IL-1)**, 3 **(IL-3)**, and 6 **(IL-6)** influence the PSC to proliferate and differentiate into the **hematopoietic stem cell (HSC).** The HSC is destined to become only a blood cell and differentiates further into the specific lymphoid or myeloid (bone marrow) cell lines. The PSC, under the influence of **myeloid growth factors,** will begin to proliferate and transform into the **colony forming unit–granulocyte, erythrocyte, monocyte, and megakaryocyte (CFU-GEMM).** This myeloid **progenitor cell** (self-renewing cell) is committed to the myeloid hematopoietic cell line. The CFU-GEMM cell is destined to become a **granulocyte, erythrocyte, monocyte,** or **megakaryo-cyte (platelet precursor).** If influenced by **lymphoid growth factors** such as IL-7 and SCF, the PSC will proliferate and differentiate into a **lymphoid stem cell (LSC),** which is found primarily in the lymphatic system of the body instead of the bone marrow. This lymphoid progenitor cell is committed to the lymphoid hematopoietic cell line. The LSC will become either a **B lymphocyte,** a **T lymphocyte,** a **killer (K) lymphocyte,** or a **natural killer (NK) lymphocyte.** The lymphoid cells are considered to be the result of **extramedullary hematopoiesis.**

The CFU-GEMM progenitor cell then responds to specific cell line growth factors listed below to become the corresponding cell shown in Figure 2–3. The **myeloid growth factors** are called colony-stimulating factors (CSFs), with a cell line designation such as G-CSF for granulocyte growth factors or M-CSF for monocyte growth factors. This balance of growth factors and cells produced is in response to the demands of the body. If an individual is anemic and in need of erythrocytes, the growth factor that increases the proliferation and differentiation of erythroid cells will be produced. If the individual has a bacterial infection, the growth factors that stimulate the granulocytic (bacterial fighting) cells to proliferate and differentiate will be produced in higher concentrations.

Depending on the specific stimulation, the CFU-GEMM will become a colony-forming unit–granulocyte monocyte (CFU-GM), colony-forming unit–eosinophil (CFU-Eo), colony-forming unit–basophil (CFU-Baso), colony-forming unit–megakaryocyte (CFU-Mega), or burst-forming unit–erythroid (BFU-E). The **CFU-GM** can be directed to differentiate into a **neutrophilic granulocyte** or a **monocyte.** Current theory suggests that only the neutrophilic granulocyte and the monocyte have a common precursor cell, the CFU-GM. The other two granulocytic cells, the eosinophilic and basophilic granulocytes, have their own committed CFU-Eo and CFU-Baso. This will be explained in more detail in Chapters 3 and 4.

Under the influence of colony-stimulating factor–granulocyte monocyte (GM-CSF), the CFU-GEMM will become the CFU-GM. This progenitor cell then responds to G-CSF to become the colony-forming unit–granulocyte (CFU-G), which is the neutrophilic granulocytic committed blast cell called the myeloblast. This cell is not classified as a progenitor cell due to the inability to reproduce itself. This cell is only capable of dividing, further differentiating into the promyelocyte, myelocyte, and metamyelocyte and maturing into a final functional **segmented neutrophilic granulocyte.** The polysegmented neutrophilic granulocyte, which is also called the polymorphonuclear (Poly, PMN, or Seg) cell, functions to **destroy bacteria** invading the body. This is discussed in detail in Chapter 3.

If the predominating growth factor influencing the CFU-GM is the M-CSF, the CFU-GM becomes the monoblast or colony-forming unit–monocyte (CFU-M). This cell is not a progenitor cell and will divide and mature into the promonocyte and final functional cell, the **monocyte.** The monocyte is an extremely important component in the body's response to infection. The monocyte is a major **phagocytic cell** of the body that not only destroys the invading organism or substance but also **relays information** about the invader to other cells of the body. This is addressed in Chapters 4 and 5.

If the CFU-GEMM responds to IL-5 and unknown eosinophil CSFs, it will become the CFU-Eo. This is a committed progenitor cell that will develop only into a promyelocyte, an eosinophilic myelocyte, an eosinophilic metamyelocyte, and a **segmented eosinophil.** Some believe that this cell derives from the CFU-GM; however, this diagram will support the evidence of a CFU unique to the eosinophil. The CFU-Eo is **involved in hypersensitivity reactions** and is seen in association with **allergies, colds, and parasitic infections.** The eosinophil is discussed in detail in Chapter 3.

In response to an unknown colony-stimulating factor–basophil (Baso-CSF), the CFU-GEMM will become the **CFU-Baso.** This is not a progenitor cell and will become a promyelocyte, a basophilic myelocyte, a basophilic metamyelocyte, and a **segmented basophil.** The basophil **mediates hypersensitivity reactions** such as **allergies and colds;** however, this mediation takes place primarily **in the tissue** rather than the blood stream. Basophils, therefore, are seen in very low numbers in the blood stream, except in some cases of abnormal granulocytic proliferation.

The **granulocytes,** neutrophils, eosinophils, and basophils, all contain **specific granules associated with their morphology and function.** For this reason they are called granulocytes. The reference to neutrophil, eosinophil, and basophil describes how those specific granules stain on the peripheral blood smear.

The megakaryocyte, in the bone marrow, is the parent cell of the platelet seen in the peripheral blood. Under the influence of a colony-stimulating factor–megakaryocyte (Mega-CSF) the myeloid progenitor cell (CFU-GEMM) will differentiate into the **CFU-Mega** or **megakaryoblast,** which will develop into a promegakaryocyte and a megakaryocyte and will eventually produce platelets. **Platelets** (PLT, thrombocytes) are **cytoplasmic fragments** of the megakaryocyte, which are a component of blood coagulation. Platelets **form the initial plug** of an injured blood vessel to contain blood flow. These cellular elements are discussed in detail in later chapters.

The PSC can be driven (by lymphoid growth factors) in the direction of the LSC. The LSC will then become a specific type of lymphocyte. The LSC is influenced by various stimulators (IL-1, IL-4, IL-6, IL-3, TNF) to proliferate and mature in the **thymus** to become a competent **T lymphocyte** or **bursa equivalent** (bone marrow?) to become a **B lymphocyte.** The K lymphocyte or NK lymphocyte develops in the lymph system. The bursa of Fabricius is an organ in chickens where the B lymphocyte was determined to gain its competency. There has been no organ equivalent to the bursa found in humans, although many believe that the bone marrow serves this function. Due to the lack of evidence to prove where the bursa equivalent is located and evidence that non–B lymphocytes originate outside of the bone marrow, the lymphocytic cells are not considered to originate from bone marrow as do the myeloid cells. Lymphocytes are produced outside the bone marrow (extramedullary) in the lymph tissue.

T cells further mature and develop into prolymphocytes and then into specific functional T cell subgroups. The T cells are instrumental, through **cell-to-cell interactions,** to the ability of an individual to produce an **immune response** and defend himself or herself against disease. **B cells** mature and develop as one population functionally; however, each clone of cells will **produce** its own **unique antibody** in an **immune response.** The B cell is capable of **developing into the plasma cell** for most efficient antibody production. **NK cells** kill target cells within the body that they recognize as foreign. **K** or **lymphocyte-activated killer (LAK)** cells are antibody dependent cell-mediated cytotoxic cells (ADCC) that destroy **invading cells** only if they are **coated with antibody.** The various lymphocytes are found in the lymph nodes, spleen, and thymus as well as transiently in the bone marrow and peripheral blood. Lymphocytes are discussed in detail in Chapter 5.

Under the influence of the hormone erythropoietin (EPO) the CFU-GEMM progenitor cell will differentiate into a **BFU-E.** This cell is called a BFU instead of a CFU, which describes how the cells grow on semisolid media. Whereas most cells form very defined colonies as they multiply, the BFU-E has irregular groupings of cells all over the culture dish. They look as though the colony has burst apart. This BFU-E will progress through five maturational stages before becoming a **mature erythrocyte** (red blood cell). Three characteristics unique to erythrocytes are the longer life span of 120 days, no nucleus in the mature cell, and only a single population. The erythrocytic cell line is discussed in detail in Chapter 7.

The life span of most of the cellular elements of the blood is a short period of time (i.e., 6 hours to 10 days). The exceptions are the erythrocytes that live for approximately 4 months and the memory lymphocytes that may live for years. Blood cell production **within the bone marrow** is termed **med-**

1. After reviewing the hematopoietic chart, draw it from memory and *do not* check your work. The various cell lines follow logically from the precursor cells with associated names. Think about the process occurring in your body as you do this exercise. It will help you to remember the cells.
2. Trade these renditions of hematopoiesis with another student. Evaluate each other's hematopoietic chart and provide questions, discussion, and feedback concerning the organization and flow. For example: Why does this cell derive from this one instead of from that one? Why is this cell given this name? What is the significance of three different stem cells?

mine the current location of cells. Not only is the cell in question enumerated and evaluated morphologically, but the cell immediately associated with this cell may also provide information about the function and kinetics of the cell.

Cell morphology includes an evaluation of any changes from the normal morphology using the basic cellular characteristics of **size, nuclear shape**, and **structure**, and **cytoplasmic contents.** This morphologic evaluation must always be done with a consideration of the quality of the specimen, the other cells seen within the same specimen, and any medications or treatments that the patient may have in progress. Each cell does not stand alone but interacts in a dynamic body environment that must be considered in the evaluation process.

ullary hematopoiesis or more specifically **myelopoiesis (granulocytes), erythropoiesis (red blood cells), monopoiesis (monocytes),** and **thrombopoiesis (platelets).** Lymphocytic cells are considered products of **lymphopoiesis,** which occurs in the lymph system and is an example of **extramedullary hematopoiesis.** Mature lymphocytes are found primarily in the lymph system (spleen and lymph nodes) but are also found in the peripheral blood and bone marrow.

CELLULAR IDENTIFICATION AND EVALUATION

The ability to identify and evaluate cells of the body at various stages is crucial to diagnosis and treatment of disease. If the cell is identified incorrectly, the treatment prescribed will not be effective. The following concepts and methods are used to accurately identify and assess the function of blood cells.

Observing the origin and current location of cells is helpful in identification. Procedures such as **bone marrow** and **lymph node** aspirations and biopsies are done to look at the **site of origin of the blood cells.** Automated **cell counter results** and **peripheral blood smears** are also evaluated to deter-

Blood cells may appear morphologically normal on routine examination although they are not functioning properly. The **function of a cell** is related directly to the **cell organelles.** Cytochemical staining is one method of evaluating the presence and function of cell organelles. When exposing cells to a stain that will only react with a specific enzyme or cytoplasmic constituent (e.g., glycogen), the presence or absence of this cytoplasmic component will aid in the **identification** of the cell or an evaluation of the **cell's function.** One such test is the leukocyte alkaline phosphatase (LAP) score. In this procedure, the cells are stained to determine the presence of the alkaline phosphatase enzyme, which is produced and utilized to defend against bacterial invasion. If the patient has a bacterial infection and the cells are functioning properly, the LAP score will be high. If the cells are not functioning properly, the score will be low. A variety of tests can be done to determine if cells are functioning properly. Most of these function-related tests are not routinely done in a clinical laboratory and are, therefore, expensive and performed by a specialty laboratory in a medical center or a reference laboratory. Some examples would be tests for cellular migration and degranulation. These tests are presented in detail in Chapters 6, 10, and 13.

The most accurate methodology that is currently in use is **flow cytometry** evaluation of **cell membrane markers, nuclear chromatin,** and **cytoplasmic components.** Cell membrane proteins are the most commonly used definitive markers for identification and function. This is done by incubating cells with monoclonal antibodies, or stains, that are specific for the marker or characteristic being evaluated. The specific monoclonal antibody is tagged with a fluorescent marker that can be detected as the cell passes through a laser beam. This method of cell identification is addressed in more detail in Chapter 6.

BONE MARROW

The **bone marrow** produces the myeloid (granulocytic, monocytic, platelet, and erythrocytic) blood cells. Although myeloid is used to refer to bone marrow–derived cells, this term may also be used to refer to only the granulocytic cells. A tool used for bone marrow evaluation is the ratio of myeloid (granulocytic) cells to erythrocytic cells. This ratio in a healthy adult bone marrow is 3 to 4:1, **myeloid:erythroid (M:E) ratio.** The M:E ratio reflects the short life span of the granulocytic cells requiring a greater commitment of the bone marrow to production of these cells. The bone marrow **stem cell pool** is made up of multipotent and unipotent stem cells. These cells have a 6- to 10-day life span before they are influenced to differentiate into a specific cell line or cell. The majority of the cell production in the bone marrow is myelocytic, specifically granulocytes. The myelocytic **proliferation and differentiation pool** consists of cells that undergo mitosis and begin developing into more mature cells. This process of differentiating into mature functional cells takes approximately 3 days. Once the myeloid cells are no longer capable of mitosis, they enter the **storage pool** where they continue to mature and are stored in large volume until needed outside of the bone marrow. Once these cells mature and enter the **peripheral blood,** they are found either in the margination granulocyte pool (MGP), which is along the blood vessel endothelial wall prepared to move through to the tissue, or in the circulating granulocyte pool (CGP), which is a method of travel to a site of bacterial invasion. When blood is drawn to evaluate the leukocytes, the CGP is the source of cells (Fig. 2–4). Fewer monocytic and thrombocytic precursor cells are present in the bone marrow. These cells and their proliferation and differentiation are discussed in Chapters 4 and 11.

Erythrocytic cells in the bone marrow are mostly immature and nucleated. The various stages of development as well as the mature erythrocytes can be identified. These cells are discussed in detail in Chapters 7 to 10.

BASIC CELL STRUCTURE AND MATURATION CHARACTERISTICS

In order to understand cell maturation, an understanding of cellular morphology is required. Figure 2–5 presents a representation of basic cell structure. This will vary from cell to cell.

The nuclear chromatin pattern, the functional organelles found in the cytoplasm, and the membrane characteristics are unique to each cell's function or stage of maturation and are useful for identification and evaluation.

The nucleus will contain **heterochromatin (dark, clumped, inactive)** if the cell does not divide and **euchromatin (light, loose, active with nucleoli)** if the cell is engaged in mitosis. The cytoplasm will be rich with RNA (blue) if a lot of protein synthesis is occurring. The RNA produces protein such as antibodies (immunoglobulins to fight off infection), cytokines (regulatory proteins produced by one cell and directed toward a leukocyte), or proteins associated with cell division and maturation. If there is an abundance of protein production, the **Golgi apparatus** (endoplasmic reticulum that prepares the protein for secretion) will be very prominent as a clear area near the nucleus. The **specific cell cyto-**

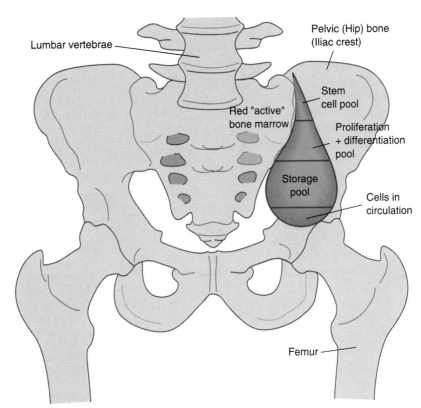

FIGURE 2-4
Bone marrow and peripheral blood pools. In the bone marrow there is a small number of the most primitive cells (stem cells), a larger proliferative/differentiation pool, and a larger storage pool of more mature cells. The cells are then released into the peripheral blood.

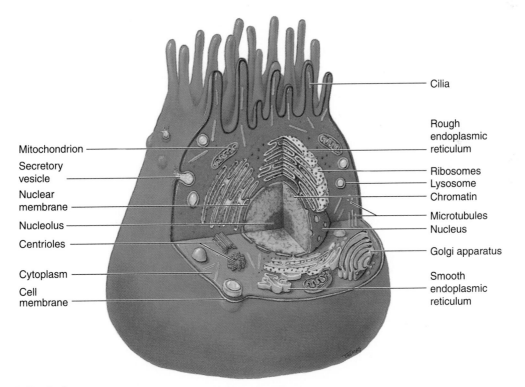

FIGURE 2-5
Basic cell structure. Every cell structure and organelle is related directly to the cell function. Identification and composition of each structure are essential for the complete understanding of the hematologic cells. (From Applegate J [ed]: The Anatomy and Physiology Learning System. Philadelphia: WB Saunders, 1995, p 44.)

plasmic organelles (e.g., granules) will have various **morphologic characteristics** and **stain a variety of colors dependent on their contents.** Knowledge of the association of the various cell structures with function results in more accurate identification and analysis of blood components as well as providing an understanding that will enhance recall of pertinent information.

The pluripotent stem cell (the earliest undifferentiated cell) is believed to be morphologically similar to the small (6 to 10 μm) resting lymphocyte. When this parent (progenitor) cell is stimulated to proliferate, it enlarges significantly. Therefore, early **immature cells** are usually very **large** (15 to 20 μm). As cells mature ("shift toward the right"), they follow a basic pattern of maturation that is important to understand in order to morphologically identify cells and determine their stage of development. The structure of the cell membrane is also important. A flow cytometry evaluation and identification of cells is dependent on the proteins within or on the surface of a specific cell membrane (Fig. 2–6).

The following criteria describe normal cellular maturation characteristics.

Keep in mind, however, that medicine is an art as well as a science, and there are exceptions to every concept. Isolated facts cannot be interpreted without looking at all circumstances and parameters involved.

CELL MATURATION

1. The **entire cell becomes smaller** in size.
2. The **nucleus:**
   A. **Becomes smaller,** is described by the nuclear: cytoplasmic (N:C) ratio, which decreases with maturity (except small lymphocytes).
   B. **Loses nucleoli** (RNA), which are associated with cell division.
   C. **DNA pattern becomes more coarse** and dense, which is called heterochromatin and indicates inactivity.
   D. **May lobe or segment.**
3. The **cytoplasm:**
   A. **Becomes less blue** due to the loss of RNA necessary for early development.
   B. Begins to **demonstrate organelles** specific to the cell function and take up stain color dependent on the organelle contents.

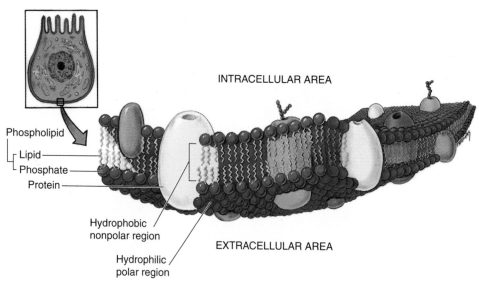

Phospholipid
Lipid
Phosphate
Protein
Hydrophobic nonpolar region
Hydrophilic polar region
INTRACELLULAR AREA
EXTRACELLULAR AREA

F I G U R E   2–6
Cell membrane. The mammalian cell membrane is a trilaminar (three-component) structure composed of two layers of lipid (a lipid bilayer) and various proteins. (From Applegate J [ed]: The Anatomy and Physiology Learning System. Philadelphia: WB Saunders, 1995, p 46.)

Review staining methodology and characteristics in Chapters 1, 6, and 10.

The automated instruments will do the initial identification of cells not fitting mature cell criteria. The specific identity of these cells must then be investigated and established. When trying to identify or evaluate a cell morphologically, the cell size, nucleus, and cytoplasm should be evaluated based on the previously presented criteria, and a decision should be made based on this information. Most cells are evaluated after staining, which accents the various cell organelles. The staining is only an additional parameter to help identification and can contribute to an incorrect evaluation if the basic cell characteristics listed earlier are not considered. The cell staining characteristics (color) may be incorrect, and only if you have accurately examined each cell characteristic would you know to ignore the erroneous color.

Cells demonstrating immature characteristics are not expected to be present in the peripheral blood. If such cells are found, they indicate: (a) a normal healthy response to a transient infection or disease such as mononucleosis, or (b) an alteration of a cell resulting in a malignancy such as leukemia or lymphoma.

Do It Now Cell Morphology

1. In a group or with one other classmate, present the cytoplasmic organelles found in a cell and ask for the cell function or current functional status. Examples are: reacting phagocytically, humorally, and so forth.
2. Draw a maturing nucleus. Be sure to show the size change as well as details of the nuclear characteristics as a cell matures.

STUDY QUESTIONS

1. Describe the characteristics of a very immature cell.
   A. Large cells, large nucleus:cytoplasmic ratio, round nucleus with loose chromatin, nucleoli, and agranular blue cytoplasm.
   B. Large cell, equal nucleus:cytoplasmic ratio, round nucleus with coarse chromatin pattern, and agranular blue cytoplasm.
   C. Medium-sized cell, low nucleus:cytoplasmic ratio, round nucleus with dark continuous nuclear chromatin, and blue cytoplasm with large prominent granules.
   D. Large cell, equal nucleus:cytoplasmic ratio, indented nucleus with light and dark areas of chromatin, and gray-blue, grainy looking cytoplasm.

2. A patient presented with fever and vomiting. A blood specimen was sent to the clinical laboratory for evaluation. Abnormal results were obtained, and you are reviewing the blood smear. Many cells have the nuclear and cytoplasmic characteristics of a segmented neutrophil cell; however, they appear in the orange color characteristic of the eosinophil cell. Which criteria would you use to make a decision with regard to which cell to report?
   A. An atypical eosinophil, because only an eosinophil would be orange and that is the most reliable characteristic.
   B. A neutrophil because the color of the cell is helpful; however, the actual cell morphology is the most significant characteristic for identification.

    C. No result can be released due to inconsistent color and morphology.

    D. The patient's blood would need to be redrawn. This is a phlebotomy error.

3. Compare and contrast a hormone, a cytokine, an interleukin, a colony-stimulating factor, and a stem cell factor. Give an example of each.

Leukocytes

In this part the origin, differentiation, and maturation of leukocytes (white blood cells) will be presented. To facilitate understanding of the material key terms and concepts are presented in bold print and Objectives and Fast Fact Sheets are available to summarize and emphasize key information. "Do It Now" exercises, which are located after each section, apply the information that is presented. Study questions can be found at the end of each chapter. Information, figures, and tables consistent with more than one chapter are repeated to allow the reader to have complete information in one chapter without the necessity of searching through other areas of the book.

In order to discuss or identify any cell or formed element of the blood, an understanding of structure, morphology, and function is important. Review Figure 2–6, which presents the cell structures, and Chapter 1 for a presentation of staining characteristics.

Leukocytes refer to white blood cells (WBCs). These cells are so-called because when they accumulate, as in the formation of "pus," or sedimentation of the blood occurs in the test tube, they exhibit a white color. The term leukocyte includes the **granulocytes** (neutrophils, eosinophils, and basophils), **monocytes/macrophages** (one population), and **lymphocytes/plasma cells** (T, B, NK, K, and LGL/LAK). All **leukocytes are nucleated** and are only **transient inhabitants** of the peripheral blood until they are required to function in the tissues. **Granulocytes and monocytes contain granules** in their cytoplasm and are produced in the bone marrow (medullary). A generic term for bone marrow–derived cells is myeloid. Some sources consider that granulocytes, monocytes, megakaryocytes, and erythrocytes are all myeloid cells because they originate in the bone marrow. The immature granulocytes have myelocytic names, whereas the other myeloid cells (monocytes, megakaryocytes, and erythrocytes) do not. This confuses the issue of rules for name associations. For this reason, **an understanding of the use of the stem "myelo-" must involve consideration of the context.** The myeloid growth factors are called colony-stimulating factors (CSFs) with a cell line designation such as G-CSF for granulocyte growth factors or M-CSF for monocyte growth factors. This balance of growth factors and cells is produced in response to the body's demands.

Lymphocytes are agranular and are produced outside of the bone marrow **(extramedullary)** in the lymph system of the body. Lymphopoiesis is influenced by the regulatory proteins called **interleukins,** followed by a number designation to identify the specific protein (e.g., IL-1, IL-3, IL-4, IL-6). The myeloid cells have a distinguishable morphology for identification. Lymphocytes all have very similar morphologic characteristics and are indistinguishable through microscopic examination. Identification is done by determining the proteins (antigens) present in the cell membrane.

Each white blood cell line is independent with different characteristics, life cycles, and functions. Leukocytes are transient inhabitants of the peripheral blood. The peripheral blood count of any white blood cell **reflects an equilibrium of the cell production, maturation, and release** from the bone marrow (movement into the peripheral blood), **migration** (within the peripheral blood or in the tissues), **sequestration** in various organs, and **destruction** or **cell death.** The term for **white blood cell production** is **leukopoiesis.** Each cell line production is also described in the same terminology, hence the terms **granulopoiesis, lymphopoiesis,** and **monopoiesis.**

Following any alterations to the body, especially injury, the leukocyte population changes not only in numbers but also in morphology. The motive for these changes is to defend the body from fatal invasion or injury; however, products of the leukocyte response may induce some secondary damaging effects. Researchers are currently looking at **this balance of a cellular response that is beneficial versus a total body (systemic) inflammation that results in tissue injury, cellular death, and secondary pathologies such as blood coagulation.** The goal is to maximize the beneficial effects of leukocyte response and function while minimizing the secondary damage.

The **leukocytes** of the blood are responsible for **defending the body** from invasion and infection. There is no cell or system within the body that can be studied or explained as a separate entity. The granulocytes, monocytes, and lymphocytes respond and interact with other cells and physiologic responses of the body.

All of these factors contribute to the data that the clinical laboratory practitioner generates. The laboratory values are essential for the health care provider (e.g., physicians, nurse practitioners, physicians' assistants) to accurately identify the patient's condition (the diagnosis) and to administer and monitor the most effective treatment.

Summaries of the leukocyte information are provided in the charts and figures throughout the chapter. Information relating the contribution of chemistry, microbiology, as well as other areas of the laboratory is included to remind the student that **hematology is not an isolated entity** but is rather one of many approaches to investigate body physiology.

By applying the knowledge of leukocytes and the associated testing, the laboratory practitioner can provide valuable pieces to the puzzle in order to complete the picture necessary for appropriate delivery of health care.

Basic Leukocyte Information

Leukocytes	Granulocytes	Myeloid Cells	Lymphocytes
WBC	Neutrophils (1)	Granulocytes	T cells (2)
	Eosinophils (3)	Monocytes	B cells (2)
WBC functions:			
1. Rid the body of	Basophils (3)	Megakaryocytes	K cells
invading organisms		Erythrocytes	NK cells
2. Immune response		Bone marrow–	LAK cells produced
3. Mediate hyper-		derived (medullary)	in the lymph system
sensitivity reactions			(extramedullary)
Protein regulators:	*Cytokines:*	*Cytokines:*	*Cytokines:*
	Colony-stimulating	Erythropoietin	Interleukins
	factors	Colony-stimulating	
		factors	
Leukopoiesis	Granulopoiesis	Myelopoiesis	Lymphopoiesis

Reference range: *4500 to 11,000 WBC/mm³ (4.5–11 × 10⁹/l)*
Granular cytoplasm: *phagocytosis (neutrophils or monocytes) or hypersensitivity (i.e., allergy) mediators through protein (histamine and antihistamine) secretion (eosinophils and basophils). The color of the cytoplasm is relative to the granule content.*
Agranular cytoplasm: *cytokine secretion (T cells), antibody production (B cells/plasma cells), physical assault (K, NK, LAK cells), or replication (blast cells). Cytoplasm is blue relative to the amount of RNA, which is relative to the amount of protein synthesis occurring.*
LAK = lymphokine-activated killer; NK = natural killer; WBC = white blood cell; RNA = ribonucleic acid.

CHAPTER 3

OUTLINE

Origin, Maturation, and Morphology of Granulocytes
Neutrophils
Eosinophils
Basophils

Physiology and Function of Granulocytes

Normal Response and Diseases of Granulocytes
Increased Neutrophil Count (Neutrophilia)
Decreased Neutrophil Count (Neutropenia)
Abnormal Neutrophil Function
Anomalies
Lupus Erythematosus Cell
Increased Eosinophils (Eosinophilia)
Decreased Eosinophils (Eosinopenia)
Increased Basophils (Basophilia)

Study Questions

Granulocytic Blood Cells

O B J E C T I V E S

Upon completion of this chapter the student should be able to:

1. Diagram and explain granulopoiesis, including neutrophils, eosinophils, and basophils from their origin through maturation.

2. Trace the kinetics of each of the granulocytes from their release in the bone marrow to cell death.

3. Apply knowledge of the function of granulocytes to case study data analysis.

4. Compare and contrast normal responses and diseases in granulocytes.

5. Correlate the appropriate leukocyte testing with granulocytes responses and disease.

6. Explain the differences among acute myelocyte leukemia (M1–M4), chronic myelogenous leukemia (CML), and myelodysplasia.

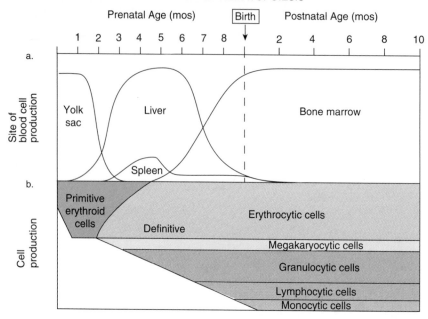

EARLY HEMATOPOIESIS

FIGURE 3–1
Production of blood cells in the fetus. Notice the location and timing of the various cells produced. The newborn has different reference ranges than has the child, adult, or elderly person.

The production of granulocytic (myelocytic) cells occurs in the bone marrow. This process is described as medullary granulopoiesis or myelopoiesis. The neutrophilic granulocyte is the first white blood cell produced in the fetus (Fig. 3–1). Eosinophils and basophils develop later on.

ORIGIN, MATURATION, AND MORPHOLOGY OF GRANULOCYTES

All of the blood cells originate from the **pluripotent stem cell (PSC),** which is under the influence of hematopoietic regulatory proteins (cytokines) and becomes the **hematopoietic stem cell (HSC)** or colony-forming unit–spleen (CFU-S). This cell is stimulated to proliferate by cytokines listed in Figure 3–2. Under the influence of specific cytokines, the HSC will become the **CFU-GEMM,** which will be influenced by various cytokines to become the **CFU-GM** (neutrophil and monocyte precursor), **CFU-Eo** (eosinophil precursor), or **CFU-Ba** (basophil precursor). The neutrophil, eosinophil, and basophil are named with re-

spect to the Romanowsky polychrome staining characteristics of the cell's cytoplasmic granules. The principle of staining, as discussed in Chapter 1, involves acid components attracting the basic stain and the basic components attracting the acid stain. The basic cell structure and organelles are discussed in Chapter 2.

The CFU-GM will become the CFU-G if stimulated by the colony-stimulating factor–granulocyte (G-CSF). Another name for the **CFU-G is the myeloblast.** The myeloblast is the first cell committed to the granulocyte cell line. The earlier cells mentioned will look morphologically similar, and only with monoclonal antibodies and techniques such as flow cytometry, fluorescent microscopy, or magnetic beads can the earliest cells be identified. The myeloblast is not easily recognized, but when considered together with location, accompanying cells, and inclusions, such as Auer rods, the identification can be fairly certain. The **myeloblast** is a **large cell** (15 μm) with a **high nuclear to cytoplasmic (N:C)** ratio due to the large, active nucleus. The nucleus is round with loose, lighter staining, euchromatin-containing nucleoli. The cytoplasm is minimal and appears blue due to the ribonucleic acid (RNA), which produces the pro-

Hematopoietic Chart
of Cell Differentiation.

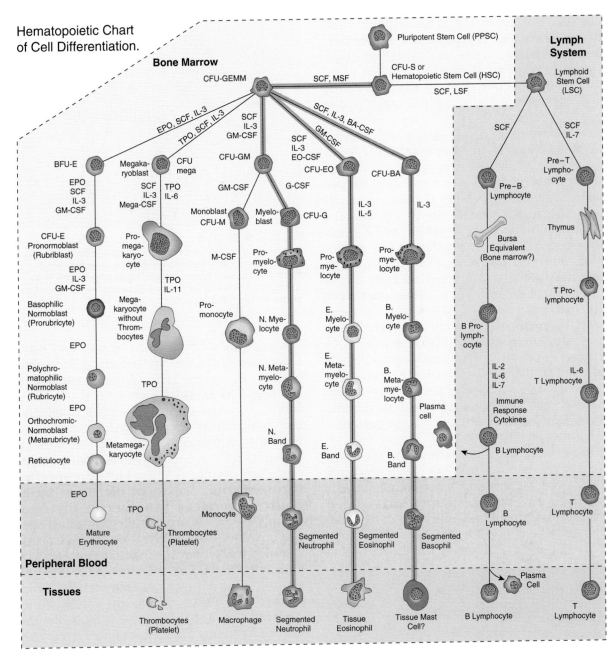

FIGURE 3–2
Hematopoiesis with granulopoiesis highlighted. The pluripotent stem cell is driven by cytokines toward the granulocytic cell lineage when these cells (neutrophils, eosinophils, basophils) are needed by the body.

teins necessary for differentiation. No granules have developed in the cytoplasm yet. This cell is primarily proliferating and begins to **differentiate by producing myeloperoxidase (MPO)** granules as it moves into the next stage of development. The myeloblast makes up about 1% of the nucleated cells in the

bone marrow and takes 18 hours to mature. In order to have a point of reference, the myeloblast (a white blood cell blast) is shown with the erythroblast (a red blood cell blast) in order to establish identification of cells through correlating their characteristics with function and contrasting the characteristics with other cells that may be in the same field. This cell **differs from the erythroblast in nuclear characteristics,** such as lighter uniform chromatin pattern and one or two nucleoli instead of three to five. There is often very little myeloblast cytoplasm, and it is a much lighter blue (Fig. 3–3).

The next stage of development in the granulocyte cell line is the **promyelocyte** (progranulocyte). This cell is an exception to the basic rule of maturation because it is **larger** than the preceding cell (myeloblast). This cell has a **high N:C ratio, loose chromatin with nucleoli, and a dark blue cytoplasm,** which is very similar to the myeloblast; however, the promyelocyte has **large granules** sparsely distributed throughout the cytoplasm of the cell and is **often seen over the nucleus** (Fig. 3–4). These are the **nonspecific granules** that contain myeloperoxidase. **Myeloperoxidase (MPO)** is a digestive enzyme produced in all early granulocytic cells and is, therefore, useful for identification. This cell makes up 3.4% of the nucleated bone marrow cells and takes 24 hours to mature. The promyelocyte is still involved in both proliferation and differentiation.

The **myelocyte** is the next cell in the granulocytic cell line. The myelocyte is a **medium size** (about 12 μm) and has a round nucleus in which the deoxyribonucleic acid (DNA) synthesis is decreasing, resulting in darker blue

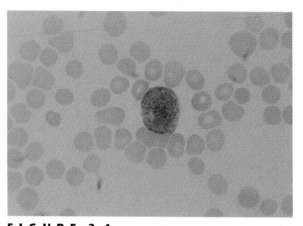

FIGURE 3–4
A promyelocyte. Notice the size; N:C ratio; loose light color; active euchromatin; nucleoli; cytoplasmic granules, which are the first or primary granules found in all granulocytes (nonspecific granules) that contain myeloperoxidase; and the blue of the RNA in the cytoplasm.

staining (heterochromatin) while the cell's functional organelles are becoming more important. This is the last cell that is capable of dividing. The myelocyte contains active RNA, which gives the cytoplasm a blue color, and the nonspecific (myeloperoxidase) granules from the promyelocyte stage are still present; however, they are much smaller. The significant characteristic of this stage is the **specific (neutrophilic, eosinophilic, or basophilic) secondary granules** in the cytoplasm. The secondary granules are called specific granules because they are the functional granules for either the neutrophilic, eosinophilic, or basophilic cell line. Each specific granule has its own **characteristic size, shape, and stain** due to the difference in contents (function), and these granules are the major identifying characteristic of each granulocytic cell. The specific granules of the neutrophil are smaller than the nonspecific granules of the promyelocyte and do not have a significant affinity for either the basic methylene blue stain or the acid eosin stain and are discretely located in the cytoplasm. The presence of these **neutral-colored specific granules** changes the color of the cytoplasm. The cytoplasm begins to demonstrate a pink or brown (neutral) color within the light blue (Fig. 3–5). This change in the color and appearance of the cytoplasm reflects the loss of

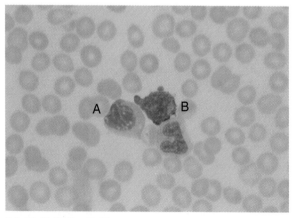

FIGURE 3–3
A myeloblast (A) and an erythroblast (B). Note the difference in size, the chromatin of the nucleus, nucleoli, cytoplasmic color, and appearance.

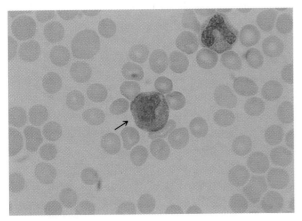

FIGURE 3–5
A neutrophilic myelocyte. Notice the size, N : C ratio, loose euchromatin with the start of some condensation to inactive heterochromatin, lack of visible nucleoli, small cytoplasmic granules that are dark blue and brown (nonspecific, primary, myeloperoxidase), and the appearance of the pink (specific, lysosomal) granules of the neutrophil (arrow). Some RNA is still present, giving a blue color to the cytoplasm.

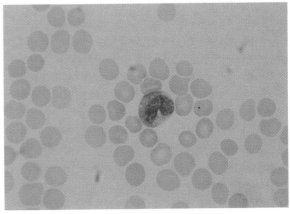

FIGURE 3–6
A neutrophilic metamyelocyte. Notice the size, the N : C ratio, the nuclear chromatin becoming more condensed and coarse, the indentation of the nucleus as it begins to mature toward segmentation. The cytoplasm has both the primary myeloperoxidase granules and the specific neutrophilic granules.

RNA in the cytoplasm and the appearance of the neutrophilic granules that contain leukocyte alkaline phosphatase (LAP), esterases, antibacterial proteins, and other digestive enzymes. The myelocyte makes up 11.9% of the bone marrow nucleated cells and takes 100 hours (4 days) to mature.

The last mononuclear stage in the granulocytic cell line is the **metamyelocyte** (Fig. 3–6). This cell is not capable of mitosis but continues to differentiate. The **nucleus** is **kidney shaped** with a fairly condensed (inactive or hetero) chromatin. The energy within this cell is directed toward production of the digestive enzymes and granule production, which is evident in the **prominent Golgi apparatus** (clear area) located at the indentation site of the nucleus. The cellular endoplasmic reticulum produces the functional lysosomal proteins, which the Golgi apparatus packages and secretes. **The cytoplasm appears very similar to the mature cell** due to the neutrophilic granules throughout. The metamyelocyte makes up 18% of bone marrow. The myeloblast, promyelocyte, myelocyte, or metamyelocyte are not seen in the peripheral blood in healthy individuals.

The final immature stage of neutrophil de-

velopment is the **band** (STAB) cell (Fig. 3–7). The band is the **same size and color as those of the mature segmented neutrophil** approximately 10 to 12 μm). The N : C ratio has reversed from the myeloblast N : C and is now 1:2 or smaller. The **nucleus** is beginning to narrow to a **sausage shape** as it progresses toward segmentation. The cytoplasm is filled with small neutrophilic granules. The classification of a neutrophil as a

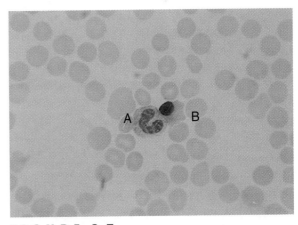

FIGURE 3–7
A neutrophilic band/stab (A) and a nucleated red blood (B). Notice the size, the N : C ratio, and the coarse heterochromatin within the band of the nucleus. The cytoplasm is visibly mature with the small neutral granules in cell A. Compare this view with the same characteristics in cell B.

band or a mature segmented neutrophil varies from one laboratory to another. There are at least three different criteria, which range from insisting on a smooth C- or S-shaped nucleus with no indentation to any cell with a filament connecting the segments that is one third or greater than the width of the segments on either side. The consistent reporting of bands is very important for accurate and efficient health care diagnosis and treatment. Every laboratory must have a written protocol that is strictly followed by the practitioners performing the test and is also known to the primary care provider. The band cell makes up about 11% of the bone marrow and about 0 to 3% of the peripheral blood. The band cell is the last immature stage and is stored in the bone marrow in 15× greater numbers than in the peripheral blood. This storage pool is still maturing but is fully functional and is only **released when there is an increased demand for neutrophils** due to exhaustion of the mature neutrophils available. An increased number of bands in the peripheral blood is suggestive of a **bacterial infection.** This is called a **leukemoid reaction** and is termed a **"shift to the left"** (toward immaturity). The band cell takes 40 to 50 hours (6.5 days) to mature.

Neutrophils

A **segmented neutrophil (seg)** is also termed a **polymorphonuclear cell (PMN or poly)** (Fig. 3–8). The mature neutrophil is 10 to 12 μm in size with an N:C of 1:3. The average nucleus has three to five segments connected by a narrow filament. If there are **less than three segments,** the cell is considered to be **hyposegmented,** which indicates **immaturity (a shift to the left).** If the cell has **more than five segments,** this indicates hypersegmentation, which is associated with **overmaturity (a shift to the right, indicative of surviving longer than usual)** as a result of specific diseases discussed later in this chapter. The cytoplasm is filled with the discrete neutrophilic granules, which become more prominent (toxic granulation) when the cell is stimulated to

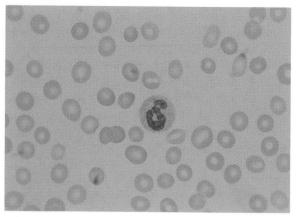

FIGURE 3–8

A segmented neutrophil. Notice the medium size (10 to 12 μm), the N:C ratio of 1:4, the coarse heterochromatin of the nucleus that has three to five segments, and the cytoplasm filled with small, neutral-colored lysosomal (digestive) granules.

function, such as in a bacterial infection. The mature segmented neutrophil makes up 10.7% of the nucleated bone marrow cells and **60 to 80% of the peripheral white blood cell population of the adult.** The PMN or seg travels briefly in the peripheral blood stream till it reaches a site outside of the blood stream where the body must be defended primarily from bacterial diseases. The average time that a PMN, or seg, spends in the peripheral blood is 10 hours. If this cell is left in the peripheral blood for long periods of time, it becomes hypersegmented, which is described as a **"shift to the right"** and is indicative of a DNA maturation problem or a problem in cell function.

Eosinophils

Eosinophils are derived from the **CFU-GEMM,** which is stimulated by IL-3, GM-CSF, and IL-5 to become the **CFU-Eo.** This cell is morphologically identical to the myeloblast and develops into a **promyelocyte** containing the primary nonspecific myeloperoxidase granules. The **eosinophilic myelocyte (E. myelocyte)** stage develops next and, as with the neutrophilic myelocyte, the specific (secondary, eosinophilic) granules begin to appear in the cytoplasm. These **large secretory granules contain a histamine-neutralizing**

substance as well as other proteins involved in hypersensitivity reactions. The **eosinophilic granules are basic and have a strong affinity for the eosin (acid) stain, appearing bright red or orange.** The **eosinophilic metamyelocyte (E. metamyelocyte)** has the characteristic **indented (kidney-shaped) nucleus** and more secondary granules. The eosinophilic band cytoplasm has only the large orange secondary granules visible, which may make it difficult to see the banded nucleus clearly. The characteristics of the **mature eosinophil are the large size** (13 μm), large **orange granules,** and usually only **two lobes of the nucleus (bilobed)** (Fig. 3–9). Eosinophils constitute approximately **3% of the peripheral blood leukocytes.**

Basophils

Basophils have not been clearly proved to develop from the same in vitro colonies containing neutrophils or eosinophils. This lack of knowledge is due to the low numbers in circulation and the lack of an efficient growth factor to stimulate greater numbers for research purposes. The current theory supports the basophil originating from the **CFU-GEMM,** which is influenced by unknown cy-

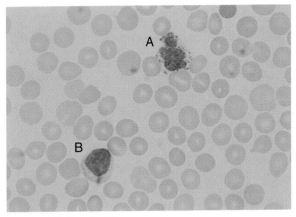

F I G U R E   3–10

A segmented basophil (A) and a lymphocyte (B). Note the smaller size than the neutrophil and the hyposegmented nucleus, if it is visible beneath the large, dark blue secondary secretory granules specific to the basophil. These secondary granules contain proteins involved in the mediation of hypersensitivity reactions such as heparin and histamine of cell A. Compare this with the characteristics of cell B.

tokines to become a **CFU-ba.** This cell is morphologically identical to the myeloblast and develops into a **promyelocyte,** containing the primary nonspecific myeloperoxidase (MPO) granules. The **basophilic myelocyte (B. myelocyte)** stage then develops and, as with the neutrophilic and eosinophilic myelocytes, the specific **(secondary, basophilic)** granules begin to appear in the cytoplasm. The basophil **granules are larger** than are the eosinophilic granules and have an affinity for the basic stain, which results in a very **dark blue color.** In a fresh rapidly stained specimen, the basophilic granules can completely **cover the cell,** masking the nucleus. Usually some of the basophilic **granules dissolve during the staining process leaving only a few large granules,** which will be found both in the cytoplasm and over the nucleus. The remaining cytoplasm will be clear and will allow recognition of the nucleus, which will usually have a few large lobes or segments. The basophil is the **smallest granulocyte** (10 μm) and makes up approximately **0.5% of the peripheral blood leukocyte population.** The **granules contain** many proteins involved in hypersensitivity reactions, including **heparin and histamine** (Fig. 3–10). The **tissue mast cell** is fixed in the tissues and is very similar to the

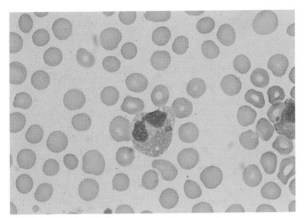

F I G U R E   3–9

A segmented eosinophil. Note the larger size than the neutrophil, the bilobed nucleus demonstrating hyposegmentation, and the large orange granules that are abundant in the cytoplasm. These granules are secondary secretory granules specific to the eosinophil, and they contain many proteins involved in mediating hypersensitivity reactions, one of which is a histamine-neutralizing substance.

Do It Now Granulocyte Origin, Maturation, and Morphology Exercise

An automated complete blood count was done on an individual patient, and some abnormal results appear. You are looking at the blood cells on a glass slide under the microscope in order to identify the cells. What characteristics need to be noted to allow you to identify the cell? List the characteristics that would tell you:

1. What stage of development is this cell (very immature, somewhat immature, mature)? Explain your decision.
2. What cell line does this cell originate from? What characteristics associate this cell with a specific cell line?
3. Get together with other individuals in your class and discuss your answers.
4. Within the group, discuss and prioritize the characteristics by numbering 1, 2, etc., in the order that your group believes to be the most reliable for identification purposes and give reasons for your answers.
5. Explain why the various cell components stain as they do. This relates to the make-up of components and properties of the stain (see Chapter 1).

basophil; however, no developmental relationship has been proved. The tissue mast cell is connective tissue of mesenchymal origin, which resembles the basophil but with a much larger size. The granular contents of the basophil and mast cell are similar with the exception of proteolytic enzymes and serotonin, which are found in mast cell granules but are not found in basophils.

PHYSIOLOGY AND FUNCTION OF GRANULOCYTES

Once the **segmented neutrophil** (PMN) is mature and released from the bone marrow, it will become part of a marginating granulocyte pool (MGP) or the circulating granulocyte pool (CGP). The MGP is along the blood vessel endothelial wall waiting to be called to function. The call to function is a **chemical signal that results in the migration or movement** of PMNs, called **chemotaxis,** throughout the blood stream and through the

endothelial cell walls of the blood vessel into the body (diapedesis) as needed. Many substances act as chemotactants, such as the **lipopolysaccharide (LPS) fragments of bacterial cell walls and various cytokines.** Once the **neutrophils** have accumulated at a site, due to chemotaxis, they begin to **phagocytize** in an attempt to rid the body of any threatening substance, such as **bacteria or toxins.** The process of phagocytosis involves engulfing the foreign substance or antigen (ingestion) due to opsonins (antibodies and other proteins). The **opsonization** will result in particles sticking together or sticking to the PMN **(immune adherence),** which encourages phagocytosis, and a membrane-enclosed phagocytic vacuole is formed. The cytoplasmic **granules containing digestive enzymes** then move to the vacuole and **fuse with the vacuole membrane** to release their enzymatic contents into the vacuole to form a lysosome containing the ingested substance that **will undergo digestion** (Fig. 3–11). The **product of digestion is hydrogen peroxide, which is bactericidal.** Following digestion, the neutrophil undergoes destruction and cellular death. In an overwhelming infection, all available PMNs will be exhausted and band cells will be released to continue to fight the invading substance. If all PMNs and band cells are used, the infection will progress to an entire body infection (sepsis). The patient will not recover but rather will succumb to the invading substance (bacteria). This is why patients whose white blood cells have been destroyed by disease or treatment of disease die more often of infections (e.g., pneumonia) rather than of the disease. These patients are given transfusions of only white blood cells to replace the destroyed cells and defend the body against infection.

In order to assess the neutrophils, their kinetics and dynamics must be considered. The distribution of mature neutrophils is 50% in the circulating granulocyte pool (CGP) and 50% in the marginating granulocyte pool (MGP). Upon activation, the marginating cells move into the tissue or into the circulating pool, and they travel to the area where they are needed. This is **chemotaxis** or directed locomotion **in response to tissue injury,**

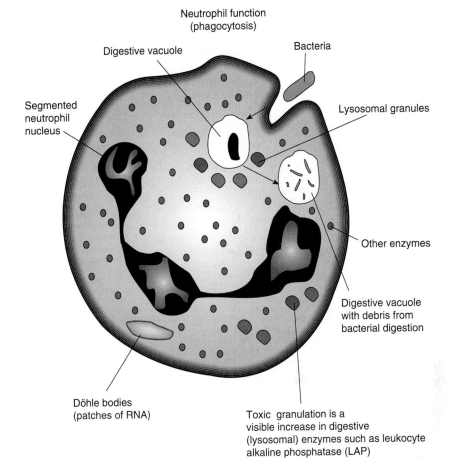

Neutrophil function
(phagocytosis)

Digestive vacuole

Bacteria

Segmented
neutrophil
nucleus

Lysosomal granules

Other enzymes

Digestive vacuole
with debris from
bacterial digestion

Döhle bodies
(patches of RNA)

Toxic granulation is a
visible increase in digestive
(lysosomal) enzymes such as leukocyte
alkaline phosphatase (LAP)

F I G U R E   3 – 1 1
Phagocytosis by a segmented
neutrophil. Note the vacuoles,
toxic granulation, and Döhle
bodies associated with a leukemoid reaction.

hormones, bacterial products, and opso-nins (substances that attract phagocytic cells). As many **neutrophils** invade the area of injury or infection, an **accumulation** occurs with the **formation of "pus"** as a result of chemotaxis and migration of cells. A **visible response to bacterial infection** includes an **increase in** azurophilic, **peroxidase-positive granules** under light microscopy and is called **toxic granulation.** This is often seen in association with **vacuolation** of the cytoplasm, the presence of **Döhle bodies** (patches of cytoplasmic rough endoplasmic reticulum, RNA), and a **shift to the left (band cells).** All or any of these characteristics are indicative of a bacterial infection (Fig. 3–12). Toxic granulation will be more visible in some neutrophils than in others, depending on the response of each individual cell. If **large prominent granulation is present in ALL neutrophils** evaluated, this indicates a **genetic abnormality (anomaly)** or inappropriate staining and not a normal response to bacterial infection (a leukemoid reaction). In order to determine if the neutrophilic cells seen in excess are normal responsive cells or abnormal unresponsive leukemic cells, they can be stained for the amount of leukocyte alkaline phosphatase (LAP) in the cytoplasmic granules. A responding cell will produce more LAP for digestion of the invading substance, whereas the leukemic cells would have no need of an increased number of digestive enzymes such as LAP. The LAP score test is discussed in Chapter 6.

Eosinophils function in the tissues throughout the body by releasing their granule contents in response to **parasitic infections and to type I hypersensitivity reactions, such as allergies, hay fever, and**

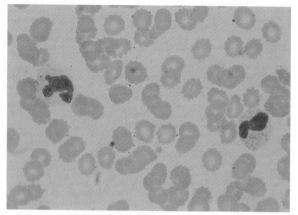

FIGURE 3–12
Segmented neutrophils responding to bacterial infection by demonstrating toxic granulation, light blue patches of RNA called Döhle bodies, and vacuoles.

eyes, runny nose, difficulty in breathing, and other symptoms of a hypersensitivity (allergic) reaction.

NORMAL RESPONSE AND DISEASES OF GRANULOCYTES

Keep in mind that laboratory data (e.g., counts, observations) on a specific cell line are a reflection of the total dynamics of each cell line. These dynamics include the **production, maturation, bone marrow release, circulation, and function or destruction,** all of which have an **impact on the numbers that we see in the clinical laboratory.**

bronchial asthma. The granules of the eosinophil release cytotoxic proteins and cytokine mediators. Eosinophil granules contain histaminase, eosinophil peroxidase, and lysophospholipase. The **IgE antibody** produced in parasitic and hypersensitivity reactions can **activate eosinophils to release cytotoxic substances that can kill parasites and destroy offending cells.** Research has suggested that eosinophils may be induced to secrete tumor necrosis factor-α (TNF-α) and transforming growth factor-β (TGF-β), which are involved in inflammation and tissue repair respectively. Adrenal corticosteroid hormones stimulate eosinophils to leave the blood stream.

We know much less about the origin and kinetics of the **basophil** than the other granulocytic cells. Basophils appear in the bone marrow and peripheral blood in small numbers and are not usually seen in the tissues. The granules contain histamine, heparin, eosinophil chemotactic factor of anaphylaxis (ECF-A), slow-reacting substance of anaphylaxis (SRS-A), and platelet-activating factor (PAF). The function of the basophil involves modulation of hypersensitivity reactions. When the antibody (immunoglobulin) **IgE** is produced in response to an allergen, it **binds to basophils causing the release of granules.** The substances in the granules of a basophil induce clinical symptoms such as watery

Increased Neutrophil Count (Neutrophilia)

The most common cause of an **increased neutrophil count** (neutrophilia, $>60\%$, $>6 \times 10^9/l$) is a good healthy response to a bacterial infection. Neutrophils will phagocytize a variety of substances; however, neutrophils are most responsive to bacteria. The significant increase in white blood cell count resembles a leukemia, thus it has been called a **leukemoid reaction.** This elevated count seen in a leukemoid reaction to a bacterial infection is transient and decreases as the patient recovers from the disease. The neutrophil leukocyte alkaline phosphatase (LAP) score, or neutrophil alkaline phosphatase (NAP) score, is used to differentiate the leukemoid reaction from **chronic myelogenous leukemia (CML).** The normal responsive neutrophils in a leukemoid reaction will have an **increase in alkaline phosphatase (125 to 400 LAP score),** whereas the abnormal nonresponsive leukemic cells will have a normal to low amount of alkaline phosphatase (NLAP) in their granules (<125 NLAP score). If a leukemoid reaction is present, some of the neutrophils will demonstrate toxic granulation, due to an increase in digestive granules and enzymes, phagocytic vacuoles, and possibly **Döhle bodies, which are light blue**

patches of RNA. To report toxic granulation, the neutrophils should demonstrate varying degrees of toxic granulation. If all neutrophils have the same appearance—that of prominent granulation—this is not toxic granulation but rather it is an artifact of staining or a genetic anomaly. Neutrophil counts may also rise due to inflammation, exercise, hormones, and various treatments. If there is a reason to believe that the patient demonstrates any of these stresses or alterations, this should be noted on the blood specimen information. The laboratory test results must reflect the patient's overall status, not just a transient change in cell count due to stress or exercise.

Other reasons for an elevated neutrophil count (neutrophilia) include **chronic granulocytic leukemia (CGL), which is also called chronic myelocytic leukemia (CML); acute granulocytic leukemia (AGL), which is also called acute myelogenous leukemia (AML); myelofibrosis; and myeloid metaplasia.**

An accurate diagnosis of leukemia is crucial to the timely administration of the correct treatment. The **quality and quantity of life for the leukemic patient depends on the accurate identification of the leukemic cell.**

Due to the proliferation of nonfunctional leukemic cells, the immune system is compromised and opportunistic infections that are not threatening to the healthy individual will overtake the leukemic patient. Chronic leukemic patients are more likely to succumb to a fatal infection than to the consequences of the leukemia. Transfusions of leukocytes may be used to avoid infections.

The **acute leukemias** are very aggressive. The **onset is rapid;** mostly **immature cells** (blasts) are seen; the **white blood cell count varies from low to high;** and the **prognosis** is often **poor** (short survival). The presence of primarily blast cells presents a cell line identification challenge. Blast cells do not have enough specific morphology to identify their cell line. For this reason **cytochemical stains** and membrane proteins recognized by the use of fluorescence and **flow cytometry**

are required for accurate identification in order to determine the most effective treatment. The French, American, and British (FAB) hematologists have categorized the acute leukemias to aid in the diagnosis and treatment of acute leukemias (Table 3–1).

Factors involved in the development of leukemia are still under investigation; however, evidence indicates that three components are in some way responsible for the development of disease. The three factors are: (1) a **genetic alteration** (normal genes to malignant genes or proto-oncogenes to oncogenes or inactivation of a gene whose protein product suppresses cancer), (2) exposure to certain **viruses** (adult T-cell leukemia and the human T-cell lymphotropic virus-I), and (3) an **initiating event,** such as exposure to a toxic substance (long-term exposure to the chemical benzene has been associated with the development of acute nonlymphoblastic leukemia [ANLL]). Leukemias are referred to as lymphocytic (lymphoid) or nonlymphocytic (myeloid). Correct diagnosis of leukemia is essential to obtain the most effective treatment. Treatment or transplantation of bone marrow may include chemotherapy, radiation therapy, or administration of peripheral blood progenitor

FAST FACTS

Acute Versus Chronic

Chronic Conditions
Slow progression (discovered secondary to an unrelated disorder such as pneumonia)
Older individuals
High white blood cell count
Usually **mature cells**
Usually not the cause of death

Acute Conditions
Rapid onset
Younger individuals
Variable white blood cell count
Anemia
Immature cells
Rapid infiltration of body organs with malignant cells resulting in death

TABLE 3–1   FRENCH-AMERICAN-BRITISH CLASS OF ACUTE MYELOID OR LYMPHOID LEUKEMIAS

FAB Class	Cells Observed	Unique Criteria	Cytochemistry/CD	%*
M1(AML)	>90% myeloblasts with minimal maturation (Pros)	Occasional Auer rods	MP, SBB, NASDC	20
M2(AML)	<90% myeloblasts; >10% more mature	Auer rods	MP, SBB, NASDC	30
M3(APL)	Predominantly promyelocytes	Often causes DIC	MP, SBB, NASDC	10
M4(AMML)	Myeloblasts and monoblasts with stages of both	Occasional Auer rods	>20% MP, SBB, NASDC; >20% NSE	12
M4eo	Same as M4 except with eosinophilia	Some with large basophilic granules	>20% MP, SBB, NASDC; >20% NSE; eos may be PAS	4
M5a(AMoL) poorly differentiated	>80% monoblasts, promonocytes, and monocytes	Later stages are poorly granulated and vacuolated	NSE (fluoride inhibitor)	5
M5b(AMoL) differentiated	<80% monoblasts, promonocytes, and monocytes		NSE (fluoride inhibitor)	6
M6(AEL)	>50% erythroblasts, also myeloblasts and monoblasts	50% Dysplastic, megaloblastic	PAS	6
M7(AMegL)	>30% megakaryoblasts		Platelet peroxidase by EM, platelet glycoprotein by immunocytochemistry	1
L1(ALL)	Small lymph cells	2–10 year olds	PAS/CD 10,19,24	71
L2(ATL)	Large irregular cells	Adult T cell associated with HTLV-I	PAS/CD 10	27
L3(ALL)	Large uniform cells	Burkitt's type	PAS/CD 10	2

*Represents the percentage of myeloid leukemias (M) or lymphoid (L) leukemias. NSE = nonspecific esterase; SBB = Sudan black B; MP = myeloperoxidase; PAS = periodic acid-Schiff; FAB = French-American-British; AML = acute myeloid leukemia; NASDC = naphthol ASD chloracetate esterase.

cells or umbilical cord blood as well as commercially made growth factors.

Chronic myelocytic leukemia (CML), also called chronic granulocytic leukemia (CGL), is typically found in individuals **older than 50 years of age** and is often discovered coincidentally when the patient is undergoing the diagnosis for a consequence of this disease, such as pneumonia or anemia. The **malignant leukemic cells** are unable to function and fight off infection, resulting in the patient being hospitalized due to a bacterial infection. If the white blood cell count has begun to increase significantly, the bone marrow may be producing excessive neutrophils instead of red blood cells, resulting in a decrease in the number of red blood cells (anemia) in which the red blood cells appear normal (normal size, shape, and color). The patient with CML may present with weight loss, enlarged spleen, fever, night sweats, and malaise. The total white blood cell count is usually greater than **$50 \times 10^9/l$ and may exceed $300 \times 10^9/l$,** most of which are **mature segmented neutrophils** (PMNs) with some bands, metamyelocytes, and myelocytes (Fig. 3–13). This cell population present in CML mimics a response to a bacterial infection (leukemoid reaction); however, the **LAP score** mentioned earlier would be **decreased.** Other myeloid cells may also be increased, such as eosinophils, basophils, monocytes, and thrombocytes. The bone marrow is hypercellular due to primarily granulocytic proliferation of all stages (Fig. 3–14). The density of the packed cells within the bone marrow may result in a "dry tap" with no sample aspirated. A diagnosis is most often made from the peripheral blood smear and a cytogenetic evaluation. Ninety to ninety-five percent of patients with CML have the Philadelphia chromosome (Ph[1]), which is a translocation of the long arm of chromosome 22 to chromosome 9. This chromosomal translocation alters the *c-abl* on-

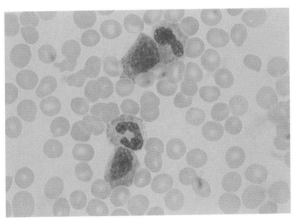

FIGURE 3–13
Chronic myelocytic leukemia as seen in the peripheral blood. Notice the abundance of mature neutrophils.

cogene (tumor-producing gene), which may be significant in the development of this leukemia.

CML is treated with busulfan (chemotherapy), which controls the disease for approximately 3 years, at which time a more aggressive disease may develop. More immature cells are seen in this blast phase, and the prognosis is poor (about 2 to 10 months). The morphology and cell populations may have inconsistent or altered characteristics as a result of the chemotherapy. This must be considered when an evaluation is made of this blood specimen.

Acute myelogenous leukemia (AML, FAB M1, and M2) is most common in the first few months of life and again in the mid to late years of life. As with any acute illness, the **onset is sudden** and aggressive, often resembling an acute infection. The patient presents with fever, malaise, and ulcers of the mouth and throat. There are two classifications of AML depending on the cells seen. Due to the similarity of acute leukemias, the French, American, and British (FAB) hematologists have devised a classification scheme presented in Table 3–1. The first type of AML is classified as **M1** (AML without maturation) by the FAB classification due to the lack of maturation seen. The predominant cell is the myeloblast, which makes up at least 90% of the nonerythroid bone marrow cells and is seen in the peripheral blood (Fig. 3–15). Some **AML myeloblasts** have cytoplasmic inclusions, called **Auer rods,** which are made of fused azurophilic peroxidase and ASD chloroacetate esterase positive granules. Auer rods appear as spindle-shaped inclusions and are seen primarily in myeloblasts and promyelocytes. They are seen less commonly in mature neutrophils and in other subtypes of AML. The presence of Auer rods is most often associated with M1 to M3. The similarity of blast cells makes cell line identification difficult; however, if Auer rods are seen, the cells are considered to be myeloblasts.

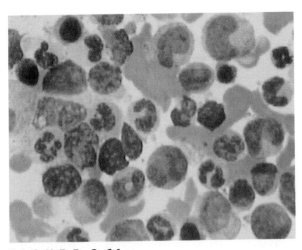

FIGURE 3–14
Chronic myelogenous leukemia as seen in the bone marrow. Notice the increase in cell proliferation called hyperplasia, which consists primarily of myeloid cells.

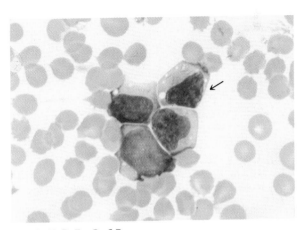

FIGURE 3–15
Acute myelogenous leukemia (AML) without maturation (M1), as seen in the peripheral blood. Notice the abundance of immature myeloblast cells (arrow), some of which contain Auer rods.

In order to **distinguish acute myelocytic leukemia (AML) from acute lymphocytic leukemia (ALL), cytochemical stains** such as myeloperoxidase (MPO), Sudan Black B (SBB), and ASD chloroacetate esterase (CAE) can be used to aid in the diagnosis (Fig. 3–16). The AML classified as **M2** (AML with maturation) demonstrates that only 30 to 89% of bone marrow cells are myeloblasts and

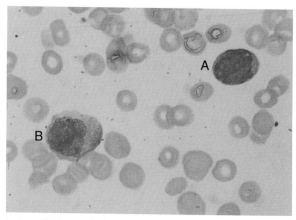

FIGURE 3–17
Acute myelogenous leukemia (AML) with some maturation of cells present (M2), as seen in the peripheral blood. Notice the abundance of myeloblasts (A) and promyelocytes (B) versus M1, which is primarily blasts.

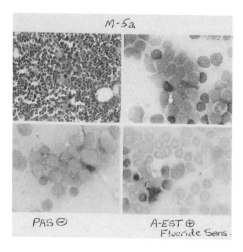

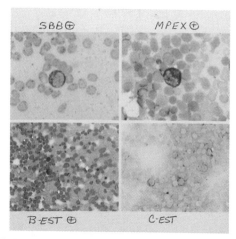

FIGURE 3–16
Acute leukemia cytochemistries. Due to the presence of primarily blasts in acute leukemias, staining the cells with specific cytochemical stains can be used to determine from which cell line the blast originates. Myelocytic cells stain with peroxidase, esterase, and Sudan black B. Monoblasts may only stain weakly with the peroxidase and strongly with esterase, which can be inhibited with fluoride. Lymphocytes would not take up any of the enzyme stains due to a lack of lysosomal cytoplasmic granules. Lymphoblasts stain with periodic acid-Schiff, which stains the cytoplasmic glycogen.

greater than 10% of the nonerythroid cells are promyelocytes, myelocytes, metamyelocytes, bands, and mature neutrophils (Fig. 3–17). Due to the presence of **primarily immature cells** and few mature PMNs in AML, there is no concern that this is a leukemoid reaction as seen with CML. The blast cells seen in AML, acute monocytic leukemia (AMoL), and acute lymphocytic leukemia (ALL) are often indistinguishable from one another. In order to identify the specific type of blast, cytochemical staining can be done (Table 3–2). Cytochemical staining is discussed in more detail in the testing section of this chapter.

Acute promyelocytic leukemia (APL, FAB M3) has hypergranular promyelocytes dominating the bone marrow (Fig. 3–18). Intensely staining azurophilic granules and Auer rods are seen in most cases of M3. There are variants (M3V) in which the promyelocyte granules are small and sparse. M3 AML is characterized clinically by severe bleeding due to procoagulants in the excessive number of promyelocyte granules initiating disseminated intravascular coagulation (DIC). Treatment consists of administration of chemotherapeutic drugs to decrease the leukemic cell numbers and heparin to avoid DIC.

Acute myelomonocytic leukemia (AMML, FAB M4) is diagnosed by the presence of a peripheral blood monocytosis of more than $5 \times 10^9/l$, 20 to 80% monocytic

TABLE 3–2   CYTOCHEMISTRIES TO DIFFERENTIATE BLAST CELLS

Leukemia	MPO	SBB	NASDC	NSE	Fluoride-Inhibited NSE	PAS
M1(AML)	+	+	+	−	−	−
M2(AML)	++	++	+	−	−	−
M3(APL)	+++	+++	+	−	−	−
M4(AMML)	++	++	++	++	−	−
M4eo	+	+	+	+	−	eos +
M5a and b(AMoL)	±	±	±	+++	++	++
M6(AEL)	−	−	−	++	−	++
M7(AMegL)	−*	−	−	−	−	−*
L1(ALL)	−	−	−	−	−	++**
L2(ATL)	−	−	−	−	−	++**
L3(ALL)	−	−	−	−	−	++**

*Positive for platelet peroxidase and platelet glycogen.
**Identified by cluster differentiation (CD) markers.
MPO = myeloperoxidase; SBB = Sudan black B; NASDC = napthol ASD chloracetate esterase (specific esterase); NSE = Nonspecific esterases (alpha-naphthyl butyrate, alpha naphthyl acetate); PAS = periodic acid-Schiff.
1+ = small amount of stain taken up; 2+ = a little more stain; 3+ = significant amount of stain; − = no stain uptake.

cells of the bone marrow nonerythroid cells (normal is 1.8%), and 30% of the total marrow cells are myeloblasts (normal is 1%). Due to the presence of both monocytic and granulocytic cells, it is important to test serum and urine lysozyme, cytochemical stain with esterase (with and without fluoride), and immunophenotype monocytes for CD14 membrane marker.

A subclass of M4 is the **M4E** which is acute myelomonocytic leukemia with eosinophilia. Most individuals with M4E are between 40 and 45 years of age, and these people present with organomegaly. More than 5% of the bone marrow nonerythroid cells are eosinophils that have abnormally large basophilic granules mixed with the eosinophilic granules. These eosinophils will stain with ASD chloroacetate esterase, unlike normal eosinophils. Also associated with M4E is a genetic inversion or deletion of chromosome 16. Treatment with chemotherapy has been quite successful.

M5 is an acute monocytic leukemia (AMoL), which is discussed later in this chapter. M6 is an acute erythroleukemia (AEL), which is discussed in Chapters 9 and 10. M7 is an acute megakaryocytic leukemia, which is presented in Chapters 11 and 13. Table 3–1 lists the FAB classification of acute leukemia.

Myelofibrosis and myeloid metaplasia are the same basic disease process, which has also been called agnogenic myeloid metaplasia and aleukemic myelosis. This disease is a chronic, progressive, panmyelosis (increase in abnormalities in all bone marrow cells). This is an uncommon disease and occurs in persons older than 50 years of age. Myelofibrosis is characterized by fibrous tissue developing in the bone marrow (fibrosis), which results in massive splenomegaly due to production of blood cells in the spleen to meet the body's need (extramedullary hematopoiesis). The infiltration of the bone marrow by the malig-

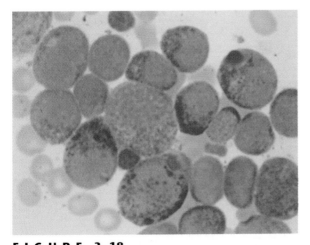

F I G U R E   3–18
Acute promyelocytic leukemia (APL, M3). Note the abundance of promyelocytes with hypergranulation.

nant fibrous tissue results in a leukoerythroblastic anemia with marked red blood cell abnormalities, circulating normoblasts, immature granulocytes, and atypical platelets. The leukoerythroblastic anemia is associated with general bone marrow replacement by any malignant disease.

Decreased Neutrophil Count (Neutropenia)

The **neutrophil count may be decreased (neutropenia or agranulocytosis)** for a variety of reasons. If an **infection has depleted** all of the available neutrophils, neutropenia should be transient until more cells can be produced and released from the bone marrow. If neutropenia is prolonged, this may indicate a severe infection that has exhausted even the bone marrow's supply of cells. This is a poor indication of the patient's ability to recover from the infection. Genetic or acquired disorders may interfere with the bone marrow (medullary) hematopoiesis. Sometimes in disease an enlarged organ such as the spleen may hold or sequester a large number of circulating cells, which will alter the cell count. **Aplasia and myeloid hypoplasia** are the failure of the bone marrow to produce cells. These can be attributed to rare genetic disorders or toxic drugs, chemicals, and radiation. Some antibiotics necessary to treat an illness may be toxic to the bone marrow and require monitoring of the blood cell count. When all cell lines are decreased, this is called pancytopenia.

Other diseases in which the neutrophils are decreased (neutropenia, $<50\%$, $<2 \times 10^9/l$) are myelodysplastic syndrome (MDS), lack of necessary vitamins such as vitamin B_{12} and folate, **leukemias, and other proliferation disorders in which the bone marrow is preoccupied with the production of the neoplastic cell** and is, therefore, not producing other cells.

Vitamin B_{12} (cyanocobalamin) deficiency, also called **pernicious anemia (PA),** is due to inadequate vitamin B_{12} absorption in the stomach. This can be due to defective production of the gastric intrinsic factor

(IF) necessary for vitamin B_{12} absorption or the production of antibodies directed against the intrinsic factor. Megaloblastic (large, immature appearing) red blood cells and hypersegmented neutrophils (>5 lobes) are seen on the peripheral blood smear (Fig. 3–19). **Folate deficiency** will have the same presentation as vitamin B_{12} deficiency. Vitamin B_{12} and folate are required for normal DNA synthesis; therefore, all dividing cells will be affected by this disorder. Serum vitamin B_{12}, serum folate, and red blood cell folate levels are performed in the chemistry and microbiology departments and should be correlated with the hematology results. Tests to determine vitamin B_{12} and folate deficiency are discussed in the granulocyte testing section of this chapter. Vitamin B_{12} and folate deficiencies are discussed in more detail in Chapters 9 and 10. The Arneth count is a method of documenting the presence of hypersegmented neutrophils. This test is described in Chapter 6.

Myelodysplastic syndrome (CMDS) is seen in individuals older than 50 years of age and presents with an anemia that is not responsive to therapy (refractory), although new treatments are improving erythropoiesis. The marrow is hypercellular with increased blast cells and abnormal maturation in one or more of the hematopoietic cell lines. This disease has been referred to as preleukemia and dysmyelopoietic syndrome due to the high proportion of cases that have progressed to overt

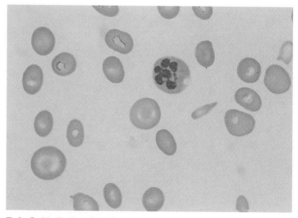

F I G U R E 3–19
Hypersegmented neutrophils. This is considered a "shift to the right" toward maturity and is seen in vitamin B_{12} deficiency.

leukemia. The French, American, and British (FAB) hematology group has classified MDS (Table 3–3). The classification of MDS is based on the cells seen in the bone marrow and peripheral blood and their morphology. **There are five types of MDS: (1) refractory anemia (RA); (2) refractory anemia with ringed sideroblasts (RARS); (3) refractory anemia with excess blasts (RAEB); (4) chronic myelomonocytic leukemia (CMML); and (5) refractory anemia with excess blasts in transformation (RAEB-T).** Refractory anemia is a decrease in red blood cells that does not respond to therapy. Ringed sideroblasts are nucleated bone marrow red blood cells with iron deposits in a ring around the nucleus. These are discussed in more detail in Chapters 9 and 10. Blasts refer to the erythroblast, which is the earliest recognizable cell of the erythroid cell line. The treatment and survival (prognosis) varies for each of the five types. Survival ranges from 3 to 52 months.

Abnormal Neutrophil Function

Beyond the quantitative disorders the number of neutrophils may be normal, but there may be **abnormal neutrophil function.** These disorders are hereditary such as chronic granulomatus disease (CGD), lazy leukocyte syndrome, Chédiak-Higashi anomaly, and vitamin B_{12} deficiency and can be diagnosed by alterations in morphology and function. A patient

Do It Now Neutrophil Exercise

A 73-year-old patient presented with a severe bacterial infection (septicemia).

1. Describe the white blood cell picture that you would expect to see in terms of total white blood cell count and any elevated or decreased individual cell counts.

The next two questions can be done individually or in small groups.

2. Is this a relative or absolute cell count (see Chapter 1)?
3. What additional tests would provide information for an accurate differential diagnosis?
4. Given the results of tests for number 3, how would you describe, in professional terms to another health care provider such as a nurse or radiologist, what was occurring in this patient?

with any one of these disorders is predisposed to infection. **Chronic granulomatous disease (CGD)** is the inability of the enzymatic digestive granules to release their contents. These individual neutrophils ingest the bacteria but are unable to destroy them. **Lazy leukocyte syndrome** is a poor response to chemotactic factors, resulting in inefficient migration and accumulation in order to destroy the bacteria. Both CGD and lazy leukocyte syndrome are diagnosed by neutrophil function tests described in the next section of this chapter.

TABLE 3–3 FRENCH-AMERICAN-BRITISH CLASSIFICATION OF MYELODYSPLASTIC SYNDROME (MDS)

| Classification | Bone Marrow Blasts (%) | Ringed Sideroblasts | Peripheral Blood (%) | |
			Blasts	Monocytes
Refractory anemia	<5	<15	<1	None
Refractory anemia with ringed sideroblasts	<5	>15	<1	None
Refractory anemia with excessive blasts	5–20	None	<5	None
Refractory anemia with excessive blasts in transformation	>20–30 Auer rods	None	<5	None
Chronic myelomonocytic leukemia	>20	None	<5	>1 × 10⁹/l

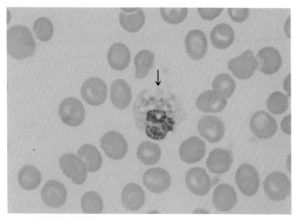

A Chédiak-Higashi white blood cell anomaly. Giant granules (arrow) are seen in the cytoplasm of all white blood cells.

Anomalies

The following four neutrophil morphologic alterations are called **anomalies,** of which three affect function. An anomaly is a marked deviation from normal, especially as a result of congenital or hereditary defects. **Chédiak-Higashi anomaly** is an autosomal recessive genetic disorder in which the neutrophils contain large inclusion granules in the cytoplasm. These abnormal granules impair the normal function of the cell (Fig. 3–20). **May-Hegglin anomaly** is a rare autosomal characterized by blue patches of RNA in the cytoplasm, resembling Döhle bodies (Fig. 3–21). This is accompanied by giant platelets and occasionally by decreased platelets (thrombocytopenia). These blue cytoplasmic patches are also seen in eo-

sinophils and monocytes. A third anomaly is the **Alder-Reilly anomaly,** which is seen in all white blood cells. Dense, azurophilic granulation resembling toxic granulation is present with no association to infection (Fig. 3–22). The fourth morphologic abnormality is the **Pelger-Huët anomaly.** Genetic hyposegmentation of the neutrophils is seen. All neutrophils will appear as band cells or will demonstrate only two lobes (Fig. 3–23). The Pelger-Huët cells are functionally normal. All four anomalies can be identified on the peripheral blood smear during morphologic evaluation.

Lupus Erythematosus Cell

The lupus erythematosus (LE) cell is an artificially developed neutrophil for the purpose of testing. These cells are not routinely seen in the peripheral blood or bone marrow of patients with LE. LE cells are only seen when blood from a patient with LE is treated, as presented in the leukocyte testing section of this chapter. The LE cell is a neutrophil that has phagocytized a mass of nucleoprotein from damaged white blood cells, which has been coated with LE protein (Fig. 3–24). Production of LE cells in peripheral blood or bone marrow specimen was a method of detecting the presence of the LE factor protein. There are now latex screening tests and fluorescent antinuclear antibody (ANA) tests that are easier, more accurate, and less expensive. If an LE preparation is done, the laboratory practi-

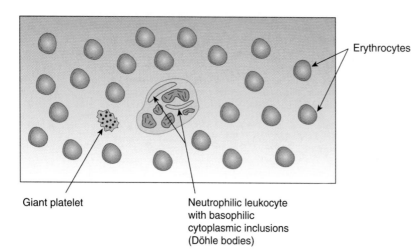

Giant platelet

Neutrophilic leukocyte with basophilic cytoplasmic inclusions (Döhle bodies)

Erythrocytes

A May-Hegglin white blood cell anomaly. The neutrophil cytoplasm contains pale blue inclusions resembling Döhle bodies. Giant platelets are also seen.

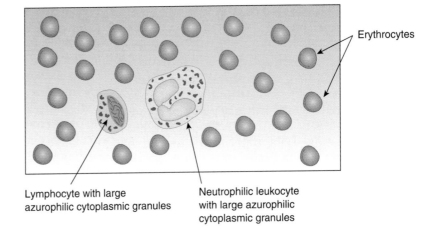

Erythrocytes

FIGURE 3-22
An Alder-Reilly white blood cell anomaly. Dense granulation resembling toxic granulation appears in all white blood cells.

Lymphocyte with large azurophilic cytoplasmic granules

Neutrophilic leukocyte with large azurophilic cytoplasmic granules

tioner must be able to distinguish the LE cell from the neutrophil, which has phagocytized an old nucleus that has not been transformed into a homogenous mass by the LE factor (tart cell). The **tart cell** is a result of a normally functioning neutrophil cleaning up debris. The contents of the tart cell will be an irregular mass of chromatin, usually smaller than the LE mass.

Increased Eosinophils (Eosinophilia)

An **increase in eosinophils (eosinophilia, $>0.35 \times 10^9/l$),** in the peripheral blood, is seen in the allergic condition such as bronchial asthma, seasonal rhinitis (hay fever), atopic dermatitis, eczema, acute urticaria (hives), parasitic infections, scarlet fever rash, uncommon pulmonary diseases, hypereosinophilic syndrome, myeloproliferative disorders (MPDs) such as chronic myelogenous leukemia (CML), following splenectomy, following administration of certain drugs such as sulfonamides, and a rare hereditary eosinophilia. The observance of eosinophils in nasal smears and sputum may aid in the diagnosis of the condition.

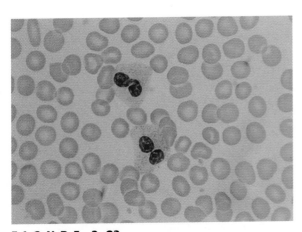

FIGURE 3-23
A Pelger-Huët white blood cell anomaly. The segmented neutrophils are hyposegmented.

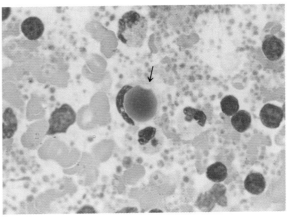

FIGURE 3-24
A lupus erythematosus (LE) cell. Note the homogeneous LE mass in the neutrophil (arrow). If this was a normal phagocytosis of an old nucleus, the chromatin would be more visible and the mass would be smaller.

Decreased Eosinophils (Eosinopenia)

Decreased eosinophils (eosinopenia, $< 0.04 \times 10^9/l$) in the peripheral blood is seen in any stressful situation resulting in the release of adrenal corticoids or epinephrine and acute inflammation. These hormones induce the marginating eosinophils into the area of inflammation in the tissues and cause the circulating eosinophils to marginate.

Increased Basophils (Basophilia)

The **increase in basophils** (basophilia, $> 0.2 \times 10^9/l$) is seen in **hypersensitivity (allergic) reactions and myeloprolifera-**

tive disorders **(MPDs)** such as chronic myelogenous leukemia (CML), polycythemia vera, hypothyroidism, chronic hemolytic anemia, and following splenectomy. A relative **transient basophilia** may be seen following **irradiation** or following administration of some **hematopoietic growth factors.**

A **decreased number of basophils** is difficult to determine. Due to the low numbers of basophils, if any, seen in peripheral blood testing, a decreased basophil count (basopenia, $< 0.01 \times 10^9/l$) is documented by counting large numbers of basophils directly. Conditions in which basopenia would be seen are sustained treatment with adrenal glucocorticoids, acute infection, acute stress, and approximately half of the patients with hyperthyroidism.

FAST FACTS

Granulocyte Information

Cell	Neutrophil	Eosinophil	Basophil
Origin:	CFU-GM	CFU-Eo	CFU-Ba
Stages:	Promyelocyte (nonspecific MPO, round nucleus, nucleoli)	Promyelocyte	Promyelocyte
	N. myelocyte (specific eo, baso, neutro granules appear with the nonspecific granules)	E. myelocyte	B. myelocyte
	N. metamyelocyte (first indentation of the nucleus)	E. metamyelocyte	B. metamyelocyte
	N. band/Stab (mature cytoplasm, band/sausage-shaped nucleus)		
		E. band/Stab	B. band/Stab
	Mature neutrophil	Mature eosinophil	Mature basophil (tissue mast cell)
Size:	Medium	Large	Small
	3–5 segments of nucleus, pinkish/brown granules	2–3 segments	2–3 segments
		Large orange granules	Large dark blue granules
Function:	Responds to bacteria, phagocytizes	Eosinophils and basophils mediate hypersensitivity reactions	Eosinophils and basophils mediate hypersensitivity reactions
		Eosinophil releases antihistamine	Basophil releases histamine and heparin
Malignancies:	M1–M4	M4e, various MPDs	Various MPDs
Stains:	LAP, MPO, CAE		
Reference:	54–62% WBC	1–3% WBC	0–1%
Values:	3000–5800/mm³	50–250/mm³	15–50/mm³

CAE = chloracetate esterase; CFU-Ba = colony-forming unit–basophil; CFU-Eo = colony forming unit–eosinophil; CFU-GM = colony-forming unit–granulocyte macrophage; LAP = leukocyte alkaline phosphatase; MPO = myeloperoxidase; MPD = myeloproliferative disorder.

STUDY QUESTIONS

1. All granulocytes originate from the same progenitor cell, which is the
   A. BFU-E
   B. CSF-G
   C. CFU-GEMM
   D. CFU-M

2. The origin of the _____ and the _____ is still not completely evident. A close association has been shown with one another and with other granulocytic cells.
   A. Basophil and tissue mast cell
   B. Eosinophil and tissue mast cell
   C. Neutrophil and tissue macrophage
   D. Monocyte and tissue macrophage

3. A 87-year-old woman who presents with a white blood cell count of $94 \times 10^9/l$, containing 90% mature neutrophils, 2% band neutrophils, and 8% lymphocytes is suggestive of:
   A. Leukemoid reaction
   B. Acute myelogenous leukemia
   C. Chronic myelogenous leukemia
   D. Parasitic infection

4. The presence of large granules in every neutrophil seen on the peripheral blood smear is most likely:

   A. Artifact of preparation

   B. A leukemoid reaction with toxic granulation

   C. A parasitic infection demonstrating Döhle bodies

   D. A genetic anomaly, such as Chédiak-Higashi syndrome

Match the Following:

5. Mediate hypersensitivity reactions by secretion of a histamine-neutralizing substance

6. Contain digestive enzymes, such as peroxidase and esterase

7. Phagocytize primarily bacteria

8. Secrete histamine and heparin when two IgE antibody molecules bind to the membrane

A. Neutrophils

B. Eosinophil

C. Basophil

True (1 or a) or False (2 or b):

9. Eosinophils are increased in the peripheral blood in allergies, colds, and parasitic infections.

10. In a leukemoid reaction, neutrophils become larger, divide, proliferate, and produce cell-secreted proteins called cytokines.

11. Band neutrophils are seen in severe bacterial infections that have exhausted the mature neutrophil supply and are demanding the bone marrow reserve of neutrophils.

12. Leukocyte alkaline phosphatase (LAP) score is elevated in chronic myelogenous leukemia (CML).

O U T L I N E

Origin, Maturation, and Morphology of Monocytes/Macrophages

Physiology and Function of Monocytes/Macrophages

Normal Response and Diseases of Monocytes/Macrophages
Increased Monocytes (Monocytosis)
Decreased Monocytes (Monocytopenia)

Study Questions

Monocyte/ Macrophage Blood Cells

O B J E C T I V E S

Upon completion of this chapter the student should be able to:

1. Diagram and explain monopoiesis from its origin through maturation.

2. Trace the kinetics of the monocyte from its release in the bone marrow to cell death.

3. List the various macrophages throughout the body and their locations.

4. Explain the following functions of a monocyte: Phagocytosis (including hemoglobin breakdown and iron storage), antigen processing and presentation, and production of interleukins and other cytokines (monokines).

5. Contrast and compare normal responses and diseases of the monocytes.

6. Correlate the appropriate leukocyte testing with monocyte responses and disease.

7. Explain the difference between the acute myelomonocytic leukemia (M4), monocytic leukemia (M5), and Gaucher's disease.

Monocytes are part of the macrophage system, also called the reticuloendothelial system (RES), which includes macrophage cells throughout the body. The macrophages are located in the tissues and have a variety of names depending on their location. Macrophage cells in the bone marrow are **histiocytes;** liver cells are called **Kupffer cells;** macrophages in the brain are called **microglial cells;** bone cells are **osteoclasts;** and skin macrophages are called **Langerhans cells.** The **monocyte is the peripheral blood macrophage.** These cells are not only the most efficient phagocytic cells that act in the body's defense but they also play a key role in relaying information about the offending cell or substance to the rest of the immune system for an effective immune response.

ORIGIN, MATURATION, AND MORPHOLOGY OF MONOCYTES/MACROPHAGES

All of the blood cells originate from the **pluripotent stem cell (PSC),** which, under the influence of hematopoietic regulatory proteins (cytokines), becomes the **hematopoietic stem cell (HSC)** or colony-forming unit–spleen (CFU–S). This cell is stimulated to proliferate by cytokines listed in Figure 4–1. Under the influence of specific cytokines, the PSC will become the **colony-forming unit–granulocyte, erythrocyte, monocyte, megakaryocyte (CFU-GEMM),** which will be influenced by various cytokines to become the **colony-forming unit–granulocyte-monocyte (CFU-GM)** (neutrophil and monocyte precursor). The CFU-GM is then stimulated to become the colony-forming unit–monoblast, which is the first committed monocytic cell. The monoblast has the basic characteristics of other white blood cell blasts with a low nuclear to cytoplasmic (N:C) ratio, no granules in the cytoplasm, and a loose chromatin pattern with nucleoli. The CFU–M then becomes the **promonocyte,** which matures into the **peripheral blood monocyte.** The monoblast is morphologically similar to the

myeloblast and the lymphoblast. The promonocyte and monocyte have only subtle differences morphologically. All three stages of monocytic development make up approximately 1.8% of nucleated bone marrow cells.

The **monocyte is the largest peripheral white blood cell,** with a diameter of 14 to 20 μm, and represents 3% to 8% of the differential white blood cell count. Monocytes are distributed in the peripheral blood between the margination monocyte pool (MMP) and the circulating monocyte pool (CMP) in a fashion similar to that of the neutrophils. There are 3.5 times as many monocytes in the MMP as in the CMP, and a large population of monocytes inhabit the spleen, which is the body's blood-filtering organ. The morphologic characteristics include a **large indented nucleus with a lacy chromatin structure.** This pattern is looser than the granulocytic nucleus and is less uniform than the smooth nucleus of the lymphocyte. The **cytoplasm is gray-blue** with a **slight pink color** appearing when the focus is adjusted slightly. This pink color is attributed to very fine azurophilic granules among the blue granules (Fig. 4–2). Monocyte primary granules contain a small amount of peroxidase activity and secondary granules with strong acid phosphatase and arylsulfatase activity.

The major monocytic characteristics for identification are the large size, the mononuclear-indented nucleus with a lacy chromatin pattern, and the very fine granular cytoplasm with a pink hue within the blue-gray (see Fig. 4–2).

The pink hue can only be seen if a fine focus is used to appreciate the various granules. The monocyte will often also display **vacuoles** and a foamy cytoplasmic appearance. The monocyte and lymphocyte are difficult to distinguish; however, the monocyte usually has a less uniform, light-colored nucleus, and the cytoplasm of the lymphocyte will never appear pink when the focus is adjusted.

Tissue macrophages analogous to the blood

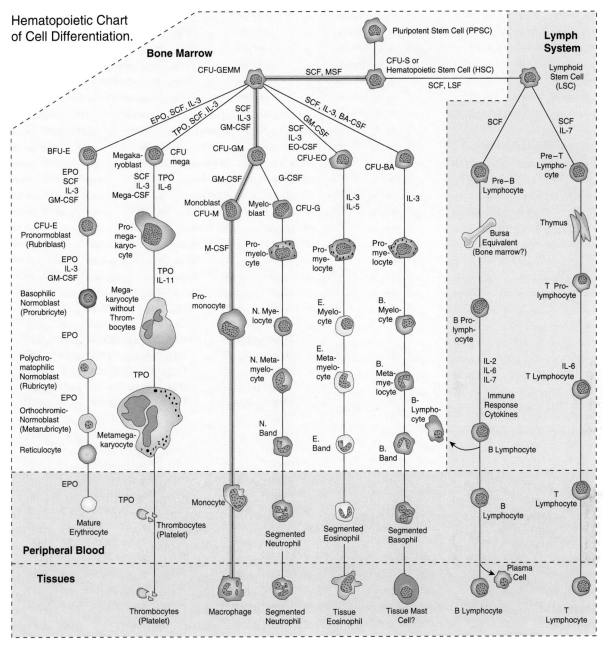

Hematopoietic Chart of Cell Differentiation.

FIGURE 4–1
Monopoiesis is highlighted in relation to hematopoiesis.

monocyte are much larger, with an eccentric round nucleus and an abundant irregular cytoplasm. The example shown here is a histiocyte from the bone marrow (Fig. 4–3). The cytoplasm of the macrophage may contain remnants of phagocytized material, such as iron or debris from red blood cell digestion.

PHYSIOLOGY AND FUNCTION OF MONOCYTES/ MACROPHAGES

The monocyte is a very important cell for development of an effective immune response to fight infection within the body. Monocytes

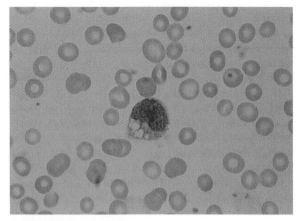

FIGURE 4–2
A monocyte. The peripheral blood macrophage. Note the twisted chromatin pattern of the nucleus, the rough, grainy-looking, gray-blue cytoplasm with a hint of pink when examined under the microscope. Vacuoles are present and common but are not diagnostic. Reactive lymphocytes may also vacuolate when exposed to anticoagulants.

spend an average of 8 hours in the peripheral blood (vascular) and much longer periods of time in the tissues (extravascular). **Three functions** are attributed to the monocyte (Fig. 4–4). The **first function is efficient phagocytosis.** The phagocytic process is the same as that described for the neutrophil; however, the monocyte/macrophage is less se-

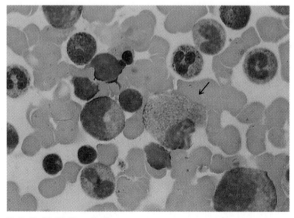

FIGURE 4–3
A histiocyte, the bone marrow macrophage, phagocytizes foreign organisms, processes the antigen phagocytized for presentation to T-helper cells, produces lymphokines, and stores the excess body iron to provide to developing erythrocytes. The histiocyte often has an irregular outline, debris from phagocytosis, and red blood cells surrounding or within the cytoplasm.

lective than the neutrophil and does not die upon digestion of foreign material. The monocyte is a scavenger cell that will ingest any cell or substance that is not a normal inhabitant of the body. An important phagocytic role of the monocyte is to break down old or abnormal red blood cells into components to be recycled within the body or excreted. Red blood cells contain **iron,** which is **stored in the macrophage** following the breakdown **(hemolysis)** of red blood cells until they are needed for new red blood cell production or for other body functions. This macrophage, iron, is observed by staining the bone marrow smear with a Prussian blue stain. Bilirubin, which is a toxic byproduct of red blood cell breakdown, is degraded further by the liver and excreted. This red blood cell lysis by macrophages is called extravascular hemolysis and is discussed in detail in Chapters 7 to 10. The **second function of the monocyte is to process the ingested material and present the antigen (also called immunogen) information on its membrane to the T-helper (CD4) lymphocyte,** which orchestrates an effective healthy immune response to fight off foreign invaders (see Fig. 4–4). This process requires the processed antigen to be presented along with the histocompatible leukocyte antigen-II (HLA-II), also called the major histocompatibility complex-II (MHC-II), membrane protein. The processed antigen and the monocyte antigen interact with the T cell receptor and the T cell MHC-II to exchange vital information for cellular defense and production of antibodies to defend the body against disease. The **third function of the monocyte is to produce and respond to interleukins (IL) and other cytokines** involved in the immune response (see Fig. 4–4). Interleukins and cytokines (regulatory proteins produced by cells) have been presented in previous chapters as part of hematopoiesis regulation and are discussed in more detail in Chapter 5 as part of the immune response. Cytokines secreted by monocytes can be more specifically called monokines and include erythropoietin (EPO), which stimulates the production of red blood cells; granulocyte/monocyte–colony-stimulating factor (GM-CSF), which stimulates the produc-

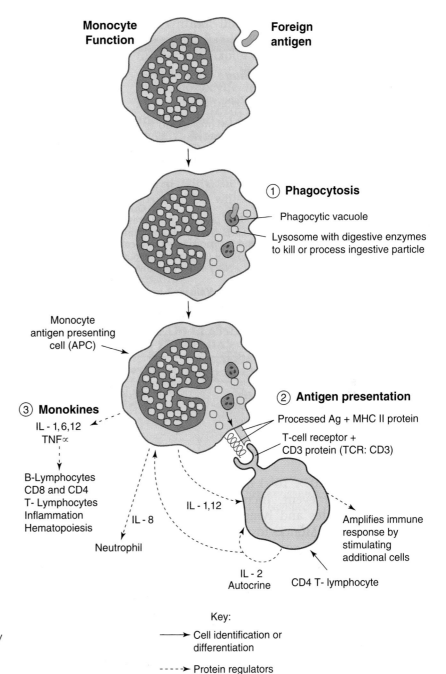

FIGURE 4–4
Functions of the monocyte: (1) phagocytosis, (2) antigen presentation (APC) to the T-helper cell, (3) secretion and response to regulatory proteins, interleukins (ILs), involved in the immune response, and (4) storage of iron (not shown).

tion of granulocytes and monocytes; monocyte–colony-stimulating factor (M-CSF), which stimulates the production of monocytes; granulocyte–colony-stimulating factor (G-CSF), which stimulates the development of granulocytes; interleukin (IL)-1 and IL-8, both of which stimulate neutrophils and lymphocytes; tumor necrosis factor-alpha (TNF-α), which is cytotoxic to tumors; tumor growth factor-beta (TGF-β), which promotes tissue repair; and interferon (IFN)-α and -β, which suppress viral replication.

uloma, **Hashimoto-Pritzker syndrome, self-healing histiocytosis, and pure cutaneous histiocytosis.** These diseases demonstrate a "foamy" cell in bone granulomas and are often found in young children, who have a very short survival rate. **Malignant histiocytosis** is characterized by malignant (life threatening) cells, showing nuclear abnormalities and abundant cytoplasm, infiltrating the body tissue. In response to infection, a benign **histiocytosis** (not life threatening) may be seen. The cells proliferating in this normal response are morphologically normal.

Testing for monocytes is distributed throughout the chapter where appropriate. Monocytes are counted, evaluated microscopically for morphology, and evaluated as histiocytes in the bone marrow for iron storage. A more comprehensive presentation of leukocyte testing is presented in Chapter 6.

Do It Now Monocyte Exercise

1. Monocytes are one of the largest peripheral white blood cells. When looking at a peripheral blood smear on a glass slide under the microscope or a drawing or photomicrograph in a book, how would you determine if a cell that you are evaluating is small, medium, or large?
2. What criteria would be used to identify a monocyte? How does this morphology relate to function?
3. In order to become familiar with the relationship of the cells in terms of amount and size, make a graph with the size of the cells on the y axis (0 to 30 units) and the relative number of cells on the x axis. How would the monocyte curve or peak pattern differ from the granulocyte curve or peak pattern?

FAST FACTS

Monocyte/Macrophage Diseases and Malignancies

Reactive Monocytosis

Acute Infection (good prognosis)
1. Bacterial = syphilis, brucellosis, subacute bacterial endocarditis
2. Protozoan/rickettsial = malaria and Rocky Mountain spotted fever

Chronic Infection
3. Collagen = rheumatoid arthritis and systemic lupus erythematosus
4. Granulomatous = Crohn's disease, ulcerative colitis, sprue, sarcoidosis
5. Fever of unknown origin, liver cirrhosis, post splenectomy

Acute Infection (poor prognosis)
6. Tuberculosis

Malignant Monocytosis

Myeloproliferation
1. Acute myelomonocytic leukemia (AMML/M4)
2. Acute monocytic leukemia (AMoL/M5)
3. Myelodysplastic syndrome (MDS)

Secondary to Lymphoproliferation
4. Lymphomas
5. Hodgkin's disease
6. Multiple myeloma (MM)
7. Polycythemia vera
8. Malignant histiocytosis
9. Various cancers, such as breast, ovarian, and stomach

Monocytopenia

Difficult to Establish Due to Low Numbers in Blood
1. Hairy cell leukemia
2. Transiently after therapy with prednisone

Miscellaneous

Abnormal Lipid Storage and Metabolism Throughout the Body Most Visible in the Macrophage Cells
1. Gaucher's, Tay-Sachs, Sandhoff's, Niemann-Pick, sea-blue histiocytosis, and Fabry's disease

STUDY QUESTIONS

1. The monocyte originates from the _____ in the bone marrow.
   A. CFU-GEMM, BFU-E
   B. CFU-GEMM, CSF-G
   C. CFU-GEMM, CFU-GM
   D. CFU-GEMM, CFU-Mega

2. The monocyte is acted upon by M-CSF and other proteins to mature in the following sequence:
   A. Pronormoblast, basophilic normoblast, polychromatophilic normoblast, monocyte, macrophage
   B. Promyelocyte, myelocyte, metamyelocyte, band, mature monocyte, tissue macrophage
   C. Promegakaryocyte, megakaryocyte, mature monocyte, tissue macrophage
   D. Promonocyte, monocyte, tissue macrophage

3. The tissue macrophage of the bone marrow is called a:
   A. Histiocyte
   B. Kupffer cell
   C. Osteoclast cell
   D. Langerhans cell
   E. Microglial cell

4. The functions of the macrophage include:
   A. Phagocytosis and antigen processing and presenting (APC) to T_h cells
   B. Secretion of monokines, such as IL-1
   C. Iron storage
   D. All of the above

5. A reactive monocytosis is associated with:
   A. Fever of unknown origin, liver cirrhosis, post splenectomy
   B. Bacterial infections such as tuberculosis, syphilis, brucellosis, subacute bacterial endocarditis, protozoan and rickettsial infections such as malaria and Rocky Mountain spotted fever
   C. Collagen disorders, such as rheumatoid arthritis and systemic lupus erythematosus
   D. All of the above

6. If the macrophages in a bone marrow slide stained extensively with Prussian blue stain, this would indicate:
   A. Antigen processing for presentation
   B. An abundance of bilirubin
   C. An abundance of iron
   D. An abundance of lipids

7. Explain the characteristics and location of the diagnostic cells present in acute myelomonocytic leukemia (M4), monocytic leukemia (M5), and Gaucher's disease.

CHAPTER 5

OUTLINE

Origin, Maturation, and Morphology of Lymphocytes and Plasma Cells

Physiology and Function of Lymphocytes and Plasma Cells
 T Lymphocytes
 B Lymphocytes and Plasma Cells
 K Lymphocytes and NK Lymphocytes

Normal Response and Diseases of Lymphocytes and Plasma Cells
 Increased Lymphocytes (Lymphocytosis)
 Decreased Lymphocytes (Lymphocytopenia)
 Malignant Lymphomas

Study Questions

Lymphocytes and Plasma Cells

OBJECTIVES

Upon completion of this chapter the student should be able to:

1. Diagram and explain lymphopoiesis from its origin through maturation.

2. Trace the kinetics of the lymphocyte from the lymphoid system and peripheral blood to cell death.

3. List the various lymphocytes throughout the body with their locations and functions.

4. Explain the following lymphocyte functions and the associated cell membrane markers, cell-mediated immunity (CMI), humoral immunity (HI), and production of interleukins and other cytokines (lymphokines).

5. Contrast and compare normal responses and diseases of the lymphocytes.

6. Correlate the appropriate leukocyte testing with lymphocyte responses and diseases.

7. Explain the difference between acute lymphocytic leukemia (ALL, L1, L2, and L3), chronic lymphocytic leukemia (CLL), miscellaneous lymphoid leukemias, Hodgkin's and non-Hodgkin's lymphoma, multiple myeloma (MM), and other lymphoproliferative disorders.

Lymphocytes are a heterogeneous family of cells with various origins, life spans, and functions. Within the lymphocyte cell line are T cells, B cells, plasma cells, K cells, and natural killer (NK) cells. The origin and the function of lymphocytes are still controversial and this is an area of ongoing research. There is no question, however, of the crucial importance of lymphocytes in our defense against disease (immune response). This is demonstrated in a very real way by the ability of the human immunodeficiency virus (HIV, which leads to the acquired immunodeficiency syndrome [AIDS]) to destroy one population of lymphocytes, which results in death due to diseases that are not life threatening to a healthy individual.

ORIGIN, MATURATION, AND MORPHOLOGY OF LYMPHOCYTES AND PLASMA CELLS

All of the blood cells originate from the **pluripotent stem cell (PSC),** which is under the influence of hematopoietic regulatory proteins (cytokines). This cell becomes the **hematopoietic stem cell (HSC)** or colony-forming unit–spleen **(CFU–S).** The HSC in the bone marrow is influenced to become a **lymphoid stem cell** (LSC) (10 to 20 μm) and migrates either to the **thymus** to become a **T lymphocyte** (6 to 10 μm) or to the **bursa equivalent (bone marrow?)** to become a **B lymphocyte** (6 to 10 μm). Birds have an organ, called the bursa of Fabricius, in which lymphocytes become competent B cells. No such organ has been discovered in humans, although humans have functional B lymphocytes. The current theory suggests that the bone marrow may function as the site of development for B cells (Fig. 5–1). The **thymus and bone marrow are considered to be the primary lymphoid organs** that influence the lymphoblast to become a competent T or B cell. The T and B lymphocytes migrate and circulate within blood and lymphoid tissue, which includes the **spleen, lymph nodes, intestine-associated lymph-**

oid tissue (Peyer's patches), and tonsils. These secondary lymphoid organs contain localized areas of T cells and B cells, where they can readily proliferate when stimulated by an antigen (immunogen). Lymphocytes recirculate between the lymphoid tissue and the blood and live from days to years.

Lymphocytes maintain a fairly consistent **basic morphology, which includes a round nucleus with a fairly continuous uniform chromosomal pattern, scant light blue cytoplasm with no visible organelles, and no granules (occasional azurophilic aggregates are seen and mistaken for granules),** hence a large nuclear to cytoplasmic ratio (Fig. 5–2). In response to stimulation, the lymphocyte may become large; the nucleus becomes less mature with visible nucleoli (for proliferation); the amount of cytoplasm increases (smaller N:C ratio); a prominent clear area (Golgi) appears next to the nucleus; and the cytoplasm becomes dark blue due to the production of proteins (RNA). This responding cell is referred to as a **reactive lymphocyte** (Fig. 5–3). Additional terms used to identify this cell are atypical lymphocyte, Turk cell, and Downey cell. The appearance of reactive lymphocytes is associated with **viral infections,** such as mononucleosis and hepatitis, which are discussed later in this section. The reactive lymphocytes indicate the active production of cytokines (lymphokines) or antibodies (Table 5–1).

T Cells. The white blood cell that migrates to the thymus is the pre–T cell. The pre–T cell is found in the thymus and expresses surface membrane markers and nuclear enzymes useful for identification (Table 5–2). The identification of cells by surface markers is called phenotyping. Accurate phenotyping is very important in the diagnosis and treatment of disease. Another important T-cell membrane family of proteins are the **major histocompatibility complex (MHC-I and -II)** antigens, also referred to as histocompatible leukocyte antigens (HLA-I and -II). MHC-I is associated with organ or graft rejection if incompatible with the host. The MHC-II antigen is essential for T_h recognition of foreign antigens presented by macrophages. The surface proteins change as the cell matures and moves

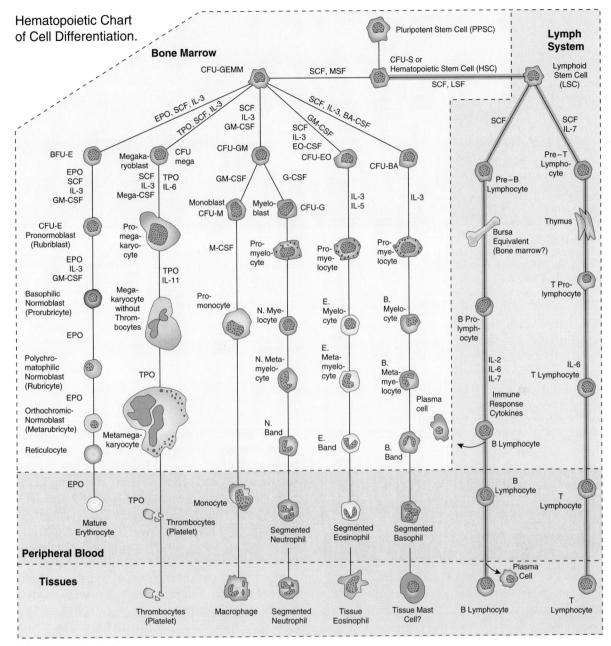

Hematopoietic Chart of Cell Differentiation.

FIGURE 5–1
Lymphopoiesis. Hematopoietic chart with lymphopoiesis highlighted.

into the peripheral lymph tissue and blood. The T lymphocyte cell makes up approximately **80% of the peripheral blood lymphocytes.**

The lymphoid cell that develops in the bone marrow is called the **pre–B cell.** The pre–B cell continues to mature and develop into the **B cell,** which is found within all lymph organs and makes up approximately **20% of the peripheral blood lymphocytes.** Due to the similarity in the morphology of lymphocytes, mature B cells are identified by surface bound (membrane) immunoglobulins, receptors, and protein markers (see Table 5–2).

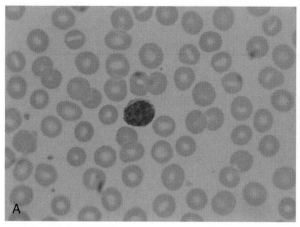
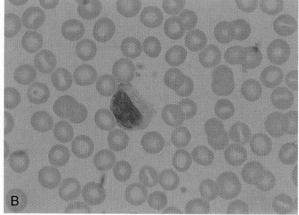

FIGURE 5-2
A and *B* are normal lymphocytes. *A* is a small lymphocyte and *B* has more cytoplasm and may be in transition to a reactive lymphocyte. Note the uniform chromatin pattern of the nucleus and the clear blue cytoplasm.

The mature peripheral blood B cell has immunoglobulins (antibodies) expressed on the outer surface of the membrane, instead of in the cytoplasm as seen in the pre–B cell. The immunoglobulins detected on the B cell membrane vary. Approximately 10 to 15% of mature B cells express IgM or IgD; less than 3% express IgG; and less than 2% express IgA. Upon antigenic stimulation, the B lymphocyte transforms into a **plasma cell,** which is the most efficient producer of antibodies.

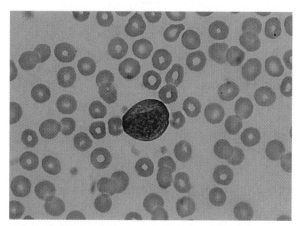

FIGURE 5-3
A reactive lymphocyte. Note the large size, the looser chromatin structure, and nucleoli, suggesting active proliferation. The dark blue cytoplasm with a prominent Golgi apparatus demonstrates increased activity of the ribosomes (RNA), which are producing antibodies or cytokines.

PHYSIOLOGY AND FUNCTION OF LYMPHOCYTES AND PLASMA CELLS

T Lymphocytes

The **T cells are responsible for cell-mediated immunity (CMI), which involves physical contact with other cells or secretion of cytokines** that stimulate, suppress, or destroy invading substances and cells within the body (see Table 5–1). This cell-mediated immunity is an important part of an immune response to defend the body against disease. Examples of cell-mediated immunity include delayed-type hypersensitivity reactions such as graft rejection, lysis of neoplastic cells (abnormal/cancerous cells), and attack of intracellular organisms. There are basically **three functions of T cells:** (1) **to be responsible for obtaining antigen (immunogen) information from antigen-presenting cells (APCs), such as monocytes, and passing this information on to other T cells and B cells;** (2) **to physically interact with a foreign or abnormal cell and destroy it;** and (3) **to produce and secrete various cytokines** to activate some cells while possibly destroying other cells (Fig. 5–4).

Various T cells carry out the aforementioned

TABLE 5–1 LYMPHOCYTE CYTOKINES* AND IMMUNOGLOBULINS

T Lymphocyte Cytokines (Part of Cell-Mediated Immunity)

Interleukin-2 (IL-2), interleukin-3 (IL-3), interleukin-4 (IL-4), interleukin-5 (IL-5), interleukin-10 (IL-10), interleukin-14 (IL-14), B-cell growth factor (BCGF), interferon gamma (IFN-γ), tumor necrosis factor-beta (TNF-β), transforming growth factor-beta (TGF-β).

B Lymphocyte Immunoglobulins (Humoral Immunity)

Immunoglobulin G (IgG)
  80% of plasma immunoglobulin, 8–16 mg/ml
  Monomer, bivalent, 7S, γ heavy chains
  Secondary response, less specific, more avid
  Incomplete or blocking = cell opsonization
  Positive direct antiglobulin test on red blood cells
  Precipitation and agglutination reactions

Immunoglobulin A (IgA)
  6% of plasma immunoglobulin, 0.4–2.2 mg/ml
  Dimer, multivalent, α heavy chains
  Secreted through endothelial cells into body fluids
  First line of defense to fight infection

Immunoglobulin M (IgM)
  13% of plasma immunoglobulin, 1.2–4 mg/ml
  Pentamer, multivalent, 19S, μ heavy chain
  Primary response immunoglobulin
  More specific, less avid
  Activates complement to C9 = cell lysis
  Hemolytic and agglutination reactions

Immunoglobulin E (IgE)
  0.002% of plasma immunoglobulin, 17–450 ng/ml
  Monomer, bivalent, ϵ heavy chain
  Binds to basophils and mast cells = granule release

Immunoglobulin D (IgD)
  1% of plasma immunoglobulin, 0.03 mg/ml
  Monomer, bivalent
  δ heavy chain, function unknown

*See Figure 5–4.

functions. The various subsets of T cells as well as other lymphocytes are morphologically very similar and are differentiated by identifying membrane proteins (antigens), which are unique to each cell. These identifying membrane markers are called **cluster differentiation (CD) markers** (see Table 5–2). The **T helper cell (T$_h$)** is the most important cell in the scheme of immunity. The T$_h$ is identified by a membrane protein called a cluster differentiation (marker) 4 **(CD4).** The T$_h$ cell receives the processed antigen information from the monocyte/macrophage by binding the T cell receptor and the HLA-II antigen (Ia, one of the major histocompatibility [MHC] antigens) to the monocyte/macrophage antigen presented along with the monocyte/macrophage MHC-II antigen. This stimulates the T$_h$ cell to proliferate and pass this information via physical surface contact to additional T$_h$ cells, T suppressor cells (T$_s$), cytotoxic T cells (T$_c$), and B cells. The antigen-presenting cell (monocyte/macrophage) also produces IL-1, which stimulates the T$_h$ cell to proliferate. The **T suppressor cells (T$_s$)** are responsible for keeping the immune response in control. The T$_s$ cell regulates the cell-mediated response of T cells as well as the humoral (antibody) response of B cells. This may be accomplished by three different T$_s$ cells, an inducer, a mediator, and an effector, all identified by the CD8 marker, which are driven by antigen and antigen-antibody interactions. This is an example of the body's system of checks and balances to maintain homeostasis and health. The **cytotoxic T cell (T$_c$)** is also called the cytotoxic T lymphocyte (CTL). The T$_c$ cell is activated by interaction with an HLA class I

TABLE 5–2 LYMPHOCYTE IDENTIFICATION MARKERS

Cell	Marker	Cell	Marker
Pre-T lymphocyte	Thy 1, TdT	Pre-B lymphocyte	Cytoplasmic μ chains (IgM)
Immature T cell	Thy 1, CD3, TdT, or Thy 1, CD4, CD8	Immature B cell	Membrane-bound IgM
Mature T cell	Thy 1, TdT, CD4/8/2/3/5	Mature B cell	Membrane-bound IgM, IgD, CD19/20/24

Thy and CD markers are membrane proteins identified by fluorescent monoclonal antibodies and flow cytometry. Fluorescent monoclonal antibodies can also be used to stain a blood or bone marrow smear if flow cytometry is not available.
Terminal deoxynucleotidyl transferase, or TdT, is a nuclear enzyme T cell marker. Peripheral blood or bone marrow smears are stained for this enzyme.

General Lymphocyte/Plasma Cell Information

Cell	T Lymphocyte	B Lymphocyte	K Cell	NK Cell
Reference Values:	56–77% lymphs 860–1880/mm³	7–17% lymphs 140–370/mm³		
Origin:	PPSC			
	Thymus	Bursa equivalent (BM?)	Unknown	Unknown
	T prolymphocyte T cell	B prolymphocyte B cell	Unknown Killer cell	Unknown NK cell
	T helper: 32–54% lymphs 550–1190/mm³ T suppressor/cytotoxic 24–37% lymphs 430–1060/mm³	Plasma cell		
Function:	Cell-mediated immunity (CMI) Delayed-type hypersensitivity reaction (DTHR)* Secretion of IL 2–6/lymphotoxin, etc.	Humoral immunity (HI) Antibody production	CMI Antibody dependent cytotoxic cell (ADCC)†	CMI surveillance of abnormal (cancerous) cells‡
Identification:	CD4/8/2/5 membrane markers; TdT nuclear stain	IgM, IgD membrane antibodies; CD 19/20/24 membrane markers		

*DTHR includes poison ivy reactions and graft rejection.
†K cells are not T or B null cells, which require antibodies on the target cell to attack.
‡NK cells are not T or B null cells, which attack any cell that is abnormal.
Stains: *Periodic acid-Schiff (PAS), acid phosphatase (AP), terminal deoxynucleotidyl transferase (TdT) nuclear stain.*
Lymphocyte Reference Value: Adult 25–33% *of the WBC differential, lymphocytes = 1500–3000/mm³, BM < 15%;* **newborn 16%** *of the WBC differential;* **pediatric** *15–50%.*
Lymphocytosis *(increase in reactive peripheral blood lymphocytes) =* **viral infection.**
Plasma Cell Reference Value: *Not seen in normal peripheral blood.* **Adult bone marrow =** *<2%, >age.*

(also called MHC) antigen and a foreign antigen that is found on a virus-infected cell or on donor cells from a transplant. The activated T_h cell then stimulates the T_c further by secretion of IL-2, which binds to IL-2 receptors on the T_c cell. The process of cell lysis by the T_c cell involves three stages. The first stage is contact and adherence to the target cell, which requires magnesium (Mg^{2+}) and involves several adhesion molecules. In the second stage, a reorientation occurs within the effector cell and a calcium (Ca^{2+})-dependent fusion of the membranes results. The third stage is cell destruction by formation of protein channels called transmembrane pores through which cytotoxic substances are released. Damage to

mitochondria and the cytoplasm leads to cell death. The T cell involved in the graft rejection, the delayed-type hypersensitivity (DTH) reaction, is noted as a **T_{DTH} cell.**

Among the cells produced after stimulation with a foreign antigen are **T memory cells.** The T memory cells remain in the body for years with the ability to respond immediately to the antigen to which they were sensitized in the first antigen exposure (**primary immune response,** Fig. 5–5). Upon a second exposure to the same antigen, the T memory cells will immediately respond and stimulate other cells to provide a rapid **secondary immune response** with a high titer of antibody produced. This is the mechanism for protec-

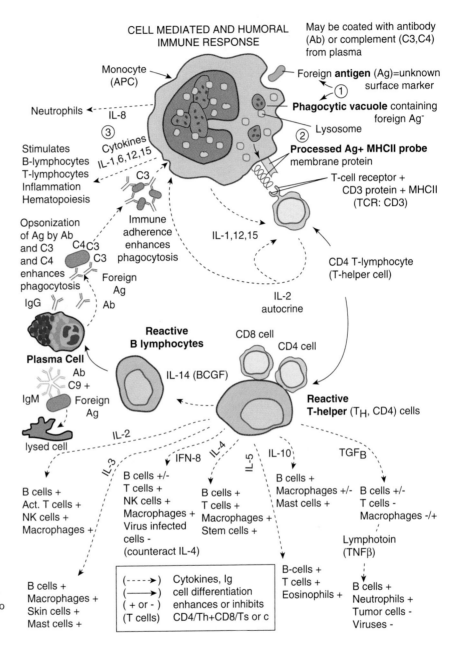

FIGURE 5–4
The cellular and humoral immune response. APC to T cells and cytokines (all T cells), other T cells to target cells to B cells to plasma cells, immunoglobulins and complement.

tion from a vaccine. Each antigenic substance or cell has many antigenic sites (epitopes) that antibodies can be produced against. Therefore, for each immune response, many antibodies are produced and many cells are sensitized—all responding to different antigenic sites of the foreign substance. This is called a **polyclonal response** due to the development of many clones of cells in response to this one foreign substance. A polyclonal response to disease is necessary to eliminate the invading substance (e.g., bacteria) from the body. Later in this chapter, diseases are presented in which there is a **monoclonal response** (only one antibody produced by one clone of plasma cells). This monoclonal antibody production is not adequate to protect against infection and inhibits normal polyclonal antibody production.

Lymphocyte identification proteins (see Ta-

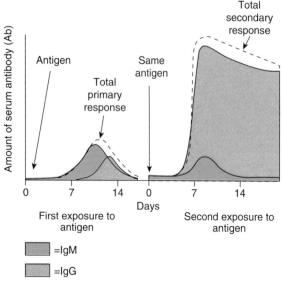

FIGURE 5–5

Primary and secondary humoral immune response. Note the slow, low titer, primarily IgM, antibody development from the first exposure to an antigen, and the rapid, high titer, primarily IgG antibody development from the second exposure to the same antigen.

ble 5–2) are detected using monoclonal antibodies and flow cytometry. This technique is described in Chapter 6.

B Lymphocytes and Plasma Cells

When **B cells are stimulated to produce immunoglobulins (antibodies), this is called humoral immunity (HI).** This terminology is derived from the original designation of proteins, which protect from diseases that were called humors. The stimulated B cell becomes large; the nucleus becomes active with visible nucleoli; the cytoplasm becomes dark blue due to increased protein production by RNA; and the Golgi apparatus enlarges to secrete antibody and is visible as a clear area near the nucleus (perinuclear halo, Hof area). This cell is then classified as a reactive lymphocyte, as mentioned earlier in this section (see Fig. 5–3), which proliferates and secretes proteins. The B cell secretes some antibodies; however, transformation into a **plasma cell** occurs, which is much more efficient at pro-

ducing and secreting immunoglobulin (see Table 5–1). The plasma cell is a little **larger than the resting lymphocyte, has abundant blue cytoplasm, an eccentric nucleus with a distinct clumped chromatin pattern, and a very prominent Golgi apparatus (perinuclear halo, Hof area, clear area) near the nucleus** (Fig. 5–6). Plasma cells make up **less than 5% of the nucleated cells of the bone marrow** and are not found in the peripheral blood. The nuclear chromatin pattern of the plasma cell is arranged in a unique way, which has been described as a "spokes in a wheel" or "clock face" pattern. The chromatin characteristics of the various white blood cells are very important and helpful in cell identification. The ability to recognize these unique nuclear patterns is obtained by repeated observation of various cell chromatin patterns over a period of time. Pictures and atlases are helpful, but each individual has his or her own comprehension of the difference in the nuclear patterns, and light microscope observation is the only way to become familiar with the characteristics of the cell. Automated instruments provide scattergrams to identify cells, eliminating the need to view normal cells under the microscope. However, there will continue to be a need to recognize the various blood cells in order to examine blood smears when unusual results are reported by the automated instruments.

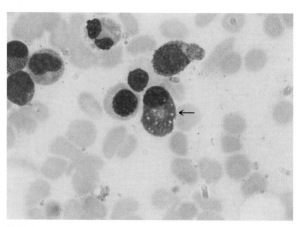

FIGURE 5–6

A plasma cell. Note the eccentric dark nucleus and the abundant dark blue cytoplasm with a very prominent Golgi apparatus.

B memory cells are produced in the primary immune response and are sensitized to the specific foreign antigen. This allows an immediate and more intense immune response (secondary) if the same antigen enters the body in the future, resulting in a secondary immune response (see Fig. 5–5). As explained earlier in relation to T cells, many clones of B cells can be stimulated by many different antigenic sites (epitopes) on an invading cell, resulting in a polyclonal response, which is the production of many antibodies (immunoglobulins) directed against the invading cell or substance.

Immunoglobulins (Ig), also called **antibodies,** are specific proteins produced by plasma cells, and to a lesser degree B lymphocytes, in response to the antigen processed by the monocyte/macrophage, discussed earlier in this chapter. The initial stimulation with a **foreign immunogen (antigen)** and production of immunoglobulins (antibodies) is a primary immune response. These immunoglobulins are produced and secreted by B lymphocytes and **plasma cells,** which are **transformed B cells.** When a **B cell receives** the immunogen (antigen) **information** from the **T helper** lymphocyte, which has received information from the **monocyte/macrophage (antigen-presenting cell/APC),** the B cell begins to proliferate, transforms into a plasma cell, and produces the specific immunoglobulin to bind to the antigen within the body to destroy it or mark it for destruction (opsonization) by phagocytic cells (see Fig. 5–4). Each parent B cell (initially activated) will give rise to many progeny, which together are called a **clone** of cells because they are all identical and will produce a single identical **immunoglobulin,** which is **specific for one antigenic determinant (epitope).** Immunoglobulins consist of two larger polypeptide chains (440 to 550 amino acids), called the heavy chains, and two smaller polypeptide chains, called the light chains (see Table 5–1 and Fig. 5–4). Every immunoglobulin (antibody) produced has a certain amount of consistent structure (homology), which is called the F crystalline (F_c) region, with every other immunoglobulin. Each immunoglobulin has an area that is unique to a specific immuno-

globulin class (IgG, IgM, IgA, IgD, IgE) and an area that is unique for the immunogen (antigen) that it was produced in response to, which is called the fragment for antibody binding (F_{ab}) region. The amino acid sequence of the heavy chain determines the class of immunoglobulin and its functional characteristics. There are five classes of immunoglobulins. Immunoglobulin gamma **(IgG)** is the most abundant (80%, 8 to 16 mg/ml) and the most important antibody to fight off infection (see Table 5–1). Many different IgGs are produced in a healthy polyclonal response to infection. Immunoglobulin M **(IgM)** is the second most important for immune defense and the third highest level in plasma (13%, 1.2 to 4 mg/ml). Immunoglobulin A **(IgA)** is the second most abundant and is mainly found in the body fluids as a first line of defense against body invasions. Plasma concentrations of IgA are 6% or 0.4 to 2.2 mg/ml. Immunoglobulin E **(IgE)** is associated with a hypersensitivity reaction, such as allergies, is responsible for the degranulation of basophils and mast cells, and makes up only 0.002% or 17 to 450 ng/ml of plasma immunoglobulin. Immunoglobulin D **(IgD)** is in very low concentration also (1%, 0.03 mg/ml) and the function is not clear.

Tests to **identify** the presence or absence of **proteins** include **immunodiffusion techniques, immunoassays, electrophoresis, and agglutination tests.** These are all addressed in more detail in the test section of this chapter; however, some aspects of **electrophoresis** are pertinent to protein (immunoglobulin) terminology. The protein electrophoresis separates the proteins by their ability to move through a medium when an **electrical charge** is applied. The chemical **(amino acid composition** of the heavy chain) and **physical makeup** (how the protein chains fold to make the three-dimensional shape) of the immunoglobulin determines the direction and how fast it will move during the incubation of the test. The various areas of protein electrophoresis migration are the alpha (slowest), beta, and gamma (fastest) regions. Most **immunoglobulins** migrate in the same basic area of the electrophoresis medium. This area is called the **gamma region of protein**

electrophoresis; thus another term for immunoglobulins or antibodies is **gamma globulins.** The electrophoresis procedure is done in the chemistry department and is correlated with hematology results. Protein electrophoresis is discussed in Chapter 6 (see also Fig. 6–18).

When a substance or cell (antigen, immunogen) enters the body for the first time, there is a 3- to 10-day period before the antibody is produced. During this initial period, the macrophage/monocyte (antigen-presenting cell) phagocytizes and processes the antigen's information and passes this information on to a T_h cell. The T_h cell proliferates and communicates the information to other lymphocytes, and the resultant activated lymphocytes produce cytokines (T cells) and immunoglobulins (antibodies, B cells) resulting in the body's **immune response** (see Figs. 5–4 and 5–5 and Table 5–1). The initial response, which is slow and produces a lower titer of primarily IgM antibody, is called the **primary immune response.** T cells and B cells produce memory cells specific for each antigen processed as a result of activation and proliferation in the primary immune response. The memory cells survive for years and are always ready to respond to the immunogen (antigen) that they were produced in response to, without the monocyte/macrophage or T_h cell involvement necessary as in the primary immune response. This is called a **secondary immune response** or anamnestic response (see Fig. 5–5). The memory cells identify and bind with the immunogen, proliferate, begin producing a high titer of primarily IgG antibody, cytokines, and perhaps, depending on the antigen, may activate T_c cells (see Table 5–1). Once the immunoglobulin is produced, it binds with the cellular immunogen (antigen) that it was produced against, resulting in lysis (destruction of the cell **intravascularly** due to antibody activation of a plasma protein called **complement)** or opsonization (coating of the particle by antibody or incomplete complement/C3), which will mark it for destruction **extravascularly** by **macrophages** (see Fig. 5–4).

K Lymphocytes and NK Lymphocytes

Some lymphocytes are classified as **null cells (neither T nor B markers)** or large granulocytic lymphocytes (LGL). These cells do, however, react with the common lymphocyte markers, which identifies their cell lineage. Three cells in this category are: (1) **killer cells (K cells),** which are activated by an antibody bound to a cell (opsonization), hence their title as antibody-dependent cytotoxic cells **(ADCC);** (2) **natural killer (NK) cells,** which are not dependent on an antibody to recognize foreign cells. These cells constantly survey the body for cells that demonstrate any surface alteration such as **cancer cells** or **virus-infected cells.** For this reason the NK cells are crucial to monitor development of tumors and other neoplasms (new or altered formation of cells); and (3) **lymphokine-activated killer (LAK) cells,** which, when activated by IL-2, lyse fresh tumor target cells that are resistant to NK cell lysis. Clinical trials are in progress involving the administration of the NK cells as treatment for patients with malignant tumors. This treatment is called immunotherapy.

A ratio of T_h to T_s in the healthy individual is **2 : 1.** These cells are identified by the cluster differentiation (CD) protein membrane markers on peripheral blood lymphocytes using fluorescently tagged monoclonal antibodies and flow cytometry. The T_h cells are **CD4 positive,** and the T_s cells are **CD8 positive.** This ratio can be used to monitor HIV-infected patients. As the AIDS virus invades and destroys the CD4 cells, this ratio will decrease and reverse.

NORMAL RESPONSE AND DISEASES OF LYMPHOCYTES AND PLASMA CELLS

At birth the lymphocytes make up 90% of the leukocytes in the blood. This number decreases gradually during the first decade of life to the adult reference value of 20 to 40%. The normal adult reference value for lymphocytes in the blood is **1.5 to 4.0 × 10^9/l, with T cells accounting for 80% and B cells 20%** of this value. Within the T cell population, the normal ratio for **CD4 (T_h) : CD8 (T_s) is 2:1.** This is reversed in patients with acquired immunodeficiency syndrome (AIDS) due to destruction of CD4 cells by the human immunodeficiency virus (HIV).

Increased Lymphocytes (Lymphocytosis)

An **increase in lymphocytes (lymphocytosis),** or any cell, can be relative or absolute. A relative lymphocytosis (an increase in the percentage of lymphocytes) may reflect neutropenia. Refer to Chapter 1 for further explanation of relative and absolute counts. Lymphocytes are involved in all immune responses; however, they are seen in increased numbers in the peripheral blood most often in response to viruses. The most common reasons for **reactive lymphocytosis are mononucleosis, cytomegalovirus infection, and infectious lymphocytosis.** These conditions are followed closely by **hepatitis, influenza, mycoplasma pneumonia, mumps, measles, rubella, varicella,** and other viral infections. A few bacterial and protozoan infections also produce lymphocytosis. These are **pertussis (whooping cough), tuberculosis, cat-scratch fever, toxoplasmosis, and malaria.** The most common reasons for **malignant lymphocytosis** are **acute lymphoblastic leukemia (ALL), chronic lymphocytic leukemia (CLL),** leukemic phase of lymphoma, and Waldenström's macroglobulinemia.

Infectious mononucleosis is an acute self-limiting (days to weeks) infection caused by **Epstein-Barr virus (EBV), which is a herpes virus.** EBV is passed by an exchange of saliva, which occurs during kissing, hence the alternate name "kissing disease." It is most common in the **17- to 25-year-old** age group and presents with lethargy (fatigue), malaise (total body discomfort), fever, pharyngitis (sore throat), lymphadenopathy (enlarged lymph nodes), and splenomegaly (enlarged spleen). The white blood cell count is usually elevated from **12 to 25 × 10^9/l** but can be as high as 80 × 10^9/l with **60 to 90% lymphocytes, more than 20% reactive.** This infection was named mononucleosis due to the prevalence of mononuclear cells, which are **reactive lymphocytes** (see Fig. 5–3), not monocytes. Abnormally **elevated liver enzyme levels** are seen in most cases due to liver infection, and occasionally a **normocytic, normochromic hemolytic anemia** is seen. Liver enzymes (aspartate aminotransferase [AST] and lactate dehydrogenase [LD]) are elevated when the liver is damaged, and they are measured in the chemistry department along with the elevated bilirubin value, which indicates increased red blood cell hemolysis from hemolytic anemia and defective liver function. The liver is responsible for the breakdown of bilirubin for excretion. The **mononucleosis test,** which indicates the presence of the infectious mononucleosis antibody, is done in the clinical immunology (serology) department of the clinical laboratory. Antibodies that may also be produced in association with the mononucleosis antibody are the rheumatoid factor and cold agglutinins.

Cytomegalovirus (CMV) infection is similar to mononucleosis. The symptoms and blood picture are the same; however, the mononucleosis test results are negative. **Large, reactive lymphocytes** make up **90% of the peripheral blood leukocytes.** The mode of transmission is multiple blood transfusions or exchange of saliva as seen with mononucleosis. A **definitive diagnosis** is made by **isolating CMV** from blood or urine or by **a rise in CMV antibody titer.** The isolation of CMV is done in the microbiology department, and the CMV titer is done in the clinical immunology, serology, or microbiology department or is sent to a reference laboratory. A **titer** is more useful if **done several times over a period of days.** The titer is significant only if a rise or a fall is seen. There are chronic cases of CMV in which the titer remains elevated and the symptoms persist for months.

Infectious lymphocytosis, which is contagious, occurs mainly in young children and has a 12- to 21-day incubation period. Children present with vomiting, fever, rashes, upper respiratory infections, abdominal discomfort, diarrhea, and signs of central nervous system involvement. An association has been made between this presentation and coxsackievirus A, coxsackievirus B6, echoviruses, and adenovirus type 12. This disease itself lasts for 3 to 5 weeks, whereas the reactive lymphocytosis in the blood may persist for up to 3 months.

Hepatitis literally means an inflammation of the liver. This inflammation can be due to various causes, such as **alcohol, toxic drugs and chemicals, and viruses.** There is a group of viruses, however, that primarily infects the liver, and these viruses are called hepatitis viruses. These diseases are identified and monitored by lymphocytosis with **reactive lymphocytes, elevated bilirubin and liver enzyme (ALT) levels, and viral markers.** Viral markers include the presence of various parts of the virus (antigens) and also the appearance of various antibodies by the individual carrying the virus. The appearance of an IgM (antihepatitis virus) antibody indicates the first exposure (a primary response), whereas an IgG antibody indicates a secondary response due to longer duration of the infection. There are several classes of hepatitis, three of which are addressed here. **Hepatitis A virus (HAV)** infection is self-limiting and is spread by **fecal-oral contamination.** This can be contracted by eating in restaurants where infected employees are not washing their hands regularly or are not wearing gloves. Incubation time for HAV is 15 to 45 days, and elevated liver enzymes precede

symptoms. **Hepatitis B virus (HBV)** is called **serum hepatitis** and is transmitted sexually (via body fluids), parenterally (via needles used for injection of drugs or blood transfusion), and perinatally (from the infected mother to the newborn infant). The incubation period following exposure to hepatitis B is 1 to 6 months. This disease is often asymptomatic. Of the 30 to 40% of individuals who do have symptoms, these symptoms include jaundice (yellow skin) due to elevated bilirubin levels, malaise, and joint pain. Approximately 1 to 3% of cases will develop into severe, fatal hepatitis. Five to 10% of patients become chronic carriers, and 25% of these individuals develop fatal cirrhosis (liver disease) or hepatoma (liver cancer). **Hepatitis C virus (HCV)** disease is also a serum hepatitis that was previously called non-A, non-B (NANB) hepatitis. HCV is similar to HBV and is the major cause of **transfusion-acquired hepatitis.**

The remaining diseases stimulating a reactive lymphocytosis are influenza, mycoplasmal (walking, primary atypical) pneumonia, pertussis, and toxoplasmosis and are addressed and diagnosed in the microbiology department. The presence of lymphocytosis with reactive lymphocytes will be an additional piece of evidence to aid the physician in making the final diagnosis.

Malignant lymphocytosis is the proliferation of neoplastic (new formation) cells. These cells become abnormal and life threatening due to a change in the genetic information or their regulatory system. The most common malignant disorders are **acute lymphocytic leukemia (ALL/L1-3), chronic lymphocytic leukemia (CLL), leukemic phase of lymphoma, and Waldenström's macroglobulinemia.** A **lymphoma** differs from a leukemia in the **primary site** of the neoplastic cells. A lymphoma is primarily in the **lymph system** and may spread (metastasize) to the bone marrow and blood, in which case it is referred to as the leukemic phase of a lymphoma.

As stated earlier in reference to the granulocytic leukemias, factors involved in the development of leukemia are still under investigation. The evidence indicates that three components are in some way responsible for the development of cancerous or malignant disease. The three factors are a **genetic predisposition,** exposure to certain **viruses** (adult T-cell leukemia and the human T-cell lymphotropic virus-I), and an **initiating event,** such as exposure to a toxic substance (which converts normal genes to malignant genes/proto-oncogenes to oncogenes or inactivation of a gene whose protein product suppresses cancer). An example is individuals exposed to the radiation from the atomic bombs in Japan who have an increased risk of acute leukemia. Correct diagnosis of leukemia is essential to obtain the most effective treatment, which may include chemotherapy, radiation therapy, or bone marrow transplant,

possibly augmented by administration of commercially made growth factors.

Acute lymphocytic leukemia (ALL) presents as three different diseases. As described earlier with the acute granulocytic and monocytic leukemias, the cells are often very similar morphologically and, therefore, other characteristics of the disease have been used by the **French-American-British (FAB)** cooperative hematology group to classify these acute leukemias (Table 5–3). Morphology, membrane protein markers, and clinical characteristics are all used to form the most accurate diagnosis possible. If the correct cell line and stage are determined, the most effective treatment can be administered. In other words, the **quality and quantity of life**

TABLE 5–3 FRENCH-AMERICAN-BRITISH (FAB) CLASSIFICATION OF ACUTE MYELOID/LYMPHOID LEUKEMIAS

FAB Class	Cells Observed*	Unique Criteria	Cytochemistry/CD	%†
M1(AML)	>90% **myeloblasts** with minimal maturation	Occasional Auer rods	Myeloperoxidase **(MP),** Sudan black B (SBB), NASDC	20
M2(AML)	<90% myeloblasts >**10% more mature**	**Auer rods**	Myeloperoxidase, Sudan black B, NASDC	30
M3(APL)	Predominantly **promyelocytes**	Often causes disseminated intravascular coagulation **(DIC)**	Myeloperoxidase, Sudan black B, NASDC	10
M4(AMML)	**Myeloblasts** and **monoblasts** with minimal maturation stages of both	Occasional Auer rods	>20% MP/SBB/NASDC >20% Nonspecific esterase (NSE)	12
M4eo	Same as M4 except with **eosinophilia**	Some with large **basophilic granules**	Same as M4; eosinophils may be shown by periodic acid–Schiff (PAS) stain	4
M5a(AMoL) poorly differentiated	>**80% monoblasts,** promonocytes, and monocytes	Later stages are poorly granulated and vacuolated	**NSE (fluoride inhibitor)**	5
M5b(AMoL) differentiated	<**80% monoblasts,** promonocytes, and monocytes		Same as M5a	
M6(AEL)	>**50% erythroblasts,** also myeloblasts and monoblasts	50% dysplastic, megaloblastic	PAS	6
M7(AMegL)	>**30% megakaryoblasts**		Platelet peroxidase by EM; platelet glycoprotein by immunocytochemistry	1
L1(ALL)	Small lymph cells	2–10 year olds	PAS/CD 10, 19, and 24	71
L2(ATL)	Large irregular cells	Adult T cell associated with HTLV-1	PAS/CD 10	27
L3(ALL)	Large uniform cells	Burkitt's type	PAS/CD10	2

* *Cells observed in the bone marrow and peripheral blood.*
† *Represents the percentage of myeloid (M) leukemias or lymphoid (L) leukemias.*

for the leukemic patient depend on the accurate identification of the leukemic cell.

ALL classified as the **FAB L1** is the most common malignancy **in children** younger than 5 years of age. Its presentation involves fever, lethargy, bone and joint pain, lymphoadenopathy, splenomegaly, and bleeding. The leukemic blasts have the membrane markers (immunophenotype) of **pre–B cells** but are common ALL antigens (CALLA/CD10) negative. Genetic translocations are common, especially t(4;11), 11q23-25, and 9p21-22. The peripheral blood may show a normocytic, normochromic anemia with nucleated red blood cells, thrombocytopenia (decreased platelets), and a white blood cell count that varies from being decreased ($< 5 \times 10^9/l$) to over $100 \times 10^9/l$. The bone marrow demonstrates more than 25% lymphoblasts, which are small and homogenous (the same appearance from one case to another) and have a high nuclear to cytoplasmic (N:C) ratio (Fig. 5–7). In the past this leukemia was fatal. Currently **more than 50% of the patients with this diagnosis are considered to be cured** after treatment. This emphasizes the importance of accurate cell identification in the laboratory to facilitate the correct diagnosis.

Each treatment is specific for a particular leukemia or cancer, and if the diagnosis is not accurate,

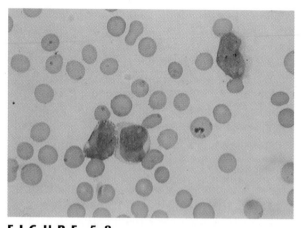

FIGURE 5–8
Adult T-cell leukemia (ATL, FAB L2). Note the large, irregular cells involved. This type of leukemia is most common in adults and is associated with the human T-cell lymphotropic virus-I (HTLV-I).

the treatment will also be inaccurate and thus remission or a cure will not occur.

FAB L2 leukemia is found most often in **adults** and is also called **adult T-cell leukemia (ATL).** The cell seen in the bone marrow and peripheral blood is a larger lymphoblast with more morphologic variation from one case to another (Fig. 5–8). The cell involved usually has a T helper (CD4) phenotype and is also positive for the CD25 and the IL-2 receptor. This leukemia is more common in southern Japan and is closely associated with the presence of the human T-cell lymphotropic virus-I (HTLV-I). HTLV-I is distantly related to the human immunodeficiency virus (HIV). Most blood banks test the units of blood for the presence of HTLV-I. Individuals with this leukemia have demonstrated genetic alterations that correlate with the prognosis (survival). The t(9;22) translocation, also called the Philadelphia (Ph[1]) chromosome, is an adverse indicator for survival for ALL in contrast with a positive prognostic indicator for chronic myelogenous leukemia (CML). The final acute stage of this disease may follow as long as 40 years after an asymptomatic carrier stage.

FAB L3 acute lymphoblastic leukemia is the leukemic phase of **Burkitt's lymphoma.** The cells in this leukemia are large

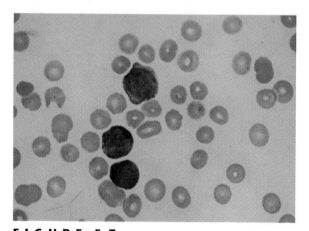

FIGURE 5–7
Acute lymphocytic leukemia (ALL, FAB L1). Note the small lymphocytes involved. ALL is most common in children younger than 5 years of age.

and uniform and have prominent nucleoli and a deeply basophilic cytoplasm with vacuoles (Fig. 5–9). These leukemic cells are determined to be mature B cells and are often common ALL antigen (CALLA/CD10) positive. Some of these cells express IgM on the membrane. Other membrane protein markers that identify these cells are Ia/HLA-DR, CD19, CD20, and CD24. The most common chromosomal translocations associated with L3 are t(8;14) and (q24;q32). These translocations produce a rearrangement of the *c-myc* oncogene. Individuals with L3 diagnosis have the poorest prognosis (survival) of the three types of acute lymphocytic leukemia.

Burkitt's lymphoma is endemic in East Africa, and can be detected in 97% of patients with the **Epstein-Barr Virus (EBV)** genome. The classic case involves children with jaw tumors, although other organs are also involved. Rappaport has classified this disorder as an undifferentiated (early cell) lymphoma, and Lukes and Collins describe it as a malignant lymphoma with small, noncleaved, follicular center cells. Burkitt's lymphoma always originates from the B cell and is a rare and aggressive disease in which an early diagnosis is important.

Chronic lymphocytic leukemia (CLL) is most common in persons older than 60 years of age and is rare in persons younger than 40 years of age. The **B cell** is the most common

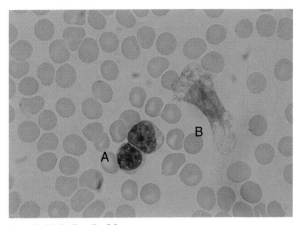

FIGURE 5-10
Chronic lymphocytic leukemia (CLL). Note the lymphocytes (*A*) and deteriorated leukemic cell (*B*) (basket [smudge] cell) that is characteristic of CLL.

phenotype. Patients present with lymphadenopathy (enlarged lymph nodes), hepatosplenomegaly (enlarged liver and spleen), anorexia (loss of appetite), and fatigue. The chronic nature of this disease results in the coincidental discovery during investigation of a problem that is unrelated to the leukemia. The average survival rate is 6 years.

The cells seen in the blood and bone marrow present a homogeneous population of **small lymphocytes** (Fig. 5–10*A*). Often there is no anemia or thrombocytopenia; however, in some cases, an autoimmune hemolytic anemia and thrombocytopenia occur due to antibodies produced by the leukemia cells. The white blood cell count is usually greater than $15 \times 10^9/l$ with an increased incidence of basket or smudge cells (Fig. 5–10*B* and 5–11). The fragile, leukemic white blood cells degenerate during the process of blood collection, preparation, and testing of patients with CLL. These degenerated cells are called **basket cells or smudge cells** (Fig. 5–11). Immunologic phenotyping (membrane marker identification) is used to determine if the leukemic cell involved is a B cell or a T cell and the stage of maturity, which is necessary for proper treatment. Lymph node biopsies show diffuse, well-differentiated cells.

Variants of CLL are **lymphosarcoma leukemia (LSL)** and **prolymphocytic leukemia (PL).** The cells seen in LSL are small

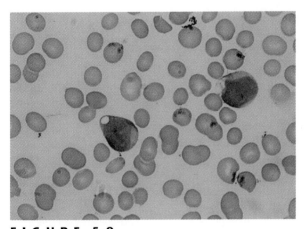

FIGURE 5-9
Acute lymphocytic leukemia (ALL, FAB L3). Note the large uniform lymphocytes involved. This is the leukemic phase of Burkitt's lymphoma.

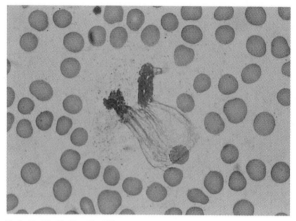

FIGURE 5–11
Basket (smudge) cell. This is a deteriorated white blood cells that are seen occasionally in healthy individuals due to normal cell death and blood smear preparation trauma. If seen in more than three fields, the basket cells should be noted.

lymphocytes that manifest deep clefts in the nuclei and variably condensed chromatin. LSL is associated with poorly differentiated lymphocytic lymphoma. A diagnosis includes observation of nodules of the poorly differentiated cells in the enlarged lymph nodes. In PL, the predominant cell is the prolymphocyte, with lymphocytosis reaching well over 100 × 10⁹/l. PL is usually less responsive to treatment (refractory) and has a poorer prognosis than does CLL.

Waldenström's macroglobulinemia is a variant of chronic lymphocytic leukemia (CLL), involving a malignancy of mature **B cells or plasma cells** from one abnormal parent cell (clone), which produce excessive amounts of a **single immunoglobulin M (IgM).** The production of excessive abnormal antibody (immunoglobulin) from one clone of cells is called a **monoclonal gammopathy** and is identified by protein electrophoresis, which is presented in Chapter 6 (see Fig. 6–18). This disease occurs in individuals **older than 40 years of age** and is found most often in 60 to 70 year olds. The excessive proliferation of cells results in hepatosplenomegaly and lymphadenopathy. The increased amount of IgM protein renders the blood hyperviscous, which is manifested by impaired kidney function, visual disturbances, neurologic symptoms, and congestive heart failure.

The abnormal protein also binds to platelets and plasma coagulation proteins inhibiting function, which results in prolonged coagulation tests and bleeding. This is considered to be a chronic disease with a good survival prognosis. Treatment with cytotoxic chemotherapy is not instituted until symptoms begin to threaten the individual.

The peripheral blood picture is a **normocytic, normochromic, or hemolytic anemia, lymphocytosis, thrombocytopenia, or pancytopenia.** There is an **elevated erythrocyte sedimentation rate (ESR)** and **rouleaux phenomena** (stacking of red blood cells like coins due to excess protein) seen on a peripheral blood smear examination (Fig. 5–12). Rouleaux do not affect the automated complete blood count (CBC) due to the dilution of the blood (protein). The bone marrow is not remarkable, with an increase in small, normal-looking lymphocytes and tissue mast cells. The bone marrow may be difficult to aspirate due to an excess of cells and protein.

Multiple myeloma (MM) is also a **monoclonal gammopathy** (an excessive pathologic production of one abnormal protein). The abnormal immunoglobulin being produced in excess is usually IgG instead of IgM. Individuals younger than 40 years of age seldom present with MM, and the average age at

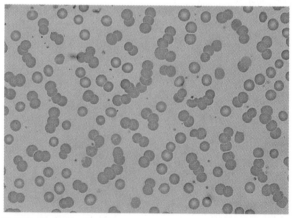

FIGURE 5–12
Rouleau phenomenon is seen on a peripheral blood smear when protein is increased in the serum. The excessive protein increases the stacking of red blood cells like coins, which is natural as sedimentation of erythrocytes occurs over several hours.

diagnosis is 62 years. The **neoplastic cell in MM is the plasma cell,** which in this disease is called a **myeloma cell.** The myeloma cell is larger than the normal plasma cell, often has multiple nuclei (Fig. 5–13), and produces large quantities of the monoclonal protein **(M protein)** associated with this malignancy. The monoclonal antibody produced in MM is not directed against any known antigen and, therefore, does not contribute to the immune defense. As a matter of fact, due to the mass production of this useless M (for myeloma) protein, two complications occur: (1) healthy antibodies that are necessary for immune defense are inhibited, resulting in increased risk of infection; and (2) the M protein binds nonspecifically to red blood cells, platelets, and coagulation factors, resulting in anemias and bleeding problems. The clinical symptoms differ from Waldenström's macroglobulinemia in the absence of organ enlargement and the presence of **bone pain and pathologic fractures due to bone pitting** from the proliferation of myeloma cells. On x-ray, the bones display punched-out osteoporotic lesions.

The blood picture with MM is usually a **normocytic, normochromic anemia,** a variable white blood cell count, and obvious **rouleaux (red blood cells stacked like coins)** on the peripheral blood smear (see Fig. 5–12). This is correlated with a protein electrophoresis (see Fig. 6–18) from the chemistry department, which will confirm a monoclonal protein, and an **elevated erythrocyte sedimentation rate (ESR)** performed in the hematology department. The myeloma protein seen on the electrophoresis is sometimes called an M spot (referring to the myeloma origin of the protein, which is usually an IgG antibody). In addition to secretion of the whole Ig molecule, excess light chains are often secreted. These chains readily pass through the kidney and appear in the urine as **Bence Jones proteins.** The bone marrow contains plasma cells and myeloma cells in the range of 10 to 90% versus <5% normally. Patients demonstrating more mature cells and less bone marrow infiltration have a better prognosis. The average survival rate is 3 years following the diagnosis, and some individuals develop sideroblastic anemia and acute leukemia. MM is treated aggressively with chemotherapy (alkylating agents and corticosteroids) to limit the myeloma cells and to improve the prognosis.

Researchers have managed to turn a malignant cell into a **useful tool** to produce much needed reagents for **clinical laboratory testing and research.** By fusing an antibody-producing B lymphocyte, which has been developed in response to a specific antigen of interest, with a myeloma cell, which has the ability to produce massive qualities of one specific monoclonal antibody, very important monoclonal antibody reagents can be produced. The resultant cell (from the fusion of a lymphocyte and a myeloma cell) is called a **hybridoma cell.**

Monoclonal gammopathy of undetermined significance (MGUS), also called benign monoclonal gammopathy, occurs in individuals with less than 10% plasma cells in the bone marrow and does not appear to affect the quality or quantity of life. MGUS mimics MM with the fortunate characteristic of not progressing. This disease is monitored but is not treated. The aggressive treatments necessary for MM could possibly induce a malignancy in the individual with MGUS and, therefore, should be avoided.

Plasma cell leukemia results from rare cases of multiple myeloma in which the peripheral blood demonstrates many plasma cells associated with tissue infiltration and a poor prognosis.

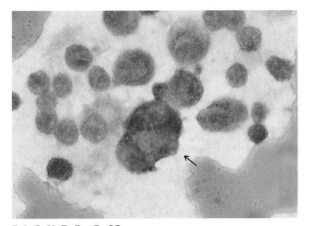

FIGURE 5–13
A myeloma cell. Note the increased size and multiple nuclei.

Decreased Lymphocytes (Lymphocytopenia)

A **decrease in lymphocytes (lymphocytopenia)** can result from **genetically impaired** lymphopoiesis, increased levels of **adrenocortical hormones, chemotherapy, or irradiation.** Lymphocytopenia has also been reported in advanced lymphomas and terminal carcinomas.

Hairy cell leukemia (HCL) is a rare disease involving a subtype of B cell. The average age of individuals with HCL is **50 years old,** and **splenomegaly** is the most common physical finding. The cells seen are medium-sized mononuclear cells of B cell origin with some nuclei notched or dumbbell-shaped. The cytoplasm is the namesake characteristic with numerous hair-like projections and irregular borders (Fig. 5–14). Cytochemically, these cells differ from other lymphocytic cells and thus can be identified by staining with **tartrate-resistant acid phosphatase stain (TRAP),** which is resistant to tartrate inhibition stain. Pancytopenia may be present, although the bone marrow will show both hypocellular and hypercellular areas with fibrosis and the hairy cell itself dominates. Splenectomy has been the traditional, most effective treatment, although effective chemotherapy has been reported.

Although hairy cell leukemia is rare, research continues due to the questionable nature of the hairy cell. Most cells involved, as stated previously, are of B cell origin; however, in some cases, the hairy cells also express T cell, granulocytic, or monocytic markers. Adding to the uncertainty of the cell involved is the ability of hairy cells to phagocytize particles. Some hematologists believe that this leukemia consists of a heterogeneous group of malignant cells instead of one cell line. **The development of this disease has been associated with irradiation and the human T-cell lymphotropic virus-II (HTLV-II).**

There are additional lymphoid disorders (lymphomas) that do not directly involve the peripheral blood or bone marrow. These disorders originate in the lymph nodes and spread to other organs as the disease progresses.

Malignant Lymphomas

Malignant lymphomas fall into two groups: Hodgkin's or non-Hodgkin's lymphoma, depending on the presence or absence of a specific cell (the Reed-Sternberg cell) found in Hodgkin's disease.

Hodgkin's lymphoma may develop early or late in life; however, there seems to be an increased frequency between **15 and 35 years of age** and again after **50 years of age.** The characteristic cell for a diagnosis of Hodgkin's disease is the presence of the **Reed-Sternberg cell in the lymph node biopsy** (Fig. 5–15). The Reed-Sternberg cell is large, binucleate or multinucleate, with large prominent nucleoli. There are several classifications of Hodgkin's lymphoma based on histologic appearance for the purpose of treatment and prognosis. The best prognosis is associated with the lymphocytic predominance classification. Other classifications include the nodular sclerosis, mixed-field type, and the lymphocyte depletion. The Reed-Sternberg cell is an activated lymphocyte that has demonstrated T cell markers in most cases of Hodgkin's dis-

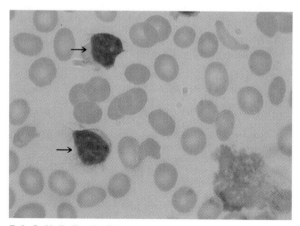

F I G U R E 5–14

Hairy cells. Note the irregular hair-like projections from the lymphocyte cytoplasm. This cell is of questionable origin. Most are B-lymphocyte associated, although development of these cells has also been associated with radiation and the human T-cell lymphotropic virus-II (HTLV-II).

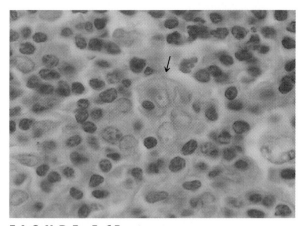

FIGURE 5–15
A Reed-Sternberg cell. Note the large size and the irregular nucleus. This activated lymphocyte is found in the lymph nodes and is diagnostic for Hodgkin's lymphoma.

ease; however, B cell markers have been found in the nodular subtype of lymphocyte predominance cases.

The peripheral blood may **show normal leukocytes and a normocytic, normochromic anemia** and **the leukocyte count** may vary **from reduced to increased.** Depending on the stage and the classification of disease, the differential count may vary significantly. Most often there is a monocytosis and lymphocytopenia, which represent the host's response to disease. Lymphopenia is a poor prognostic indicator. The disease is divided into stages, determined by the areas of the body that are infiltrated with malignant cells. This staging is used to direct the radiation therapy that accompanies the chemotherapy. The current therapy has increased the life expectancy of, and in some cases cured, the individual with Hodgkin's disease.

Non-Hodgkin's lymphomas are classified by their pattern within the lymph node (follicular or diffuse) and the type of cell involved. The Working Formulation of Non-Hodgkin's Lymphoma for Clinical Use was established by expert hematologists from several institutions to classify these disorders (Table 5–4). The follicular pattern has a better prognosis independent of the cell involved. An extensive regimen of chemotherapy is given to treat the non-Hodgkin lymphoma, which varies from one institution to another and from one patient to another.

Mycosis fungoides and Sézary syndrome are cutaneous T-cell lymphomas (CTCL) that appear in mid to late years of life and involve cells within cerebriform nuclei (Sézary cells), which may occasionally appear in the peripheral blood (Fig. 5–16). Mycosis fungoides is characterized by a dermatitis resembling eczema and psoriasis in which the lesions form ulcerous plaques. A biopsy of the skin lesion reveals abscesses of lymphocytic cells. A prolonged chronic course is often followed by infiltration of many organs, which terminates within 2 years, with death due to infection. The presence of peripheral blood lymphocytosis is called Sézary syndrome. Genetic, environmental, and infectious agents have been implicated. Treatment includes topical application of chemotherapy, radiation, and light and laser therapy as well as systemic chemotherapy if the disease progresses.

TABLE 5–4 THE INTERNATIONAL WORKING FORMULATION OF MALIGNANT NON-HODGKIN'S LYMPHOMA FOR CLINICAL USE

Low Grade
Small lymphocytes, consistent with chronic lymphocytic leukemia, plasmacytoid
Small cleaved cell, follicular, diffuse areas, sclerosis
Mixed small cleaved and large cell, diffuse areas, sclerosis

Intermediate Grade
Large cell, follicular, diffuse areas, sclerosis
Small cleaved cell, sclerosis
Mixed small and large cell, diffuse, epithelioid cell component, sclerosis
Large cleaved and noncleaved cell, diffuse, sclerosis

High Grade
Large immunoblastic cell, plasmacytoid, clear cell, polymorphous, epithelioid cell component
Lymphoblastic convoluted and nonconvoluted cell
Small noncleaved cell, Burkitt's, follicular areas

Miscellaneous
Composite
Mycosis fungoides
Histiocytic
Extramedullary plasmacytoma
Unclassified
Other

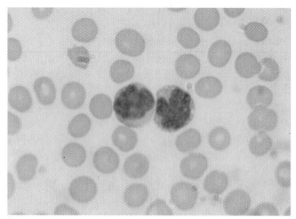

FIGURE 5–16

Sézary cells. These cutaneous T-cell lymphoma (CTCL) cells are seen in a skin biopsy taken from a person who has the disease mycosis fungoides. Note the cerebriform (indented) nucleus.

FAST FACTS

Lymphocyte and Plasma Cell Diseases

Reactive lymphocytosis:	Mononucleosis (Epstein-Barr virus [EBV])
	Cytomegalovirus (CMV) infection
	Infectious lymphocytosis
	Hepatitis (HAV, HBV, HCV)
	Influenza
	Mumps, measles
	Rubella, varicella
	Mycoplasmal pneumonia
	Pertussis (whooping cough)
	Tuberculosis
	Cat-scratch fever, toxoplasmosis, and malaria
Malignant lymphocytosis:	Acute lymphoblastic leukemia (ALL)
	Chronic lymphocytic leukemia (CLL),
	Leukemic phase of lymphoma
Malignant B/ plasma cells:	Waldenström's macroglobulinemia
Malignant plasma cells:	Multiple myeloma
	Waldenström's macroglobulinemia
	Plasma cell leukemia

Do It Now Leukocyte Disease Exercise

Fill in the chart below to contrast and compare some of the myelocytic and lymphocytic disorders:

	AML(M1-4)	CML	MDS	ALL	CLL	MM	Mono
Onset							
Average Age							
Cell(s)							
Diagnostic Tests							
Miscellaneous Notes							

ALL = acute lymphocytic leukemia; CLL = chronic lymphocytic leukemia; CML = chronic myelogenous leukemia; MDS = myelodysplastic syndrome; MM = multiple myeloma.

STUDY QUESTIONS

1. Lymphopoiesis occurs in which of the following orders?
   A. CFU-GEMM, CFU-L (lymphoblast), pre-T or -B (prolymphocyte), mature T or B lymphocyte

   B. CFU-L (lymphoblast), pre-T or -B (prolymphocyte), mature T or B lymphocyte, plasma cell from B cell

   C. BFU-E, CFU-E (lymphoblast), T or B prolymphocyte, T or B metalymphocyte, mature T or B lymphocyte, plasma cell from B cell, helper cell from T cell

   D. CFU-L (lymphoblast), prolymphocyte, thymocyte (T cell) or bursa equivalent (B cell), mature T or B cell

For questions 2 to 6 choose true (1/A) or false (2/B)

2. The life cycle of the lymphocyte begins in the lymph tissue and circulates within the lymph tissue, only inhabiting the peripheral blood and bone marrow transiently.

3. A reactive lymphocyte is a large cell with a dark lacy nucleus that is indented.

4. Reactive lymphocytes are seen in response to viral infections.

5. Lymphomas originate and predominate in the lymph tissue.

6. Nucleoli are seen in both reactive lymphocytes and acute lymphocytic leukemia blasts.

Match the following:

7. Small mature lymphocytes and basket cells

8. Large heterogenous lymphoblasts

9. Small dark lymphoblasts

10. Large lymphoblasts with vacuoles

A. L1

B. L2

C. L3

D. CLL

11–16. List the names, morphology, identification proteins, and functions of all lymphocytic cells, including subsets and plasma cells.

CHAPTER 6

OUTLINE

Leukocyte Counts
Automated Complete Blood Count (CBC)
Manual Leukocyte Count

Microscopic Leukocyte Evaluations
Leukocyte Differential and Peripheral Blood Smear
Evaluation Procedure
Cytochemical Stains
Leukocyte (Neutrophil) Alkaline Phosphatase
(LAP/NAP) Score
Arneth Count for Neutrophil Segmentation
Buffy Coat Preparation for Leukocyte Evaluation

Special Leukocyte Tests

White Blood Cell Function Tests

**Related Methodologies for Protein and Vita-
min Identification and Quantitation**

Study Questions

Leukocyte Testing

OBJECTIVES

Upon completion of this chapter the student should be able to:

1. Describe the acceptable specimen for leukocyte testing.

2. Explain the routine leukocyte test methodology.

3. Correlate the various leukocyte tests and their significance.

4. When given a testing scenario, determine if there are reasons to question the validity of the results.

5. State the various diseases in terms of the cells involved and the relevant testing.

LEUKOCYTE COUNTS

The equipment required for most leukocyte testing is an ethylenediaminetetra-acetic acid **(EDTA) tube (with the purple top) at least one-third full, fresh, and well mixed to prevent clotting.** If the specimen cannot be tested upon return to the laboratory, it should be **refrigerated at 4° C until needed** and allowed to reach room temperature before testing.

Once the **EDTA tube** is filled with blood, the tube should be **inverted completely six to eight times** to adequately mix the blood with the anticoagulant that will inhibit clotting. The liquid portion of the whole blood (plasma) must be pale yellow and fairly clear. **If the plasma is dark yellow, milky, or red, this will interfere with accurate testing** and must be redrawn or dealt with accordingly in testing. The causes of this unacceptable plasma are explained in Chapter 1. Some procedures described later in this section require the use of a heparinized specimen (green top tube) or serum (red top tube) and may be performed in areas of the laboratory other than hematology.

EDTA is the anticoagulant of choice for cellular testing because it **preserves the cell function and morphology better than do any of the other anticoagulants.** For most accurate results, the counts should be performed within 2 hours, because in time all cells begin to change. However, some individuals' cells become altered immediately after exposure to the anticoagulant. **If a patient's cells are altered by EDTA, sodium citrate (Na citrate) can be used if the blood is tested within a few hours.** Some special tests such as cytochemical staining and lupus erythematosus preparations require alternate anticoagulants, which are discussed later in this section along with the specific test.

Our mission in the clinical laboratory is to: (1) provide test results that reflect the condition within the body (in vivo), not changes that took place once the blood was removed from the patient and placed into a glass tube (in vitro), and (2) correlate results from all test information (puzzle pieces)

---

available to provide the primary health care provider with a clear and accurate picture of the patient's state of health. If the laboratory practitioner is not correlating results, fragmented information is provided that can hamper the efficiency of health care and prove detrimental to the patient.

Automated Complete Blood Count (CBC)

The most common test performed is the **complete blood count (CBC).** This test is part of a routine examination when a patient is admitted to the hospital. The cells are automatically counted and evaluated with a cell counting instrument, and other hematology tests are included. The **CBC** includes a **total white blood cell count and differentiates the various white blood cells,** determining percentages and absolute values for each type. The other components of a CBC are the **red blood cell count with histogram and scattergram, platelet count with histogram and scattergram, hemoglobin, hematocrit, red blood cell and platelet indices, reference ranges, and flags for out-of-range values.** The typical reference value for a **total leukocyte count** is **5 to 10 × 10⁹/l.** The normal reference value for a neutrophil count is approximately $6.8 \times 10^9/l$ or 68% (see the absolute cell counts in Chapter 1). The reference value for eosinophils is $0.2 \times 10^9/l$. A basophil reference value is approximately $0.04 \times 10^9/l$ and $0.6 \times 10^9/l$ for monocytes. Keep in mind that normal reference values are given for the adult general population. If only the black population or infants are of interest, they would both have slightly higher reference values. On the other hand, if only European adults were of interest, the normal reference value would be slightly lower.

Each laboratory must establish its own normal reference values, due to variances in instrumentation, procedures, and local populations, which may render the generic normal reference values less accurate for the specific laboratory involved in the testing.

There are several **instruments that perform the complete blood count.** Electronic impedance, laser light scatter, light absorbance, and staining characteristics are the various principles utilized by various instruments. **Electronic impedance** is used to count cells by the Coulter Cell Counters, a modified version by the Cell-Dyn 3000 marketed by Abbott, the Sysmex NE 8000 Cell Counter by Baxter, and the COBAS Cell Counter by Roche. Some of these also use light scatter (described later) to differentiate the cells for the automated differential.

The following **basic procedure** is an outline used for the methodology just described.

---

1. **Dilution of the EDTA whole blood specimen in an electrolyte solution** such as saline. The cells that are suspended in this fluid are poor conductors of electricity, whereas the solution is a good conductor of electricity. The dilution must allow an adequate number of cells to count without a concentration so high that more than one cell goes through the aperture at once (coincidence error). If more than one type of cell (particle) is present in the sample, it may be necessary to lyse or remove one of them to get an accurate count on the other.
2. The instrument will have electrodes located on either side of the counting orifice or path. An electrolyte solution is placed between the electrodes, and **a flow of electrical current is established.**
3. **A specific amount of solution is pulled through the aperture. Any particle (cell) that passes through the aperture will momentarily increase the resistance of (or interrupt) the electrical flow between the electrodes generating a pulse, which can be counted, measured, and displayed on a screen.** The size of the resistance is proportional to the size of the cell. From this information the counter computer can provide an accurate count and size of the particle.
4. A **background** (quality assurance) check is obtained by first counting any miscellaneous particles within the vial of saline that may be erroneously counted as cells. This background should be very low.

---

5. **Controls or standards must also be counted** to ensure accuracy of the data generated. This should be a specimen with a known value.
6. **All specimens should be run at least in duplicate,** and most instruments do three to five determinations on each specimen to ensure the precision of the data generated.

The specific procedure for each cell instrument is provided by the company manufacturing the instrument.

Laser light scattering is the methodology utilized by some Coulter instruments to characterize cells for the scattergrams. Laser light scatter is utilized for cell counts as well as cell characterization by **flow cytometers,** such as the Technicon H-3, Abbott Cell-Dyn 3000, and Serono Diagnostics System 9000. There are also flow cytometers that are not primarily cell counters but rather identify cellular membrane protein markers using monoclonal antibodies and fluorescence. The flow cytometers used to identify, sort, and collect cells using monoclonal antibodies and fluorescence are discussed later in this section. In these routine laboratory blood cell evaluation systems, the following procedure must be followed.

---

1. The sample is **diluted** in the instrument into a stream of fluid containing the cells to be counted **in a single cell flow (hydrodynamic focusing).**
2. These **cells pass through a flow cell on which a light is focused.** As the cell passes through the light path, **it scatters the light in all directions.** A photodetector senses and collects **this light scatter information** and transforms it into digital information, which **provides characteristic information about the specific cell** as it passes through the flow cell. Traditional flow cytometers utilize forward light scatter (0 degrees) and orthogonal light scatter (90 degrees) to differentiate lymphocytes, monocytes, and granulocytes.

The Cell-Dyn 3000 uses two additional dimensions of light scattering to more accurately separate the cell characteristics. This new technique is called multiangle polarized scatter separation (MAPSS) and involves the use of narrow-angle light scatter (10 degrees) to resolve basophils and depolarized light scatter (90 degrees) to resolve eosinophils. This additional information eliminates the need for cytochemical staining or monoclonal tagging to identify these cells.

Light absorbance is used along with light scatter by the Sysmex 8000, the COBAS, and the Technicon H-3. Another use of the light scatter techology is to specifically stain the cells of interest. This requires a darkfield optical system to count and classify leukocytes. The procedure is similar to that of light scatter, but the detection system is different. The light is scattered through the opening around a darkfield disk as cells pass through the sensing zone, one at a time. The light scatter is measured with a photodetector and is related to the cell number. If the cell is stained, some of the light will be absorbed proportional to the amount of staining. By using various specific cell stains, a leukocyte differential can be done.

The automated instruments provide histograms and scattergrams that will identify an alteration in cell number, size, and some internal characteristics (Fig. 6–1). The histograms provide the number on one axis and the cell size on the other axis. The scattergrams plot various degrees of light scatter on the vertical and horizontal axes to classify cells based on the nuclear and cytoplasmic characteristics of light scatter. Any alteration in these two parameters can be recognized. The scatterplots are obtained by plotting the cell size, nuclear structure and surface, and internal characteristics within a three-dimensional matrix. The cell distribution is not a factor in the scatterplot information but rather cell identification and any alteration in specific cell characteristics. An evaluation of the blood smear is indicated if the automated instrument reports any unusual cells or an abnormal cell count. The white blood cell differential and peripheral blood smear evaluation are important to correlate with the automated histogram or scattergram in order to note morphologic alterations that may indicate a specific disorder.

Correlation Factors. Many of the results will appear within the normal reference range and, although they must still be reviewed for appropriateness, can be verified and sent to the patient's chart without additional correlation. If there is a special mark or "flag" near a result to alert the laboratory practitioner to an abnormal value, **other tests should be considered to support and validate this result.** The white blood cell count should correlate with a white blood cell estimate from looking at a **peripheral blood smear** made on the specimen. If specific cell characteristics are not seen, such as with blast cells, **cytochemical stains** may be used to differentiate a myeloblast from a monoblast or a lymphoblast. Specific identification of the cell is important for proper treatment. If the patient is diagnosed and treated correctly, many leukemias have a good prognosis for survival and possibly a cure. If a patient is not given the correct treatment due to an incorrect diagnosis, the prognosis would be poor. If the white blood cell evaluation indicates **increased neutrophils,** characteristics such as toxic granulation, Döhle bodies, and vacuoles would help to associate this elevation with a **bacterial infection.** If these characteristics are absent, a **malignancy** may be indicated. If the white blood cell count demonstrates an increase in lymphocytes, the presence of **reactive lymphocytes** would support a **viral infection.** The absence of reactive lymphocytes may indicate a malignancy.

Sources of Error. An appropriate blood specimen is essential to perform an accurate white blood cell count. If the specimen **clots** or is physically damaged or tested at a **temperature** other than room temperature, or the tube is **inappropriately filled,** the blood must be redrawn or, if the problem only involves temperature, brought to the correct temperature. When a whole blood (WB) specimen is refrigerated, the white blood cells and platelets stick together. Alterations that are artifacts or secondary to a primary disease (e.g., **hemolysis, lipemia, cold agglutinins**) can result in incorrect automated cell counts.

If the white blood cell **count is greater than 10 × 10⁹/l,** the incidence of two cells passing through the aperture at once increases with an increasing count. This results in a

Volume Histograms

White blood cell normal histogram

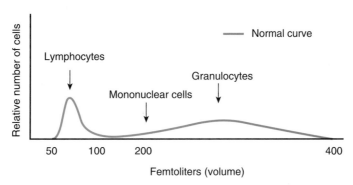

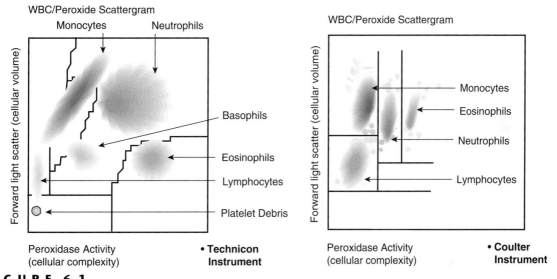

FIGURE 6–1

A typical leukocyte histogram and Coulter and Technicon scattergrams. The histograms represent the quantity and size. The scattergrams present the quantity and size in a less obvious manner, but separate individual cells (i.e., neutrophils, lymphocytes, monocytes, eosinophils, and basophils) by nuclear and cytoplasmic characteristics and complexity.

count that is low due to the two cells passing through together being counted as one large cell. The computerized cell counting instruments automatically correct for this, and older cell counters have a "coincidence correction chart" provided from the manufacturer that must be used to **correct any count over 10×10^9/l.** This correction will always increase the observed count. If the cell count is excessively high, resulting in cells that are too numerous to count, additional dilutions can be made to bring the count within counting limits of the procedure.

Pyknotic cells are dead, deteriorated white blood cells that may be included in the wrong count because they will have a different character than when the cell was intact (Fig. 6–2). Additional abnormalities that will alter a white blood cell histogram and scattergram are: (1) **nucleated red blood cells** (NRBCs), which would be counted as white blood cells and are discussed further in Chapter 10; (2) **basket and smudge cells,** which are dead, fragmented white blood cells, (3) the presence of **micromegakaryocytes** (platelet precursors), which would be counted as white blood

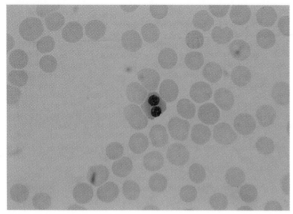

FIGURE 6–2
A pyknotic cell. This is a cell that is deteriorating and the nucleus has lost its characteristics.

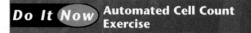

Do It Now — **Automated Cell Count Exercise**

1. Draw your own histogram and scattergram of a normal white blood cell (WBC) differential.

Draw a histogram that demonstrates the presence of:

2. Nucleated red blood cells (NRBC)
3. Immature white blood cells
4. Chronic lymphocytic leukemia
5. Using your laboratory's cell counting instrument or one at a local facility, draw your own diagram following the sample from entry to exit (waste) and generation of the result. Exchange this diagram with that of another class member who used the same instrument at a different time and see if you can follow that person's diagram. Check to see if he or she missed any steps in the process.

cells, and (4) a **poorly mixed specimen** that provides a less than random count (this is less likely because the newer instruments rotate the blood before sampling).

Manual Leukocyte Count

A manual white blood cell count is rarely performed unless the cell count is too low for accuracy on the automated instruments. Other instances in which a manual leukocyte count may be performed are when the automated instrument is not functioning (although most laboratories have a smaller back-up automated instrument) or the laboratory is so small and

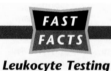

FAST FACTS

Leukocyte Testing

Methodology	Instrument	Company
Cell Counting		
Electronic impedance	STKS	Coulter Corporation
Modified	Cell-Dyn 3000	Abbott Laboratories
Electron impedance	Sysmex NE 8000	Baxter Scientific
	COBAS	Roche Diagnostics
Cell Counting or Characterization for Differentiation		
Laser light scatter	STKS	Coulter Corporation
	Technicon H-3	Bayer Corporation
	Cel-Dyn 3000	Abbott Laboratories
	System 9000	BioChem ImmunoSystems
Light absorbance	Sysmex NE 8000	Baxter Scientific
	COBAS	Roche Diagnostics
	Technicon H-3	Bayer Corporation
Fluorescence	FACSCalibur	Becton Dickinson

remote that an automated instrument is not feasible. Extremely low white blood cell counts occur occasionally in patients with severe myelodysplastic disorders and after chemotherapy or radiation treatments. Body fluids, other than whole blood, have very few cells in them and are counted manually. Examples of these body fluids are cerebrospinal fluid (CSF), joint fluid, pleural fluid, and peritoneal fluid.

The **hemocytometer method** is used for manual cell counts as well as for sperm counts on seminal fluid. The variation in the calculation is dependent on the specimen, the procedure (dilution), and the cells that are counted. A hemocytometer is a thick glass slide with a central area that is 0.1 mm lower than the sides. A special thick glass coverslip, ground to a perfect plane,

unlike ordinary coverslips, which have uneven surfaces, rests on the higher sides of the central counting area, and the diluted specimen is delivered under this coverslip (Fig. 6–3B). The center area of the hemocytometer is engraved with squares to allow accurate counting of the cells. The Neubauer ruling on the central counting area is 9 mm², and these squares are divided into smaller squares to facilitate counting (see Fig. 6–3A).

Safety Precautions

1. Wear or use personal protective equipment, such as gloves, shields, etc., when performing manual counts.
2. Never pipette by mouth. Use a suction apparatus to draw up a specimen into a pipette.

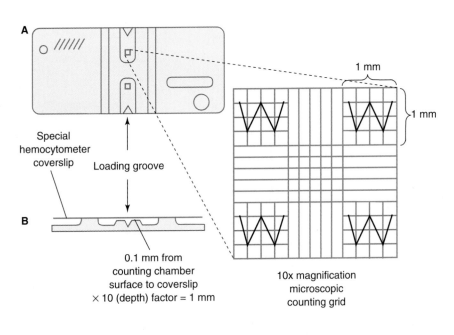

Calculate the cell count as follows:

$$\frac{\text{No. of cells counted}}{\text{No. of 1 mm}^2 \text{ counted}} \times \text{dilution} \times \underset{10^*}{\overset{\text{(depth factor)}}{}} = \text{No. of WBC/mm}^3 \text{ or } /\mu l$$

*The hemocytometer chamber is only 0.1 mm deep; therefore, to report mm³ the 0.1 mm depth must be multiplied by 10 to equal 1 mm.

F I G U R E   6–3
A top view of the improved Neubauer Hemocytometer Counting Chamber (A). Note there are nine large 1 × 1-mm squares. The four large corner squares are used for counting white blood cells (W). A side view of a hemocytometer (B).

GLASS WHITE BLOOD CELL PIPETTE (THOMA) DILUTION METHOD FOR MANUAL COUNTS

1. Obtain a fresh whole blood sample (usually EDTA), but the sample can be capillary blood from a finger puncture.
2. Using an appropriate suction device (Fig. 6–4A), dilute the sample 1:20 with a white blood cell pipette (Fig. 6–4B). The diluting fluid for the white blood cell pipette method must lyse the red blood cells that would obscure the white blood cells (due to greater number of red blood cells than white blood cells) and provide some color to the white blood cells. An appropriate diluting fluid is:

Distilled water	100 ml
Glacial acetic acid	2 ml
1% solution of gentian violet	1 ml (optional)

   Well mixed blood is drawn to the 0.5 mark; the pipette is wiped off; and diluting fluid is drawn to the 11 mark. This results in a 1:20 dilution in the bulb of the pipette. If the count is extremely low, a 1:10 dilution can be made by drawing blood to the 1 mark and diluting fluid to the 11 mark.
3. Mix the glass pipette for about 5 minutes on a mechanical mixer. During this time, clean the hemocytometer and the coverslip (Fig. 6-4C) with a mild, dilute, liquid detergent followed by distilled water and alcohol. Dry with a soft lint-free cloth (e.g., cheesecloth) to avoid scratching the surface of the chamber or leaving particles on the counting surface.
4. Discard the first 2 or 3 drops from the pipette to allow the dilution in the glass bulb to reach the delivery end of the pipette.
5. Touch the delivery end of the pipette to the groove on the side of the counting area of the hemocytometer chamber, and fill one side of chamber at a slow steady pace (Fig. 6–5). Overfilling (flooding) or underfilling the chamber will result in erroneous counts. Repeat this process on the opposite side to obtain a duplicate count. Lay the pipette down or place it back on the mixer to use for additional counting if the first two counts do not agree. Always remix the pipette and drop out the first 2 or 3 drops before refilling the chamber.

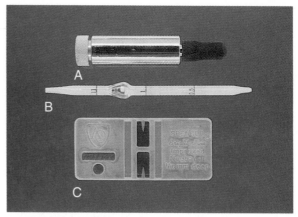

FIGURE 6–4
A, A pipette suction device. *B,* A white blood cell counting pipette. *C,* A hemocytometer.

6. Once the chamber is filled, place it in a moist Petri dish unless counting is performed immediately. If the specimen on the hemacytometer chamber begins to evaporate, the count will not be accurate.

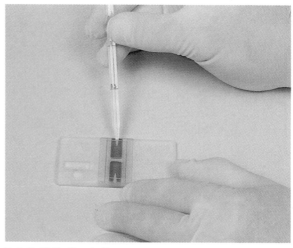

FIGURE 6–5
Delivery of a diluted specimen to a hemocytometer chamber with a glass white blood cell pipette.

UNOPETTE DILUTION METHOD FOR LEUKOCYTE COUNTING

1. Obtain a fresh whole blood sample from an EDTA tube or a finger puncture.
2. Dilute the specimen with an unopette reservoir and pipette (Fig. 6–6A and B). The

pipette is allowed to fill by capillary action to the inside of the first cuff.

3. Wipe the outside of the pipette tip clean to remove excess blood.

4. Place a finger over the large end of the pipette; squeeze the reservoir; and insert the pipette into the reservoir without removing the finger from the pipette or releasing the reservoir.

5. Simultaneously release the finger from the opening of the pipette and the reservoir by squeezing, which will pull the blood from the pipette into the diluent reservoir. The reservoir contains 1.98 ml of ammonium oxalate, which will lyse the red blood cells and render the white blood cell characteristics more visible.

6. Gently squeeze the reservoir to force the diluent up into the pipette to rinse the blood out. Do this two or three times.

7. Remove the pipette from extending inside the reservoir; turn it in the opposite direction; fit it into the reservoir; and cover the pipette with the cap.

8. Mix the solution and allow it to sit for 10 to 15 minutes in order for the red blood cells to lyse.

9. Remix the unopette; discard the first two or three drops by squeezing the reservoir; and fill a clean hemocytometer chamber by dispensing drops into the groove (Fig. 6–7).

10. Once the chamber is filled, place it in a moist Petri dish unless counting is performed immediately. If the specimen on the hemacytometer chamber begins to evaporate, the count will not be accurate.

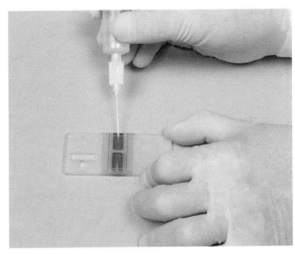

FIGURE 6–7
Delivery of a diluted specimen to a hemocytometer chamber with an unopette.

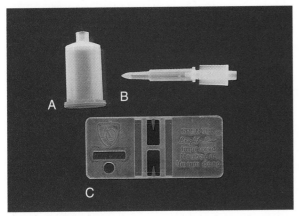

FIGURE 6–6
Unopette reservoir (A), pipette (B), and hemocytometer (C).

HEMOCYTOMETER CELL COUNTING OF DILUTED CELLS

1. With the light off, place the loaded hemocytometer chamber on the microscope stage.

2. Center one of the two chambers under the shortest (5× or 10×) objective.

3. Turn the light on; limit exposure to the light to avoid evaporation of the specimen.

4. **Looking from the side,** move the lowest (shortest) objective and the hemocytometer as close to each other as possible. This is important to prevent the objective from breaking the chamber.

5. Looking through the oculars, **move** the objective and the specimen **away** from each other until the counting grid comes into focus (see Fig. 6–3A).

6. Center to the upper left corner 1-mm square (which contains 16 smaller squares).

7. Rotate the nosepiece of the microscope to the 10× objective. At this point there may appear to be no cells on the chamber due to an excessive amount of condensed light.

8. **Lower the condenser,** and adjust the light to provide maximum contrast for enhancing the visibility of the unstained white blood cells.

Box continued on page 118

9. Begin in the upper left hand corner of the upper left (a) 1-mm square and record, with a counter, the number of white blood cells seen. To avoid counting some cells that fall on a line more than once, count only cells on the same two adjacent lines of each small square (Fig. 6–8).
10. Progress back and forth across the 1-mm square until the entire square has been counted.
11. Record your results.
12. Move over to the next 1-mm corner square (b, then c, then d), and repeat steps 9 to 11.
13. Continue this procedure until all four 1-mm corner squares have been counted. If one of the large squares has an inconsistent count, it may be discarded and the center 1-mm square can be counted instead.
14. Upon completion of one of the chambers, move immediately across to the other chamber and repeat steps 9 to 12. Excessive exposure to the light will evaporate the specimen and alter the results.
15. Calculate the white blood cell count as follows:

$$\frac{\begin{array}{c}\textit{No. of White Blood}\\\textit{Cells Counted}\end{array} \qquad \textit{Depth Factor}}{\begin{array}{c}\text{No. of 1-mm squares counted} \times \text{dilution}\\ \times 10^* = \text{No. of WBC/mm}^3\end{array}}$$

* The hemocytometer chamber is only 0.1-mm deep; thus, to report mm³, the depth must be equal to 1 mm. $0.1 \times 10^* = 1$ mm $\times$ the 1 mm by 1 mm square (as counted on the chamber).

Correlation Factors. The **manual cell count** should reflect the peripheral blood smear **white blood cell estimate.** All 1-mm squares counted should agree within 10% of each other. If a significant difference exists between the four squares counted, the large cen-

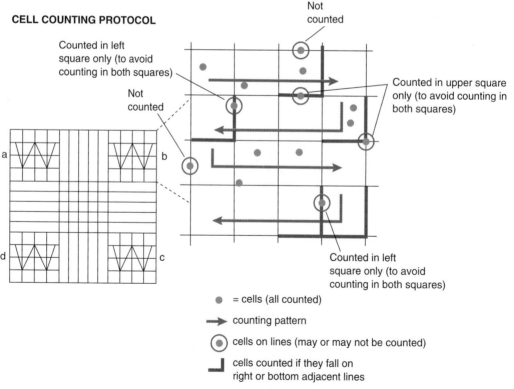

CELL COUNTING PROTOCOL

Not counted

Counted in left square only (to avoid counting in both squares)

Not counted

Counted in upper square only (to avoid counting in both squares)

Counted in left square only (to avoid counting in both squares)

● = cells (all counted)

→ counting pattern

◉ cells on lines (may or may not be counted)

⌐ cells counted if they fall on right or bottom adjacent lines

Count = # ● (8) + # ◉ (4) = 12 cells recorded for this 1-mm square.

F I G U R E 6–8
A diagram of a hemocytometer grid demonstrating a method of counting and an adjacent line procedure to avoid counting a cell twice, once in each square on either side of the line.

ter square can be counted. This value would replace the original square that was not in agreement, or the hemocytometer can be cleaned and refilled from the same pipette after mixing and release of the first two drops.

Sources of Error. Errors can be made due to an **incorrect** or **inadequate specimen; inadequate mixing** of the specimen prior to sampling; **incorrect dilution, diluting fluid,** or **calculation** of the count; and **incorrect counting** or counting some cells twice, or not counting all cells. If **nucleated red blood cells (NRBCs)** are present in the specimen, they will resemble white blood cells on the manual counting chamber. The following calculation must be done to correct this erroneously high count.

$$\frac{\text{Total number of white blood cells counted}}{\text{Number of NRBC/100 white blood cells* } + 100}$$
$$= \text{corrected WBC/mm}^3$$

MICROSCOPIC LEUKOCYTE EVALUATIONS

The best peripheral blood smear is a fresh specimen collected at bedside, avoiding blood exposure to anticoagulants such as EDTA. This

---

Do It Now Manual Cell Counting Exercise

1. Draw the hemocytometer (both sides) and the counting grids while actually looking at one (not from the text figures).
2. Randomly place some cells throughout the counting grids.
3. Count your cells. Do the duplicate counts (both sides) agree within acceptable limits? If they do not agree, what procedure would you follow to correct this lack of precision?
4. Exchange drawings with another student, and count each other's chambers.
5. If your counts do not agree, try to determine the problem and correct it.

---

* This is the number of NRBC counted throughout the peripheral blood smear 100 cell differential.

can be done by collecting a capillary specimen via a finger stick or by forcing the blood remaining in the needle following a venipuncture onto a slide at the bedside and making the slides immediately. Bedside slide preparation is not very practical; thus most peripheral blood smears are prepared in the laboratory from the EDTA tube specimen. The slides are then stained with a Romanowsky polychrome type of stain such as **Wright-Giemsa,** which will differentiate the various components of the cell. A peripheral blood smear for evaluation is prepared and stained as explained in Chapter 1. The following procedure is followed to evaluate the white blood cells.

Leukocyte Differential and Peripheral Blood Smear Evaluation Procedure

1. Examine the smear before placing it on the microscope. Look to see if it is long enough and if the feathered edge is straight or curved (Fig. 6–9). This will provide information about determining an adequate reading area and an accurate pattern of movement discussed later (Fig. 6–10). Scan the slide on the low-power microscope objective (10×). **Determine the direction** toward the thick area and the thin feather edge; look for any abnormal distribution of cells; and assess the quality of the stain and the size of the good reading area to perform the differential. The **good reading area** (Fig. 6–11) is defined as the monolayer area between the feathered edge, where the cells are distorted with large gaps (Fig. 6–12), and the thick area of the blood smear in which the cells are overlapping (Fig. 6–13). The cells in the monolayer area are evenly distributed with little distortion or artifact.
2. Using the **high dry (40×) objective,** count the number of white blood cells per 5 to 10 random fields in the good monolayer reading area. This reading is an average and is correlated with the expected total white blood cell count. This **white blood cell estimate** represents a normal count if the **average number of white blood cells** seen per 40× field averages

Box continued on page 120

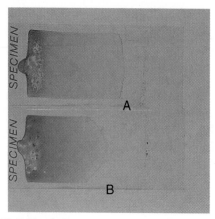

FIGURE 6–9
Peripheral blood smears with a straight edge (A) and a curved edge (B).

between 2 and 7. Only **five or more high dry (40×) objective fields** are necessary if a consistent number of cells is seen; however, if an abnormal value or an inconsistent value is seen, then 10 fields may be required to obtain a more accurate average. The randomness of the fields is essential. If consecutive fields are counted, a bias may be introduced. If this estimate includes fields that are too far out into the feathered edge or too far into the thick area of the smear, inaccurate values will be generated. The monocytes and neutrophils are in higher concentration at the feathered edge, and lymphocytes are in higher concentration in the thicker area of the blood smear.

FIGURE 6–10
The peripheral blood smear evaluation movement pattern. The best smears have a fairly straight edge (A). Note that the movement from the end of one vertical line to the beginning of the next represents one 100× field. Moving farther than one field will result in reaching the thick area before 100 white blood cells have been classified. If the peripheral blood smear does not have a straight edge, note the modification of the pattern of movement (B). The initial vertical pattern may only be a few fields. As the width of the monolayer area increases, the length of the vertical movement and the number of fields available for evaluation will increase.

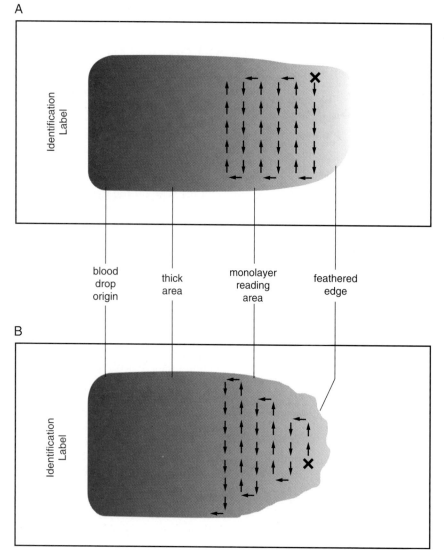

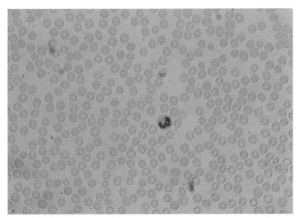

FIGURE 6-11
A peripheral blood smear monolayer. Note the uniformly spaced cell population with random cell distribution, no cells on top of one another, and expected cell characteristics without artifact.

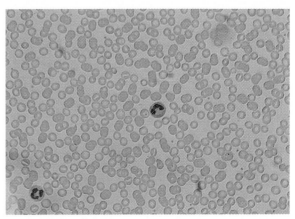

FIGURE 6-13
A thick area of a peripheral blood smear. Note the erythrocytes layered on top of each other, obstructing the clear cellular morphology evaluation. There are artifacts, such as enhanced central pallor in the erythrocytes and distortion of the leukocyte morphology.

3. Find the outermost good reading area of the blood smear, and move to the top or bottom of the smear in order to begin the evaluation in an orderly manner (see Fig. 6-10).

4. Rotate the microscope nosepiece objectives between the high dry (40×) objective and the oil (100×) objective; place a large drop of immersion oil on the slide; turn the oil immersion objective (100×) into the oil; and bring the cells into focus with the **fine focus adjustment control.**

5. Begin moving through the smear as shown in Figure 6-10, classifying each white

blood cell seen and entering these data into a counter, until 100 white blood cells have been classified. In several (five) fields, count and average the number of platelets and evaluate the red blood cells and the platelets for morphology and size. The red blood cell morphology and evaluation are discussed in Chapters 7, 9, and 10. The platelet morphology and evaluation are discussed in Chapters 11 and 13.

Correlation Factors. The peripheral blood smear **estimate of** the number of **white blood cells,** performed as described earlier, should correlate with the actual white blood cell count. This estimate of the number of white blood cells is dependent on a well mixed, properly prepared blood smear to obtain an accurate random WBC estimate. The cellular characteristics are also important to differentiate the cause of an abnormal cell count. These characteristics are described in the white blood cell count correlations.

Sources of Error. An **inappropriate specimen** results in the inability to obtain an accurate peripheral blood smear. EDTA (purple top tube) is the specimen of choice because it preserves the cells. If the EDTA tube is **at least one third full, well mixed** to ensure no clotting has occurred, maintained between 25° C and 4° C, and the plasma is acceptable

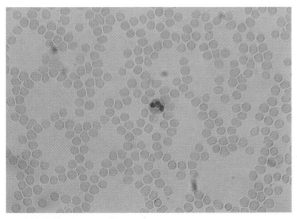

FIGURE 6-12
The feathered edge of a peripheral blood smear. Note the large spaces between groups of cells, distorted shapes of erythrocytes, and no central pallor.

(not demonstrating **hemolysis = red; lipemia = white cloudy; or icterus = dark yellow),** the tests can be performed accurately. Other options that may be available are Na citrate (sodium citrate in a blue top tube), which can be used for a complete blood cell count, if used immediately, before the cells begin to change.

The ability to determine the best reading area on a peripheral blood smear is a valuable skill necessary to obtain accurate results. The blood smear should have a straight edge; however, if it is necessary to perform an evaluation on a blood slide with a curved edge, adjustments must be made in the procedure to avoid reaching the thick area of the slide before 100 white blood cells have been evaluated (see Figs. 6–9, 6–10, and 6–13).

Cytochemical Stains

Staining of cells for cytoplasmic substances useful for identification was discussed earlier and is presented in association with acute leukemia classification in Table 6–1. These cytochemical stains are used primarily to differentiate cells of granulocytic origin from cells of monocytic or lymphocytic origin. The most commonly used cytochemical stains for cell line classification are myeloperoxidase (MPO), Sudan black B (SBB), specific esterase (SE) or nonspecific esterase (NSE), and periodic acid-Schiff (PAS).

TABLE 6–1   FRENCH-AMERICAN-BRITISH (FAB) CLASSIFICATION OF ACUTE MYELOID/LYMPHOID LEUKEMIAS

FAB Class	Cells Observed	Unique Criteria	Cytochemistry/CD* Markers	%†
M1(AML)	>90% **myeloblasts** with minimal maturation	Occasional Auer rods	Myeloperoxidase **(MP)**, Sudan black B (SBB), NASDC	20
M2(AML)	<90% myeloblasts >**10% more mature**	**Auer rods**	Myeloperoxidase, SBB, NASDC	30
M3(APL)	Predominantly **promyelocytes**	Often causes disseminated intravascular coagulation **(DIC)**	Myeloperoxidase, SBB, NASDC	10
M4(AMML)	**Myeloblasts** and **monoblasts** with stages of both	Occasional Auer rods	>20% MP/SBB/NASDC >20% Nonspecific esterase (NSE)	12
M4eo	Same as M4, except with **eosinophilia**	Some with large **basophilic granules**	Same as M4; eosinophils may be shown by periodic acid–Schiff (PAS) stain	4
M5a(AMoL) poorly differentiated	>**80% monoblasts,** promonocytes, and monocytes	Later stages are poorly granulated and vacuolated	**NSE (fluoride inhibitor)**	5
M5b(AMoL) differentiated	<**80% monoblasts,** promonocytes, and monocytes		Same as M5a	6
M6(AEL)	>**50% erythroblasts,** also myeloblasts and monoblasts	50% dysplastic, megaloblastic	PAS	6
M7(AMegL)	>**30% megakaryoblasts**		Platelet peroxidase by EM, platelet glycoprotein by immunocytochemistry	1
L1(ALL)	Small lymph cells	2–10 year olds	PAS/CD 10, 19, and 24	71
L2(ATL)	Large irregular cells	Adult T cell associated with HTLV-1	PAS/CD 10	27
L3(ALL)	Large uniform cells	Burkitt's type	PAS/CD 10	2

*Cluster differentiation markers to identify cells.
†Represents the percentage of myeloid (M) leukemias or lymphoid (L) leukemias.

Leukocyte (Neutrophil) Alkaline Phosphatase (LAP/NAP) Score

Another type of cytochemical staining is useful when a patient presents with a **high white blood cell count** and the differential demonstrates **mostly neutrophils.** The physician may choose to determine if this is a normal healthy response to a bacterial infection or a malignant disease such as leukemia. The **leukocyte alkaline phosphatase (LAP) score,** also called the neutrophil alkaline phosphatase (NAP) score, is the test to examine the **amount of digestive enzyme in the cells.** If the process that is occurring is a normal healthy response to infection, the LAP score should be high, demonstrating the cells' attempt to increase digestive enzymes and destroy the bacteria. If the LAP score is low, this demonstrates an increase in cells for no biologically normal reason, because they are not functioning properly and merely proliferating to the detriment of the patient. The LAP score is also elevated in the erythrocyte disorder polycythemia, which is discussed in Chapters 9 and 10.

The LAP score requires fresh capillary blood or venous blood in a **heparinized (green stopper) tube,** due to stain inhibition by EDTA. A drop of blood is spread onto a slide as described in the procedure for preparing a peripheral blood smear in Chapter 1. Positive and normal **control specimens** must be prepared and stained also to ascertain the validity of the procedure. A positive result can be obtained by using the blood of a pregnant or postpartum woman and a negative control can be obtained from a healthy volunteer or by placing a blood smear from a normal control in boiling water for 1 minute after it has been fixed to inactivate enzymes. The blood smears are fixed in citrate buffered acetone, incubated with a naphthol phosphate alkaline solution, counterstained with hematoxylin, and examined and scored for the amount of stain with a light microscope (Fig. 6–14). The evaluation involves observing 100 neutrophil cells, which are scored on the amount of LAP that they contain. The LAP score can range from 0 (no LAP stain seen in the cell) to 4+ (dark stain throughout the entire cell). This scoring is done on 100 neutrophils, which taken times the total number for each cell provides a LAP score of 0 to 400. A normal healthy adult's LAP score ranges from 30 to 150. If there is an increase in PMNs and **a low LAP score** (0 to 15), **chronic myelocytic leukemia** is suspected. A **high LAP score** indicates a **bacterial infection.** An erythrocyte disorder, polycythemia vera, also demonstrates an elevated LAP score. The blood smears for the LAP score should be prepared immediately and stained within 8 hours or fixed and frozen.

Arneth Count for Neutrophil Segmentation

In order to objectively determine if there is an increased number of hypersegmented neutrophils (Fig. 6–15), as seen in vitamin B_{12} deficiency, the Arneth count is done. The number of segments in the nucleus of each neutrophil

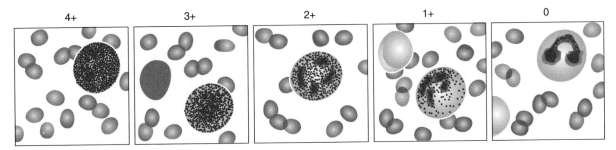

FIGURE 6–14
A leukocyte alkaline phosphatase (LAP) score or neutrophil alkaline phosphatase (NAP) score. For scoring, 100 neutrophils are scored from 1+ to 4+ for the amount of stain uptake. A normal score is 30 to 150.

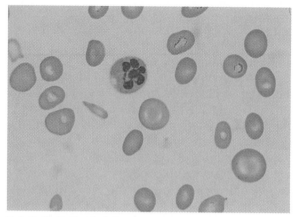

FIGURE 6–15
A hypersegmented neutrophil with six lobes. The Arneth count is done by counting the number of lobes in 100 neutrophils on a blood smear specimen and averaging the number of lobes per neutrophil. An average higher than five segments is hypersegmentation. An average of less than three segments is hyposegmentation.

examined, during a differential count of 100 cells, is recorded and an average is calculated. An average greater than 5 confirms hypersegmentation, and an average less than 3 would be reported as hyposegmentation. The presence of hypersegmented neutrophils is considered a "shift to the right" towards maturity, as opposed to a "shift to the left" toward immaturity with the presence of hyposegmented neutrophils or bands.

Buffy Coat Preparation for Leukocyte Evaluation

In some instances, the white blood cell count is too low to be accurately evaluated by the automated instruments or on the peripheral blood smear. In order to concentrate the white blood cells, a buffy coat preparation must be made. This is done by the following procedure.

1. Using a 5¾″ Pasteur transfer pipette, fill a Wintrobe tube with whole blood, from an EDTA tube. Cap to avoid evaporation, and centrifuge for 30 minutes at 2500 g.
2. After removing the plasma, carefully remove the white layer (buffy coat) of cells and drop them onto a series of clean, dry

glass slides. Prepare and stain the buffy coat smear in a similar fashion as a routine peripheral blood smear, described in Chapter 1. More than 100 (200 to 500) cells should be examined and evaluated due to the lack of random distribution of cells in this modified technique.

Correlation Factors. If the buffy coat is concentrated and collected properly, there should be **very few red blood cells** on the blood smear. More than one slide should be examined in order to ensure that a random distribution of white blood cells has been evaluated. If the **duplicate slides** vary significantly, additional slides should be prepared and examined.

Sources of Error. Errors include **not mixing the original blood specimen**, which would bias the results due to lack of a random sampling from the whole blood specimen; **mixing** the original specimen **too vigorously**, thus damaging some of the cells; and **not centrifuging** the Wintrobe tube **for the specified period of time** or at the specified velocity.

SPECIAL LEUKOCYTE TESTS

Lupus Erythematosus (LE) Preparation. Lupus erythematosus is an autoimmune collagen-vascular disease. The presence of antibodies directed against nuclear proteins (among other antigens) provides a marker for diagnosis. The LE preparation involves damaging the white blood cells in the patient's blood or bone marrow specimen to expose the nuclear proteins and allowing the LE antibody to transform the nucleoprotein into a homogeneous (LE) mass. This attracts neutrophils, which will surround the cell and form an LE rosette. Phagocytosis by a neutrophil follows, and an **LE cell is formed** (Fig. 6–16). This method has been used for diagnosis in the past. After the normal death and normal phagocytosis of the nucleus (not a homogeneous mass) of a degenerated leukocyte, a "tart" cell is formed. This cell must not be mistaken for an LE cell. The LE preparation is

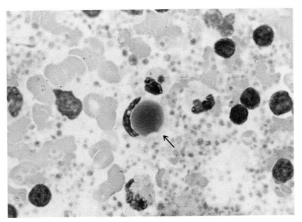

FIGURE 6–16
A lupus erythematosus (LE) cell. Note the large LE mass that has been phagocytized by the neutrophil and is taking up most of the cytoplasm of the cell. The cell nucleus has been pushed to the side.

not performed often due to the ability to **diagnose LE** by **latex agglutination screening tests** and **fluorescent antibody confirmatory tests.**

Flow Cytometry. As explained earlier, the basic concept of flow cytometry is used in many counting instruments; however, a flow cytometer is used primarily to **identify and sort cells** by marking surface proteins as well as by collecting the light scatter characteristic information (Fig. 6–17). This instrument is also called a **fluorescence activated cell sorter (FACS).** The cells of interest are tagged with fluorescent dyes that bind to the cell component of interest (e.g., RNA, DNA) or are bound to antibodies directed against a membrane protein (e.g., CD markers, receptors). The fluorochrome-tagged cells intersect the laser beam in the flow cytometer (Fig. 6–17A), and are detected along with light transmitted to the detectors of both forward-angle light scatter (FALS) (Fig. 6–17B) and 90-degree light scatter (providing cell characteristics for scattergrams). The fluorescence (Fig. 6–17C) is attached to a protein that is specific for the cell or component of interest. The number of cells emitting a specific fluorescence (Fig. 6–17D) is demonstrated by the histograms (Fig. 6–17E). The flow cytometer not only identifies specific cells but can also sort these cells and collect a specific cell population into a separate container for further testing and research (Fig. 6–17F). The flow cytometer can be programmed to place a positive or negative charge on the drop containing a cell, which transmits a specific fluorescent dye and will direct that cell into a separate container from the other drops containing other cells. This technology is capable of detecting up to four different fluorescent dyes in one sample, thus allowing more specific identification of a variety of cells. Flow cytometers are expensive and require a specially trained technician to perform and assist in interpretation of the cell analysis.

The CD, Ig, and other membrane markers are used to classify blood cells and identify leukemic or abnormal cells. The normal healthy individual has a CD4 (T helper cell) : CD8 (T suppressor cell) ratio of 2:1. A patient with AIDS, however, has an inverse ratio of 1 : 2 due to the destruction of the CD4 cell by the human immunodeficiency virus (HIV).

WHITE BLOOD CELL FUNCTION TESTS

The following **tests for neutrophil function** are performed less often and usually in special hematology or chemistry laboratories. The **lack of ability of neutrophils to degranulate** is an inherited disease called chronic granulomatous disease (CGD) and is tested for with the **nitroblue tetrazolium reduction test (NBT).** In this test, the patient's cells are incubated with bacteria and then stained with NBT. If the granules are functioning properly, the NBT will turn blue, being reduced by the granule contents. The inability of neutrophils to respond to **chemotaxis and migrate** to the area of need is measured by a test using the **Boyden chamber.** In this technique a glass chamber is fitted with a semipermeable membrane. The patient's neutrophils are placed on one side of the chamber, and a chemotactic substance is placed on the other side. If the cells are functioning properly, they will migrate toward the chemotactant and thus accumulate on the membrane in an attempt to reach the other

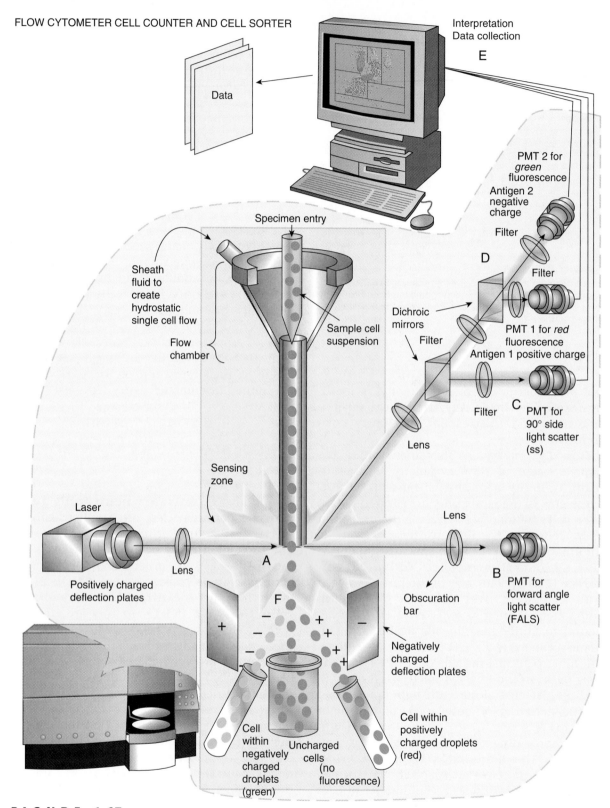

FLOW CYTOMETER CELL COUNTER AND CELL SORTER

Interpretation
Data collection

E

Data

PMT 2 for *green* fluorescence

Antigen 2 negative charge

Filter

D

Dichroic mirrors

Filter

Filter

PMT 1 for *red* fluorescence

Antigen 1 positive charge

Filter

C PMT for 90° side light scatter (ss)

Specimen entry

Sheath fluid to create hydrostatic single cell flow

Flow chamber

Sample cell suspension

Sensing zone

Lens

Lens

Laser

Lens

Positively charged deflection plates

A

F

Obscuration bar

B PMT for forward angle light scatter (FALS)

+ − + −
− +
+
+

Negatively charged deflection plates

Cell within negatively charged droplets (green)

Uncharged cells (no fluorescence)

Cell within positively charged droplets (red)

F I G U R E 6–17

A Flow Cytometer Particle Counter and Cell Sorter. This instrument, also called a Fluorescence Activated Cell Sorter (FACS) is used to identify and count cells (A), collect or sort specific cells (F), evaluate the amount of DNA or RNA, and detect platelet aggregation and platelet factor release.

side. The number of cells that respond can then be counted. Other methods are also available using agarose gel or a microscopic slide. A disease called lazy leukocyte syndrome can be diagnosed in this way. A patient with any of the aforementioned diseases is predisposed to **bacterial infection.**

RELATED METHODOLOGIES FOR PROTEIN AND VITAMIN IDENTIFICATION AND QUANTITATION

Protein identification and quantitation are related to leukocyte function. The procedures for protein identification and quantitation are **performed in the chemistry area** of the laboratory or sometimes in an area designated for special techniques. **The specimen of choice for protein testing is clear, fresh serum (red top tube).** The related methodologies section describes protein and vitamin quantitation and identification procedures associated with diseases presented here.

The protein chemistry test methodology is presented here because it relates to hematologic diseases and testing. The perspective of the entire laboratory is essential for the best health care of the entire person. In order to keep the big picture in perspective, it is important for the clinical laboratory professional to be aware of the tests done in other areas of the laboratory that may validate or correlate with tests done in hematology. This information is then much more accurate and useful to the clinician.

Protein electrophoresis separates and quantitates proteins as a result of each protein's unique physical characteristics. A serum sample is dispensed onto a support medium, such as cellulose acetate or agarose, which is placed in contact with a negative electrode (cathode) on one end and a positive electrode (anode) at the other end in the electrophoresis chamber with the ends of the cellulose strip extending into a buffer (Fig. 6–18*A*, steps 1 & 2). An electrical charge is applied. The proteins will migrate at various rates in various directions based on: (1) the **net charge of the molecules** (the greater the net charge, the greater will be the movement), (2) the **size of the molecules** (larger molecules move slower), (3) the **support medium** used (small pores slow the movement of larger proteins), (4) the **strength of the electrical field,** (5) the **ionic strength** of the buffer, (6) the **pH of the buffer** (a lower pH increases the rate of movement), (7) the **temperature** (the greater the temperature, the faster will be the movement), and (8) **endosmosis,** which is the flow of solute and solvent particles against the flow of the separating molecules in association with the support medium that the sample is moving across. (This occurs when the support medium becomes negatively charged because of the adsorption of hydroxyl ions from the buffer, which retards or reverses the protein migration). This procedure separates into five general groups of proteins: albumin, alpha-1, alpha-2, beta, and gamma globulins. Protein electrophoresis is used to determine the absence of a normal protein, the elevation of a normal protein, or the presence of an abnormal protein (Fig. 6–18*B*).

High-resolution agarose protein electrophoresis is more useful for quantitation of serum protein. This technique allows a more specific separation of proteins for evaluation of subgroups, such as various types of haptoglobin. The agarose bands are read by nephelometry (light scatter) to provide quantitative values to be reported. No graph is generated as seen with a densitometer reading from the cellulose acetate electrophoresis (Fig. 6–18*B*).

Immunoelectrophoresis (IEP) involves first **electrophoresing the serum proteins** in the patient's sample (unknown antibodies) **through a gel medium** in a Petri dish or on a glass slide that does not contain any antibody. Once the various serum proteins have been separated, **known (reagent) antibodies** are added to a well that extends the length of the gel. This reaction dish or slide is then incubated in a moist chamber at 37° C overnight to allow **the antibody (known reagent) to diffuse into the medium and precipitate with the corresponding anti-**

Protein Electrophoresis

Step 1. Application of serum.

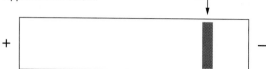

A.

Step 2. Electrophoresis of serum on a strip of cellulose acetate connecting two buffer baths.

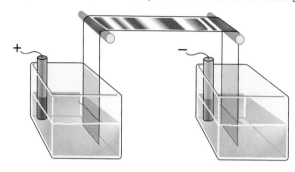

B.

Step 3. Serum protein staining part of application.

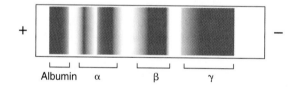

Albumin α β γ

Step 4. Densitometer scan of stained proteins on cellulose acetate strip from protein electrophoresis.

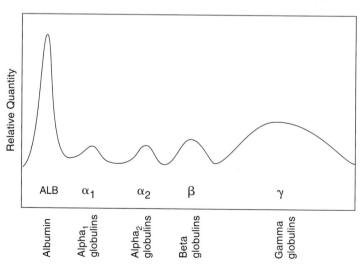

Relative Quantity

ALB α₁ α₂ β γ

Albumin Alpha₁ globulins Alpha₂ globulins Beta globulins Gamma globulins

F I G U R E 6–18

An electrophoresis specimen application and chamber (A). This type of equipment is used to separate proteins for identification and quantification. The serum protein electrophoresis pattern is presented here (B). Hemoglobin electrophoresis is discussed in Chapters 8 and 10.

gen (patient serum, unknown), which has been electrophoresed in the medium, if present. The known reagent antibody is diffusing to the antigen that has been separated by electrophoresis (Fig. 6–19).

Disorders in which these tests aid in diagnosis and monitoring of treatment are: gammopathies such as multiple myeloma (MM) and Waldenström's macroglobulinemia, or hypogammaglobulinemia (the decrease or absence of normal immunoglobulins or antibodies necessary to defend the body against infection). The electrophoresis procedure is performed in the chemistry area of the laboratory and should be correlated with the hematology results.

Radial immunodiffusion (RID) is one method of immunoassay that utilizes the principle of immunoprecipitation. Serum proteins bind to the specific immunoglobulins (antibodies) produced against them and produce an insoluble complex that is visible. Some proteins that can be identified and quantitated by this method are: immunoglobulins (antibod-

ies), complement components (plasma proteins involved in inflammation and the immune response), acute phase reactants (associated with inflammation), and some coagulation factors such as fibrinogen.

The protein of interest is the **(unknown, patient) antigen.** If the protein of interest is an antibody (e.g., IgG, IgM), that antibody now becomes the antigen in this test system, reacting with an antibody (antiglobulin) directed against it. A specific amount of the patient's fresh, clear serum (containing the Ag, Ab, or protein of interest) is added to a well in a Petri dish, or similar container, filled with a semisolid medium (gel) containing the specific **antibody (known reagent),** which will react only with the Ag, Ab, or protein (antigen) of interest, if it is present. The reaction dish is placed in a 37° C incubator for a specified period of time, and the patient's serum sample (antigen, antibody, or protein of interest) begins to diffuse out of the well in a radial fashion (Fig. 6–20). Initially, the concentration of antigen diffusing out of the well is greater

FIGURE 6–19
Immunoelectrophoresis (IEP). The unknown patient serum is electrophoresed through a gel, which does not contain any antibodies, to separate the proteins. A trough is then cut in the agar, and antibodies are added. These proteins are allowed to diffuse together, and any antigens coming into contact with the corresponding antibody will produce a visible precipitation arc.

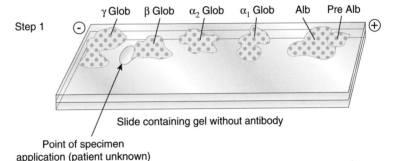

Step 1

γ Glob   β Glob   α₂ Glob   α₁ Glob   Alb   Pre Alb

Slide containing gel without antibody

Point of specimen application (patient unknown)

Electrophoresis to separate proteins (unknown antigens)

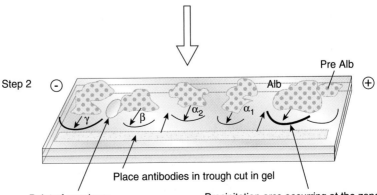

Step 2

Pre Alb

Alb

γ   β   α₂   α₁

Place antibodies in trough cut in gel

Point of specimen application (patient unknown)

Precipitation arcs occurring at the zone of equivalence or at optimal concentrations of Ag and Ab

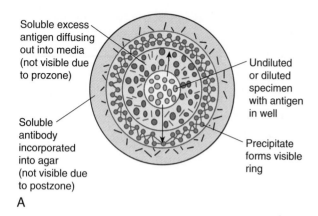

A

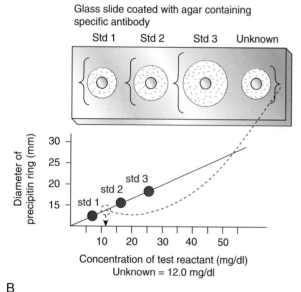

B

F I G U R E 6–20

Radial immunodiffusion (RID). Note the diameter of visible antigen-antibody complexes at the zone of equivalence. The circle diameter is proportional to the concentration of the unknown.

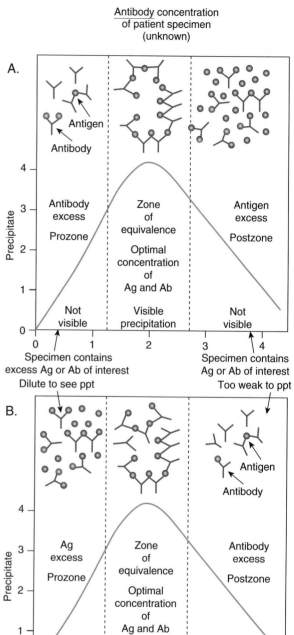

F I G U R E 6–21

A diagram of precipitation reactions. A prozone exists when the specimen is too concentrated. A zone of equivalence is visible precipitation when optimal concentrations of antigen and antibody are reached, and a postzone occurs when the specimen is too dilute from diffusion or dilution or the original concentration of the specimen is low.

than the antibody in the medium (prozone) (Fig. 6–21*B*). This does not allow visible insoluble complexes to form, because all of the antibody binding sites are bound to antigen and therefore unable to crosslink other antibody-antigen complexes. **As the antigen diffuses through the medium, it becomes more and more dilute. At the point at which the concentration of antigen, which is diffusing from the well, and the concentration of antibody in the gel are optimal (i.e., the zone of equivalence or** optimal concentration), **insoluble complexes form that are visible.** If the antibody concentration in the medium is greater than the antigen concentration diffusing from the well, all of the antigen-binding sites will be blocked by antibody and no crosslinking can occur to form insoluble complexes that are visible (postzone) (Fig. 6–21).

The **visible precipitation** confirms the **presence of the unknown protein,** and the **diameter of the ring** produced indicates the **quantity of the protein** that corresponds to the reagent antibody in the medium. If there is no visible precipitation, the corresponding protein is not present or is present in too high a concentration (prozone reaction) or is present in a concentration that is too weak (Fig. 6–21). The reagent (known) antibody concentration in the medium is determined by the manufacturer to be the concentration equivalent to the average concentration of the antigen (unknown) expected in a serum sample. Samples suspected of having **too much of the antigen or antibody** of interest (prozone reaction) **should be diluted,** and the test should be performed again on the diluted sample. A specimen suspected of not containing enough of the antigen or antibody of interest should be drawn again at a later date when more antibody or antigen production is expected.

The **diameter of the precipitation ring is proportional to the amount of unknown antigen (protein of interest in the patient's serum)** (Fig. 6–20A). Controls are run, and diagrams of precipitin rings are provided to determine the antigen concentration by comparing the diameters of these rings (Fig. 6–20B).

The radial immunodiffusion (RID) technique just described is a single diffusion procedure. Only the antigen (the patient's unknown serum sample) is diffusing. The antibody is distributed in an equal concentration throughout the gel medium. Immunoprecipitation assays are performed in the chemistry area of the laboratory and are correlated with hematology data.

The principles of immunoprecipitation, just explained in reference to RID, have been modified in many ways in order to provide more versatility,

accuracy, and convenience. The choice of a test method (for any clinical laboratory analysis) is determined by the availability, specificity, sensitivity, and cost as well as the laboratory equipment and personnel available.

Other methods utilizing immunoprecipitation follow.

Electroimmunodiffusion (EID). In this method, the unknown agent is electrophoresed into the gel containing the known antibody reagent instead of allowing natural diffusion. The result is a rocket-shaped precipitation rather than a circle. The **height of the rocket is proportional to the amount of unknown agent.** This technique is called single diffusion. The antibody is distributed in an equal concentration throughout the gel medium, and the antigen diffuses through the medium precipitating when equivalence or optimal concentrations are reached.

Ouchterlony Double Immunodiffusion Technique. This technique is used to compare the similarities and differences of various antigens and antibodies. A neutral (without antigen or antibody) agar gel medium in a Petri dish or on a glass slide has various wells cut into it. The known reagent antibody is placed into one well, and the unknown fresh, clear serum sample from the patient is added to another well. Several different preparations or samples are used in various wells to compare the antigen characteristics. The antigen and antibody are allowed to diffuse toward each other into the medium for a specified amount of time at a specified temperature. If the antigens in the two wells are identical and demonstrate complete antigenic **identity,** a **solid arc line of precipitation** will be visible (Fig. 6–22A). If there is more than one antigenic determinant in the patient's sample and some of the antigens are identical and some are not, a **fused arc with a spur** is visible, demonstrating **partial identity** (Fig. 6–22C). Any antigen in the test scenario has more than one antigenic determinant (i.e., many areas of the antigen have a unique structure that will bind with an antibody specific for only that one area of the molecule.) Therefore two antigens may have some antigenic sites in common and others none in

DOUBLE DIFFUSION

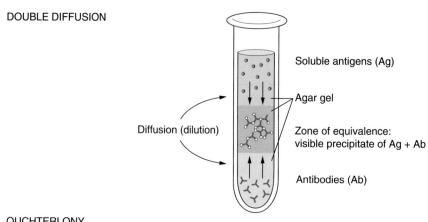

Soluble antigens (Ag)

Agar gel

Diffusion (dilution)

Zone of equivalence:
visible precipitate of Ag + Ab

Antibodies (Ab)

OUCHTERLONY
DOUBLE IMMUNODIFFUSION
(Two-Dimensional)

(A) IDENTITY

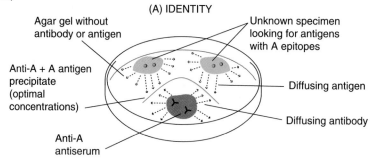

Agar gel without
antibody or antigen

Unknown specimen
looking for antigens
with A epitopes

Anti-A + A antigen
precipitate
(optimal
concentrations)

Diffusing antigen

Diffusing antibody

Anti-A
antiserum

(B) NONIDENTITY

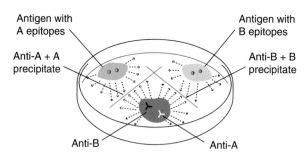

Antigen with
A epitopes

Antigen with
B epitopes

Anti-A + A
precipitate

Anti-B + B
precipitate

Anti-B

Anti-A

(C) PARTIAL IDENTITY

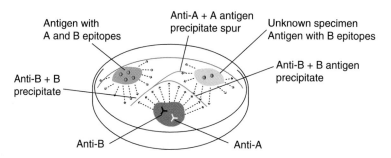

Antigen with
A and B epitopes

Anti-A + A antigen
precipitate spur

Unknown specimen
Antigen with B epitopes

Anti-B + B
precipitate

Anti-B + B antigen
precipitate

Anti-B

Anti-A

F I G U R E 6–22
Double immunodiffusion methods of protein identification and quantitation. The antigen and antibody are migrating through a neutral gel toward each other. In the tube a precipitin line will form if equivalences of Ag and Ab are met. Using the Ouchterlony method, if the two specimens are the same, a solid arc will form; if they have some of the same antigens, an arc with a spur will form; if they are not related, two distinct lines will be observed.

common. If the two antigens are not antigenically identical, the precipitin lines will cross to **make an X,** with no precipitating characteristics alike, indicating **non-identity** (Fig. 6–22B).

Immunoprecipitin Tests. When light is directed at particles (e.g., antigen-antibody complexes) within a liquid medium, the light is transmitted, absorbed, scattered, and reflected and this information can be detected and utilized to measure the particles of interest. This methodology is similar to the cell counting and evaluation explained earlier in this chapter. The characteristics of the light alteration are dependent on the wavelength of the incident light and the size and shape of the particles. Two methods for light measurement follow.

Turbidimetric Immunoprecipitin Assay. This assay involves measurement of direct light transmission by a photodetector, such as a photometer or spectrophotometer. The solution in which the antigen and antibody have been allowed to react is placed in the spectrophotometer, and the amount of light that passes through the solution and reaches the photodetector on the other side is measured. The **greater the amount of antigen-antibody complexes, the more light will be absorbed;** therefore, less light is transmitted through to the photodetector. This method is of limited use because of a lack of sensitivity (unable to detect small changes in light transmission). This test is performed in the chemistry area of the laboratory.

Nephelometric Immunoprecipitin Assays. These assays involve the measurement of light scattered at an angle to the incident light. Nephelometers that measure scattered light at a more forward angle are more sensitive (detect lower levels of light scatter). Nephelometry is the method of choice for determination of relatively abundant serum proteins. The **more antigen-antibody reaction** occurring, the **more unknown protein is present** and the **more light scatter to indicate and quantitate the protein** of interest.

If proteins or any substance of interest can be tagged with a detectable label, such as fluorescence, radioisotopes, or color, this provides a method of detection and measurement. Some examples of labeled immunoassay follow.

Radioimmunoassay (RIA). This assay is one of the earliest labeled immunoassay techniques. In this technique, an unlabeled antibody, antigen, or other protein that will bind specifically to the antigen or substance of interest is fixed to a microtiter well or latex bead within a well (Fig. 6–23). There are two different approaches to attaching an indicator, in this test a **radioisotope,** to the unknown Ag or Ab of interest, in order to measure the amount present. The first is the **noncompetitive immunoassay** (also known as the indirect, "sandwich," or "solid phase" technique) in which the patient's sample with the unknown is allowed to bind to the known Ab (or other specific protein) (corresponding Ag) attached to the microtiter well. The well is washed, then a **second antibody** (or other specific protein) usually an anti-antibody (antiglobulin) that can be used tagged with a radioisotope indicator, is added to the microtiter well. This tagged, known reagent is allowed to incubate and binds only to any of the patient's unknown Ab that is bound to the first reagent fixed in the well. The well is then washed to remove any unbound, tagged reagent protein (antiglobulin) and read for amount of radioactivity, which is reported in counts per minute (cpm). The amount of **cpm is proportional to the amount of unknown** substance that was bound. Therefore, a high cpm indicates a large amount of the unknown substance, and a low cpm indicates a very small amount of the unknown substance.

The second RIA technique is the **competitive immunoassay.** In this technique (Fig. 6-23B), the known reagent protein (antigen) is bound to the microtiter well or plastic bead, as described earlier; however, the patient's sample with the unknown protein of interest (antibody) is added to the well at the same time as the radioisotopically tagged known reagent antibody analogous to the patient's unknown antibody. These two antibodies compete for binding sites on the original reagent antigen attached to the well. The wells are washed to remove any unbound proteins, and the microtiter dish is read for the amount of radioactivity (cpm). The amount of **cpm is inversely proportional** to the amount of unknown Ab in the patient's sample. If the

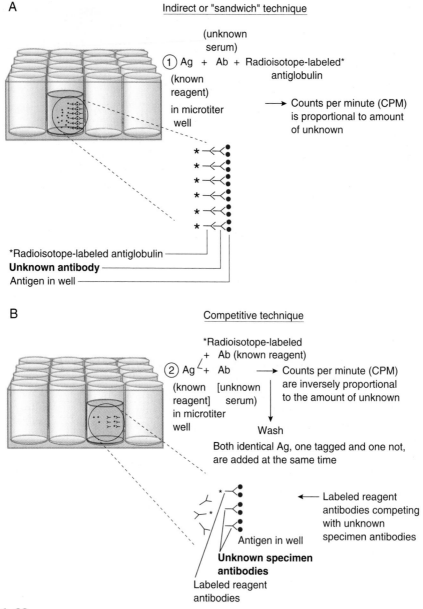

A Indirect or "sandwich" technique

(unknown
serum)
① Ag + Ab + Radioisotope-labeled*
(known   antiglobulin
reagent)

in microtiter
well

⟶ Counts per minute (CPM)
is proportional to amount
of unknown

*Radioisotope-labeled antiglobulin ————
Unknown antibody ————
Antigen in well ————

B Competitive technique

*Radioisotope-labeled
+ Ab (known reagent)
② Ag + Ab ⟶ Counts per minute (CPM)
(known [unknown   are inversely proportional
reagent] serum)   to the amount of unknown

in microtiter
well   Wash

Both identical Ag, one tagged and one not,
are added at the same time

⟵ Labeled reagent
antibodies competing
with unknown
specimen antibodies

Antigen in well ————
**Unknown specimen
antibodies** ————
Labeled reagent
antibodies ————

F I G U R E 6–23
A radioimmunoassay (RIA). Note the two different procedures. The indirect (solid phase) technique results in counts per minute if radioisotopes are directly proportional to the unknown. In the competitive technique counts per minute are inversely proportional to the amount of unknown.

patient's sample has a high level of the Ab of interest, it will compete more with the radioisotope tagged analogous reagent Ab and less of the tagged reagent will be able to bind, resulting in a lower cpm. If the patient's sample has a low level of the Ab of interest, there will be less competition with the tagged reagent and more radioisotope tagged Ab will bind, resulting in more cpm. Therefore, the higher the cpm, the lower will be the amount of the patient's unknown Ab; conversely, the lower the cpm, the greater will be the amount of the patient's unknown Ab. RIA is used to quantitate a variety of proteins including antibodies, antigens, and hormones. This technique is performed in the chemistry area of the laboratory or a specialized area of testing.

Enzyme Immunoassay (EIA). This assay,

which is sometimes called enzyme-linked immunosorbent assay (ELISA), is a technique that utilizes the same basic technique just described for the RIA, differing only in the method of detection. Instead of counting radioisotope counts per minute (cpm) (attached to the second known reagent), an enzyme is attached to this reagent, which is then incubated with a chromogenic substrate to produce a color that is proportional to the amount of unknown protein of interest (Ag or Ab) that is bound (Fig. 6–24). EIA is widely used to quantitate a variety of proteins, including antibodies, antigens, and hormones. This technique is performed in the chemistry area of the laboratory or a specialized area involved in special testing procedures.

Serum vitamin B_{12} and folate levels are measured using radioimmunoassay (RIA) or enzyme immunoassay (EIA) techniques previously described. Normal reference range for B_{12} is **160 to 1000 ng/l.** The normal reference range for **folate is 6 to 21 μg/l.** Vitamin B_{12} and folate are necessary for synthesis of DNA. Therefore, with this disorder, fewer cells are produced and cells seen may have abnormal DNA patterns or abnormal maturation (asynchronous). These tests are performed in the chemistry area of the laboratory.

Erythrocyte folate concentrations are

| Do It Now | Leukocyte Test Methodology Exercise |

1. Using immunoglobulin G (IgG) as your antigen, make a diagram of this test done by RID, RIA, and EIA to determine the presence and quantity of IgG (e.g., reagent or unknown Ag or Ab in gel or gel well or microtiter plate well, + unknown reagent Ag or Ab + indicator such as precipitation (ppt) or reagent antibody with radioisotope or enzyme + substrate or fluorescent microscope = result reported in proportion to the amount of unknown present, using appropriate units).
2. Note where there could be problems in the test procedure and possible corrections.

more reliable than the serum folate levels. This test is performed on erythrocyte hemolysates, and the normal reference range is **166 to 640 μg/l.** This test is performed in the chemistry department of most laboratories.

The **Shilling urinary excretion test** is the most common method for testing B_{12} absorption. In order to first saturate body binding sites, 1000 μg of nonradioactive B_{12} is injected intramuscularly; simultaneously the patient is given 0.5 to 2 μg of radioisotope labeled B_{12} orally. Urine specimens are collected for 24 to 72 hours after ingestion and

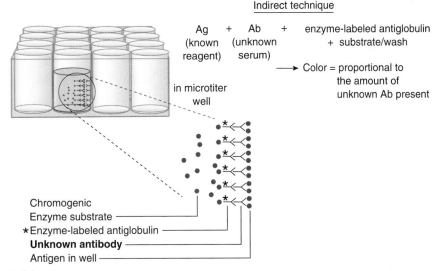

Indirect technique

Ag   +   Ab   +   enzyme-labeled antiglobulin
(known   (unknown   + substrate/wash
reagent)   serum)

→ Color = proportional to
the amount of
unknown Ab present

in microtiter well

Chromogenic
Enzyme substrate
*Enzyme-labeled antiglobulin
Unknown antibody
Antigen in well

FIGURE 6–24

An enzyme immunoassay (EIA). Note the same basic methodology as a radioimmunoassay with an enzyme indicator attached to the reagent protein, resulting in color development of the chromogenic substrate in proportion to the amount of unknown.

assayed for radioactivity. If the patient is absorbing the oral vitamin B_{12}, the radioisotope will be excreted in the urine as a by-product of vitamin B_{12} metabolism. This test is performed in a special area of chemistry or a separate radionuclide area.

STUDY QUESTIONS

1. The anticoagulant of choice for routine leukocyte testing is:
   A. EDTA
   B. Heparin
   C. Na citrate
   D. No anticoagulant required

2. The Coulter cell counter basic counting principle is:
   A. Light scatter
   B. Laser light absorbance
   C. Electrical impedance
   D. Radioisotope counts/min (cpm)

3. The automated white blood cell count was 22,000/mm³ and the peripheral blood smear demonstrated a white blood cell estimate within a normal reference range. The most appropriate interpretation of these results is:
   A. These results correlate. Report the results.

   B. This does not correlate. The peripheral blood smear should be evaluated for random distribution.

   C. This does not correlate. Run a control or standard to check the accuracy of the counting instrument.

   D. This does not correlate. The peripheral blood smear is the least accurate of the two. Report the automated result, and disregard the peripheral blood smear estimate.

4. If the white blood cell count demonstrates 100% lymphocytes with 80% reactive cells:
   A. This represents a transient viral infection.

   B. This represents a leukemia or lymphoma.

   C. This represents a bacterial infection.

   D. This could be a, b, or c.

Which of the Following Tests Can Be Correlated to Validate Results:

5. White blood cell count

6. White blood cell differential

7. Toxic granulation in white blood cells

A. Scattergrams and histograms

B. Leukocyte alkaline phosphatase score (LAPS)

C. Buffy coat layer percentage of sedimented whole blood

Describe and Explain Three Sources of Errors in Leukocyte Testing Due to the Specimen Collection and Preparation:

8.

9.

10.

PART III

Erythrocytes

The following pages will reveal the origin, maturation, function, diseases, and testing of erythrocytes. To facilitate understanding of the material there are objectives, key terms and concepts, and critical thoughts. "Fast Facts" summarize and emphasize key information; "Do It Now" exercises are located after each section to apply what was presented; and study questions are located at the end of each chapter. Each person has a different capacity for and perspective on learning. All possible presentations have been inserted in this text to facilitate learning for a diverse group of learners.

Other areas of the clinical laboratory are incorporated into the text when appropriate to help develop the whole picture of laboratory medicine. It is very important that, while reading this book, the patient is never forgotten. Every aspect of hematology involves a dynamic body process that is not isolated or absolute. The human body is a complex balance of production, metabolism, destruction, stimulation, inhibition, and constant dynamic change. In order to maintain the best perspective, this information is presented in terms of the entire body, not just the blood.

Erythrocytes differ from leukocytes significantly. There is only **one population of erythrocytes** compared with at least five diverse populations of white blood cells. The erythrocyte's function requires the **loss of the nucleus,** while the leukocyte maintains and in some cases utilizes the nucleus throughout the life of the cell. The erythrocyte **does not require cytoplasmic granules** to function, while the granulocytic and monocytic leukocyte function is dependent on the presence of abundant functional cytoplasmic granules. The mature erythrocytes spend their **entire life span within the circulatory system** (e.g., blood vessels or vasculature) in contrast with the leukocytes, which are transiently in the extravascular (tissue) as a means of transportation to the area in which they are needed. Erythrocytes **live for 120 days,** and their sole purpose is to **transport oxygen (via the hemoglobin protein)** to the body, while the leukocytes' life span ranges from hours to years, depending on the cell type, and their functions vary to defend the body from harmful organisms, cells, and other invaders.

Adequate oxygen throughout the body is necessary to maintain life. If brain tissue is **deprived of oxygen (hypoxia, anoxia), a stroke occurs,** leaving some of the brain **tissue dead (cerebral necrosis).** If the heart is deprived of oxygen, a **heart attack occurs** and results in the death of heart tissue **(cardiac necrosis)** and a **myocardial infarct (MI).** The stroke and heart attack are well known examples; however, any cell in your body, such as kidney cells, liver cells, or skin cells will die if oxygen is not adequate. This is why cardiopulmonary resuscitation (CPR) is so crucial for individuals deprived of oxygen after incidents such as smoke inhalation and drowning. Restoration of oxygen flow to the body minimizes the cellular damage.

An understanding of erythrocytes will increase the chances of correct (accurate) correlation and reporting of results to aid the physician in diagnosis and treatment.

FAST FACTS

Basic Erythrocyte (Red Blood Cell)

Structure	Function	Peripheral Blood Reference Values
Biconcave disk	Transports O_2 from the lungs to the body tissue via hemoglobin	$4.2–6.2 \times 10^{12}/l$
No nucleus 6–8 μm diameter 80–95-femtoliter (fl) volume		120-day life span Visible central pallor (pale center) with Wright-Giemsa stain

O U T L I N E

Origin, Maturation, and Morphology of Erythrocytes

Metabolism, Physiology, and Function of Erythrocytes

Study Questions

Erythrocytic Blood Cells

O B J E C T I V E S

Upon completion of this chapter the student should be able to:

1. Diagram and explain erythropoiesis from its origin through maturation.

2. Trace the kinetics of the erythrocyte from its origin in the bone marrow and release to cell death.

3. Recognize the Embden-Meyerhof, hexose monophosphate shunt, methemoglobin reductase, and Rapoport-Luebering metabolic pathways responsible for erythrocyte viability and function.

4. Be able to apply knowledge of erythrocyte physiology when given a clinical scenario and asked to analyze the situation.

5. Diagram and explain the synthesis and breakdown of hemoglobin.

6. Correlate the appropriate erythrocyte testing with erythrocyte response and disease.

7. Explain the following erythrocyte disorders: hemoglobinopathy related anemias, anemias other than hemoglobinopathies, polycythemia, and erythroleukemia

8. Contrast and compare intravascular and extravascular hemolysis.

ORIGIN, MATURATION, AND MORPHOLOGY OF ERYTHROCYTES

Prenatal erythropoiesis occurs first **outside of the embryo** in the mesenchyme tissue of the yolk sac during the first month of prenatal life. The cells produced are primitive undifferentiated cells called mesoblasts, which are believed to migrate to the yolk sac and form blood islands. The **fetal yolk sac** begins producing a large nucleated cell called a hemocytoblast or primitive erythroid cell. At this time the blood vessels are formed, and plasma is secreted to begin the formation of whole blood. The primitive erythroblast retains its nucleus and contains a very primitive hemoglobin (oxygen-carrying protein). The primitive hemoglobin begins as **Gower 2**, which is followed by the production of **Gower 1, HbF, HbA, and finally HbA$_2$** near the time of birth. As the earlier hemoglobins begin to decrease, the later hemoglobins increase in quantity within the cell as the fetus matures (Fig. 7–1). The differences between the various hemoglobins are discussed later in Chapter 8.

Hepatic (liver) hematopoiesis begins at about 6 to 8 weeks from gestation, peaks at 3 to 4 months, and continues until a few weeks before birth. **Definitive erythroblasts,** which will lose their nucleus **and synthesize hemoglobin F and A,** are formed extravascularly (outside the blood vessels) in the liver. Granulopoiesis (production of granulocytes) and megakaryopoiesis (production of platelets) are also evident, but to a lesser degree (see Fig. 7–1).

Hematopoietic activity begins in the **spleen,** and to a lesser degree in the **lymph node,** at 4 months' gestation and ceases prior to birth. The involvement of the spleen in hematopoiesis is controversial and debatable.

Both the liver and spleen have the ability to revert to hematopoietic activity in response to extreme stress and demand for hematopoietic cells due to bone marrow failure. This **production of hematopoietic cells outside of the bone marrow is called extramedullary hematopoiesis.**

The lifelong **hematopoiesis** begins about the sixth month of fetal development in the **bone marrow** and is called **medullary hematopoiesis.** At birth there is **active red marrow** in all bones, including the shafts of the long bones. Gradually as the body grows, and the marrow cavities enlarge, not all the marrow is needed, thus **inactive fatty (adipose) white or yellow marrow** develops in the long bones of the body, leaving red marrow in the **pelvis, ribs, skull, and sternum** of the adult. This fatty marrow can be replaced by active red marrow as needed.

Erythropoiesis, as well as hematopoiesis in general, results from a unique interaction of the early bone marrow cells, the bone marrow's microenvironment of stromal cells, which are made up of fibroblasts, macrophages, endothelial cells, adipocytes/fat cells, cell adhesion molecules (CAMs) for anchored growth in the bone marrow, and the extracellular matrix and cytokines (growth factors and regulatory proteins). These components of hematopoiesis work in a unique balance to produce normal healthy blood cells (see Fig. 2–1). **At birth, 90%** of the bone marrow is hematopoietically active **red marrow; by 20 years of age, 50%** of the marrow is red; and by **70 years of age, only 30%** remains active red marrow (Fig. 7–2). As the demand for blood cell production decreases with age, the inactive bone marrow becomes filled with fat cells (adipocytes) and is called white marrow.

Regulation of erythropoiesis is influenced by many body proteins, such as cytokines and hormones. The greatest **erythropoietic**

Do It Now Early Hematopoiesis/ Erythropoiesis

1. Dissect the early hematopoietic chart provided and recreate this information in as many different ways as possible. Brainstorm with other classmates.
2. Share all of the different presentations developed by this exercise. Determine which one is the most useful to learn and understand the content.

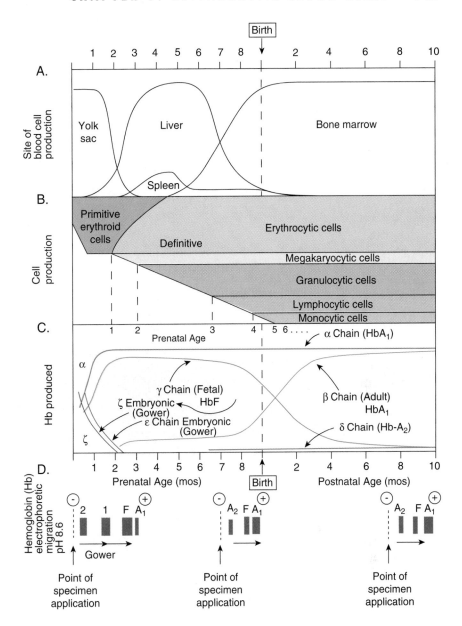

FIGURE 7–1
Early hematopoiesis and erythropoiesis. Note the interrelationship of: (A) cells produced, (B) site of production, (C) hemoglobin produced in erythrocytes, and (D) migration of various hemoglobins on electrophoresis for identification.

stimulator (growth factor) is **erythropoietin (EPO),** a glycoprotein hormone that is primarily produced in the kidney. Erythropoietin is produced in response to decreased oxygen (O_2) in the body (hypoxia), which may progress to no oxygen in the tissues (anoxia). There is an increased production and release of EPO by the peritubular cells of the kidney when the body's oxygen is low. A decrease in the oxygen available for body tissue or organ use depends on the atmospheric availability

(higher altitudes have less oxygen), the respiratory (lung) capacity and function, and the body's metabolism and pH. A variety of other body cells, such as liver cells, secrete small amounts of EPO and are capable of increasing production in the event of renal (kidney) failure. The **kidney produces 90% of the EPO,** and approximately 10% is produced by the liver and other cells of the body.

Additional erythropoietic regulators include stem cell factor (SCF, also called *c-kit* ligand

Young
Child

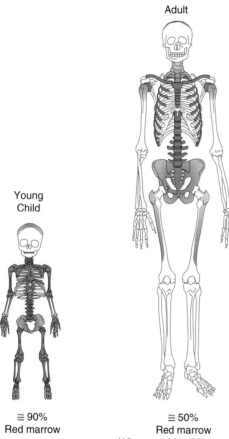

Adult

Older Adult

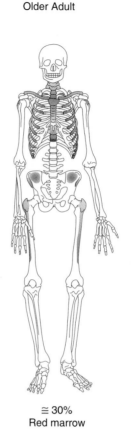

≅ 90%
Red marrow

≅ 50%
Red marrow
(18 years old to 60 years old)

≅ 30%
Red marrow

F I G U R E   7–2
Sites of bone marrow blood cell production. As the bone marrow mass increases and demand decreases (from a child to an adult to an elderly person), the active red marrow becomes inactive white marrow.

and Steele factor), interleukin (IL)-1, IL-3, IL-4, IL-9, granulocyte macrophage colony-stimulating factor (GM-CSF), granulocyte colony-stimulating factor (G-CSF), macrophage colony-stimulating factor (M-CSF), androgen, and thyroid hormones. **IL-3 and GM-CSF synergize with SCF to exert the second strongest erythropoietic influence after EPO.** The effect of unbalanced endocrine activity will alter erythropoiesis and may be striking. This is not a direct effect but rather an indirect effect on erythropoiesis due to the changes in metabolism that the hormonal imbalances elicit. Imbalances and alterations in body metabolism (endocrine) or breathing (respiration) are often the cause (etiology) of abnormal blood gas results. Under these conditions the abnormalities are described as metabolic or respiratory acidosis (low pH), res-

piratory alkalosis (increased pH), or metabolic alkalosis. When the metabolic or respiratory problem is corrected, the blood gases and pH will also return to normal. This is demonstrated by the oxyhemoglobin dissociation curve discussed in the function section of this chapter (see Fig. 7–15).

Hypoxia and anoxia (loss of oxygen to the body tissues) will result in cell death. If there is enough cell death in one area or organ of the body, this may initiate organ failure consequences such as a stroke (brain damage), respiratory failure (lung damage), or heart attack (heart damage), and ultimately death.

Maturation. All of the blood cells originate from the *pluripotent stem cell* (PSC), which is under the influence of hematopoietic regulatory proteins (cytokines) and becomes the **hematopoietic stem cell** (HSC) or colony-forming unit–spleen (CFU–S). The HSC is stimulated to proliferate by specific cytokines to become the **CFU-GEMM** (Fig. 7–3). The CFU-GEMM is influenced by various cytokines to become the **burst forming unit–ery-**

throid (BFU–E), the first definitive erythroid cell. The erythrocyte is named with respect to the naturally red color of the cells and the Romanowsky polychrome (Wright-Giemsa) staining characteristics. The principle of stain-

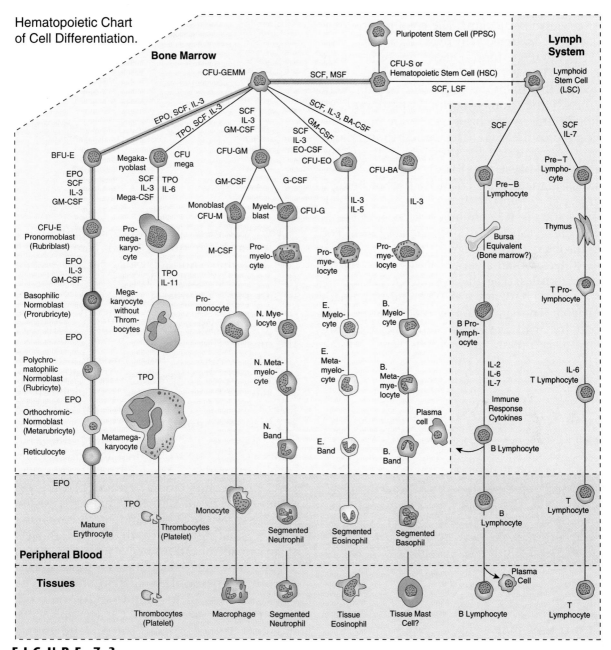

Hematopoietic Chart of Cell Differentiation.

F I G U R E 7–3
Hematopoiesis with erythropoiesis highlighted.

ing, as discussed in Chapters 1 and 10, involves acid components of the cell attracting the basic stain and the basic components attracting the acid stain. The basic cell structure and organelles are discussed in Chapter 2.

The BFU-E matures into the **colony-forming unit–erythroid (CFU-E).** The BFU-E derives its name from the growth characteristics on a semisolid medium. The colonies are irregular and scattered all over the plate. The CFUs, however, form a more uniform colony of cells. The erythroid cell maturation stages beyond this point are subject to two different names. Either nomenclature is appropriate, although the normoblast terms are more descriptive of the stage. The earliest morphologically recognizable erythrocytic cell is the **pronormoblast** (rubriblast). This cell follows the basic maturation characteristics of being a large cell (20 μm) with a large nucleus (high N:C ratio, 6:1), containing 2 to 5 nucleoli, and the cytoplasm is deep blue (RNA). The erythroblast (pronormoblast, rubriblast) is visibly different than a white cell blast due to two characteristics. The nucleus has a unique appearance of dark areas of DNA and prominent nucleoli. The cytoplasm is much darker blue than the white cell blasts, and the RNA renders the cytoplasm more visible (Fig. 7–4).

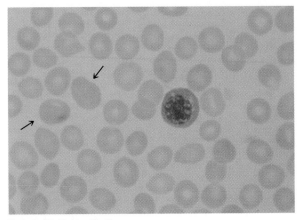

FIGURE 7–5
A basophilic normoblast or prorubricyte in a peripheral blood smear stained with Wright-Giemsa stain. Arrows point to stress reticulocytes.

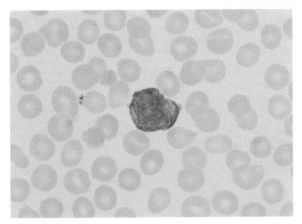

FIGURE 7–4
A pronormoblast (also called a rubriblast or an erythroblast). Note the greater N:C, dark blue cytoplasm, and unique nuclear texture with nucleoli. This is bone marrow with Wright-Giemsa stain.

The next stage of erythrocytic maturation is the **basophilic normoblast** (prorubricyte). The basophilic normoblast is slightly smaller than the blast with a centrally located nucleus within more cytoplasm (decreased N:C ratio of 4:1). The cytoplasm is slightly less blue, and there is still a looser chromatin pattern in the nucleus (Fig. 7–5).

As the basophilic normoblast matures, the cytoplasmic RNA decreases (less blue color), the cell begins to synthesize hemoglobin (oxygen-carrying protein), and the **polychromatophilic normoblast** (rubricyte) is formed. This stage is polychromatophilic (takes up many colors) due to the first recognizable hemoglobin production, which results in a gray, blue, pink combination of color in the cytoplasm (polychromasia). The nucleus is smaller (decreased N:C of 1:1) and more condensed (darker staining) (Fig. 7–6). This is the last stage capable of mitosis.

The final nucleated stage is the **orthochromic normoblast** (metarubricyte). This cell is smaller (10 to 12 μm) and is only one third nucleus (decreased N:C). The chromatin has lost all recognizable pattern and thus is pyknotic. The cytoplasm may appear red but is most often pale blue or gray due to increasing amounts of hemoglobin and decreasing

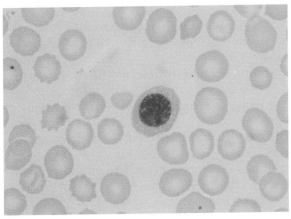

F I G U R E 7 – 6
A polychromatophilic normoblast or rubricyte. A peripheral
blood smear stained with Wright-Giemsa stain.

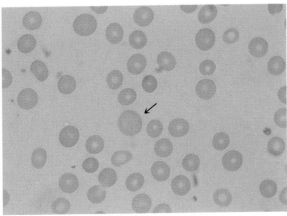

F I G U R E 7 – 8
A polychromatic red blood cell or stress reticulocyte. A peripheral blood smear stained with Wright-Giemsa stain demonstrating the slightly blue color and larger size of the cell.

amounts of polyribosomes (RNA), which is
still described as polychromasia (Fig. 7–7).

The last immature erythrocyte stage is the
reticulocyte, which has slightly less than a
full complement of hemoglobin and no nucleus. The reticulocyte is the last erythrocyte
stage in the bone marrow before release of the
mature erythrocyte into the peripheral blood.
The normal amount of slightly immature
erythrocytes **(late reticulocytes)** is **0.5%** of
the peripheral blood erythrocytes, and these

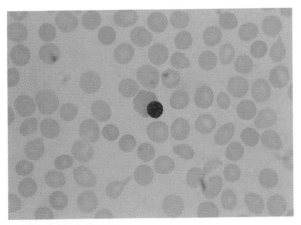

F I G U R E 7 – 7
An orthochromic normoblast or metarubricyte. This is the last
nucleated red blood cell stage. A peripheral blood smear
stained with Wright-Giemsa stain. The cell pictured is extrud-
ing its nucleus to become a reticulocyte.

cells are **not visibly immature** on a Wright-
Giemsa stained peripheral blood smear. If released into the peripheral blood earlier in the
maturation process, the **larger size** of the reticulocyte may contribute to a macrocytic
blood picture. The **blue color of the cytoplasm** is noted on a blood smear evaluation
as **polychromasia** to indicate the presence
of these larger, blue, immature, red blood
cells, which are called **stress reticulocytes**
(Fig. 7–8; see also Fig. 7–5). The term stress
reticulocyte refers only to the **large blue
cells** that are released from the bone marrow
under erythropoietic stress, such as a decrease
in circulating red blood cells (anemia). This
occurs **when all of the mature erythrocytes and most mature reticulocytes
have been released and there is still a
demand for more erythrocytes to carry
oxygen to the tissue,** resulting in release of
the stress reticulocytes. To count and report
the percentage of reticulocytes in the peripheral blood, a reticulocyte vital stain (buffered
new methylene blue) is used to demonstrate
the RNA reticulum that confirms the reticulocyte stage (Fig. 7–9). The **reticulocyte
count** is the **best indicator of bone marrow function,** and the procedures are discussed in Chapter 10.

The **mature erythrocyte** is small (6 to
8 μm) and round with a biconcave shape and

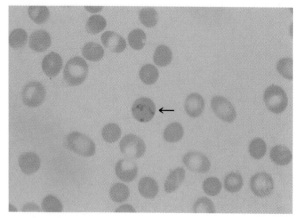

F I G U R E 7–9
A reticulocyte. A peripheral blood smear stained with reticulocyte stain to demonstrate the RNA reticulum in these slightly immature red blood cells.

appears red with slight clearing in the center (central pallor) when stained with Wright-Giemsa stain. The central pallor is due to the biconcave shape of the cell resulting in an uneven distribution of hemoglobin (Figs. 7–10 and 7–12). The erythrocyte takes 5 to 7 days to mature from the blast in the bone marrow and spends 120 days in the peripheral blood picking up oxygen (O_2) in the lungs, distributing this oxygen to the body tissues, and assist-

ing in the elimination of carbon dioxide (CO_2). The normal reference values for erythrocytes are 4.2 to $5.4 \times 10^{12}/l$ for females and 4.6 to $6.2 \times 10^{12}/l$ for males. The glycoprotein hormone **erythropoietin (EPO)** influences the late BFU-E and CFU-E to proliferate, **increasing the numbers** and **maturation** of erythroid cells as well as **stimulating synthesis of hemoglobin** and **preventing programmed cell death (apoptosis)**. As mentioned earlier, EPO is **produced primarily by the kidney** in response to low oxygen pressure ($<$Po$_2$ levels) in the tissues, which is called **hypoxia**. The most common causes of hypoxia are **anemia** (lack of erythrocytes or hemoglobin within the erythrocytes), cardiac or pulmonary disorders, or low atmospheric oxygen tension found at high altitudes. This erythrocyte physiology is discussed in other sections of this chapter.

The fate of erythropoietic cells is influenced by many factors. Developing erythroid cells do not roam freely, but rather they adhere to **specific cell adhesion molecules (CAMs) within the microenvironment of the bone marrow** (see Fig. 2–1). Some of the protein factors that enhance the early erythroid cells (erythroprogenitor cells) are **interleukin-3 (IL-3), interleukin-4 (IL-4), interleukin-9 (IL-9), colony-stimulating factor (CSF), and EPO.** Other proteins, such as **activin,** are produced by several cells including macrophages and influence early hematopoiesis by induction of mesoderm in the

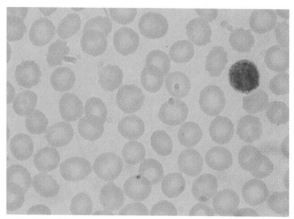

F I G U R E 7–10
Normal red blood cells described as normocytic/normochromic. A peripheral blood smear stained with Wright-Giemsa stain. Note the central pallor due to their biconcave shape, and compare the size to the small lymphocyte in the upper right.

Do It Now Erythrocyte Morphology/ Maturation

1. Draw each stage while looking at it through the microscope or on a Kodachrome slide. Note details of the N:C ratio, the nuclear texture, the cytoplasmic contents, and how this determines the color after staining with Wright-Giemsa stain.
2. Think about the function and morphology of each stage, and list as many associations as possible with basic chemistry and biology from past prerequisite classes.

FAST FACTS

Erythrocyte (Red Blood Cell) Development

Origin
Bone marrow
Normoblast terminology refers to a nucleated erythrocyte (NRBC) and is more descriptive.
The rubriblast nomenclature is the previous terminology, which does not describe the cell.

Maturation
Pronormoblast (rubriblast)—large, with large nucleus containing nucleoli; minimal dark blue cytoplasm; nuclear to cytoplasm (N:C) ratio of 6:1.
Basophilic normoblast (prorubricyte)—slightly smaller than the previous cell; large nucleus with no visible nucleoli; more dark blue cytoplasm; N:C of 4:1.
Polychromatophilic normoblast (rubricyte)—medium-sized cell; a smaller, more condensed nucleus; first identifiable hemoglobin (Hb) synthesis that results in a light blue-gray abundant cytoplasm.

Orthochromic normoblast (metarubricyte)—smaller size; small pyknotic (degenerated) nucleus; and abundant cytoplasm that is slightly blue-gray. This is the last nucleated stage of erythrocyte maturation.
Reticulocyte—slightly larger than the mature red blood cell; may be blue; polychromasia, due to remnants of RNA and less Hb; no nucleus; confirmed as a reticulocyte only if stained with a reticulocyte stain.
Mature erythrocyte—6 to 8 μm in diameter; 80 to 95-fl volume; biconcave; no nucleus; most dense of all blood cells due to hemoglobin content.

Function
Transport oxygen from the lungs to the body tissues.

Major Regulatory Factor
Erythropoietin (EPO)

Reference Range
4.2 to 6.2 × 10^6 mm^3 or 4.0–5.0 × 10^{12}/l

---

embryo. **Inhibition** of erythropoietic activity has been demonstrated by cytokines released during inflammation, such as **interleukin-1 (IL-1)** and **tumor necrosis factor (TNF).** One observation that can explain preferential production of one hematopoietic cell over another is the competition of cytokines for the stem cell membrane receptors. The **cytokine in highest concentration** would bind an increased number of hematopoietic stem cell receptors and **influence the direction of lineage-specific differentiation** into an erythroid cell, for example. Another mechanism of erythropoietic regulation may be production of **protein regulators** that stimulate an **increased responsiveness of the early erythroid cells to cytokines and growth factors.** All of these mechanisms of cell production and differentiation not only play a crucial role in erythropoiesis but may also be

critical for a programmed cell death (apoptosis) at approximately 120 days.

Research has demonstrated a unique difference in fetal, newborn, and adult erythroid progenitor cells in terms of erythropoietin sensitivity, growth rate, number of colonies of cells produced, and production of hemoglobin. The **fetal and newborn** erythroid progenitor cells were **more sensitive to EPO;** the fetal cells demonstrated peak growth significantly earlier than did the newborn or adult cells. Fetal erythroprogenitor cells produced twice as many colonies as did the newborn cells and ten times as many as did the adult cells. The relatively high numbers of erythroprogenitor cells in the fetus and newborn infants may be due to the demand for rapid expansion of erythropoiesis in a small amount of bone marrow present in the fetus and newborn.

The early pluripotent stem cell is the essential cell necessary for bone marrow transplant success. Several laboratories have demonstrated the presence of approximately 5% of these cells in a bone marrow donation and approximately 80% PSCs in cord blood cells. The placenta and **cord blood** cells from delivery, which are routinely discarded, would be **an excellent source of erythroprogenitor cells for bone marrow transplant.**

METABOLISM, PHYSIOLOGY, AND FUNCTION OF ERYTHROCYTES

Erythrocyte Metabolism. The developing erythroid bone marrow cell (still a nucleated normoblast) derives energy from oxidative phosphorylation and the Krebs cycle. The lack of mitochondria in the more mature erythrocytes (bone marrow reticulocyte and peripheral red blood cell) requires a shift to **glycolysis,** utilizing different metabolic pathways as the primary energy source. Two closely linked pathways are responsible for glycolysis within the mature erythrocyte. The **Embden-Meyerhof pathway** (EMP) provides 90% of the energy molecules (ATP) from anaerobic metabolism of glucose to lactic acid. The remaining 10% comes from the reduction of glutathione (GSH) by the aerobic **hexose monophosphate shunt** (HMPS), which generates NADPH (Fig. 7–11). These energy molecules are needed for: (1) synthesis of DNA, RNA, lipids, proteins, and heme in the maturing erythrocyte; (2) active membrane ion transport (intracellular K^+ and extracellular Na^+); (3) maintaining membrane flexibility and shape; and (4) maintaining functional hemoglobin within the cell.

The ability to understand the anemias (decreased oxygen transport due to decreased number of erythrocytes or decreased hemoglobin within the red blood cells) derived from deficiencies within these pathways is dependent on a familiarity with this aspect of erythrocyte metabolism. It is not necessary to memorize the entire pathways, but rather to have an overall sense of the pathways and understand how the marked enzymes, substrates, or products result in disease if they are altered or deficient (see Fig. 7–11). The diseases associated with these metabolic alterations will be discussed in Chapter 9.

Erythrocyte Physiology. In order to maintain the **surface:volume ratio** necessary for adequate exchange of blood gases and flexibility to travel through small blood vessels (vasculature such as capillaries), it is important for the erythrocyte to remain in the biconcave shape (Fig. 7–12). The characteristic erythrocyte shape is maintained by the continuous generation of energy molecules by the metabolic pathways discussed in the previous section. The ATP energy produced from erythrocyte glucose metabolism maintains the correct concentration of K^+ inside the cell and keeps high levels of Na^+ out of the cell. This is accomplished by a **Na^+/K^+ membrane pump,** which must be functional to maintain the characteristics of the cell.

The red blood cell membrane, like other cell membranes, is 50 to 60% composed of a double layer (bilayer) of lipids (mostly phospholipids, some cholesterol, and glycolipids), and the rest is a heterogeneous group of proteins. The proteins are categorized by their location in association with the membrane. There are extracellular membrane proteins, intramembranous proteins embedded in the membrane with extensions into or out of the cell, and intracellular proteins, such as spectrin and actin, that make up the membrane skeleton (Fig. 7–13). The extracellular and intramembrane/intracellular proteins function as receptors, functional proteins, and identifying antigens. Although many of the membrane proteins present are genetically determined, they are not stationary or inert. The **cell membrane is fluid,** and various **membrane proteins** may move about the cell membrane and may **increase or decrease in number as needed** for cell function. Beyond the cell membrane proteins' role in cell function, they are important in the immunohematology department (blood bank) of the clinical laboratory. The erythrocyte membrane proteins

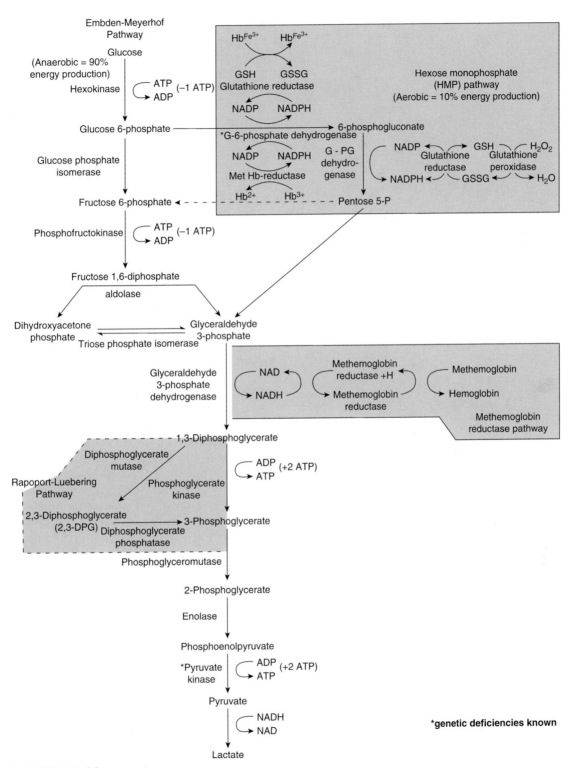

F I G U R E   7–11

Mature erythrocyte glucose metabolism. The Embden-Meyerhof anaerobic pathway, the hexose monophosphate shunt (HMPS), the methemoglobin reductase pathway, and the Rapoport-Luebering pathway are all sources of energy molecules to keep the red blood cell membrane and hemoglobin functional. (From Rodak BF: Diagnostic Hematology. Philadelphia: WB Saunders, 1995, p 103.)

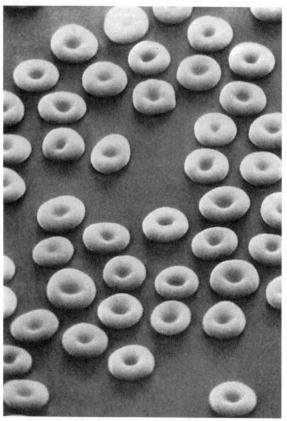

FIGURE 7–12
Normal biconcave-shaped red blood cells. This shape increases the flexibility and surface to volume ratio for maximum ability to deliver oxygen to the tissues. (From Rodak BF: Diagnostic Hematology. Philadelphia: WB Saunders, 1995, p 83.)

(blood group antigens) of the donor unit of blood are compared with those of the patient receiving the blood. This is referred to as typing and crossmatching of blood for transfusion.

As mentioned earlier, the **semipermeable erythrocyte membrane** must allow movement of fluids (osmosis), ions, and nutrients in and out of the cell. If this flow is altered, the erythrocyte will shrivel up (crenate) or will swell, become spherocytic, and burst. The cell membrane is crucial in normal cell metabolism to maintain cell function.

The erythrocyte receives oxygen in the lungs and carries it to the body tissue. The O_2 **is exchanged for CO_2, which is a waste product of cellular metabolism.** The CO_2 is returned to the lungs for release. The **CO_2 is not carried in the same capacity as O_2** and is not associated with the Fe^{2+} molecule. Oxygen sensors in the kidney and liver stimulate increased production of the hormone erythropoietin (EPO), which is necessary for healthy production of red blood cells. EPO is primarily produced by the kidney cells in hypoxia (low oxygen pressure). The fibroblastic cells, which are peritubular capillary lining cells of the kidney, continuously produce EPO and recruit additional kidney cells into EPO production when more is needed. EPO reacts with erythroprogenitor cells (BFU–E and CFU–E) (see Fig. 7–3) in the bone marrow to produce more erythrocytes, and EPO also prevents programmed cell death (apoptosis). The erythropoietin receptor (EPO-R) is a member of the cytokine receptor family.

The sensitivity of the oxygen sensors is reduced in chronic inflammation. In the presence of carbon monoxide in the blood, EPO production is inhibited. The **blood gases and ions (O_2, CO_2, H_2CO_3, and HCO_3^-) have a direct effect on blood pH, which in turn affects the oxygen affinity** (ability to bind and release O_2 associated with 2,3-DPG levels) of the hemoglobin molecule within the erythrocyte (Figs. 7–14 and 7–15). This balance of blood gases and pH can be a result of respiratory alkalosis or acidosis (poor lung function) or metabolic alkalosis or acidosis due to metabolic errors such as impaired kidney function. Measurement of EPO and laboratory diagnosis of disease are discussed in Chapter 10.

Erythrocyte Function. The function of erythrocytes is to **transport oxygen (O_2),** to **maintain functional hemoglobin,** and to **maintain cell shape.** Hemoglobin carries O_2 from the lungs to the body organs and tissues of the body, where it must release the O_2 and carry small amounts of carbon dioxide (CO_2) back to the lungs where the process repeats itself. The erythrocytes are able to perform this function due to the oxygen-carrying protein hemoglobin (Hb), which is synthesized within the erythrocyte and influenced by

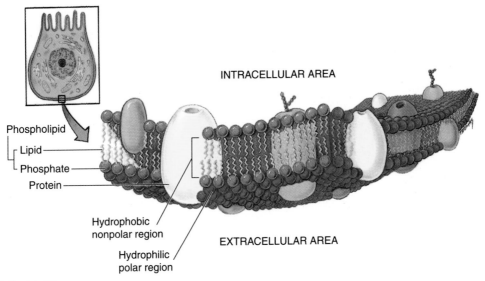

INTRACELLULAR AREA

Phospholipid
  Lipid
  Phosphate
Protein

Hydrophobic
nonpolar region

Hydrophilic
polar region

EXTRACELLULAR AREA

FIGURE 7–13
An erythrocyte membrane. A three-dimensional model to illustrate the relationship of the fluid membrane lipids with the proteins and glycoproteins necessary for cell function. (From Applegate EJ: The Anatomy and Physiology Learning System. Philadelphia: WB Saunders, 1995, p 46.)

metabolic environment of the body. Hemoglobin is presented here as one aspect of erythrocyte function within the whole cell. Refer to Chapter 8 for a more detailed discussion of hemoglobin.

The blood gas level within the body, which has a direct influence on oxygen transport, is measured most accurately by obtaining arterial blood (via radial [wrist] or brachial [arm] syringe technique) and analyzing the partial

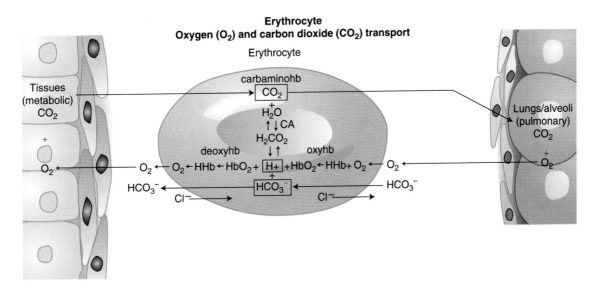

Erythrocyte
Oxygen (O_2) and carbon dioxide (CO_2) transport

Erythrocyte

Tissues (metabolic) CO_2

carbaminohb
CO_2
+
H_2O
↑↓CA
H_2CO_2

deoxyhb ↓↑ oxyhb

O_2 ← O_2 ← HHb ← HbO_2 + H+ + HbO_2 ← HHb + O_2 ← O_2
+
HCO_3

HCO_3^- ←   Cl⁻   ←   Cl⁻   → HCO_3^-

Lungs/alveoli (pulmonary) CO_2

O_2

FIGURE 7–14
Oxygen and carbon dioxide transport. Blood gases are a major factor in the body's acid-base balance. The tissue production and lung excretion of CO_2 are equal under normal circumstances.

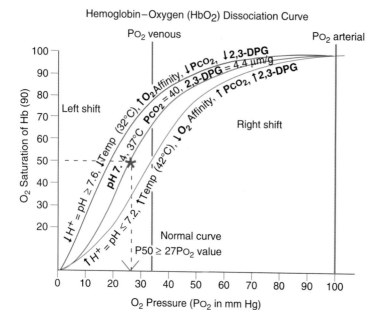

Hemoglobin–Oxygen (HbO$_2$) Dissociation Curve

F I G U R E 7–15

The hemoglobin-oxygen (HbO$_2$) dissociation curve. Changes in pH, temperature, and CO$_2$, and 2,3-DPG levels affect the availability of O$_2$ (HbO$_2$ affinity) to the body tissues.

pressures of the **blood gases (PO$_2$, PCO$_2$)** and blood gas ions (**H$_2$CO$_3$/carbonic acid, HCO$_3^-$/bicarbonate).** The process of oxygen exchange in the body as well as the chloride ion (Cl$^-$) concentration are associated with the blood pH and O$_2$ affinity for Hb (see Fig. 7–15). The blood gas dynamics and ionization determine the **acid-base balance** of the body. At erythrocyte intracellular and extracellular equilibrium, the **blood pH** reference value is **7.4.** For this reason pH is also measured and reported as part of blood gas testing. Imbalances and alterations in body metabolism or respiration (breathing) are often the cause (etiology) for abnormal blood gas results. Under these conditions, the abnormalities are described as metabolic or respiratory acidosis (low pH), respiratory alkalosis (increased pH), metabolic acidosis, or metabolic alkalosis. When the metabolic or respiratory problem is corrected, the blood gases will also return to normal. Acid-base balance is usually taught in clinical chemistry, and diagnostic testing is performed in the chemistry department of the laboratory.

Hemoglobin exists alone or in association with various blood gases. Hemoglobin associated with O$_2$ is called **oxyhemoglobin (HbO$_2$).** Arterial blood has the highest con-centration of oxyhemoglobin and is a red color. Once the O$_2$ has disassociated from the hemoglobin in the tissue, it is described as **deoxyhemoglobin (Hb)** and is found primarily in the venous circulation and is a dark red/blue color. Oxyhemoglobin and deoxy-hemoglobin are normal functional states of hemoglobin associated with oxygen transport from the lungs to the body tissue.

Under certain circumstances the oxygen-carrying capacity of hemoglobin may be altered. If carbon monoxide (CO) is present, this gas will preferentially bind to hemoglobin in place of O$_2$ to form **carboxyhemoglobin (HbCO).** Carbon monoxide has a 210× greater affinity for the hemoglobin molecule and manifests a bright cherry red color in the blood. The inability of the HbCO to carry O$_2$ results in body tissue anoxia and ultimately death. Pure O$_2$ administration will enhance the O$_2$ binding to form HbO$_2$ instead of the formation of only HbCO. If sulfur is present during the oxidation of hemoglobin, it will be incorporated into the heme ring of the hemoglobin, producing a green color. This form of hemoglobin is **sulfhemoglobin (HbS),** which is not capable of O$_2$ transport and is irreversible. Additional oxidation denatures the hemoglobin to form **Heinz bodies.** The structure of hemoglobin and formation of Heinz bodies is discussed in detail in Chapter 8. A variety of drugs (e.g., sulfonamides or aromatic amines) as well as severe constipation, *Clostridium perfringens* infection, and a condition known as enterogenous **cyanosis (blue skin due to poor oxygenation of the blood)** result in the formation of HbS. The sulfhemoglobin level seldom reaches more than 10% of total hemoglobin and, therefore, is usually not life threatening. The iron (Fe) molecule associated with hemoglobin, and the actual binding of O_2, is functional in the reduced ferrous state (Fe^{2+}). When oxidized to the ferric state (Fe^{3+}), hemoglobin is unable to bind with O_2 and is, therefore, nonfunctional. This oxidized state of hemoglobin is called **methemoglobin (Hi).** Increased levels of Hi result in cyanosis and anemia (decreased oxygen transport). Methemoglobin is being formed in the blood at a low level throughout the process of normal oxygen transport. For

this reason, the Embden-Meyerhof pathway and the hexose monophosphate shunt glycolytic pathway in the red blood cell provide systems to reduce the Fe back to a functional state. The **methemoglobin reductase pathway** associated with the Embden-Meyerhof pathway is the primary Fe reduction mechanism. A second Fe reduction mechanism is the **hexose monophosphate shunt pathway,** which depends on **glucose-6-phosphate dehydrogenase (G-6-PD)** to reduce glutathione which in turn reduces the hemoglobin iron. Genetic anemia associated with G-6-PD deficiency and test methodology are discussed in Chapter 10.

As mentioned earlier, the combination of certain compounds with hemoglobin will result in a **detectable color.** For this reason, hemoglobin is oxidized to **methemoglobin** and **bound to cyanide** (HiCN) in vitro in order to produce a color that can be measured photometrically for assessing the concentra-

Erythrocyte Metabolism and Physiology

Glycolytic Pathway	Disorder	Notes
Embden-Meyerhof	Pyruvate kinase (PK) deficiency	90% of red blood cell energy Na^+/K^+ energy = cell shape
Hexose monophosphate shunt (HMPS)	Glucose-6-phosphate dehydrogenase (G-6-PD)	10% of red blood cell energy reduces glutathione/HbFe
Methemoglobin reductase	None known	Reduces oxidized Hb
Rapoport-Luebering	2,3-Diphosphoglycerate	Increased O_2 affinity Less exchange in the body

Organ	Disorder	Gas or Ion Physiology
Lungs	Respiratory acidosis if pH < 7.4, $P_{CO_2} > 40$ Respiratory alkalosis if pH > 7.4, $P_{CO_2} < 40$	O_2 and HCO_3^- into RBC CO_2 and Cl^- out of RBC Retention of CO_2 or excessive loss of CO_2
Tissues	Metabolic acidosis if pH < 7.4, $P_{CO_2} < 40$ Metabolic alkalosis if pH > 7.4, $P_{CO_2} > 40$	CO_2 and Cl^- into RBC O_2 and HCO_3^- out of RBC Kidney regulates reabsorption of HCO_3^- and excretion of H^+

The human body and, therefore, clinical laboratory science cannot truly be separated into hematology, chemistry, blood bank, clinical immunology, and microbiology. As shown here, hematology and chemistry are intimately related at the physiologic and metabolic levels in the red blood cell.

tion. This method of measuring hemoglobin levels is discussed in the erythrocyte testing section in Chapter 10.

The **arterial blood gas** analysis is performed most often by respiratory therapists in the **respiratory therapy department** of the hospital, not in the clinical laboratory. **Venous blood gas** evaluation can be done by respiratory therapy or in the **clinical chemistry department of the laboratory.** If the phlebotomist is drawing a venous blood gas, a heparin (green stopper) tube is drawn, and it is very important not to remove the cap from the tube or expose the blood to room air in any way prior to testing. The quantity of oxygen combined with erythrocyte hemoglobin in the blood, reported as oxygen saturation (SO_2) level, is evaluated by noninvasive co-oximetry at the bedside to obtain a general idea of O_2 and to monitor treatment. This is done by placing a device on the finger that measures capillary O_2. This SO_2 is compared with the oxygen content, which is the amount of oxygen that could combine with hemoglobin in that blood. The amount of O_2 combined with hemoglobin is related to the oxygen pressure available (PO_2). An oxyhemoglobin dissociation curve has been established for normal adult hemoglobin at the **standard pH of 7.4 and normal body temperature (37° C)** (Figs. 7–14 and 7–15). Notice that the other parameters that influence oxygen exchange are the oxygen pressure (PO_2), the carbon dioxide pressure (PCO_2), the 2,3-diphosphoglycerate level (2,3-DPG) or 2,3-biphosphoglycerate (2,3-BPG). These all affect oxygen affinity and, therefore, determine the curve and any **shift to the left or shift to the right** of normal. If hemoglobin with increased oxygen affinity (e.g., HbF) is present, the curve will also shift to the left. Hemoglobin is presented in detail in Chapter 8.

STUDY QUESTIONS

1. The correct order for erythropoietic maturation is:
   A. Pronormoblast, basophilic normoblast, polychromatophilic normoblast, orthochromic normoblast, reticulocyte, mature erythrocyte

   B. Pronormoblast, polychromatophilic normoblast, basophilic normoblast, orthochromic normoblast, mature erythrocyte

   C. Rubriblast, prorubricyte, rubricyte, metarubricyte, reticulocyte, mature erythrocyte

   D. Erythroblast, proerythroblast, metaerythroblast, orthoerythroblast, reticulocyte, mature erythrocyte

   E. Both A and C are correct.

2. The erythrocyte originates in the _____.

3. The erythrocyte survives in the peripheral blood for _____.

Match the Following (4–6):

4. Glucose-6-phosphate dehydrogenase (G-6-PD) reduction of glutathione, which in turn reduces Hb Fe from the ferric (Fe^{3+}) to the ferrous (Fe^{2+}) state

5. Anaerobic glycolysis to lactate, providing 90% of the cell energy molecules (ATP, NADH)

6. Produces 2,3-diphosphoglycerate (2,3-DPG) or 2,3-biphosphoglycerate (2,3-BPG), which are directly related to the Hb oxygen affinity

   A. Embden-Meyerhof pathway   C. Rapoport-Luebering pathway

   B. Hexose monophosphate shunt   D. Methemoglobin reductase pathway

Choose the Best Answer:

7. The following hemoglobin state is virtually irreversible because the molecule involved has 200× greater affinity for hemoglobin than for oxygen.

   A. Carboxyhemoglobin   C. Sulfhemoglobin

   B. Methemoglobin   D. All of the above

8. The hemoglobin dissociation curve can be shifted due to:

   A. pH   D. P_{CO_2} levels

   B. Temperature   E. All of the above

   C. 2,3-DPG levels

O U T L I N E

Hemoglobin Structure, Synthesis, and Breakdown

Hemoglobin Iron Kinetics

Classification and Function of Hemoglobin

Study Questions

Hemoglobin

OBJECTIVES

Upon completion of this chapter the student should be able to:

1. Diagram the structure of hemoglobin.

2. Explain the synthesis and breakdown of the various hemoglobin components.

3. Contrast and compare intravascular and extravascular hemolysis.

4. Follow the kinetics of iron, including ingestion, use, storage, and loss.

5. Describe how hemoglobins are classified and the significance of the types.

Hemoglobin is the oxygen-carrying protein within the erythrocytes of the blood. It is made of heme and globin, and the red pigment of the **heme provides the red color of blood.** If there are not enough erythrocytes to carry the necessary hemoglobin or the hemoglobin itself is decreased, abnormal, or nonfunctional, the body will be deprived of oxygen and the body tissues will begin to die. The amount of oxygen delivered to the body is also dependent on respiratory (lung) function, atmospheric oxygen, and body metabolism. For this reason, an evaluation of a patient's oxygen status is dependent not only on the clinical laboratory erythrocyte count and hemoglobin value but also on the arterial blood gas (ABG) values from respiratory therapy and values reflecting the metabolic status of the patient, which are part of the chemistry profile.

HEMOGLOBIN STRUCTURE, SYNTHESIS, AND BREAKDOWN

The molecular structure of hemoglobin consists of **four globin (polypeptide) chains** (two pairs) and **four heme (protoporphyrin) groups,** each containing one atom of iron, hence **four iron (Fe^{2+}) molecules** (Fig. 8–1). Each heme group is located precisely in a pocket or fold of the globin chain near the surface of the molecule. The heme reversibly combines with one molecule of O_2 in the lungs and delivers it to the body tissues where needed. The ability of the hemoglobin to carry oxygen efficiently is influenced by many factors, which include respiratory (lung) function, presence of atmospheric oxygen, and body metabolism. The specific amino acid sequence of the **globin chain determines the classification** or type of hemoglobin present and the way in which the chain folds to create the heme pocket. A molecule from the Embden-Meyerhof pathway in the mature erythrocyte, **2,3-diphosphoglycerate (2,3-DPG) or 2,3-biphosphoglycerate (2,3-BPG),** becomes associated with the molecule of hemoglobin simultaneously with a change in the shape of the globin chains so that they will more readily take up oxygen. The ability of the hemoglobin molecule to bind with O_2 is the oxygen affinity. The 2,3-DPG level may be used in the blood bank area of the laboratory to determine the oxygen-carrying capacity of the stored units of blood. When O_2 is unloaded, the B chains of the hemoglobin molecule pull apart, permitting entry of the metabolite 2,3-diphosphoglycerate and resulting in a lower affinity for O_2. The interaction of 2,3-DPG and other factors, which are listed in Figure 8–2, influence the sigmoid shape of the hemoglobin O_2 dissociation curve. In vivo, O_2 exchange is 95% saturation for arterial blood and 70% for venous blood. The position of the curve is dependent on the concentrations of 2,3-DPG, H^+, and CO_2. Fetal hemoglobin (Hgb F) cannot bind 2,3-DPG, which changes the configuration of the hemoglobin molecule to enhance the release of O_2. This shifts the oxygen dissociation curve to the left due to the inability to give up O_2 (see Fig. 8–2).

The structure of hemoglobin is directly related to the function (uptake and release of O_2); therefore, one change in the amino acid sequence of a polypeptide globin chain may affect the function. The best example of this is a change in a single amino acid (one glutamic acid is replaced by valine) in the beta globin chains, resulting in the sickling of the erythrocytes and the inability to carry oxygen. Normal responses and diseases of erythrocytes are presented in Chapter 9.

Sixty-five percent of **hemoglobin synthesis** occurs in the immature nucleated red blood cell, and 35% occurs in the reticulocyte (immature anucleate red blood cell). This synthesis occurs in the **mitochondria (heme)** and in the **ribosomes (globin)** in the **cytoplasm** (Fig. 8–3). The condensation of glycine and succinyl co-A is **the first step in heme synthesis, and this is limited by the action of amino levulinic acid (ALA) enzyme.** Pyridoxal phosphate (vitamin B_6) is a cofactor for this reaction, which results in the **synthesis of the protoporphyrin ring, which combines with iron (Fe^{2+})**

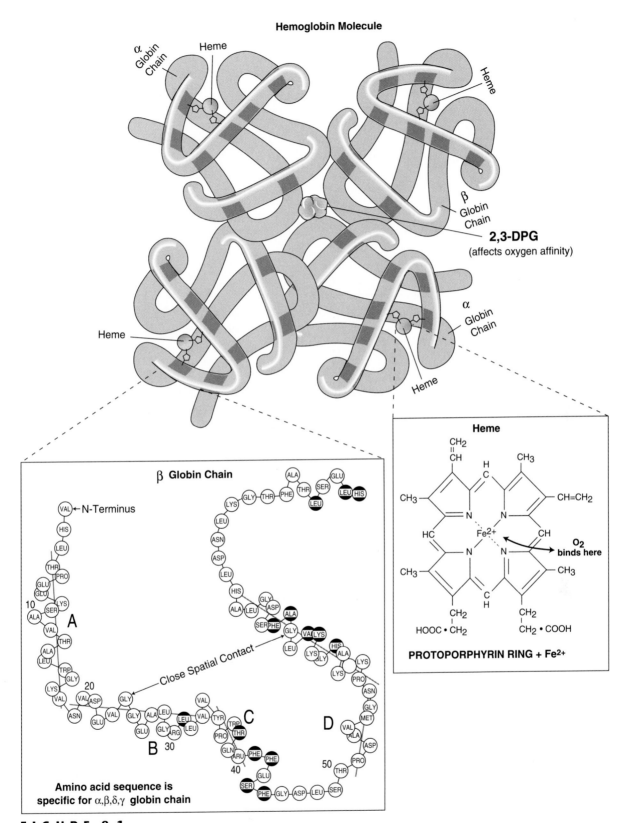

FIGURE 8-1

Hemoglobin structure. Note the arrangement of the specific globin chains, heme molecules with iron and O_2, and 2,3-diphosphoglycerate (DPG).

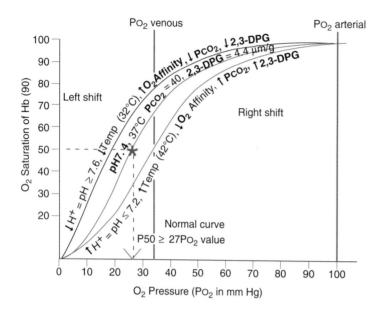

FIGURE 8–2
Hemoglobin-oxygen dissociation curve.

to form heme. **Heme synthesis is stimulated by EPO and inhibited by heme.** A test to aid in the diagnosis of abnormal hemoglobin diseases is the **free erythrocyte protoporphyrin (FEP).** Diagnostic tests and diseases are discussed in Chapters 9 and 10.

The heme is then combined with the globin (amino acid) chains produced by the polyribosomes in the plasma. Four globin chains combine with four heme to become the hemoglobin molecule. The classification or type of globin chain present determines the specific hemoglobin produced. This is discussed in detail in a later section of this chapter.

Hemoglobin (Hb) catabolism or breakdown occurs through two types of hemolysis (red blood cell breakdown or lysis). **Intravascular hemolysis** occurs within the blood stream. This hemolysis results in the immediate release of **free hemoglobin** into the plasma, making it appear **red** (Fig. 8–4). In order not to lose this hemoglobin via excretion through the kidney (renal system) into the urine, free hemoglobin will bind to various proteins within the plasma such as **haptoglobin,** hemopexin, or albumin and will eventually be phagocytized by macrophages

for breakdown. Haptoglobin is the major free hemoglobin transport protein with hemopexin and albumin to rescue the free Hb when all of the haptoglobin has been saturated. Once the red blood cell is phagocytized by a macrophage, the breakdown process is the same for all types of hemolysis. **Extravascular hemolysis** occurs when a damaged or abnormal red blood cell is phagocytized by a macrophage (usually in the liver or spleen) and the product of heme catabolism is a **yellow,** toxic substance called **bilirubin** (see Fig. 8–4). The bilirubin is further catabolized in the liver and excreted through the kidneys in the urine and through the digestive tract in the feces. The globin chains are broken down and returned to the amino acid pool of the body. When heme is broken down, the **iron** (Fe^{2+}) is bound to a protein, **transferrin,** and is carried to the bone marrow (BM) for the ongoing production of new erythrocytes (erythropoiesis) or is stored for future use in the macrophage as **ferritin** or in other organs as **hemosiderin.** The serum ferritin test is the best indicator of iron stores in the body. Other tests for an evaluation of iron are the serum iron, total iron-binding capacity (TIBC), which measures the free transferrin level that is not

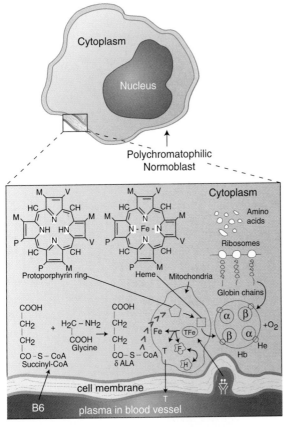

> = 6 forms of porphyrins
H = hemosiderin
T = transferrin
Fe = iron
F = ferritin - 20-50 μg/ml
He = heme
Hb = hemoglobin
α = alpha globin chain
β = beta globin chain

FIGURE 8–3
Hemoglobin synthesis. Note that all components (globin chains, porphyrins, and iron) must be available and assembled properly. Heme is synthesized in the mitochondria, and the globin chains are synthesized by the ribosomes.

bound to iron. The percent saturation of transferrin with iron can also be measured. These tests are explained in Chapter 10. Keep in mind that iron is not used only for hemoglobin; a small percentage is required for certain metabolic functions within the body involving enzymes. The chemical portion of

heme is further broken down into urobilinogen, which is excreted by the gastrointestinal tract (fecal) or the renal system (kidneys, urine).

HEMOGLOBIN IRON KINETICS

Iron in the ferrous state (Fe^{2+}) is a key component of hemoglobin, and the majority of iron in the body is in hemoglobin. The nonhemoglobin iron, used by enzymes and other body processes, is negligible. The iron molecule in the reduced **ferrous (Fe^{2+})** state binds to the oxygen for transportation from the lungs to the body tissues. When the iron becomes oxidized to the **ferric state (Fe^{3+})** due to chemicals or reactions in the body, oxygen is unable to bind to the hemoglobin molecule; therefore, to be functional, hemoglobin must contain iron in the reduced state.

Iron is not synthesized in the body but must be ingested regularly as well as retained and not lost through the intestinal or urinary tract (see Fig. 8–4). Once iron is in the body, it is transported by the carrier protein **transferrin** to the bone marrow for use in new red blood cells or is utilized to a lesser degree for metabolic processes throughout the body. Tests to determine iron status are the serum

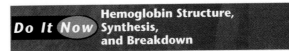

Do It Now Hemoglobin Structure, Synthesis, and Breakdown

1. Create flash cards that depict the origin, synthesis, catabolism (breakdown), and testing of hemoglobin. Write the explanation on the back of the card with the event drawn on the front. Include the various regulators (e.g., EPO, Fe, genes). This activity will require *at least* eight cards. It does not take an artist to do this.
2. Use your flash cards with other classmates to share knowledge of the kinetics of hemoglobin. You will all learn from this experience.

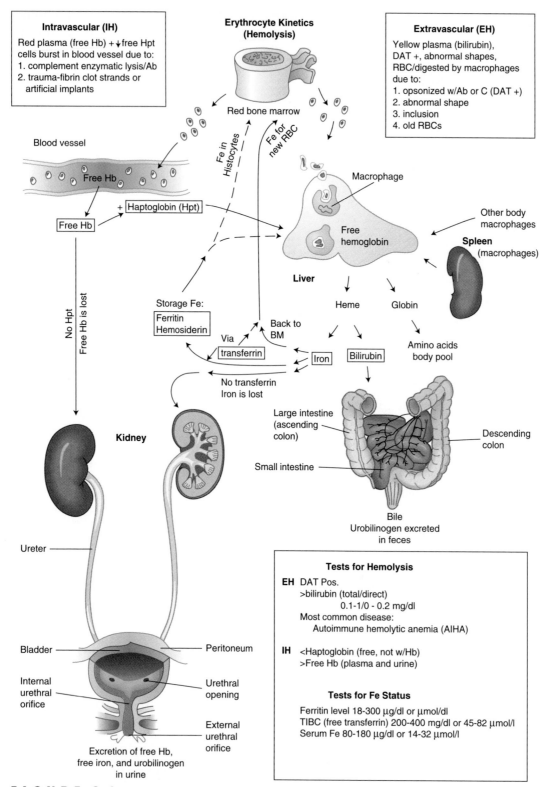

Intravascular (IH)

Red plasma (free Hb) + ↓free Hpt
cells burst in blood vessel due to:
1. complement enzymatic lysis/Ab
2. trauma-fibrin clot strands or
   artificial implants

**Erythrocyte Kinetics
(Hemolysis)**

Red bone marrow

Extravascular (EH)

Yellow plasma (bilirubin),
DAT +, abnormal shapes,
RBC/digested by macrophages
due to:
1. opsonized w/Ab or C (DAT +)
2. abnormal shape
3. inclusion
4. old RBCs

Blood vessel

Fe in
Histiocytes

Fe for
new RBC

Free Hb

Macrophage

Free Hb

+ Haptoglobin (Hpt)

Free
hemoglobin

Other body
macrophages

Spleen
(macrophages)

No Hpt
Free Hb is lost

Liver

Storage Fe:

Ferritin
Hemosiderin

Via
transferrin

Back to
BM

Heme

Globin

Iron

Bilirubin

Amino acids
body pool

No transferrin
Iron is lost

Kidney

Large intestine
(ascending
colon)

Descending
colon

Small intestine

Ureter

Bladder

Peritoneum

Internal
urethral
orifice

Urethral
opening

External
urethral
orifice

Excretion of free Hb,
free iron, and urobilinogen
in urine

Bile
Urobilinogen excreted
in feces

Tests for Hemolysis

EH DAT Pos.
   >bilirubin (total/direct)
       0.1-1/0 - 0.2 mg/dl
   Most common disease:
       Autoimmune hemolytic anemia (AIHA)

IH <Haptoglobin (free, not w/Hb)
   >Free Hb (plasma and urine)

Tests for Fe Status

Ferritin level 18-300 μg/dl or μmol/dl
TIBC (free transferrin) 200-400 mg/dl or 45-82 μmol/l
Serum Fe 80-180 μg/dl or 14-32 μmol/l

FIGURE 8-4

Intravascular hemolysis versus extravascular hemolysis. Note the difference exists in the cause, tests, and condition prior to liver breakdown of hemoglobin.

Hemoglobin Structure, Synthesis, and Breakdown

	Heme	**Globin**
Hb Structure:	4 protoporphyrin rings $+Fe^{2+}$	4 amino acid chains
Synthesis:	Mitochondria	Polyribosomes
Catabolism:	Protoporphyrin: in macrophage to bilirubin (yellow); liver degrades bilirubin for excretion Iron (Fe^{2+}): in macrophage as ferritin, hemosiderin for storage, or bound to transferrin in the plasma	In macrophage to amino acids
Regulation:	Less O_2 stimulates erythropoietin (EPO), which stimulates Hb synthesis. Excess heme and more O_2 inhibit Hb synthesis.	
Miscellaneous:	Intact hemoglobin molecules outside of the red blood cell (intravascular hemolysis) bind to the haptoglobin carrier protein in the plasma until phagocytized by a macrophage for further degradation.	

iron, ferritin level, total iron-binding capacity (TIBC) of transferrin, and iron stain of bone marrow and peripheral blood smears. These tests are explained and discussed in Chapter 10. If the diet is deficient in iron, less hemoglobin will be produced, resulting in less oxygen to the tissues. The disease associated with this state is iron deficiency anemia. Additional diseases involving inappropriate utilization of iron in red blood cells are discussed in Chapter 9.

CLASSIFICATION AND FUNCTION OF HEMOGLOBIN

Classification of hemoglobin is determined by the globin chain present. Each glo-

Hemoglobin Iron

Origin:	Diet and stored in macrophages of the body; histiocytes in the bone marrow	
Loss:	Bleeding; excretion in feces and urine if not bound to a carrier	
Iron States:	*Reduced Iron:*	*Oxidized Iron:*
	Ferrous (Fe^{2+})	Ferric state (Fe^{3+})
	Able to bind O_2	Unable to bind O_2
	Maintained by the hexose monophosphate shunt, glucose-6-phosphate dehydrogenase, and gluta-thione (GSH)	Developed by oxidative molecules (i.e., prima-quine drugs)
Carriers:	*Free Iron:*	*Stored Iron:*
	Transferrin	Ferritin
		Hemosiderin

Do It Now Hemoglobin Iron

1. List foods that contain iron.
2. Draw an *original* diagram of the kinetics of iron. Begin with the ingestion of iron and end with the incorporation of iron into new erythrocytes or the loss of iron through excretion. Emphasize the points at which iron is measured by tests. Exchange your diagram with a classmate, and let your classmate critique your chart for completeness and accuracy.

bin chain has a different **amino acid sequence,** which determines how it will **function** and how it will **migrate on electrophoresis** (Fig. 8–5). This procedure is presented in more detail in Chapter 10. The amino acid sequence of the globin chain is **genetically determined.** In other words, the DNA codes for a specific sequence of amino acids in the globin chain and, therefore, a specific hemoglobin. The most common globin chains are the alpha, beta, delta, and gamma chains (Fig. 8–6C, D, and E).

The embryo has very primitive hemoglobins—Gowers 1, Portland, and Gowers 2. These contain two sigma and two epsilon globin chains in each molecule of Gowers 1; hemoglobin, two sigma and two gamma globin chains in the Portland hemoglobin molecule; and two alpha and two epsilon globin chains in the Gowers 2 hemoglobin molecule. The fetus develops **hemoglobin F (HbF),** which contains two alpha and two gamma ($\alpha_2\gamma_2$) globin chains in each molecule. This fetal hemoglobin **functions well in the low O_2 environment** in the uterus, because the oxygen affinity is higher. The HbF can reach the very low O_2 environment of the fetus before giving up its O_2. The switch to adult hemoglobin A begins shortly before birth and is not complete for 3 to 6 months. Adult **hemoglobin A (HbA)** consists of two alpha and two beta ($\alpha_2\beta_2$) globin chains (see Fig. 8–6C, D, and E).

Adult hemoglobins in the erythrocytes contain **96 to 98% HbA, also referred to** as **HbA$_1$,** which contains two alpha and two beta chains ($\alpha_2\beta_2$), **0.5 to 0.8% HbF** (two alpha and two gamma chains [$\alpha_2\gamma_2$]), and **1.5 to 3.2% HbA$_2$,** made up of two alpha and two delta ($\alpha_2\delta_2$) chains (see Fig. 8–6D and E). HbA$_1$ is subdivided into various glycosylated fractions—A$_{1a}$, A$_{1b}$, and A$_{1c}$. The A$_{1c}$ is the one of interest for monitoring glucose metabolism in diabetic patients. The amount of glycosylation (sugar molecules) of the hemoglobin A$_1$ reflects the sugar metabolism of the body over several days. The serum glucose level is subject to immediate diet, exercise, and other transient factors. The HbA$_{1c}$ is a steady-state measure of the average amount of

Hemoglobin Electrophoresis

Cellulose Acetate Method (pH 8.4)

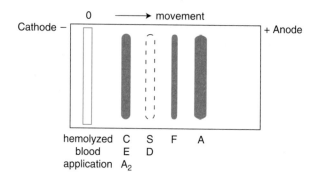

Citrate Agar Method (pH 6.0 - 6.2)

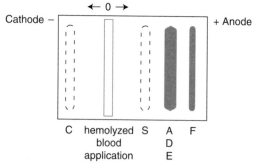

FIGURE 8–5

Cellulose acetate and citrate agar hemoglobin electrophoresis. Solid bars represent the normal hemoglobins; broken bars represent the abnormal hemoglobins.

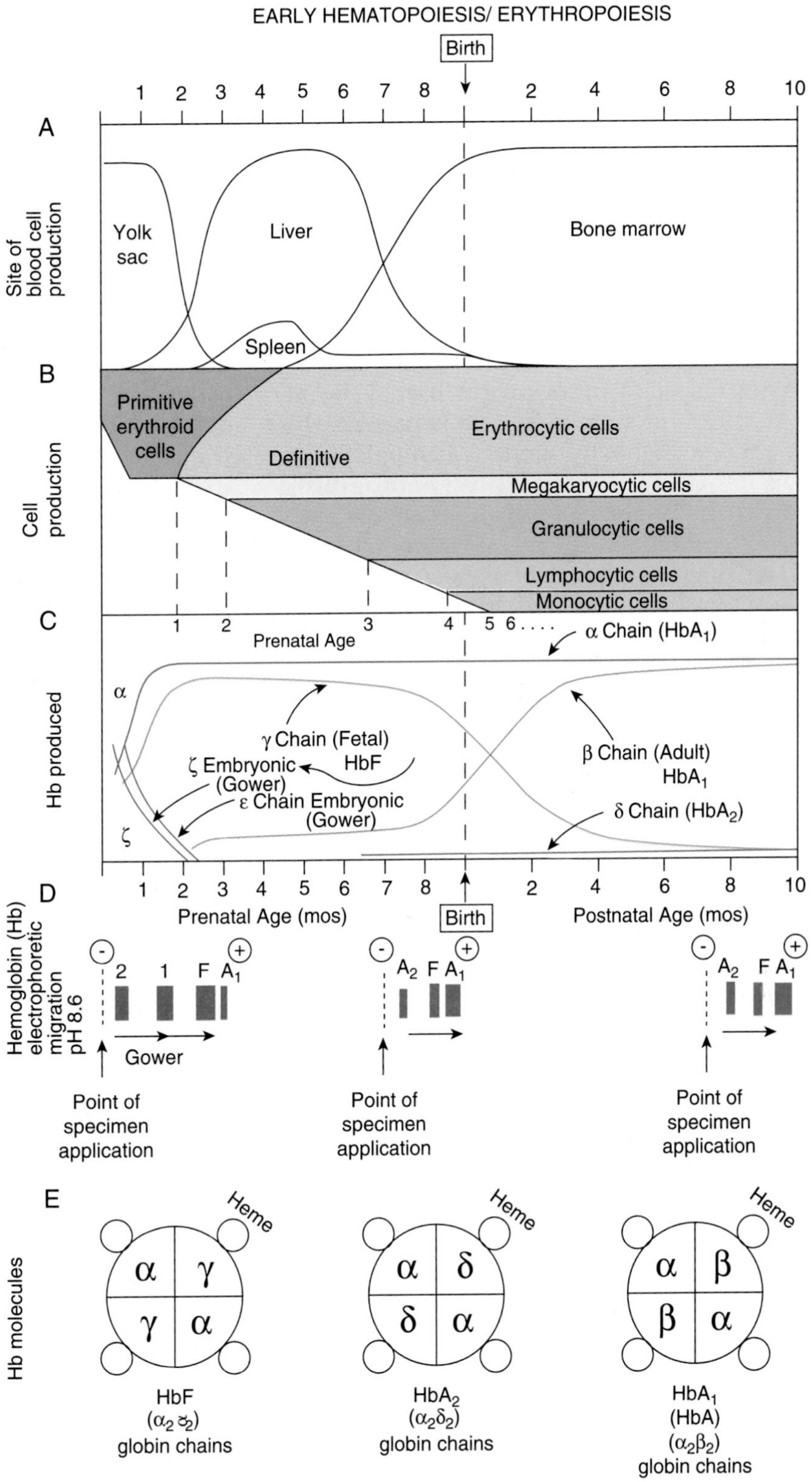

EARLY HEMATOPOIESIS/ ERYTHROPOIESIS

FIGURE 8–6
Fetal and adult hemoglobins (C, D, and E). Note the difference between HbA, A_2, and F is the class of globin chain present. HbF has two α and two γ chains, HbA_2 has two α and two δ chains, HbA_1, also called HbA, has two α and two β chains (E).

sugar in the body. For this reason, **HbA$_{1c}$ is a more reliable method of monitoring a diabetic diet** and therapy.

Hemoglobin is capable of binding with substances other than O$_2$ **oxyhemoglobin (HbO$_2$).** Once the O$_2$ has dissociated with the hemoglobin in the tissue, it is described as **deoxyhemoglobin (Hb)** and is found primarily in the venous circulation. Oxyhemoglobin and deoxyhemoglobin are normal functional states of hemoglobin and are associated with oxygen transport from the lungs to the body tissue.

Under certain circumstances, the oxygen-carrying capacity of hemoglobin may be altered. If carbon monoxide (CO) is present, this gas will preferentially bind to hemoglobin in place of O$_2$ to form **carboxyhemoglobin (HbCO).** Carbon monoxide has a 210× greater affinity for the hemoglobin molecule and manifests a bright cherry red color in the blood. The inability of the HbCO to carry O$_2$ results in body tissue anoxia and ultimately in death. Pure O$_2$ administration will enhance the O$_2$ binding to form HbO$_2$ instead of the formation of only HbCO. If sulfur is present during the oxidation of hemoglobin, it is incorporated into the heme ring of the hemoglobin, producing a green color. This form of hemoglobin is **sulfhemoglobin (SHb),** which is not capable of O$_2$ transport and is irreversible. Additional oxidation denatures the hemoglobin to form Heinz bodies. The structure of hemoglobin and the formation of Heinz bodies are discussed in detail in Chapters 9 and 10. A variety of drugs (e.g., sulfonamides or aromatic amines) as well as severe constipation, *Clostridium perfringens* infection, and a condition known as enterogenous **cyanosis (blue skin due to poor oxygenation of the blood)** result in formation of SHb. The sulfhemoglobin level seldom reaches more than 10% of total hemoglobin and, therefore, is usually not life threatening. The iron (Fe) molecule associated with hemoglobin and the actual binding of O$_2$ is functional in the reduced ferrous state (Fe^{2+}). When oxidized to the ferric state (Fe^{3+}), hemoglobin is unable to bind with O$_2$ and is, therefore, nonfunctional. This oxidized state of hemoglobin

is called **methemoglobin (Hi).** Increased levels of Hi result in cyanosis and anemia (decreased oxygen transport). Methemoglobin is formed in the blood at a low level throughout the process of normal oxygen transport. For this reason the Embden-Meyerhof pathway and the hexose monophosphate shunt glycolytic pathway in the red blood cell provide systems to reduce the Fe back to a functional state. The methemoglobin reductase pathway associated with the Embden-Meyerhof pathway is the primary Fe reduction mechanism. A second Fe reduction mechanism is the **hexose monophosphate shunt** pathway, which depends on **glucose-6-phosphate dehydrogenase (G-6-PD)** to reduce glutathione, which in turn **reduces the hemoglobin iron.** Genetic anemias associated with G-6-PD deficiency and test methodology are discussed in Chapters 9 and 10.

As mentioned earlier, the combination of certain compounds with hemoglobin will result in a detectable color. For this reason, hemoglobin is oxidized to methemoglobin and is bound to cyanide (HiCN) in vitro in order to produce a color that can be measured photometrically for assessing the concentration. This method of measuring hemoglobin levels is discussed in the erythrocyte testing section in Chapter 10.

Abnormal hemoglobins may result from **genetic alteration of the amino acid sequence** during synthesis of one of the globin chains, such as in sickle cell disease, or **the rate of synthesis of one chain is altered,** as demonstrated by a disease called thalassemia. Although a normal sequenced chain is produced, a decreased rate of synthesis results in disease. A decreased amount of hemoglobin is produced and any excess chains will form inclusions that will mark the cells for destruction by the macrophages. These abnormal hemoglobins are identified and confirmed by **hemoglobin electrophoresis** (see Figs. 8–5 and 8–6D). Hemoglobin electrophoresis is performed in the chemistry area of most laboratories. This procedure is similar to the protein electrophoresis methodology described in Chapter 6. Hemoglobin electrophoresis separates the hemoglobins by physical characteristics, which vary depending on the globin chain sequence. An example of two variations of hemoglobin electrophoresis is shown in Figure 8–6 and explained in Chapter 10. The **cellulose acetate** method at a **pH of 8.4** is the most commonly used; however, some hemoglobins migrate together (i.e., S and D) and, therefore, cannot be accurately identified. A second method available for the identification of hemoglobin is **citrate agar** hemoglobin electrophoresis, which is performed at an acid **pH of 6.0 to 6.2.** The change in pH and medium (agar instead of acetate sheet) results in a different movement (migration) pattern, which separates the hemoglobins differently. An analysis of both patterns will increase the chance of identifying the abnormal hemoglobin. Screening kits, currently available for the most common hemoglobin abnormalities, such as sickle cell disease, are explained in Chapter 10.

There are hundreds of abnormal hemoglobins, most of which do not result in a noticeable difference in hemoglobin function. Only if the genetic substitution of amino acids occurs in a crucial area of the globin chain will the function of hemoglobin be compromised. Hemoglobin abnormalities may **also be caused by problems in heme synthesis or iron supply and utilization.** Diseases associated with abnormal hemoglobins are discussed in Chapter 9.

Do It Now — Classification and Function of Hemoglobin

1. Build a model of hemoglobin. This can be done by cutting all of the parts out of colored construction paper or felt and then assembling and disassembling the parts to produce the various classifications and functional states of hemoglobin. The necessary components are: normal globin chains (make the alpha, beta, delta, gamma); abnormal globin chains (these would be folded differently); protoporphyrin rings (without Fe, but with a space for iron); iron molecules (in both Fe^{2+} and Fe^{3+} states); 2,3-DPG molecules; and oxygen, carbon monoxide, sulfur, and carbon dioxide molecules. (Be sure to determine the size relationship of the components before constructing the model.)
2. Construct the various states of hemoglobin, and explain the function, malfunction, method of correction to a functional form, etc. (This can be done in small groups, as an entire class, or as a homework assignment. If felt and a felt board are available, this model would be easier to construct.)
3. Explain how the structure made will affect electrophoresis migration and oxygen affinity.

FAST FACTS

Classification and Function of Hemoglobin

Hemoglobin	Globin Chain Classification	%, Function, or Association
Fetal hemoglobin F	$\alpha_2\gamma_2$	100% fetus:1% adult; $> O_2$ affinity
Adult hemoglobin A	$\alpha_2\beta_2$	97%, $A_{1a,b,c}$: A_{1c} to monitor diabetes
Adult hemoglobin A_2	$\alpha_2\delta_2$	2% $>$ associated with thalassemia

Hemoglobin	Gas or Molecule Bound	Comments and Notes
Oxyhemoglobin	O_2 (HbO$_2$)	Primarily in the arteries and lungs Red blood, normal
Deoxyhemoglobin	No O_2 (Hb)	Primarily in the veins and tissues Dark red blood, normal
Carboxyhemoglobin	Carbon monoxide (HbCO)	210× greater affinity Bright cherry red blood
Sulfhemoglobin	Sulfur (SHb)	Incorporated into the heme ring Green blood, Heinz bodies
Methemoglobin	Oxidized (Hi) ferric state (Fe^{3+})	Unable to bind with O_2; nonfunctional Embden-Meyerhof and hexose monophosphate shunt (G-6-PD) reduce the Fe

STUDY QUESTIONS

1. Given the following possible structures for hemoglobin, identify the correct structure (see Fig. 8–6E).

Match the Following:

2. Genetic disorders or pathway interference results in brown-colored urine and reduced Hb.

3. Genetic disorders result in the abnormal function of Hb, such as in sickle cell anemia.

4. Increased amounts of ferritin and hemosiderin

A. Globin synthesis

B. Protoporphyrin synthesis

C. Iron utilization

Choose the Best Answer from the Choices Provided to Complete the Sentence Below:

5. Engulfing of an erythrocyte by a _____,

6. with resultant production of _____ from the breakdown of heme,

7. which produces a _____ color in the plasma,

8. is called _____.
   A. Yellow   B. Bilirubin   C. Macrophage   D. Extravascular hemolysis

9. Iron transportation in the blood is accomplished by which of the following proteins?
   A. Haptoglobin

   B. Transferrin

   C. Bilirubin

   D. Ferritin

10. The hemoglobin present is determined genetically and results in a:
    A. Specific porphyrin ring formation

    B. Specific heme production

    C. Random binding of four globin chains

    D. Specific amino acid sequence of globin chains

CHAPTER 9

OUTLINE

Physiologic Decreases in Erythrocyte Count

Abnormal Decreases in Erythrocyte Count or Hemoglobin (Anemia)

Physiologic Increases in Erythrocyte Count

Abnormal Increases in Erythrocyte Count (Polycythemia and Erythroleukemia)

Study Questions

Normal Responses and Diseases of Erythrocytes

O B J E C T I V E S

Upon completion of this chapter the student should be able to:

1. Explain the mechanisms involved in an elevated or decreased erythrocyte count due to physiologic processes.

2. Differentiate between polycythemia and erythroleukemia.

3. Classify the anemias by both erythrocyte morphology and etiology.

4. Correlate the appropriate erythrocyte testing and results with erythrocyte response and disease.

It is very important that as this book is read the patient is never forgotten. Every aspect of hematology involves a **dynamic body process that is not isolated or absolute. The human body is a complex balance of production, metabolism, destruction, stimulation, inhibition, and constant dynamic change.** As with leukocytes, thrombocytes, coagulation factors, erythrocytes, or any body component, meeting the needs of the body requires a **sufficient quantity (amount)** of each component, and the **quality (function)** of the component must be adequate for normal function. Erythropoiesis (the production of red blood cells) is stimulated in response to decreased oxygen in the body tissues **(hypoxia)** by the hormone erythropoietin **(EPO),** which induces erythropoiesis and the release of erythrocytes from the bone marrow. Erythrocytes may transiently become increased or decreased in response to a normal physiologic body response. They may proliferate excessively due to a malignancy (e.g., cancer, abnormal growth), or they may lack the components necessary for their production or the genetic ability to function properly.

In order to maintain the best perspective, consider this information in terms of the entire body, not just the blood, and the entire laboratory, not just hematology.

PHYSIOLOGIC DECREASES IN ERYTHROCYTE COUNT

The erythrocyte morphology provides an insight into the mechanism or etiology of erythrocyte disorders. The morphology is associated with various cell components and processes and can be observed through a microscope or interpreted from the erythrocyte histogram, values, indices, and calculations generated from the automated instruments. The **erythrocyte morphology,** seen in various anemias, can be used for classification of disease. The various morphologies are **normocytic, normochromic, microcytic, hypochromic,** **or macrocytic.** Each morphology is associated with the possible **etiology (cause)** (Figs. 9–1 and 9–2 and Fast Fact Sheets). **Hemoglobin** renders the red blood cell color and, therefore, determines the described **chromicity (color).** This morphology correlates with the erythrocyte indices, the mean corpuscular hemoglobin (**MCH,** i.e., the average hemoglobin per cell), and the mean corpuscular hemoglobin concentration (**MCHC,** i.e., the concentration of hemoglobin per cell considering cell size). **Normochromic** erythrocytes are medium **red with a slightly lighter center (central pallor)** due to a thinner area of their biconcave shape (Fig. 9–3). Erythrocytes are **hypochromic (very little color, large central pallor)** if they are not carrying an adequate volume of hemoglobin (Fig. 9–4). If erythrocytes are **uniformly dark red with no central pallor;** become round and are not maintaining their biconcave shape; they are called **spherocytic (round in shape)** (Fig. 9–5). This relates to the examination of a manual blood smear, keeping in mind that the erythrocytes on the outer edges of the smear will not demonstrate a central pallor and that the erythrocytes in the thicker area of the smear may demonstrate an artificially pronounced central pallor due to the preparation. The examination of the **polychrome (Wright-Giemsa) stained peripheral blood smear** must take place **in the monolayer** area between the thick area of the smear and the feathered edge, where the cells are not distorted by artifacts of preparation (see Fig. 9–3). There is also the issue of **stain quality.** Look at many different fields of the smear before making a judgment on chromicity. Inaccurate staining may render the erythrocytes **all** dark red or **all** pale, which is **an artifact of the preparation** and is not relevant to the patient's condition. A peripheral blood smear manual evaluation of erythrocyte morphology is performed when the automated results suggest an abnormality.

If the entire erythrocyte evaluation is kept in perspective rather than making decisions based on one cell, one field, one slide, or one laboratory value, an accurate assessment can be made and reported

Erythrocyte Morphologies

Name	Morphology	Correlation	Name	Morphology	Correlation
Normocyte (discocyte)	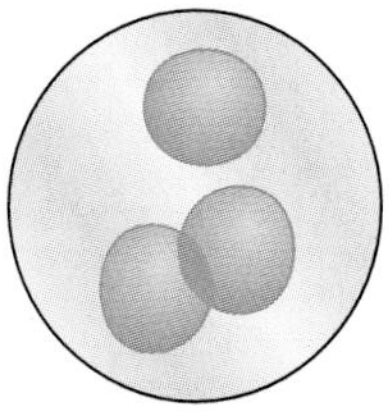	Healthy erythrocytes	Teardrop cells (dacryocytes)	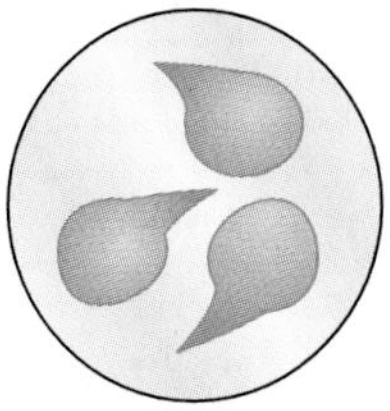	Extramedullary hematopoiesis, myelofibrosis (myeloid metaplasia)
Echinocytes, burr cells (crenated)	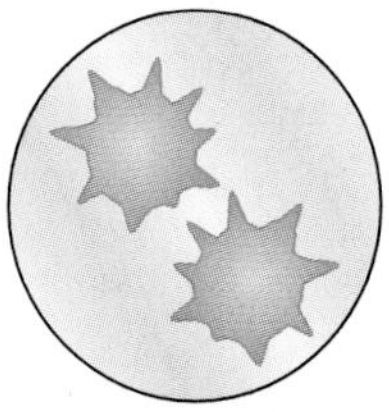	Uremia, artifacts (alkaline glass effects), hypotonic environment	Sickled cells (drepanocytes)	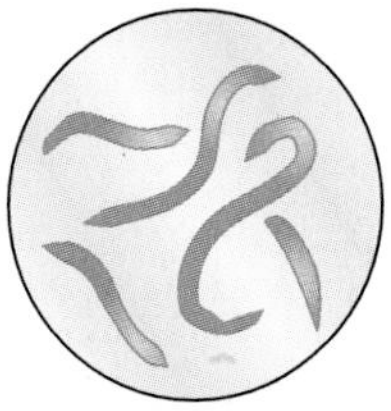	Hemoglobin S
Acanthocytes	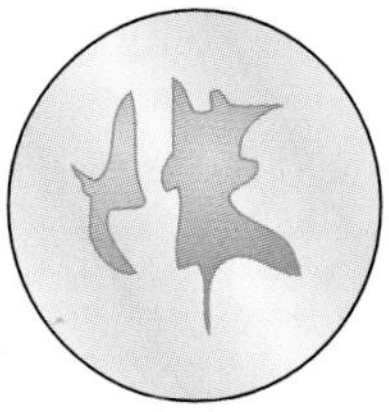	Abetalipoproteinemia, severe liver disease	Helmet cells	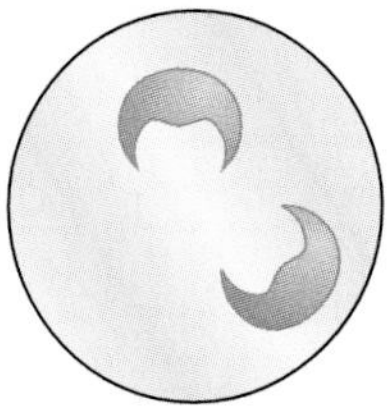	Hemolytic process
Target cells (leptocytes)	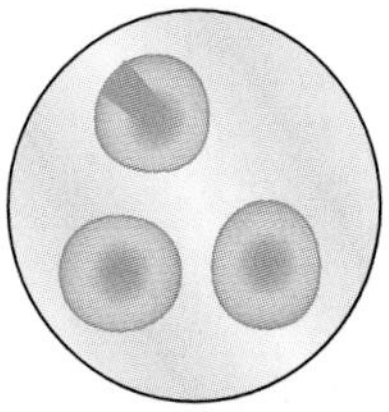	Liver disease, hemoglobinopathies	Schistocytes (rbc fragments)	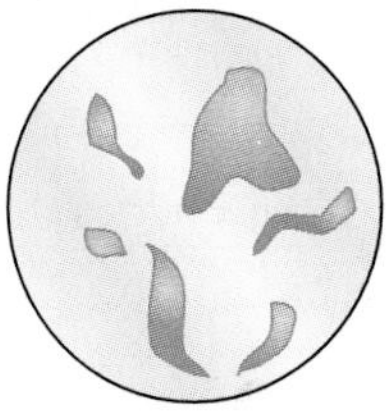	Disseminated intravascular coagulation (DIC), thrombotic thrombocytopenic purpura (TTP), hemolytic processes
Spherocytes	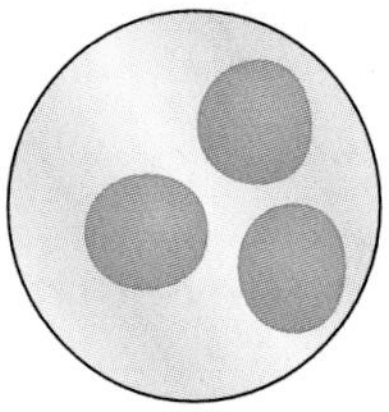	AIHA, HDN, and other extravascular hemolytic processes; hereditary spherocytosis	Stomatocytes (mouth cells)	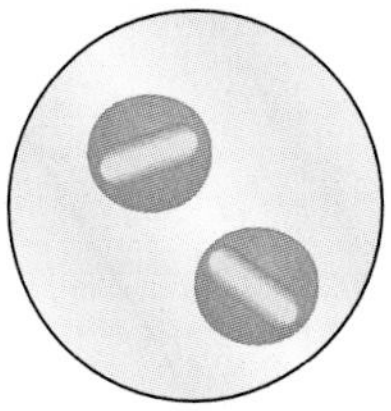	Liver disease, hereditary stomatocytosis
Elliptocytes	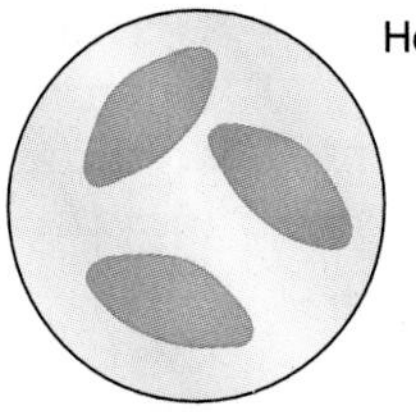	Hereditary elliptocytosis			

FIGURE 9–1
Various erythrocyte morphologies associated with disease.

Erythrocyte Shapes

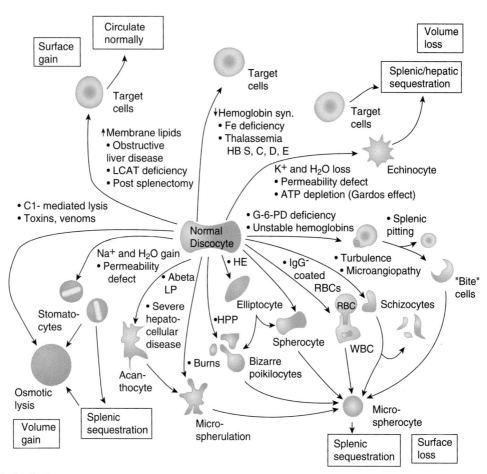

FIGURE 9–2

Erythrocyte shapes, membrane abnormalities, and associated disorders in terms of their effects on surface area and blood cell volume. (Adapted from Beck WS [ed]: Hematology. Cambridge, MA: MIT Press, 1977, pp 269–298.)

to the nurse, physician, or other health care practitioner to facilitate the rapid and efficient diagnosis and treatment of the patient.

Anemia is defined as a **decrease in** the **number of erythrocytes** in circulation or a **decrease in** the **hemoglobin** level or **function** of the erythrocytes. If the erythrocyte count is low or if the hemoglobin is not adequate to carry oxygen, **hypoxia** (decreased oxygen [O_2] in the body tissues) occurs. The decreased O_2 in the body tissues triggers the **production (synthesis) of the glycopro-**

tein hormone erythropoietin (EPO) by the kidney. EPO stimulates the bone marrow to **release** immature erythrocytes such as **reticulocytes,** capable of carrying a significant amount of O_2, and also **increases** the rate of erythroid cell production and maturation **(erythropoiesis).** Stress erythropoiesis is when the level of erythropoiesis is greater than normal and large blue reticulocytes are released. A normal reference range for erythrocytes is 4.0 to 5.0 million/mm³ (4.0 to 5.0×10^6/mm³ or 4.0 to 5.0×10^{12}/l). A normal reference range for hemoglobin is 12 to 16 g/dl; however, this range varies from a

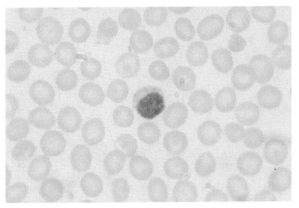

FIGURE 9–3
A normocytic, normochromic stained peripheral blood smear. Note the monolayer area of the slide where the cells are individually spaced. The cells have a uniform size (compared with the small lymphocyte), shape, and central pallor in the center of the erythrocytes.

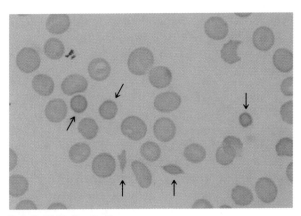

FIGURE 9–5
Spherocytes and schistocytes on a stained peripheral blood smear *(arrows)*.

newborn to an adult to the elderly and between female and male individuals. Refer to Chapter 8 for details about hemoglobin.

Relative Anemia. This category, also called pseudoanemia, represents situations in which the red blood cell count is normal; however, due to a **shift of fluid** within the body, the red blood cells are diluted and appear as an anemia. This appearance of anemia, which is secondary to an unrelated condition, is usually transient until the primary problem is no longer present. Conditions in which there would be an increase in the amount of plasma, thus decreasing the number of red blood cells per volume of whole blood, would include **pregnancy, cirrhosis of the liver** (degeneration), **nephritis** (renal disease), and **congestive heart failure.** All of these disorders require tests to be performed in the chemistry or clinical immunology area of the laboratory for diagnosis. Pregnancy involves the shifting of fluids between various locations in the body tissues, as does cirrhosis of the liver due to decreased protein production and nephritis, which results in a loss of protein through the damaged kidneys. In order to **maintain the osmotic gradient** (adequate level of water in the blood vessels), there must be a specific level of plasma protein. This normal **plasma protein level is a balance of liver protein production and renal retention of proteins.** The hemoglobin and hematocrit may appear to be transiently decreased due to less red blood cells per aliquot of whole blood. The **reticulocyte count** (indicating bone marrow erythrocyte production) would be **normal (<1.5%)** and the red blood cells would be **normocytic, normochromic** (normal size, shape, and color).

Another category of relative anemia is **intravenous (IV) fluid dilution anemia.** When an individual arrives in the hospital and intravenous fluids are used, there may be a temporary relative anemia until the body adjusts to the additional fluid. The laboratory hematocrit and hemoglobin values will be temporarily decreased, as seen in the physiologic fluid shift described earlier.

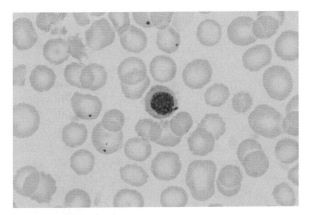

FIGURE 9–4
Hypochromic erythrocytes. Notice the larger central pallor and pale color.

ABNORMAL DECREASES IN ERYTHROCYTE COUNT OR HEMOGLOBIN (ANEMIA)

A **decreased number of erythrocytes** (red blood cells) can be due to a **lack of bone marrow production (aplasia), abnormal production (dyserythropoiesis), or increased rate of destruction (hemolysis) after their release from the bone marrow. A decrease in hemoglobin may be due to a lack of production, or the quantity of hemoglobin produced may be sufficient; however, the quality (function) of the hemoglobin produced is not adequate. Hemoglobin** renders the red cell color and, therefore, determines the **chromicity (color).** This morphology correlates with the erythrocyte indices, mean corpuscular hemoglobin (**MCH,** i.e., average hemoglobin per cell), and the mean corpuscular hemoglobin concentration (**MCHC,** i.e., concentration of hemoglobin per cell considering cell size). **Normochromic** erythrocytes are medium **red with a slightly lighter center (central pallor)** due to the thinner area of their biconcave shape (see Fig. 9–3). Erythrocytes are **hypochromic (very little color and large central pallor)** if they are not carrying an adequate volume of hemoglobin (see Fig. 9–4). If erythrocytes are **uniformly dark red;** have no central pallor; have become round; are not maintaining their biconcave shape; they are called **spherocytic (round in shape)** (see Fig. 9–5). This is only relevant if a manual blood smear is examined, keeping in mind that the erythrocytes on the outer edges of the smear will not demonstrate a central pallor and the erythrocytes in the thicker area of the smear may demonstrate an artificially pronounced central pallor due to their preparation. The examination of the **polychrome (Wright-Giemsa) stained peripheral blood smear** must take place **in the monolayer** area between the thick area of the smear and the feathered edge, where the cells are not distorted by artifacts of preparation (see Fig. 9–3). There is also the issue of **stain quality.** Look at many different fields of the smear before making a judgment on chromicity. The stain may render the erythrocytes **all** dark red or **all** pale. If the entire evaluation of the erythrocytes is kept in perspective (rather than making decisions on one cell, one field, one slide, or one laboratory value), an accurate assessment can be made and reported to the nurse or physician to facilitate a rapid, efficient diagnosis and treatment of the patient.

Absolute Anemia. The diagnosis and treatment of anemia relate to the **etiology (cause)** and whether the anemia is **inherited or acquired.** Due to the variety of anemias there is no specific age association, although certain age groups are more susceptible to anemia secondary to a primary etiology. In the clinical laboratory, observation of changes in erythrocyte morphology aids in the diagnosis and monitoring of treatment. Keep in mind that knowledge of the cause of the morphology will result in the meaningful performance of additional tests to support the reason for the morphology. The subsequent tests can determine the etiology in order for the physician to make an accurate diagnosis and prescribe the appropriate treatment (Fig. 9–6). The morphology and associated etiologies are listed in Fast Fact sheets (see also Figs. 9–1 and 9–2).

Acute posthemorrhagic anemia is the term for **loss of blood** from the blood stream over a **short period of time.** This blood may be lost into the tissue spaces, the gastrointestinal tract, a body cavity, or the blood may be lost outside the body. The immediate symptom is **decreased blood volume (hypovolemia),** which is manifested by a rapid pounding pulse, low blood pressure, faintness, and pallor (pale skin). If a hematocrit or hemoglobin is drawn immediately, before an IV line has been started, the results will be normal. Although the blood has been lost, it is lost in equal proportions, thus the hematocrit and hemoglobin values will be normal. One indicator in this situation, however, would be a **low thrombocyte (platelet) count due to the activation** of the platelets to close the site of blood loss and also the fact that they are being consumed in their clotting function. The reference thrombocyte count is 150 to $400 \times 10^{12}/mm^3$ or 150 to $400 \times 10^9/l$. Once an IV has been started and the IV fluid

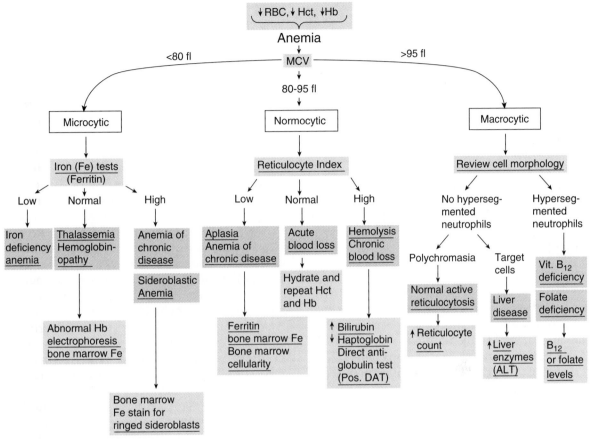

FIGURE 9–6
Test flow chart to determine the etiology of anemia in an organized, efficient manner.

fills the space in the circulation, anemia is easily detected by the decrease in hematocrit and hemoglobin. This would happen physiologically, even without an IV, over a period of hours due to fluid shifts within the body; therefore, if the patient is seen several hours after the bleeding has occurred, anemia will be evident in the laboratory results. Within 1 hour of blood loss the **platelet count, which dropped initially, will become elevated** as the platelets are released and mobilized to the site of injury. This will be followed a few hours later by a **neutrophilic leukocytosis with a slight shift to the left** (the appearance of band cells) to defend the body against bacterial invasion at the site of injury. The **reticulocyte count would be normal** due to the **acute nature** of this event. The bone marrow would not have

enough time to release and generate additional reticulocytes. The erythrocyte morphology would be **normocytic, normochromic** demonstrating normal production, just not enough present.

Chronic posthemorrhagic anemia is a **slow loss of blood** over an extended period of time. Only if the decreased erythrocyte count results in tissue hypoxia ($<O_2$) will increased amounts of erythropoietin (EPO) be synthesized by the kidney to increase red blood cell synthesis and release. This increased synthesis and release of erythrocytes is **stress erythropoiesis,** which is usually reflected by increased reticulocytes that are large and polychromatic (blue) (Figs. 9–7 and 10–3). Anemia may not be detectable in the erythrocyte count initially, and the **reticulocyte count may be normal or slightly increased.**

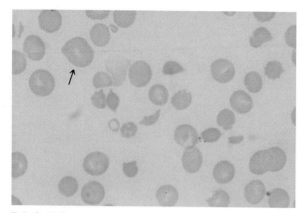

FIGURE 9-7
Polychromasia (large blue cell, arrow), anisocytosis (variation in size from small to large), and poikilocytosis (variation in shape, sickle cells, and target cells) on a stained peripheral blood smear.

The erythrocyte morphology is generally **normocytic, normochromic;** however, if there is an increase in reticulocytes, the morphology may appear **macrocytic** due to the larger size of the **reticulocytes.** This is considered to be a **normal temporary responsive macrocytosis** in response to the need for more red blood cells. When the anemia has depleted all of the body's iron stores, hematocrit and hemoglobin results will become abnormal, and at this point an iron deficiency anemia may be detected. If the **chronic hemorrhage** results in **iron-deficient erythrocytes,** the erythrocyte morphology will become **microcytic, hypochromic.**

Anemias, other than hemorrhagic anemias, are due to one of three mechanisms: **(1) decreased production; (2) abnormal production; or (3) increased destruction.** The first two mechanisms involve the bone marrow, and the third involves an etiology outside of the bone marrow.

Anemia of decreased production can be genetic or acquired. Two rare genetic **hypoplastic** (decreased formation) or **aplastic** (without formation) anemias are known. **Diamond-Blackfan syndrome** affects only production of erythrocytes, and **Fanconi's** anemia results in the decreased production of all bone marrow cells. Acquired aplastic anemias also occur. Some **antibiotics, chemicals, certain viruses, and radiation** are known to be **toxic to the bone marrow.** Examples

are the antibiotic chloramphenicol; the drug benzene; excessive consumption of alcohol; and viral infections with human parvovirus (B19) secondary to hepatitis. Chemotherapeutic drugs given to treat malignancies such as leukemia are chosen for their aplastic effect on the leukemic cells. If an individual is exposed to, or given, a known bone marrow toxicant, the blood cell count should be checked regularly. If the blood cell count begins to decrease significantly, the individual should no longer be in contact with this chemical or drug.

The **hemoglobin and hematocrit will be decreased;** the erythrocytes will be **normocytic and normochromic;** and the **reticulocyte count will be normal to decreased. The reticulocyte is the best indicator of bone marrow function.** In aplastic anemia, the cells produced are normal, but not enough cells are produced.

When anemia is present, tissue hypoxia occurs and results in increased synthesis of the hormone **erythropoietin (EPO),** which in turn stimulates **increased synthesis** and **release of bone marrow erythrocytes.** In the aplastic anemias there is no response to the EPO present. An inappropriate EPO response appears to play a role in the development of some anemias. **Cytokines** (regulatory proteins such as interleukin 1[IL-1], tumor necrosis factor [TNF], and gamma interferon [INF]) may also be involved by **inhibiting erythropoiesis.** EPO levels can be measured by immunoassay techniques in a special area of the chemistry section of the laboratory. EPO, as well as various cytokines, are not often measured routinely in the laboratory because of time, expense, and limited requests. If EPO or cytokine levels are necessary, they can be sent to a reference laboratory where the tests can be performed efficiently and economically.

Anemia of abnormal production ranges from **genetically defective production of** the hemoglobin molecule, **lack of or inhibition of vitamins, minerals, or enzymes** necessary for adequate production of hemoglobin and cell function, to **abnormal membrane production.**

Hemoglobinopathies are **genetic** and involve an **abnormal production of globin**

chains (e.g., sickle cell anemia), a **decreased quantity of globin** chains produced (e.g., thalassemia), or a **deficiency that interferes with heme synthesis** (e.g., porphyria). There are hundreds of variant hemoglobins: Some do not change the function of the hemoglobin and, therefore, are only discovered secondary to another problem. Others, such as the ones discussed here, result in a change in hemoglobin function that is readily apparent and may be life threatening. The hemoglobin molecule and its synthesis are presented in Chapter 8. A characteristic cell seen in association with any **hemoglobinopathy** is the presence of **target cells** (Fig. 9–8). Target cells are also associated with **liver disease.**

Sickle cell trait and sickle cell disease result from genetic substitution of glutamic acid for valine at the sixth position on the beta hemoglobin chain produced in these individuals. If one of the two hemoglobin genes is the S gene, this is sickle cell trait. The other hemoglobin gene or corresponding allele is the normal adult A gene. Sickle cell trait is noted as HbAS, indicating a heterozygous inheritance, one A gene and one S gene. **Sickle cell disease** results from the homozygous inheritance of both S genes and is noted as HbSS. This single amino acid **substitution** results in a change in the charge on the surface of the Hb molecule, which **decreases the solubility or function** of the molecule and changes the electrophoretic charge resulting in

a **different migration pattern on electrophoresis.** The insolubility of the molecule when it is in the deoxyhemoglobin form (without O_2) results in crystallization of the hemoglobin, giving the red blood cell a **sickled shape.** The **rigid cells** also become trapped in small blood vessels, forming plugs that **block blood flow (infarcts)** and result in tissue death (necrosis) due to **lack of oxygen (anoxia).** Any organ can be affected; however, joint swelling with pain, asplenia (death of the spleen due to lack of blood flow), and kidney failure are the most commonly seen manifestations of sickle cell disease.

Sickle cell disease is found **most often** in the **African population;** however, studies using molecular biology techniques have found the **sickle cell gene in all populations.** Today, almost 10% of the patients in urban centers with sickling disorders are non-black. Sickle cell disease is first **seen in early childhood** and is usually fatal by 30 years of age. Although gene therapy is in developmental stages, there is currently no cure for sickle cell disease, and treatment remains supportive, such as **blood transfusions** administered to provide normal oxygen transport to the tissues. In the disease, **sickling** of the erythrocytes occurs in the tissue blood circulation resulting in **hemolysis** of the cells by trauma (rigidity resulting in tearing of the cell) or removal and lysis by macrophages (extravascular hemolysis) due to the abnormal shape. The destruction of the abnormal erythrocytes will decrease the erythrocyte count significantly. The erythrocyte indices (MCV and MCHC) described a **normochromic and normocytic** erythrocyte morphology that could be observed on a Wright-Giemsa–stained peripheral blood smear of an individual with sickle cell disease. However, this blood smear often demonstrates a **polychromatic, poikilocytic (sickle cells/drepanocytes and target cells)** picture (see Figs. 9–7 and 9–8). Polychromasia (blue erythrocytes that are stress reticulocytes) may be present due to the bone marrow response to the anemia, releasing more reticulocytes capable of carrying oxygen to the tissues. Erythrocytes containing **Howell-Jolly bodies of aberrant DNA** (Fig. 9–9) may be seen if the **spleen has been ren-**

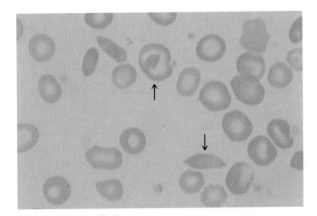

FIGURE 9–8
Target cells seen in association with hemoglobinopathies and liver disease. Note the arrow pointing to the sickled cell.

RBC Inclusion	Morphology	Stain	Correlations
Hemoglobin C crystals	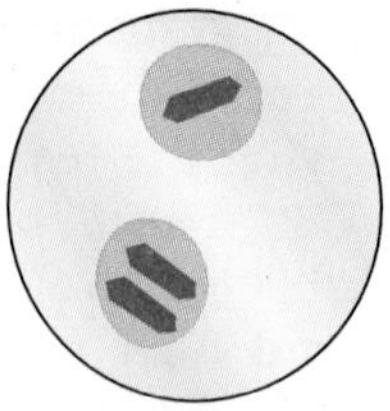	Wright-Giemsa	HbC Post splenectomy
Howell-Jolly body DNA	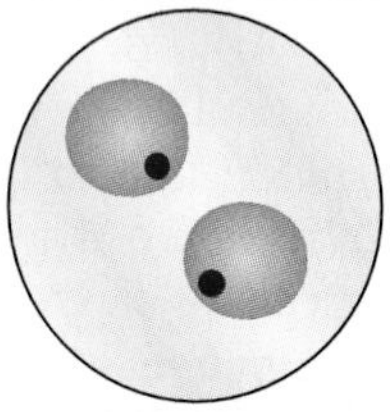	Wright-Giemsa	Abnormal erythropoiesis Vitamin B$_{12}$ deficiency
Basophilic stippling RNA	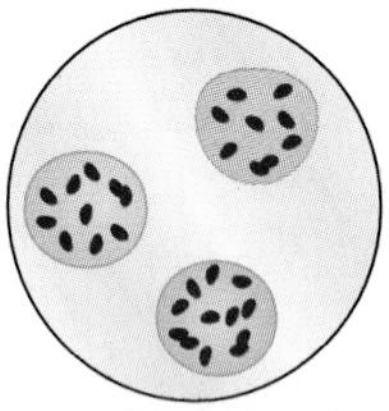	Wright-Giemsa New methylene blue	Lead poisoning Thalassemia
Pappenheimer bodies Pale blue patches Siderotic granules Iron	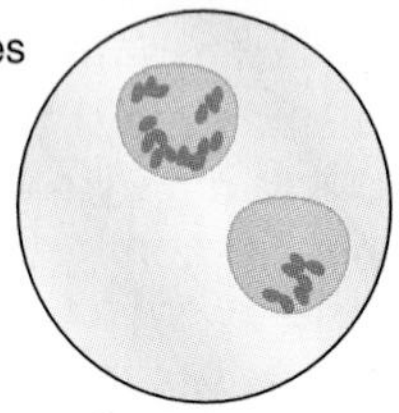	Wright-Giemsa Prussian blue	Sideroblastic anemia Hemoglobinopathies
Heinz bodies Denatured hemoglobins	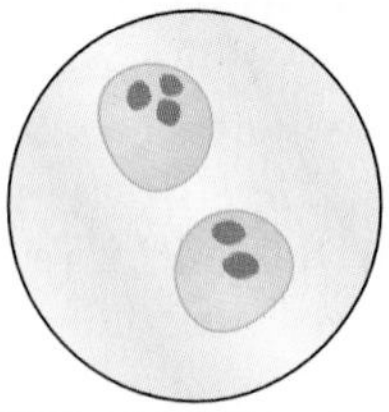	Supravital stain such as cresyl blue (NOT seen with Wright's stain)	Unstable hemoglobins G-6-PD deficiency Thalassemia
Cabot rings Nuclear remnants	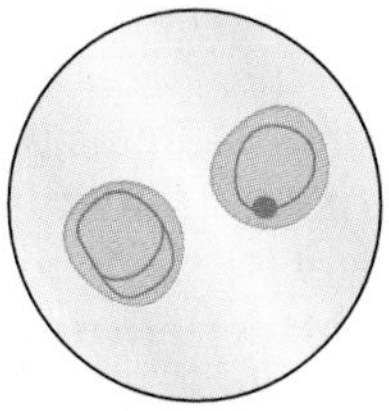	Wright-Giemsa	Megaloblastic anemia
Parasites Malaria	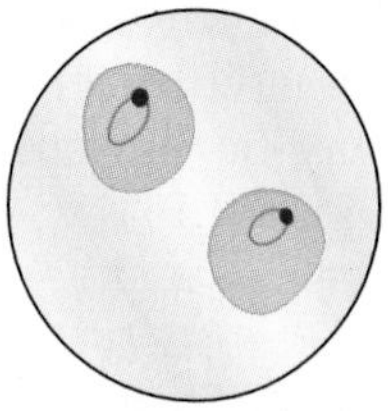	Wright-Giemsa	Parasitic infection Malaria Babesia Trypanosomes

FIGURE 9–9
Various erythrocyte inclusions.

dered **nonfunctional** because of splenic infarcts. The macrophages within the spleen normally remove any cells with inclusions, abnormal shapes, or abnormal surface proteins.

Sickle cell trait presents a **normochromic, normocytic** peripheral blood smear picture with Wright-Giemsa stain. Only in extreme situations of oxygen reduction, such as the screening test environment in vitro, travel to high altitudes, or stress resulting in less oxygen intake into the body, will sickling of the erythrocytes occur. The sickle cell trait is believed to have evolved as a protection against endemic malaria in Africa and Eastern countries. These parasites are unable to infect erythrocytes that contain HbS.

Several **screening tests** are available to test quickly and inexpensively **for insoluble hemoglobins.** The most common insoluble hemoglobins are **S, D, and C.** The screening test uses **dithionite reduction** to reveal hemoglobin insolubility. These tests are explained in detail in Chapter 10. If the result of the screening test is positive, a **hemoglobin electrophoresis is done to confirm** the specific hemoglobin present. The hemoglobin electrophoresis is described in Chapters 8 and 10.

Less common hemoglobinopathies, which also involve a change in the sequence of amino acids in the globin chain, include **HbC disease** and **HbD disease.** Most hemoglobinopathies demonstrate target erythrocytes that relate to abnormal distribution of hemoglobin within the cell. **HbC** also demonstrates **dark red crystals** within some of the red blood cells (see Fig. 9–9). Sickle cell disease and HbC disease are the only two diseases associated with a specific erythrocyte morphology other than target cells.

Occasionally, an individual will be genetically programmed to continue the production of high levels of hemoglobin F, which results in less production of hemoglobin A. This **adult persistence of hemoglobin F** creates an anemia due to the difference in oxygen affinity (ability to bond to or release O_2) of the fetal hemoglobin. In the fetal environment of the mother's body, there is no exposure to the high levels of oxygen that exist in the mother's lungs. The mother's adult hemo-

globin A picks up O_2 in the lungs and, due to a lower oxygen affinity, readily releases this O_2 in the lower oxygen environment of the body tissues, such as in the uterus at which point the soluble O_2 diffuses through to the placenta for fetal use. The fetal blood, however, must have the ability to pick up the O_2 near the placenta and carry it to the even lower oxygen environment of the fetal tissue for release. The primary hemoglobin in the fetal erythrocytes is **HbF,** which has a **higher O_2 affinity,** thus it will readily pick up the low levels of placental or uterine O_2 and distribute it throughout the even lower oxygenated fetal tissues. As an adult, the **HbA,** with a **lower O_2 affinity,** combines with the O_2 in the very high oxygen level of the lungs and readily releases this oxygen to the body tissues. As a matter of fact, the level of oxygen in the tissue environment of the adult would be equivalent to the O_2 level in the placental or uterine environment in which the HbF would pick up oxygen and not release oxygen. For this reason hemoglobin F does not provide enough oxygen to adult tissue, and **anoxia** results in a functional anemia. The adult persistence of HbF can be confirmed only by **hemoglobin electrophoresis,** which is described in Chapter 10.

During **pregnancy** the maternal blood and fetal blood should never come into contact with one another. All substances move through membranes to and from the mother. If a pregnant woman experiences bleeding of the fetal blood into her blood stream, there is the potential for an **immune response.** If the fetal cells carry strong antigens inherited from the father that differ from the mother's antigens, they will be recognized as foreign invaders and antibodies will be produced against these fetal cells. The most common scenario is a **mother** without the Rh antigen on her erythrocytes **(Rh negative)** and a **baby** with the Rh antigen on his or her erythrocytes **(Rh positive)** inherited from the father. The Rh antibody produced by the mother will pass through the placenta into the fetal circulation and destroy the baby's cells, resulting in **hemolytic disease of the newborn (HDN),** which may be severe enough to cause a still birth. In order to try to avoid such a fatal outcome, the blood bank area of the laboratory needs to measure how many of the fetal cells entered the mother in order to provide the correct amount of **Rh immune globulin (RhIg)** to prevent an immune response. The diagnosis and treatment of HDN is dependent on tests performed in the blood bank area of the laboratory. Hemoglobin electrophoresis is not adequate for fetal hemoglobin quantitation owing to the small quantity of **fetal erythrocytes in the mother's blood** and, therefore, a small quantity of **HbF.** Tests used to quantitate a fetal bleed into the mother are the **cell agglutination test, resistance to acid elution (Kleihauer-Betke method),** and **alkali denaturation resistance test.** These tests utilize the fact that HbF is resistant to acid elution and alkali denaturization, and the mother's HbA is not and will be destroyed. A mother with persistence of HbF would need to have a baseline test done early in pregnancy, and she may not be able to be evaluated accurately by these techniques. These procedures are explained in more detail in Chapter 10.

Thalassemia disease or trait is seen primarily in the **Mediterranean population.** Individuals of Italian descent often have the trait, which was first described by Cooley and Lee and resulted in the original name of Cooley's anemia. The globin chains are normal in terms of the amino acid sequence, thus function is not the issue. The problem is the **decreased production of one of the chains,** resulting in less hemoglobin produced and lysis of some of the red blood cells due to the inclusion of excess unaffected chains. There are several classifications of thalassemia based on the chain affected and whether this affects all hemoglobin produced (homozygous) or only half of the hemoglobin produced (heterozygous). The name describes the character of the disorder. *α*-**Thalassemia major** is the most severe type. All hemoglobin produced is missing a significant number of α-globin chains and, therefore, cannot form an adequate number of hemoglobin molecules. The excess unused beta chains form inclusions and mark or opsonize the cell for phagocytosis by the macrophages. α-Thalassemia minor is less

severe with an adequate, but decreased, amount of hemoglobin production. β-Thalassemia is less common and involves a decreased production of the β-globin chain instead of the α chain. The stained smear will demonstrate **target cells, polychromasia,** and, in severe cases, a **microcytic, hypochromic** blood picture (Fig. 9–10). Since microcytic, hypochromic erythrocytes are most commonly associated with iron deficiency anemia, **testing for iron is recommended for the differential diagnosis of** thalassemia. In thalassemia, the iron level would be normal to increased because of the decreased production of hemoglobin using iron and increased lysis of red blood cells releasing iron. There is no screening test in addition to the peripheral blood smear or automated blood count observations. The **confirming test is the hemoglobin electrophoresis** in which the hemoglobin A_2 **level is increased (>2%)** to compensate for the decreased hemoglobin.

There are incidences in which a **combination of hemoglobinopathies** are present. For example, a 22-year-old Asian woman presented to a clinic with headaches. Through hemoglobin electrophoresis and family genetic studies it was found that she had inherited an HbE gene from one parent and a β-thalassemia gene from the other parent, both of which affect the β-globin chain. The resultant **thalassemia was characterized by severe microcytic, hypochromic anemia with**

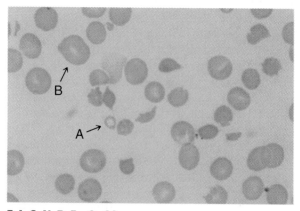

FIGURE 9–10
Thalassemia showing a microcytic, hypochromic blood picture (A) with polychromasia (B).

poikilocytosis of targets, schistocytes (fragmented cells), spherocytes, nucleated red blood cells, and a resulting splenomegaly (enlarged spleen) due to excessive phagocytosis of the abnormal cells. Another severe dual hemoglobinopathy is the inheritance of an HbS gene and an HbC gene. This combination of hemoglobin genes is found as often in the American black population as the HbSS (sickle cell disease) combination. The resultant HbSC disease is less severe than sickle cell disease but is more severe than is sickle cell trait. There have been many **hemoglobinopathy combinations** published, some of which are found coincidentally and **show very little effect on the erythrocyte morphology, erythrocyte function, or health of the patient.**

Gene therapy is in an experimental stage; there is currently no treatment for any of the hemoglobinopathies other than **supportive transfusion** to increase the normal hemoglobin present to carry O_2 to the body. In the future perhaps we will be able to replace the abnormal gene in the fetus or neonate's (newborn) own cells with a normal hemoglobin gene. Currently **transplantation of stem cells to the bone marrow,** from discarded cord blood of patients with severe thalassemia is the **only curative procedure.** This has been done primarily in Asian countries, such as in Thailand.

A rare **genetic deficiency of enzymes** necessary for the production of heme from porphyrin results in a disease called **porphyria.** Photosensitivity, abdominal pain, and neuropathies result from increased porphyrins. Laboratory investigation of porphyria includes screening for an **increased level of porphyrins** or their precursors, such as α-**aminolevulinic acid (α-ALA)** in urine, feces, and blood. **Free erythrocyte protoporphyrin (FEP)** is also used to measure the excess protoporphyrin in the cell that is not synthesized properly and is, therefore, not part of the hemoglobin molecule. The ALA and FEP are measured in the chemistry area of the clinical laboratory. Excretion of protoporphyrin products in urine will make the **urine dark.** Hematology will detect the **anemia** due to a low hemoglobin level; however,

chemistry and urinalysis indicators of porphyrin levels will be the key results for diagnosis.

Glucose-6-phosphate dehydrogenase (G-6-PD) deficiency is associated with the X chromosome and is found in 10% of the black male population. G-6-PD is necessary for the reduction of glutathione (GSH), which in turn reduces the hemoglobin iron from the +3 (ferric) to the +2 (ferrous) state. This process is part of the hexose monophosphate shunt (HMPS) glycolytic pathway in the erythrocyte. The anemia is **normochromic and normocytic.** If the patient's blood specimen is treated with a vital stain such as **cresyl green** (as described in Chapter 10), **Heinz bodies,** which consist of **denatured Hb,** can be seen in the cells. G-6-PD anemia can be a result of drugs such as primaquines and other oxidizing chemicals. The **G-6-PD level** can be measured by special chemistry tests.

Decreased red blood cell production may be due to an **acquired,** not genetic, deficiency of a necessary factor for normal erythrocyte production. The most common of these anemias is **iron (Fe) deficiency anemia.** Iron is stored in the body as ferritin or hemosiderin within cells of the body such as macrophages of the bone marrow (histiocytes), which are part of the monocyte/macrophage system formerly called the reticuloendothelial system (RES). Various forms of iron, or iron-associated proteins, can be measured in the plasma to determine the iron status in the body. The **serum iron** can be measured; however, this is less reliable than alternative tests due to the transient nature of this form of iron in the blood. Iron is transported in the blood by a protein called **transferrin.** Transferrin keeps the iron from passing out of the body through the kidney and also makes it attractive to the macrophage cells that will phagocytize the iron for storage. The amount of transferrin that is not bound to iron can be measured with the **total iron-binding capacity (TIBC)** test. The results are inversely proportional to the amount of iron available. The **percent saturation** of iron to transferrin can be calculated. The best indicator of iron stores is the serum **ferritin** test. Ferritin is a storage form of iron that is soluble and is found in the plasma and macrophage cells. **Ferritin levels are directly proportional to the iron stores in the body** and reflect the steady state of iron, which is not affected by diet, activity, or transient body physiology. The iron tests are performed in the chemistry area of the clinical laboratory and are discussed further in Chapter 10.

A **bone marrow smear** can be stained with a **vital iron stain (Prussian blue)** and examined for iron inclusions, in the form of **ferritin or hemosiderin, in the cytoplasm of the histiocytes.** The bone marrow procedure is not done routinely to measure iron but rather as a special test if other test results do not provide clear information. The chemistry tests for iron, ferritin, serum iron, and TIBC are much more accurate and reproducible than are bone marrow smears. Diagnostic of **iron deficiency anemia is a hypochromic and microcytic erythrocyte picture, and all iron test results are decreased except the TIBC,** which would be **elevated** to indicate no iron bound to the transport protein transferrin (Fig. 9–11). Iron deficiency anemia is most common in young women who are not eating properly or who are losing excess blood during the menstrual cycle, in old women as a result of poor diet, and in pregnant women owing to increased demand by the fetus.

Sideroblastic anemia is less common and encompasses a heterogenous group of disorders characterized by **hypochromic, and of-** **ten microcytic, erythrocytes mixed with normochromic cells resulting in a dimorphic peripheral blood smear picture.** The diagnostic cell is an immature nucleated erythrocyte with iron granules surrounding the nucleus **(ringed sideroblast),** which is found in the bone marrow. The extreme excess of iron may result in **iron (siderotic) granules** in the erythrocytes, iron deposition in the body tissues **(hemochromatosis),** including the skin, which gives the individual a bronze skin cast. Siderotic granules on a **Wright-Giemsa** peripheral blood-stained smear would look like blue patches called **Pappenheimer bodies,** and these cells are referred to as siderocytes (see Fig. 9–9). A blood smear stained with **Prussian blue iron stain** would reveal several **irregular-shaped granules** together within the erythrocyte. All iron within the normal erythrocyte should be incorporated into the hemoglobin and, therefore, would not be visible upon staining.

Treatment of sideroblastic anemia involves the use of various **chemicals to bind the iron (chelation therapy)** for removal, and the administration of **supportive transfusions** if the hemoglobin drops below 8 g/dl. Keep in mind that patients receiving multiple transfusions for severe anemia may develop transfusional hemosiderosis and require administration of drugs that will chelate (bind to) the iron for removal. In some patients, a **unit of blood may need to be removed** to relieve iron overload. There is a limited association of sideroblastic anemia developing into leukemia. The various sideroblastic anemias have been classified by the French-American-British classification as part of the **myelodysplastic syndrome** (Table 9–1).

Anemia of chronic disease (ACD) is becoming more commonly recognized as our population ages and more and more patients present with chronic diseases. The anemia results from a combination of **shortened red blood cell survival** and an **insufficient bone marrow response** to anemia **(decreased reticulocyte count).** Iron-associated testing reveals a **decreased serum iron, decreased total iron-binding capacity (TIBC) of transferrin, and decreased**

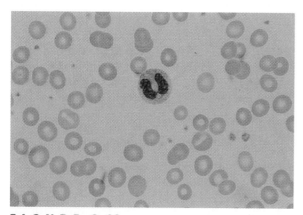

FIGURE 9–11
Iron deficiency anemia demonstrating a microcytic, hypochromic blood picture.

TABLE 9–1   FRENCH-AMERICAN-BRITISH (FAB) CLASSIFICATION OF MYELODYSPLASTIC SYNDROME

| Classification | Bone Marrow (%) | | Ringed Siseroblasts | Peripheral Blood (%) | |
	Blasts			Blasts	Monocytes
Refractory anemia (RA)	<5		<15	<1	None
Refractory anemia with ringed sideroblasts (RARS)	<5		>15	<1	None
Refractory anemia with excessive blasts (RAEB)	5–20		None	<5	None
Refractory anemia with excessive blasts in trans-formation (RAEB-t)	>20–30 Auer rods		None	<5	None
Chronic myelomonocytic leukemia (CMML)	>20		None	<5	$>1 \times 10^9/l$

percent saturation. **Increased free erythrocyte protoporphyrin (FEP) and serum ferritin reflect increased iron stores in the macrophages (reticuloendothelial cells). The erythrocytes appear normochromic and normocytic** or occasionally hypochromic and microcytic. The anemia will improve if the primary problem (chronic disease) is treated successfully.

Vitamin B$_{12}$ (cobalamin) deficiency was called pernicious anemia before the etiology (cause) was determined. This anemia usually results from the **inability of the gastric mucosa to secrete intrinsic factor (IF) or production of an autoantibody that inactivates the IF.** Intrinsic factor is necessary for absorption of **vitamin B$_{12}$, which is required for normal synthesis of DNA.** A normal diet provides adequate intake of B$_{12}$, and body stores will last for several years if the intake is cut off, thus nutritional deficiencies are extremely rare. Other rare causes of vitamin B$_{12}$ deficiency are malabsorption syndromes, such as celiac disease, and tapeworms or bacteria in the host that compete for the vitamin. Symptoms **include jaundice (yellow skin), sore tongue, and gastrointestinal and central nervous system abnormalities.** The erythrocyte peripheral blood smear morphology appears as **macrocytic erythrocytes** and **hypersegmented neutrophilic granulocytes** (Fig. 9–12). The

bone marrow **nucleated erythrocytes (red blood cells)** show **asynchronous maturation,** with the nucleus less mature than the cytoplasm. These cells are described as having a **megaloblastic nucleus.** The genetic predisposition for this disease is inherited but does not usually manifest until an individual is older than 40 years of age. This disease can be found in very strict vegetarians (e.g., Hindus) but is seen most often in association with gastrointestinal plasma transport or cellular metabolic disorders.

Another vitamin, **folic acid,** is also required **for normal DNA synthesis,** which, if deficient, will produce an **anemia very**

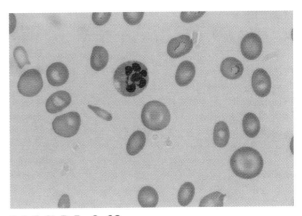

FIGURE 9–12
Vitamin B$_{12}$ deficiency (pernicious anemia) with macrocytes and a hypersegmented neutrophil.

similar to that of the vitamin B$_{12}$ deficiency. Folic acid deficiency anemia is usually **secondary to a poor diet** and an **increased demand (pregnancy).** Folic acid is not stored on a long-term basis in the body like vitamin B$_{12}$ and must be ingested daily.

Macrocytic anemias can occur that are **not megaloblastic** (demonstrating immature nuclei), and these are most often associated with **alcoholic liver disease.** The membrane lipids are inappropriately synthesized in liver disease, resulting in **macrocytic and target red blood cells** (Fig. 9–13).

Toxic levels of lead result in **lead poisoning,** which causes gastrointestinal and central nervous system abnormalities as well as **interfering with heme synthesis.** This poisoning is not limited to lead. Other substances, such as benzene and pesticides, will also interfere with body processes. Lead poisoning and other chemical heme inhibitors cause an **acquired porphyria.** One classic hallmark of lead poisoning is **basophilic stippling** inclusions in some of the erythrocytes (Fig. 9–14; see also Fig. 9–9). Basophilic stippling is dark blue aggregates, of retained RNA, throughout the entire cell. Basophilic stippling is seen in heme synthesis problems, other than lead poisoning, and is **very discrete and easily missed.** If the **fine focus of the microscope** is not utilized during blood smear examination, the stippling will not be visible. A confirmatory diagnosis requires that a **lead level** be performed in the chemistry area of the clinical laboratory.

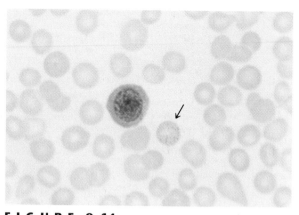

FIGURE 9–14
Basophilic stippling seen in erythrocytes as small blue dots throughout the cell associated with hemoglobin synthesis disorders, such as lead poisoning.

Some **anemias** are **due to the increased destruction of the cells** after their production. This can be **secondary to shape change, inclusions, antibodies, or complement** associated with the membrane. The term for these is **hemolytic anemias.** Erythrocytes can be destroyed **(lysed) within the blood stream (intravascular hemolysis)** or **phagocytized by macrophages** that destroy the cells **(extravascular hemolysis).**

Intravascular hemolysis is caused by **trauma,** which is tearing of cells producing schistocytes, **abnormal membranes** that break, or production of **antibody** proteins that activate a plasma protein termed **complement. Mechanical trauma** due to fibrin strands in clots that tear the cells as they pass through and artificial valves that tear cells can also be the cause of intravascular hemolysis. Abnormal membranes, such as occur in hereditary spherocytosis and rigid sickled cells, rupture and break easily. Antibodies, that activate complement enzymatically produce holes in the erythrocyte membrane; this is presented in more detail in Chapters 5 and 8. Disorders in which complement is fully activated usually involve antibodies that are produced as part of an immune response to **antigens within your own body (autoimmune)** or **antigens on the cells of another member of the species (alloimmune).** An example of autoimmune intravascular hemolysis is **paroxysmal nocturnal hemoglobinuria**

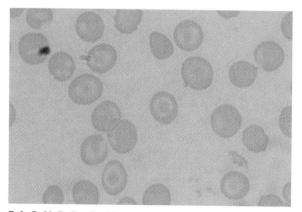

FIGURE 9–13
Liver disease demonstrating macrocytes and target cells.

(PNH), demonstrating a sensitivity of the red cells to complement hemolysis in an acid pH environment that occurs during long hours of sleep. The first morning void of urine is red with free hemoglobin. A second anemia is **paroxysmal cold hemoglobinuria (PCH),** which results from activation of certain cold antibodies that activate complement. An example of alloimmune intravascular hemolysis is the reaction to a transfusion of incompatible donor red cells. This hemolysis results in immediate release of **free hemoglobin** into the plasma, making it appear **red** (Fig. 9–15). In order not to lose this hemoglobin through kidney (renal) excretion into the urine, free hemoglobin binds to various proteins within the plasma (**haptoglobin,** hemopexin, or albumin) and eventually is phagocytized by macrophages for breakdown. Once the red cell is phagocytized by a macrophage, the breakdown process is the same for all types of hemolysis.

Extravascular hemolysis resulting in anemia can be autoimmune or alloimmune also. Examples of **autoimmune hemolytic anemia (AIHA)** are seen secondary to other autoimmune diseases, such as **rheumatoid arthritis and lupus,** as well as sometimes occurring in the **elderly** whose immune system becomes overzealous and produces unwarranted autoantibodies. **If cells are altered by viruses or contain antigens similar to viral antigens,** the antibodies produced to attack the viral infected cells may cross-react with normal red blood cells. When an erythrocyte has antibodies or partially activated complement bound to the membrane, these **opsonize** the cell, marking it for phagocytosis by a macrophage (usually in the liver or spleen). The test to detect the presence of immunoglobulin G (IgG) and C3 and C4 complement components acting as opsonins is the **direct antiglobulin test (DAT)** performed in the blood bank. The product of heme catabolism by the **reticuloendothelial (RE, macrophage)** cells is a **yellow,** toxic substance called **bilirubin** (see Fig. 9–15). The bilirubin is further broken down and **detoxified by the liver and excreted in the urine and feces.**

Tests to diagnose hemolytic anemia and **differentiate between intravascular and** **extravascular hemolysis** are discussed in more detail in Chapter 10.

Free plasma hemoglobin and free hemoglobin in the urine can be measured and are directly proportional to the amount of **intravascular hemolysis.** The test for the free hemoglobin plasma transport protein, **haptoglobin,** is done by measuring the haptoglobin that is not bound to free hemoglobin. The **haptoglobin result is inversely proportional to the level of free hemoglobin.**

A result indicative of **extravascular hemolysis** is a positive **direct antiglobulin test (DAT).** This indicates the presence of antibody or partially activated complement on the erythrocyte membrane, and an elevated **plasma bilirubin** value indicates an extravascular hemolysis as seen most often in **autoimmune hemolytic anemia (AIHA).** If antibody production is the mechanism involved, **steroids,** which destroy the lymphocytes and therefore antibody production, are administered to **inhibit antibody synthesis.** Since most of the extravascular hemolysis takes place in the spleen, a **splenectomy** can also be considered as a treatment to **reduce the destruction of the red blood cells.** The tests presented here are described in detail in Chapter 10.

Abetalipoproteinemia is a **rare genetic lipid metabolism disease** resulting in abnormal formation of the erythrocyte membrane. Lipids are metabolized in the liver; therefore, certain **liver diseases may mimic the genetic abetalipoproteinemia.** The abnormal morphology seen in abetalipoproteinemia is poikilocytosis in the form of **irregular spicules off of the erythrocyte membrane.** These cells are **acanthocytes** and are unique to this disease. It is very important to differentiate the pathologic acanthocyte with irregular erythrocyte membrane projections from the **more regular membrane projections of the echinocyte (crenated normal red blood cell)** (see Figs. 9–1 and 9–2).

Spherocytosis can be the result of a **rare genetic anemia** caused by a **defective sodium/potassium (Na+/K+) pump mechanism within the red blood cell mem-**

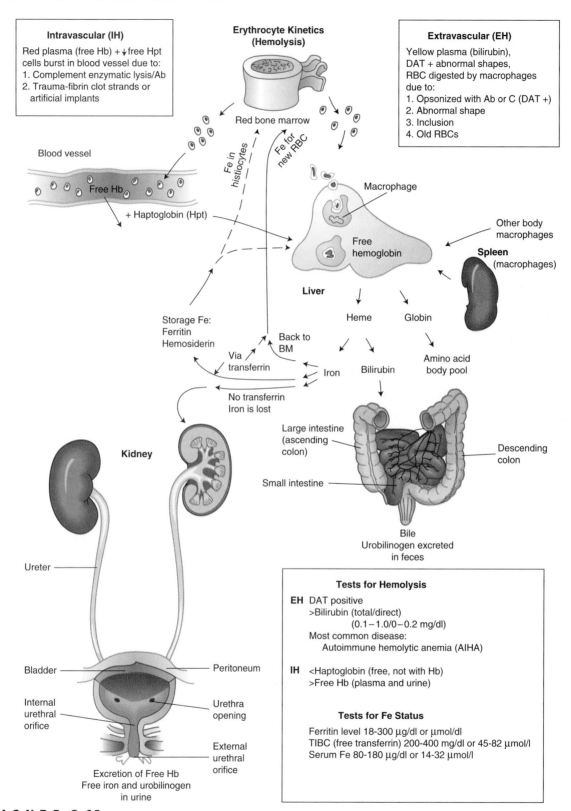

Intravascular (IH)

Red plasma (free Hb) + ↓free Hpt
cells burst in blood vessel due to:
1. Complement enzymatic lysis/Ab
2. Trauma-fibrin clot strands or
   artificial implants

**Erythrocyte Kinetics
(Hemolysis)**

Extravascular (EH)

Yellow plasma (bilirubin),
DAT + abnormal shapes,
RBC digested by macrophages
due to:
1. Opsonized with Ab or C (DAT +)
2. Abnormal shape
3. Inclusion
4. Old RBCs

Red bone marrow

Blood vessel

Fe in histiocytes

Fe for new RBC

Free Hb

+ Haptoglobin (Hpt)

Macrophage

Free
hemoglobin

Other body
macrophages

Spleen
(macrophages)

Liver

Storage Fe:
Ferritin
Hemosiderin

Back to
BM

Via
transferrin

Iron

Heme

Globin

Bilirubin

Amino acid
body pool

No transferrin
Iron is lost

Kidney

Large intestine
(ascending
colon)

Descending
colon

Small intestine

Bile
Urobilinogen excreted
in feces

Ureter

Bladder

Internal
urethral
orifice

Peritoneum

Urethra
opening

External
urethral
orifice

Excretion of Free Hb
Free iron and urobilinogen
in urine

Tests for Hemolysis

EH DAT positive
>Bilirubin (total/direct)
(0.1−1.0/0−0.2 mg/dl)
Most common disease:
Autoimmune hemolytic anemia (AIHA)

IH <Haptoglobin (free, not with Hb)
>Free Hb (plasma and urine)

Tests for Fe Status

Ferritin level 18-300 µg/dl or µmol/dl
TIBC (free transferrin) 200-400 mg/dl or 45-82 µmol/l
Serum Fe 80-180 µg/dl or 14-32 µmol/l

FIGURE 9–15

Breakdown of the erythrocyte into its components following intravascular hemolysis.

brane. This results in round erythrocytes that are likely to burst in the blood stream (**intravascular hemolysis**) and also be removed by macrophage (RES) cells (primarily in the spleen) due to the abnormal shape (**extravascular hemolysis**). If the macrophage manages to engulf only a small piece of the erythrocyte membrane, instead of the entire cell, the remaining membrane will stretch and close around the full complement of hemoglobin. Due to the inability to correct the etiology (cause), the most common treatment is **splenectomy, which eliminates cells responsible for the majority of hemolysis.** Once the spleen has been removed, various shapes and inclusions will remain in the circulation and will be visible on a stained peripheral blood smear. This then is a microspherocyte (MCV <80 fl), which will be dark red and fragile and show no central pallor (MCHC >36%). The spherocytes can still carry oxygen if they are not destroyed by the spleen. **Spherocytes and schistocytes** occur occasionally in the blood due to **extravascular hemolysis** of normocytic opsonized red blood cells, such as in hemolytic disease of the newborn. The schistocytes are small (MCV <80 fl), irregular pieces of red blood cells after a partial phagocytosis by a macrophage of the RES or a result of cell trauma. The presence of both **spherocytes and schistocytes suggests an extravascular hemolytic anemia** that involves antibodies from an immune response (see Fig. 9–5). Not only would the mean cell hemoglobin concentration (MCHC) be decreased, but the red blood cell distribution width (RDW >14.5%) will be elevated, indicating an abnormal variety of cell sizes. Hemolytic disease of the newborn (HDN) and hemolytic transfusion reactions (HTRs) may demonstrate spherocytes as a result of the extravascular hemolysis that is occurring. A positive direct antiglobulin test (DAT) would confirm an autoimmune hemolysis.

In Figures 9–1 and 9–2, the various red blood cell shapes are listed. Refer to a hematology atlas for more examples of **poikilocytosis** (variation in shape) and **anisocytosis** (variation in size).

Do It Now Anemias

1. Draw the following tubes of blood in which the component parts (erythrocytes, leukocytes, thrombocytes, and plasma) have separated and settled.
   A. Normal percentage of each component. Think about and write your explanation for the maintenance of these percentages. What body processes move fluid in and out of the blood vessels? Where do the formed elements come from and go to? What regulators are there for these processes? Be creative and represent this clearly, but briefly. (Examples: Draw diagrams, make up index cards showing each process.) The more creative the examples, the better. Share these examples with classmates. You will learn from one another.
   B. Decreased percentage of erythrocytes. List the three basic mechanisms resulting in anemia. Under each mechanism, list diseases associated with these mechanisms.
2. List the diagnostic tests associated with the three basic mechanisms of anemia.
3. Explain the consequences of anemia. What body functions are affected first and why?

PHYSIOLOGIC INCREASES IN ERYTHROCYTE COUNT

Polycythemia is the term used to describe an increase in the concentration of red blood cells within the body. Polycythemia is also described as an **increase in red blood cell mass.** The term **polycythemia** is used instead of erythrocytosis, because in some cases all hematopoietic cells are increased, but the **large number of erythrocytes** creates the problems observed. The significantly increased number of red blood cells results in a very thick, viscous blood that is sluggish and difficult for the heart to pump. The increased volume of blood results in **high blood pressure,** which increases the risk of stroke and myocardial infarction ([MI] and heart attack, (cardiovascular accident [CVA]). **Elevated hematocrit and hemoglobin values** are often, but not always, seen in this disorder. The

Anemias Classified by Morphology

Morphology	Synonyms	Etiology/Treatment	Comments/Tests
Microcytic, hypochromic	Small size, less color	Iron deficiency >Iron intake Thalassemia/transfusion	Pregnancy, diet, chronic bleeding Ferritin test to diagnose
Microspherocytic	Small size, more color	Hereditary spherocytosis	Osmotic fragility Family genetics
Macrocytic, normochromic	Large size, normal color	Vitamin B_{12} deficiency Folate deficiency Liver disease	Autoimmune B_{12} level Pregnancy folate level Alcohol, virus Liver enzymes
Macrocytic, polychromatic	Large size, blue color	Stress reticulocytes	Anemia (chronic) Reticulocyte count
Normocytic, normochromic	Normal size and color	Hemolytic anemia	Autoimmune (AIHA) DAT positive, reticulocyte count okay
		Lead poisoning	Basophilic stippling
		Aplastic anemia	Bone marrow toxicity Reticulocyte count <0.5%
		Hemoglobinopathies	Unless in crisis Hb electrophoresis
		G-6-PD deficiency	G-6-PD level Heinz body stain
		Hemorrhage	Acute, no reticulocytes <Hematocrit
		Porphyrias	Genetic Reticulocyte count okay
Anisocytic, poikilocytic	Abnormal size and shape	Hemoglobinopathies	Severe or in crisis Sickle cells, crystals, etc Hb electrophoresis
		Hemolytic anemias	Spherocytes and schistocytes DAT positive
		Biologic trauma Mechanical trauma	Burns, clots, artificial valves, etc. Schistocytes

Normocytic = normal size = mean cell volume (MCV) = 80–100 femtoliters (fl).
Normochromic = normal color = normal hemoglobin content = mean cell hemoglobin concentration = 30–36%.

increase in red blood cell mass may be due to a normal physiologic shift of fluids with resultant concentration or dilution of the red blood cell mass. Polycythemia can also be due to an increase in the production of red blood cells.

Relative, secondary, or stress polycythemia is due to a normal physiologic process of fluid movement in the body stimulated by an unrelated problem. The movement of fluid out of the blood vessels results in an increase in red blood cells **relative to the plasma volume.** This polycythemia is **transient and secondary to the primary problem.** The best examples of this occur in the emergency room situation. If a child comes in after having had prolonged diarrhea and vomiting, dehydration will be evident. This **loss of body fluid** will result in a relative concentration of the red blood cells, which have not changed in numbers. If the scenario is a 90-year-old woman who has a chronic decrease in red blood cells and has been vomiting and losing fluid, this transient concentration of red blood cells will result in the erroneous appearance of a normal red blood cell volume due to the relative lack of plasma. The opposite phenomenon will occur

FAST FACTS

Anemias Classified by Etiology

Classification	Synonyms	Etiology/Morphology	Comments/Tests
RELATIVE	Pseudoanemia	Shift of fluid into the vasculature; normocytic and normochromic	Normal reticulocyte count, pregnancy Liver cirrhosis (degeneration), nephritis (renal disease), and congestive heart failure
ABSOLUTE: Inherited/genetic	Fanconi's anemia	<Production Normocytic, normochromic	<Reticulocyte count Aplastic anemia
	Diamond-Blackfan syndrome	<Production Normocytic, normochromic	<Reticulocyte count Aplastic anemia
	Glucose-6-phosphate dehydrogenase deficiency (G-6-PD)	<G-6-PD to reduce HBFe Normocytic, normochromic	Heinz bodies form in erythrocytes
	Hemoglobinopathies (abnormal production)	Altered amino acid sequence of the globin chain; normocytic, normochromic (abnormal shapes in disease crisis) Decreased production of one of the globin chains; microcytic, hypochromic, targets	Sickle cell anemia (sickle cells, targets) HbC disease (crystals in cells, targets) Hb electrophoresis >300 Hemoglobinopathies known Thalassemia: major or minor; alpha or beta < Howell-Jolly bodies Hb electrophoresis
	Porphyrias	Deficiency of enzyme for heme synthesis	Dark urine, urine levels of: δ-Aminolevulinic acid (ALA) Porphobilinogen level (PBG)
Acquired	Acute posthemorrhagic anemia	Sudden excessive loss	Trauma injury, aneurysms, ulcers <Hematocrit, reticulocyte count okay
	Iron deficiency anemia	Microcytic and hypochromic	Deficient diet Excessive use (pregnancy) <Iron and ferritin
	Anemia of chronic disease (ACD)	Iron trapped in histiocytes; normocytic and normochromic	2° to chronic disease Reticulocyte count okay >Iron and ferritin
	Sideroblastic anemia (myelodysplastic syndrome)	Excess iron Hypochromic Dimorphic	Ringed sideroblasts in bone marrow Hemochromatosis
	Vitamin B$_{12}$ def. anemia (pernicious anemia [PA])	<Vitamin B$_{12}$ macrocytic (megaloblastic)	Antibodies to intrinsic factor in the stomach to absorb vitamin B$_{12}$ (autoimmune disease)
	Folate deficiency anemia	<Folate, macrocytic	Pregnancy, diet
	Lead poisoning	Inhibition of heme synthesis	Basophilic stippling in erythrocytes
	Hemolytic anemia (autoimmune hemolytic anemia, AIHA, PNH, PCH)	Destruction of red blood cells	Autoimmune Alloimmune
Genetic/acquired	Abetalipoproteinemia	Irregular spiculated red blood cells	Membrane lipid abnormal
Genetic	Spherocytosis	Small, dark, round red blood cells	Defective Na+/K + membrane pump

Diagram of a normal hematocrit. Refer to Chapter 1 for the proportions of blood components.

1. Draw pictures of hematocrits taken from the individuals in the scenarios described earlier (p. 192). Explain your drawings to another classmate and ask your classmate to describe his or her drawing to you. Work with a different individual for each scenario.
2. Think about how the body functions and produces erythrocytes when needed. An individual arrived in the emergency room after an automobile accident with severe blood loss. The phlebotomist, who was nearby, was contacted and collected the specimen immediately. What would the blood component proportions look like? Draw a sedimented tube of blood demonstrating the results that you would predict.

if a patient with a normal red blood cell count has an intravenous line (IV) providing excess fluid to the blood vessels. In this case the red blood cell mass is diluted, which results in the appearance of a lower red blood cell mass. In the case of a polycythemic patient, this would dilute the red blood cell mass to an erroneously normal volume.

ABNORMAL INCREASES IN ERYTHROCYTE COUNT (POLYCYTHEMIA AND ERYTHROLEUKEMIA)

Absolute benign polycythemia results from the **production of red blood cells in response to increased erythropoietin (EPO) levels due to a decreased supply of oxygen from the lungs to the tissues.** This is a second mechanism for a transient polycythemia as discussed earlier. Scenarios here include a patient with severely compromised lungs, such as a **smoker or a person with emphysema,** or an individual from the midwest traveling to a **high altitude** in Colorado. In both of these situations there is **not an adequate amount of oxygen from**

the lungs and the body compensates by producing more cells in order to carry more oxygen. In all of these situations, polycythemia will disappear if the primary problem is eliminated.

Absolute Malignant Polycythemia. Excessive erythropoietin (EPO) production will result in an inappropriate increase in red blood cell production. Conditions that have resulted in **increased EPO levels** are **tumors** (neoplasms), which secrete EPO, **kidney (renal) disorders,** and familial disorders due to the presence of a **high oxygen affinity for hemoglobin** (will not release O_2 to the tissues), a **decrease** in the number of **EPO-responsive erythroid progenitor cells,** or **genetically defective EPO production.** Absolute malignant polycythemia may also represent a **clonal myeloproliferation** (bone marrow proliferation originating from one cell). In the case of polycythemia vera, the cell is an **early undifferentiated progenitor cell** (not committed to only one cell line) that gives rise to red blood cells, white blood cells, and platelets. Therefore, all of these cells are elevated, with the increased concentration of red blood cells creating the physiologic problem of **hypervolemic blood flow.** This disorder is more common in individuals older than **40 years of age.**

Diagnosis and Treatment of Polycythemia. A 60%, or greater, hematocrit is often seen at diagnosis. This increase in hematocrit results in increased viscosity of the blood, which places stress on the heart and blood vessels. A hematocrit greater than 46% has been associated with decreased cerebral blood flow, resulting in decreased cerebral (brain) function. A definitive diagnosis requires a **blood cell mass determination of equal to or greater than 0.36 ml/kg in males and 0.32 ml/kg in females.** A test to determine the cause of polycythemia is the **erythropoietin (EPO) level,** which may be determined from urine or from a specimen of plasma. **Erythrocyte counts are high** in addition to other changes in laboratory values, such as an **elevated leukocyte alkaline phosphatase (LAP) level** and shifts in the white blood cell differential. These tests are explained in Chapter 10. Also contributing to the diagnosis are splenomegaly (enlarged spleen) and an arterial blood oxygen saturation of greater than 92%. The oxygen saturation rules out polycythemia due to a lack of oxygen in the cells. If left **untreated,** patients have a **6- to 18-month survival rate.** When **properly treated** throughout their lifetimes, a **normal life expectancy can be predicted. Polycythemia is treated by** periodic **removal of a unit of blood.** The frequency of phlebotomy is determined by the physician, based on the hematocrit value. It is recommended to remove a unit of blood when the hematocrit exceeds 46%. This **therapeutic phlebotomy** is often performed in the blood bank (immunohematology) area of the clinical laboratory. The unit of blood is discarded, and the patient must pay for the procedure. **Chemotherapy** is also used to treat primary malignant polycythemia. Chemotherapeutic treatment includes use of myelosuppressive agents such as radioactive phosphorus (^{32}P), hydroxyurea, and alkylating agents such as busulfan.

Malignant Erythrocytosis. Erythroleukemia (FAB M6), also called acute erythroleukemia **(AEL),** previously called di Guglielmo's disease, is a clonal (originating from one cell) myeloproliferation (rapid production within the bone marrow) of an early hematopoietic cell. Classified by the French, Americans, and British, an **M6 leukemia** (Table 9–2) demonstrates more than **50% erythroid dysplasia** (abnormal formation) in the bone marrow with **megaloblastic normoblasts containing diffuse blocks of cytoplasmic glycogen** when stained with periodic acid–Schiff (PAS) stain and more than 30% nonerythroid (myelo) blasts. Only about 5% of acute leukemias are M6. Some individuals have developed M6 following myeloproliferative syndromes and myelodysplastic syndromes. **Howell-Jolly bodies** (DNA aggregates in mature red blood cells) and **ringed sideroblasts** (bone marrow normoblasts with a ring of iron around the nucleus visible with iron stain) are present. **Differentiation** of M6 **from myelodysplastic syndrome** is difficult. Use of **monoclonal antibodies** (anticarbonic anhydrase I, CAI, and FA6-152) and **flow cytometry** allows more accurate identification of the multipotent stem cell associated with M6. This disease is seen most often in individuals **older than 40 years of age.**

FAST FACTS

Polycythemia

Type	Synonym	Etiology	Example
Relative	Secondary Stress Transient	Secondary to the primary problem Loss or shift of body fluids	Diarrhea and vomiting
Absolute	Benign Transient	Production of red blood cells in response to increased erythropoietin (EPO) due to decreased O_2 from the lungs to the tissues.	Smokers Emphysema High altitudes
	Malignant Primary	Increased EPO levels	Tumors (neoplasms) Kidney/renal disorders High O_2 affinity Hb <EPO responsive erythroid progenitors Genetically >EPO

Diagnosis: Hematocrit and red blood cell mass.
Reference values: >60% hematocrit, >46% increases the risk of decreased cerebral blood flow; red blood cell mass > 0.36 ml/kg in males and >0.32 ml/kg in females.
Treatment: Therapeutic phlebotomy.

TABLE 9-2   French-American-British (FAB) Class of Acute Myeloid or Lymphoid Leukemias

FAB Class	Cells Observed	Unique Criteria	Cytochemistry/CD*	%†
M1(AML)	**>90% myeloblasts** with minimal maturation (Pros)	Occasional Auer rods	Myeloperoxidase (MP), Sudan Black B (SBB), NASDC	20
M2(AML)	**<90% Myeloblasts; >10% more mature**	**Auer rods**	Myeloperoxidase, Sudan black B, NASDC	30
M3(APL)	Predominantly **promyelocytes**	Often causes disseminated intravascular coagulation	Myeloperoxidase, Sudan black B, NASDC	10
M4(AMML)	**Myeloblasts and monoblasts** with stages of both	Occasional Auer rods	>20% MP/SBB/NASDC >20% Nonspecific esterase (NSE)	12
M4eo	Same as M4 except **with eosinophilia**	Some with large **basophilic granules**	Same as M4; eos may be PAS	4
M5a (AMoL) poorly differentiated	**>80% monoblasts,** promonocytes, and monocytes	Later stages are poorly granulated vacuolated	**NSE (fluoride inhibitor)**	5
M5b(AMoL) differentiated	**<80% monoblasts,** promonocytes, and monocytes		Same as M5a	6
M6(AEL)	**>50% erythroblasts;** also myeloblasts and monoblasts	50% Dysplastic, megaloblastic	Periodic acid–Schiff stain (PAS)	6
M7(AMegL)	**>30% megakaryoblasts**		Platelet peroxidase by EM, platelet glycoprotein by immunocytochemistry	1
L1(ALL)	Small lymph cells	**2–10 yr olds**	PAS/CD 10, 19, 24	71
L2(ATL)	Large irregular cells	**Adult T cell associated** with **HTLV-1**	PAS/CD 10	27
L3(ALL)	Large uniform cell	**Burkitt's** type	PAS/CD 10	2

* *Cluster differentiation markers for flow cytometry identification of cells.*
† *Represents % of acute myeloid leukemias (M) or acute lymphoid (L) leukemias.*

When a patient presents with an erythrocyte abnormality, the morphology seen may suggest additional tests to support the cause (etiology). The subsequent tests can determine the etiology in order to aid in the diagnosis and to monitor the success of the treatment. Flow charts are established to provide logical directional testing and to avoid random testing or misdiagnosis and consequent treatment (see Fig. 9–6).

STUDY QUESTIONS

Match the Choices With the Best Causative Mechanism.

1. Increased levels of erythropoietin (EPO)

2. Increase in plasma volume

3. Acute hemorrhage

4. Vomiting and diarrhea

5. Bone marrow aplasia

A. Increased erythrocyte count

B. Decreased erythrocyte count

C. No change

Choose the Best Answer for the Following Questions:

6. A 66-year-old white male patient presented with what appears to be polycythemia. The erythrocyte morphology would be:
   A. Normocytic, normochromic
   B. Macrocytic, normochromic
   C. Microcytic, normochromic
   D. Microcytic, hypochromic

7. The most conclusive test to confirm polycythemia is the:
   A. Hematocrit
   B. Hemoglobin
   C. Radioisotope whole blood volume
   D. Radioisotope red blood cell mass

8. In order to differentiate hemolytic anemia from aplastic anemia, the least expensive yet most conclusive test is:
   A. Direct antiglobulin test (DAT)
   B. Reticulocyte count
   C. Erythrocyte count with differential
   D. Red blood cell survival test

9. A test done to differentiate iron deficiency anemia from thalassemia would be:
   A. Red blood cell count   B. PB smear evaluation   C. Ferritin   D. Hemoglobin

10. For confirmation of a hemoglobinopathy such as sickle cell trait, the best test is:
   A. Hb electrophoresis   B. PB smear evaluation   C. Hb solubility test   D. DAT

CHAPTER 10

OUTLINE

Complete Blood Count

Hemoglobin and Hematocrit

Microscopic Evaluation of Erythrocytes

Special Erythrocyte Tests

Study Questions

Erythrocyte Testing

OBJECTIVES

Upon completion of this chapter the student should be able to:

1. Describe the acceptable specimen for erythrocyte testing.

2. Explain the routine erythrocyte test methodology.

3. Correlate the various erythrocyte tests and their significance.

4. When given a testing scenario, determine if there are reasons to question the validity of results.

5. State the various erythrocyte disease states in terms of cells involved and relevant testing.

COMPLETE BLOOD COUNT

The **specimen** required for most erythrocyte testing is in an ethylenediaminetetraacetic acid **(EDTA)** tube **(purple top)** at least one-third full, fresh, and well mixed to prevent clotting. The whole blood specimen should be inverted (not shaken) completely six to eight times for adequate mixing.

If the specimen is shaken, the erythrocytes may be damaged and hemolysis will occur, interfering with an accurate complete blood count (CBC).

EDTA is the anticoagulant of choice for cellular testing because it **preserves the cell function and morphology** better than do any of the other anticoagulants. For the most accurate results, the counts should be performed within 2 hours, since with time in vitro, all cells begin to change. However, some individuals' cells become altered immediately (i.e., platelets attach to the white blood cells in EDTA) after exposure to the anticoagulant. If a patient's cells are altered by EDTA, sodium citrate (Na citrate, blue top tube) anticoagulant can be used. **If Na citrate anticoagulant is used,** the blood must be well mixed, **tested within a few hours** after collection, and **tested before any coagulation testing** has been performed on the Na citrate specimen. The **quantity of Na citrate** in the specimen collection tube may be a greater volume than the EDTA, **requiring that a dilution factor be taken into account for accurate results.** Some special tests, such as cytochemical staining, osmotic fragility testing, and lupus erythematosus preparations, require alternate anticoagulants that are discussed later in this section along with the specific test.

Once the EDTA tube is filled with blood, the tube should be **inverted (not shaken) completely six to eight times** to adequately mix the blood with the anticoagulant, which will inhibit clotting. If the **CBC results do not correlate,** the quality of the specimen may be in question. Allow the components in the tube of blood to separate by setting the tube in a rack to sediment or **centrifuge the**

specimen at 60 to 100g or 10 minutes in order to **examine the liquid (plasma)** portion of the whole blood (which **should be pale yellow and slightly hazy**). If the **plasma is dark yellow, milky, or red,** this will interfere with accurate testing and the **specimen must be redrawn or dealt with using the manufacturer's protocol** to correct the test results. The causes of this unacceptable plasma are explained in Chapter 1.

If the laboratory practitioner is not correlating results to see if the test data "make sense," fragmented information can hinder the efficiency of health care and be detrimental to the patient.

CBC testing must be **done at room temperature** with **well-mixed EDTA** anticoagulated blood to obtain accurate results. If the specimen cannot be tested for several hours after collection, the specimen may require **refrigeration at 4° C to maintain the cells** as they were in vivo. Refer to the protocol established in your facility for transport and storage of a specimen. Before testing, it is important for the specimen to be allowed to equilibrate to room temperature for 20 to 30 minutes.

Our mission in the clinical laboratory is: (1) to provide test results that reflect the condition within the patient's body (in vivo), requiring the knowledge and ability to maintain the specimen and perform the testing with minimal change in the specimen after the blood has been removed from the patient and placed into a glass tube (in vitro); (2) to provide accurate test information (puzzle pieces) to the primary health care provider with a clear and accurate picture of the patient's state of health. The laboratory practitioner must be able to **correlate** and **validate** the results that are being reported.

The most common test is the **complete blood count (CBC).** This test is part of a routine examination that is done at the time of the patient's admission to the hospital. The formed elements (erythrocytes, leukocytes, and thrombocytes) of the blood are counted in triplicate by the cell-counting instruments in most laboratories.

The CBC performed using a large hospital laboratory instrument includes a red blood cell count with a histogram and morphologic indices; a total white blood cell count with a histogram; a scattergram (for differentiation of the various white blood cells); a platelet count with a histogram; a morphologic index; hemoglobin level; hematocrit; indices; reference ranges; and markers for out-of-range values.

Smaller hematology instrumentation, used in small laboratories and physician office laboratories (POLs), may only generate the count and hemoglobin information without histograms and scattergrams. The average reference range for an **erythrocyte count is 4 to 5 ×** 10^{12}**/l.** Keep in mind that normal reference values are given for the average adult population. Male values are slightly higher than are female values, and the geriatric (elderly) population may demonstrate lower values due to decreased erythropoiesis and effects of chronic disease. **Each laboratory must establish its own normal reference values,** due to variances in instrumentation, procedures, and local populations that may render the textbook reference values less accurate for the specific laboratory population involved in the testing.

Automated Complete Blood Count (CBC) Procedure. There are several instruments that perform the complete blood count. Electronic impedance, laser light scatter, light absorbance, and staining characteristics are some of the principles utilized by various instruments.

Electronic impedance is used to count cells by the Coulter Cell Counter, the Sysmex NE 8000 Cell Counter by Baxter, and the COBAS Cell Counter by Roche, and a modification of electrical impedance is used by the Abbott Cell-Dyn 3000. Some of these machines also use light scatter (described later) to differentiate the cells for the automated differential. The following procedure is used for the electronic impedance CBC.

1. **Dilution of the EDTA whole blood specimen in an electrolyte solution** such as saline must first be done to allow a smaller, but significant, number of cells to be counted.

The cells suspended in this fluid are poor conductors of electricity, whereas the solution is a good conductor of electricity. The dilution must allow an adequate number of cells to be counted without a concentration so high that more than one cell goes through the aperture at the same time (coincidence error). If more than one type of cell (particle) is present in the sample, it may be necessary to lyse or remove one type to get an accurate count of the other (i.e., erythrocytes must be lysed in order to count the leukocytes). The leukocytes do not need to be removed from the erythrocyte dilution due to the insignificantly low numbers of leukocytes present once they are dispersed in the high dilution used for an erythrocyte count.

2. The instrument will have electrodes located on either side of the counting orifice or path. An electrolyte solution is placed between the electrodes, and a **flow of electrical current is established.**

3. **A specific amount of solution is pulled through the aperture. Any particle (cell) that passes through the aperture will momentarily increase the resistance of (or interrupt) the electrical flow between the electrodes and will generate a pulse that can be counted, measured, and displayed on a screen.** The amount of the resistance is proportional to the size of the cell. From this information, the counter-computer can provide an accurate count of particles and their size.

4. **Instrument background** (quality assurance check) values are obtained by counting the isotonic diluent without blood present to detect any miscellaneous particles within the vial or diluent that may be erroneously counted as cells. This background test must demonstrate very low, insignificant values.

5. **Controls and standards** must also be tested to ensure accuracy of the data generated. This should be a specimen with a known value that is tested exactly the same as the unknown patient's specimen to verify the accuracy and precision of the test system.

6. The test **results** for each specimen must be **reproducible.** In order to demonstrate the consistency of the value obtained, **each specimen must be run at least twice** to

ensure a similar value each time. Most large hematology instruments perform three to five determinations on each specimen to ensure the precision of the data generated.

The specific procedure for quality assurance protocol and acceptable values for each instrument will be provided by the company manufacturing the instrument.

Laser light scattering is the methodology utilized by some Coulter instruments to characterize cells for the scattergrams. Laser light scatter is utilized for cell counts as well as cell characterization by **flow cytometers,** such as the Technicon H-3, Abbott Cell-Dyn 3000, and BioChem ImmunoSystem 9000. The detection of the light scatter is a method of obtaining information relevant to the counting and classification of cells in a specimen. As discussed previously, there are flow cytometers that are not primarily cell counters but rather they identify cellular membrane protein markers using monoclonal antibodies and fluorescence. These more sophisticated flow cytometers are used to identify, sort, and collect cells for accurate diagnosis and treatment of previously determined disease.

The routine laboratory blood cell evaluation systems follow this procedure:

1. The sample is **diluted** in the instrument into a stream of fluid containing the cells to be counted in a **single cell flow (hydrodynamic focusing).**

2. These **cells pass through a flow cell on which a light is focused.** As the cell passes through the light path, it **scatters the light in all directions.** A photodetector senses and collects this **light scatter information and transforms it into digital information, which provides characteristic information about the specific cell** as it passes through the flow cell. Traditional flow cytometers utilize forward light scatter (0 degrees) and orthogonal light scatter (90 degrees) to differentiate lymphocytes, monocytes, and granulocytes.

The Cell-Dyn 3000 uses two additional dimensions of light scattering to more accurately separate the cell characteristics. This new technique is called multiangle polarized

scatter separation (MAPSS) and involves the use of a narrow-angle light scatter (10 degrees) to resolve basophils and depolarized light scatter (90 degrees) to resolve eosinophils. This additional information eliminates the need for cytochemical staining or monoclonal tagging to identify these cells.

Light absorbance is used along with light scatter by the Sysmex 8000, the COBAS, and the Technicon H-3. Another use of the light scatter technology is to specifically stain the cells of interest. This requires a darkfield optical system to count and classify leukocytes. The procedure is similar to light scatter, but the detection system is different. The light is scattered through the opening around a darkfield disc as cells pass through the sensing zone, one at a time. The light scatter is measured with a photodetector and related to the cell number. If the cell is stained, some of the light will be absorbed proportional to the amount of staining. By using various specific cell stains, a leukocyte differential can be done.

Indices are values calculated from the erythrocyte count, the hemoglobin, and the hematocrit and are useful measurements to predict the morphology of the cell, which is directly related to the disease mechanism. Erythrocyte counting by automated methods provides the information on indices in addition to the erythrocyte count, hemoglobin, and hematocrit. The **mean corpuscular volume (MCV)** provides the average cell size, which is measured by the automated methods. If there is an equal population of large and small erythrocytes, the average would be normal; thus, other indices were established to provide the percentage of variation in red blood cell size. This is equivalent to the coefficient of variation discussed in Chapter 1. The **red blood cell distribution width (RDW)** is the standard deviation of the erythrocyte cell size divided by the average erythrocyte cell size (MCV), which provides the percentage of erythrocytes outside of the reference range. Each manufacturer explains the calculation for RDW relative to the instrument. The **mean corpuscular hemoglobin (MCH)** provides the average hemoglobin per cell. This, however, does not take into account an abnormal cell size. The **mean corpuscular hemoglobin concentration (MCHC)** factors in the hematocrit in order to account for cell size and provides a more accurate value of the hemoglobin level of each cell. The calculations for these indices are in Chapter 1.

The automated instrument provides a red blood cell **histogram that depicts any alteration in cell number and size** (Fig. 10–1). The histogram provides the relative number of cells present on the vertical axis and the cell volume in femtoliters on the horizontal axis. Histogram A is a normocytic (MCV of 83.4 fl), normochromic (MCHC of 32.8 g/dl) erythrocyte population with an acceptable distribution of erythrocyte size variation (RDW of 13.8%). The complete blood count (CBC) results for histogram B appear normocytic

F I G U R E 10–1

A–C, Erythrocyte cell counts and indices with histograms.

CBC Results

RBC: 5.69 M/μl
HGB: 15.6 g/dl
HCT: 47.4%
MCV: 83.4 fl
MCH: 27.3 pg
MCHC: 32.8 g/dl
RDW: 13.8%

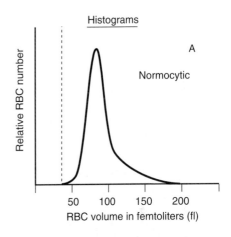

RBC: 3.00 M/μl
HGB: 9.3 g/dl
HCT: 28.2%
MCV: 94.0 fl
MCH: 31.1 pg
MCHC: 33.1 g/dl
RDW: 17.8%

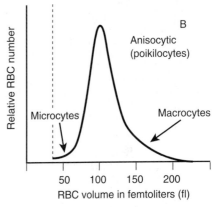

RBC: 3.71 M/μl
HGB: 5.6 g/dl
HCT: 19.3%
MCV: 52.2 fl
MCH: 15.2 pg
MCHC: 29.2 g/dl
RDW: 20.7%

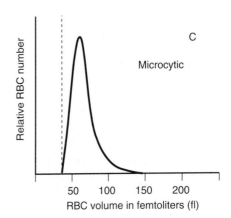

(MCV of 94.0 fl), which is misleading when compared with the RDW of 17.8%, suggesting a significant number of erythrocytes outside the reference range for cell size. The histogram suggests a range of sizes and possibly shapes, including some microcytes and macrocytes that have provided the deceiving average erythrocyte size (MCV) value falling within the acceptable reference range. Histogram C depicts primarily a microcytic cell population, such as seen in iron deficiency anemia; however, the abnormally elevated RDW (20.7%) rules out a single population of small cells. A bimorphic (two cell populations) or even trimorphic (three distinct cell populations) erythrocyte picture may be present due to bone marrow release of large stress reticulocytes and the administration of a unit of packed (normocytic) erythrocytes to treat the anemia. A unit of blood may be administered when the hemoglobin value dips to 7 g/dl or lower if symptoms of anemia (e.g., faintness, weakness) are present.

Scattergrams would not be helpful for erythrocyte evaluation. Scattergrams provide information concerning the nuclear and cytoplasmic characteristics of light scatter from the nucleus of cells, and red blood cells are a single anucleate cell population. Evaluating the blood smear is indicated and performed only if the automated instrument reports any unusual cell size or an abnormal cell count.

It is important to correlate the peripheral blood smear evaluation, as well as other test results, even from other areas of the laboratory, with the automated hematology results.

Correlation Factors. Many of the results will appear **within the normal reference range** and, after being **reviewed for appropriateness and validity,** can be verified and sent to the patient's chart. If there is a **special mark or "flag"** near a result to alert the laboratory practitioner to an abnormal value, **other tests should be considered to support and validate** this result. Examples of test correlation are the erythrocyte indices correlating with the peripheral blood smear morphology evaluation of the same specimen.

The erythrocyte count, if accurate, will correlate with the hemoglobin and hematocrit values, which are discussed later. If the cells appear visually to be decreased in hemoglobin (hypochromic), the hemoglobin value should be low. If the erythrocyte count is low, the hematocrit should be low. If the histogram and indices indicate large erythrocytes, these macrocytes should be observed on a peripheral blood smear. By correlating the automated results with additional tests, the validity of the result is established.

Sources of Error. An **appropriate blood specimen** is essential to perform an accurate erythrocyte count. If the specimen is **clotted, hemolyzed** (physically damaged due to shaking and so forth), maintained or tested at an **inappropriate temperature, or incorrectly collected,** or if the specimen **container is inappropriately filled,** the **blood must be collected again or the problem corrected before testing.** When a whole blood (WB) specimen is **refrigerated, the white blood cells and platelets stick together;** however, the red blood cells maintain very well. Very small red blood cells **(microcytes) may fall within the platelet count** area due to their similar size with large platelets, which may result in incorrect interpretation of results. All blood components, but especially erythrocytes, are very sensitive to an altered environment and, therefore, will lyse, crenate, or die if not maintained in an isotonic solution. Alterations that are artifact or secondary to a primary disease **(hemolysis, lipemia, cold agglutinins, rouleaux)** can result in incorrect automated cell counts. **Hemolysis,** due to specimen collection technique, would result in fewer intact red blood cells yielding an **erroneously low count.** If cold agglutinins are present, the erythrocytes will agglutinate and pass through the counter in groups rather than individually. The resultant count will reflect a **low number of very large cells** due to the agglutinates. If this specimen is warmed, the cells will disperse and an accurate count can be determined. **Rouleaux phenomena** occur when there is an excessive amount of protein in the plasma, which increases stacking of erythrocytes like coins (see Fig. 5–12). This is visible on a peripheral blood smear but **should not affect the automated cell count** because the dilution of the specimen also dilutes the protein and the cells become free flowing. The rouleaux phenomenon is the basis for the erythrocyte sedimentation rate (ESR) test to monitor excessive or abnormal protein production.

The erythrocyte count is always greater than $10 \times 10^9/l$; therefore, **the coincidence of two cells passing through the aperture of the instrument at once increases as the count increases.** This results in a count that is low due to the two cells passing through together being counted as one large cell. The **computerized cell-counting instruments automatically correct for this,** and older cell counters have a "coincidence correction chart" provided from the manufacturer that must be used to correct any count over $10 \times 10^9/l$. This correction will **always increase the observed count.** If the cell count is excessively high, resulting in cells that are too numerous to count, additional dilutions can be made to bring the count within counting limits of the instrument and procedure.

Erroneous measurements will be made, and **incorrect data and histograms** will be generated if any of the following conditions is present: (1) **nucleated red blood cells** (NRBCs) counted as white blood cells; (2) pieces of **fragmented white blood cells** counted as red blood cells; (3) **cold agglutinins** are present; (4) a **poorly mixed specimen** providing a less than random count (this

---

Do It Now Automated Cell Count Exercise

1. Draw your own histogram of a normal RBC differential.

Draw histograms that demonstrate the presence of each of the following:

2. Nucleated red blood cells (NRBC) in the specimen
3. Macrocytic anemia
4. Normocytic anemia
5. Cold agglutinins present
6. Using your laboratory's cell counting instrument or one at a local facility, draw your own diagram following the sample from entry to exit (waste) for an erythrocyte count and generation of the results.

Exchange this diagram with that of another class member who did the same instrument at a different time, and see if you can follow your class member's diagram and check to see if he or she missed any steps in the process.

FAST FACTS

Erythrocyte Counting Instruments

Methodology	Instrument	Company
Cell Counting		
Electronic impedance	STKS	Coulter Corporation
Modified	Cell-Dyn 3000	Abbott Laboratories
Electron impedance	Sysmex NE 8000	Baxter Scientific
	COBAS	Roche Diagnostics
Cell Counting or Characterization for Differentiation		
Laser light scatter	STKS	Coulter Corporation
	Technicon H-3	Bayer Corporation
	Cell-Dyn 3000	Abbott Laboratories
	System 9000	BioChem ImmunoSystems
Light absorbance	Sysmex NE 8000	Baxter Scientific
	COBAS	Roche Diagnostics
	Technicon H-3	Bayer Corporation
Fluorescence	FACSCalibur	Becton Dickinson

is less likely because the newer instruments rotate the blood before sampling).

HEMOGLOBIN AND HEMATOCRIT

The **specimen of choice for the automated instruments** found in the laboratory is a **lavender top EDTA.** This anticoagulant preserves the formed elements better than does any other anticoagulant. If a small **point of care instrument** (bedside) or a **manual hematocrit** is done, **fresh whole blood from a finger puncture,** drawn into a tube containing heparin (noted by a red band on the tube), may be used if an EDTA specimen is not available.

A capillary specimen (finger puncture) must be drawn into a tube containing an anticoagulant (usually heparin, noted by a red band on the tube) to inhibit clotting. If an alternate source is drawn for any specimen (capillary versus arterial versus venous), this must be noted on the test report form due to the variation in reference values.

The automated cell counters also perform hemoglobin and cell (particle) size measurements and calculate the hematocrit and indices. The specimen for the red blood cell count is divided into three samples and diluted with a cyanmethemoglobin reagent, which lyses the red blood cells and **forms a color compound in proportion to the amount of hemoglobin present.** This specimen, in triplicate, is measured by a spectrophotometric method to determine the amount of color change that provides a hemoglobin value. The erythrocytes being counted are measured for their size, and this information is recorded for **calculation of the hematocrit** and generation of the histogram. The number of cells and the size of the cells are used to calculate the hematocrit. The **manual hematocrit may be 2% higher** than the automated hematocrit due to plasma trapped between the cells tested.

Manual **hemoglobin estimates** can be done by placing a drop of blood, from a finger

puncture, in a **copper sulfate solution (CuSO₄)** with a **specific gravity of 1.054.** This solution allows a drop of whole blood containing at least 12.5 g/dl of Hb to fall to the bottom in less than 15 seconds. Anemic (low Hb) blood will take longer or will float on top. The accuracy of the result can be checked by the microhematocrit method; the value obtained should be approximately 3× the Hb value desired. This procedure is used most often by blood banks to screen donors.

MICROSCOPIC EVALUATION OF ERYTHROCYTES

EDTA is the anticoagulant of choice for peripheral blood smear preparation and evaluation. The EDTA **preserves the cell morphology** better than do any of the other anticoagulants.

The **peripheral blood smear evaluation** is not done routinely in most large laboratories but is used to confirm or clarify any un-

---

FAST FACTS

Erythrocyte Complete Blood Count (CBC) Values

Erythrocyte count = $4–5 \times 10^{12}$/dl
Hemoglobin = Hb = 11–18 g/dl
Hematocrit = Hct = 33–54%

Keep in mind that the values will vary depending on the age and sex of the patient. Women and the elderly have values on the low side of normal, whereas men and children have higher values.

Size of red blood cells = mean corpuscular volume = **MCV** = 80–100 femtoliters (fl)
% Variation in size = red blood cell distribution width = **RDW** = 11.5–14.5%
Average Hb in the cell = mean corpuscular hemoglobin = **MCH** = 27–31 picograms (pg)
Concentration of Hb in the cell = mean corpuscular hemoglobin concentration = **MCHC** = 30–36%

usual automated results. Smaller laboratories without the ability to perform automated differentials on their cell counting instruments must continue to evaluate peripheral blood smears on a regular basis. A fresh peripheral blood smear fixed and stained with a non-vital polychrome stain such as Wright-Giemsa can provide a wealth of information.

A fresh whole blood specimen is smeared onto a glass slide and stained with a Wright-Giemsa stain. The methodology for slide preparation is presented and explained in Chapter 1. The acceptability of the smear and the examination protocol are discussed in Chapter 6 and demonstrated with the use of slides and figures of peripheral blood smears. The **erythrocyte evaluation is usually done while performing a white blood cell evaluation (differential).** In every field in which a white blood cell is evaluated, the red blood cells are also evaluated and, after **assessing several fields,** the **size, shape, color,** and visible **inclusions** are recorded. The normal **(normocytic)** size and shape of an erythrocyte are about those of a small lymphocyte nucleus (6 to 8 μm), and the normal **(normochromic)** color appears pink with a slight light area **(central pallor)** in the center of the cell (Fig. 10–2; see also Figs. 7–10 and 7–12). Any variation in size **(anisocytosis),** shape **(poikilocytosis),** Hb content **(chromicity),** or **inclusions** will suggest or confirm additional testing to aid in the patient's diagnosis.

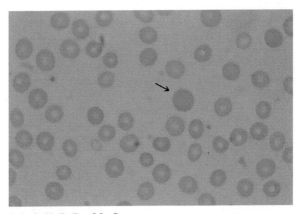

FIGURE 10–3
A stress reticulocyte on a Wright-Giemsa stained peripheral blood smear. Note the larger size and blue color compared with the mature erythrocytes.

Stress reticulocytes will appear large and blue on a Wright stain. This is described as **polychromatic** (Fig. 10–3; see also Figs. 7–8 and 9–7).

Anisocytosis, poikilocytosis, chromicity (Fig. 10–4), and inclusions (Fig. 10–5) of erythrocytes are listed in association with the stain used and the disease process.

Special stains are utilized to make one aspect of interest in the cell visible for evaluation. One of these is used for the **reticulocyte count.** The reticulocyte stain is a **monochrome vital stain** (buffered new methylene blue). Monochrome refers to the use of only one stain component (color) and an equal quantity of blood and stain (i.e., one drop each), which are mixed for cell staining prior to preparing the slide and fixing the cells. Thus, the cells are still "vital" or alive when they are stained versus the non-vital Wright-Giemsa stain, which is used after the smear has been made and the cells have been fixed. The reticulocyte stain is used to determine the number of **reticulocytes** (young erythrocytes indicating the appropriate bone marrow response to anemia) in the peripheral blood by precipitating the excess RNA to make it visible microscopically (Fig. 10–6).

Manual reticulocyte counting method:

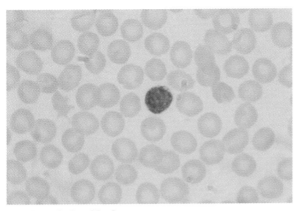

FIGURE 10–2
Normocytic, normochromic peripheral blood smear erythrocytes stained with a Wright-Giemsa polychrome stain. The small lymphocyte can be used for size relativity.

1. Reagent stain:

Methylene blue N	0.5 g
Potassium oxalate	1.4 g
Sodium chloride	0.8 g

Erythrocyte Morphologies

Name	Morphology	Correlation	Name	Morphology	Correlation
Normocyte (discocyte)	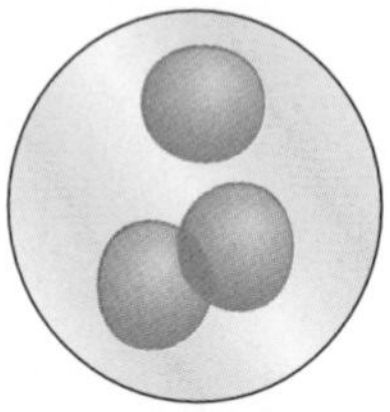	Healthy erythrocytes	Teardrop cells (dacryocytes)	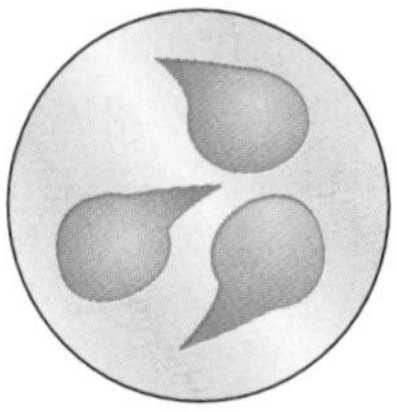	Extramedullary hematopoiesis, myelofibrosis (myeloid metaplasia)
Echinocytes, burr cells (crenated)	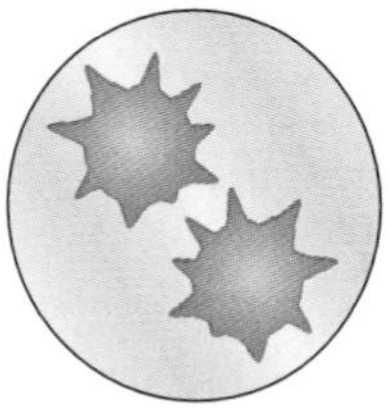	Uremia, artifacts (alkaline glass effects), hypotonic environment	Sickled cells (drepanocytes)	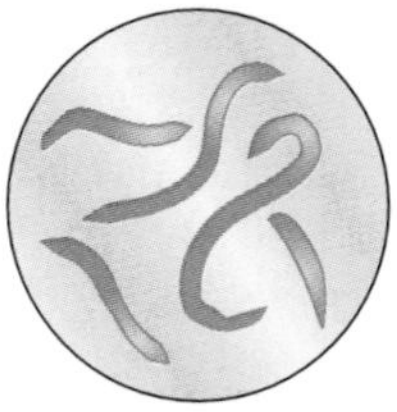	Hemoglobin S
Acanthocytes	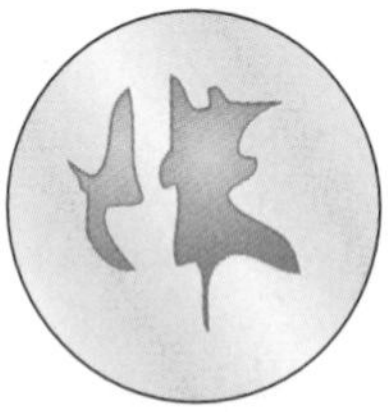	Abetalipoproteinemia, severe liver disease	Helmet cells	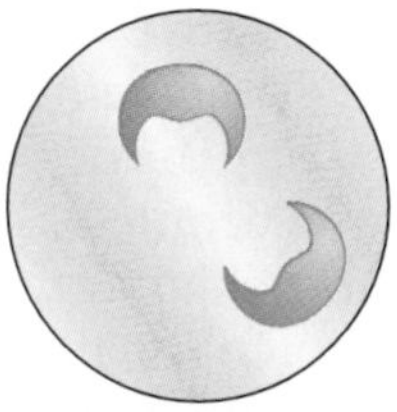	Hemolytic process
Target cells (leptocytes)	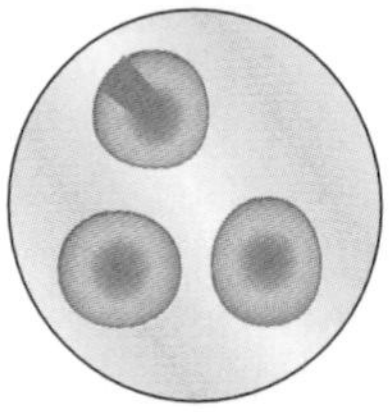	Liver disease, hemoglobinopathies	Schistocytes (RBC fragments)	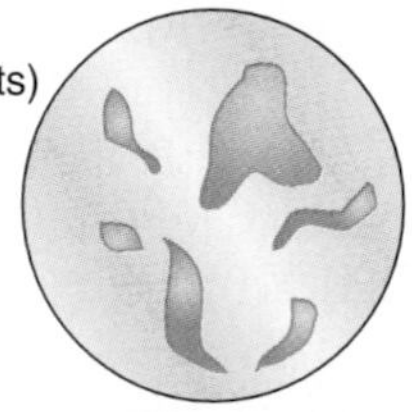	Disseminated intravascular coagulation (DIC), thrombotic thrombocytopenic purpura (TTP), hemolytic processes
Spherocytes	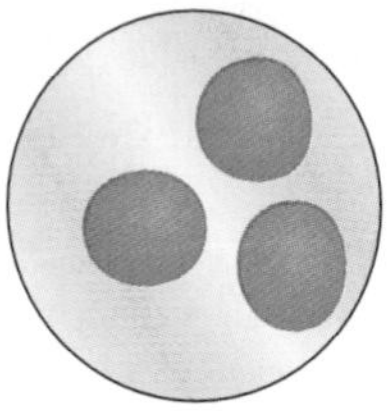	AIHA, HDN, and other extravascular hemolytic processes; hereditary spherocytosis	Stomatocytes (mouth cells)	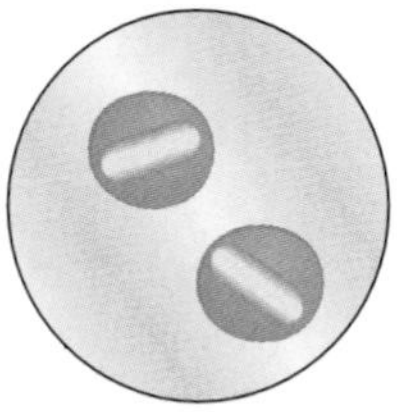	Liver disease, hereditary stomatocytosis
Elliptocytes	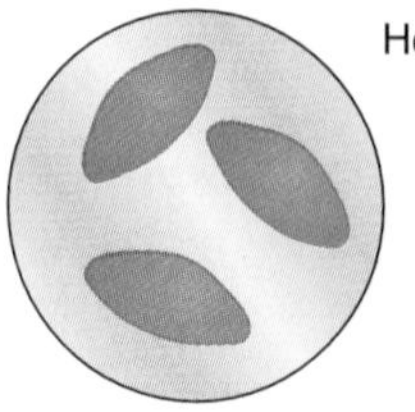	Hereditary elliptocytosis			

FIGURE 10–4
Erythrocyte morphology and the associated abnormality.

RBC Inclusion	Morphology	Stain	Correlations
Hemoglobin C crystals		Wright-Giemsa	HbC Post splenectomy
Howell-Jolly body DNA		Wright-Giemsa	Abnormal erythropoiesis Vitamin B_{12} deficiency
Basophilic stippling RNA		Wright-Giemsa New methylene blue	Lead poisoning Thalassemia
Pappenheimer bodies Pale blue patches Siderotic granules Iron		Wright-Giemsa Prussian blue	Sideroblastic anemia Hemoglobinopathies
Heinz bodies Denatured hemoglobins		Supravital stain such as cresyl blue (NOT seen with Wright's stain)	Unstable hemoglobins G-6-PD deficiency Thalassemia
Cabot rings Nuclear remnants		Wright-Giemsa	Megaloblastic anemia
Parasites Malaria		Wright-Giemsa	Parasitic infection Malaria Babesia Trypanosomes

F I G U R E 10–5
Erythrocyte inclusions and the associated abnormality.

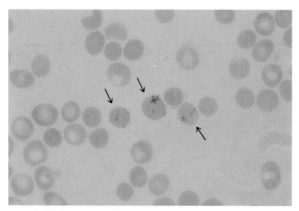

F I G U R E 10–6
Reticulocyte preparation. Note the three cells in the center with a visible precipitated RNA reticulum. All red blood cells are counted, and the total number of reticulocytes is recorded until approximately 1000 red blood cells have been counted.

2. Place the stain components in a 100-ml volumetric flask and dilute with distilled water to the calibration mark. Mix well.

3. Store in a clean, dark bottle at room temperature (approximately 25° C), labeled with the name of the reagent, the date, time, and name of the individual preparing the solution.

4. Filter the stain before each use.

5. Add equal volumes of whole blood and reticulocyte stain and mix.

6. Allow to stain for at least 2 minutes. Be consistent and always stain the same amount of time once the laboratory procedure has been established.

7. Mix the solution and prepare at least two peripheral blood smears with adequate monolayers for evaluation of individual red blood cells. Air dry the smears.

8. Routine light microscope method of counting reticulocytes:

   a. Bring the reticulocyte smear into clear focus in the good monolayer area with a 100× (oil immersion) objective in place (care and use of the microscope are presented in Chapter 1).

   b. In a consistent fashion with a counter, count the red blood cells in an area of the monolayer containing approximately 100 cells (see Fig. 10–3).

   c. Any of the red blood cells counted that contain visible reticulum (see Fig. 10–6) are recorded as reticulocytes. (Reticulocytes are included in both counts: once in the red blood cell count and again in the reticulocyte count.)

   d. Repeat b and c until approximately 1000 red blood cells have been counted microscopically in the monolayer area of the smear. Do not stop in the last field of cells (closest to 1000). Complete the field, and record the total number of erythrocytes counted.

   e. The following calculation is done to determine the observed level of reticulocytes in the peripheral blood.

   $$\frac{\text{Number of reticulocytes recorded}}{\text{Number of erythrocytes counted}}$$
   $$= \% \text{ of reticulocytes in peripheral blood}$$

   f. The reticulocyte reference range is approximately 0.5 to 1.5%. There are modifications of this technique that include placing a calibrated optical device in one ocular of the microscope to allow a more accurate reproducible count.

9. The Miller disk (Fig. 10–7) procedure is as follows:

   a. A reticulocyte peripheral blood smear is prepared.

   b. A Miller disk is placed in one ocular of the light microscope.

   c. A good monolayer area of the smear,

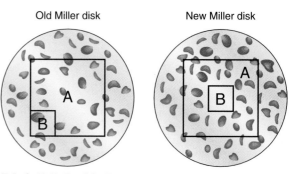

Old Miller disk   New Miller disk

F I G U R E 10–7
The Miller disk counting ocular device for reticulocyte counting.

with approximately 100 cells/field, is located.

d. The red blood cells in the smaller square are counted with a counter.

e. The reticulocytes in the larger square (A) are recorded. Any reticulocytes that appear in the small square (B) are counted twice: once in the red blood cell count and again in the reticulocyte count.

f. Repeat d and e until approximately 500 red blood cells have been counted microscopically in the monolayer area of the smear. Do not stop in the last field of cells (closest to 500). Complete the field and record the total number of erythrocytes counted.

g. Duplicate slides must be examined for demonstration of precision and quality control of the procedure. Options are counting 500 on each of two slides, or another laboratory practitioner can count 500 cells on the duplicate slide.

h. The following calculation is done to determine the observed level of reticulocytes in the peripheral blood.

$$\frac{\text{Number of reticulocytes in square A}}{\text{Total erythrocytes counted in square B} \times 9}$$
$$\times 100 = \% \text{ of reticulocytes}$$

i. The reticulocyte reference range is approximately 0.5 to 1.5%.

Corrective calculations for a patient's abnormal hematocrit, severity of the anemia, and so forth are presented later in this chapter.

Sources of Error. The manual reticulocyte count has many sources of error: the **randomness of the slide prepared;** the **quality of the stain;** incorrect **calculations;** and the **personal bias** of the individual performing the count, which compromises accuracy and precision.

Correlation. The reticulocyte count will correlate roughly with the appearance of stress reticulocytes **(polychromatic cells)** with a Wright-Giemsa stained peripheral blood smear. However, many reticulocytes are not visible with Wright's stain if they are more mature. An awareness of the correlation of the appearance of stress reticulocytes on a Wright-Giemsa stained peripheral blood smear with a significantly elevated reticulocyte count is a method of validating elevated reticulocyte results, although this is not a quantitative correlation. The **reticulocyte count** is the best **index of bone marrow function.** If a patient is anemic and the bone marrow is functioning properly, the reticulocyte count will be elevated in response.

Automated methods for reticulocyte counting are also available, two of which are offered by the Coulter and Sysmex instruments. Standardization of the method must be done, and laboratory reference values may need to be reassessed, as with any new procedure. The advantage of the automated system is the **reproducibility of results** and the **ability to analyze a greater number of cells (30,000** compared with 1000 manually). An example of the methodology for reticulocyte counting is flow cytometry using forward light scatter for a size indicator and **fluorescence for a more accurate RNA content,** hence **reticulocyte identification.** A fluorescent dye that binds to the RNA reticulum allows the laser in the instrument to quantitate the number of reticulocytes within a given number of erythrocytes. Several manufacturers produce automated reticulocyte counting instruments or have developed modifications to their cell counting instruments that offer the advantage of reticulocyte counting in addition to the CBC results without purchasing a separate instrument.

There are also **additional reticulocyte calculations** that may be reported in order to more accurately reflect the true, thus accurate, reticulocytosis. The **absolute count** (number of reticulocytes × erythrocyte count) can be determined and used for further calculations. The absolute value can be **corrected** (compared with the reference value) to determine how many more reticulocytes are in this patient's blood than are normally present. The average absolute reticulocyte count is $50 \times 10^9/l$, which is divided into the patient's absolute count. The **reticulocyte production index (RPI)** accounts for the 2 days required for the average reticulocyte to mature in the peripheral blood.

The reticulocyte calculations are as follows:

Patient values:
Erythrocyte count
$$2.40 \times 10^{12}/l \text{ (ref. } 4\text{–}5 \times 10^{12}/l)$$
Reticulocyte count   8% (ref. 0.5–1.5%)
Hematocrit
$$0.22 \text{ g/dl } (0.33\text{–}0.54\text{g/dl})$$

Absolute reticulocyte count:
$$8\% \times 2.40 \times 10^{12}/l = 192 \times 10^9/l$$

Comparison to reference count:
$$\frac{192 \times 10^9/l}{50 \times 10^9/l} = 4 \text{ times as many reticulocytes}$$

Correction for anemia:
$$\frac{8\%(\text{patient's reticulocytes})}{1\%(\text{reference reticulocytes})}$$

$$\times \frac{0.22(\text{patient's hct})}{0.45(\text{reference hct})} = 4\%$$

reticulocytes after considering less erythrocytes due to anemia.

Reticulocyte production index (RPI) $\dfrac{4}{2} = 2\%$

reticulocyte production by bone marrow.

Correction for a shift to the left (immature cells)

Reticulocytes take 2 days to mature. In this example, the reticulocyte release from the bone marrow is only 0.5% above normal after correcting for the anemia.

The calculations are necessary to assess the **accurate bone marrow response to the anemia.** The bone marrow can produce twice the normal red blood cells within 1 week if the hematocrit decreases to 0.35 and the iron supply is adequate. If the hematocrit decreases to 0.25, the normal healthy bone marrow can produce three times as many red blood cells as usual. If additional iron is available, the bone marrow can produce up to eight times as many red blood cells to meet the body's demand for oxygen.

An **iron stain** is a **monochromatic** (one color), nonvital (applied after cells have been fixed on a slide) stain that is also called **Prussian blue** iron stain. The majority of iron (Fe) in the body is incorporated into the hemoglobin molecule. The rest is in storage forms such as ferritin or hemosiderin, and a small amount is necessary for various metabolic body functions. Any extra HbFe in red blood cells is seen on Wright's stain as **Pappenheimer bodies** (**blue patches** within the red blood cells) and with Prussian blue iron stain as a **few irregular granules** within the mature red blood cell (see Fig. 10–5). These cells are called **siderocytes.** The Fe stain is primarily used for bone marrow (BM) smear preparations to determine the amount of storage Fe available in the macrophages of the **BM (histiocytes)** for use in erythropoiesis. A moderate amount of iron should be observed in most of the histiocytes in the bone marrow if iron is not the cause of anemia. If **no iron** is seen in the histiocytes using an iron stain, **iron deficiency** is suspected; if **excess iron** is observed, **anemia of chronic diseases** is suspected.

Heinz body stains such as brilliant cresyl blue or methyl violet are vital stains for the purpose of demonstrating **unstable hemoglobin** in the erythrocytes. Individuals who are **deficient in the enzyme glucose-6-phosphate dehydrogenase (G-6-PD)** are unable to maintain their hemoglobin in the reduced (ferrous, +2) state that is required for transport of oxygen. This enzyme functions in the hexose monophosphate shunt (HMPS), which is presented in Chapter 7 (see Fig. 7–11), to reduce glutathione, which in turn reduces the HbFe. If hemoglobin is not functional, it becomes unstable and will precipitate into Heinz bodies when stained with the Heinz body stain and examined microscopically (Fig. 10–5).

A **cytochemical stain** to aid in diagnosis of acute erythroleukemia is the periodic acid-Schiff (PAS) stain (see Table 9–2). The PAS stains glycogen in the cell cytoplasm, which appears as red blocks. Polycythemia does not involve a leukemic cell, and the normoblasts in the bone marrow do not demonstrate the visible cytoplasmic glycogen as seen in the acute erythroleukemic (AEL, FAB M6) blasts.

SPECIAL ERYTHROCYTE TESTS

Sickle cell screening tests subject an aliquot of lysed, reduced blood to a high molarity phosphate buffer, which will form polymers and become turbid if HbS is present. The **insolubility of HbS** is compared with a reference specimen that is soluble, producing a clear suspension (Fig. 10–8). The lysed red blood cells are treated with **dithionite** (sodium hydrosulfite), which reduces the **HbS** and renders it **insoluble** in the concentrated inorganic buffers present in the test system, resulting in an **opaque (cloudy) solution.** If only HbA is present, the solution will remain clear enough to read newsprint through the tube containing the test specimen. **Confirmation** of a positive solubility screening test result requires an **Hb electrophoresis** to specifically identify the presence of an abnormal hemoglobin.

Hb solubility screening tests are inexpensive, and the reaction takes only 5 minutes. The Hb electrophoresis confirmatory test is more expensive and takes over 1 hour. The screening tests are available from several laboratory supply companies under various names. A crude, but interesting, procedure to determine the presence of **HbS** is the **wet prep.** A small drop of whole blood is placed on a glass slide; a drop of sodium metabisulfate (reducing agent) is added; a coverslip is placed over the two drops and sealed with petroleum jelly. This slide is examined under light microscopy at 40× magnification, and the shape of the erythrocytes is observed and recorded. The slide is placed in a moist chamber and examined at intervals of 30 minutes and again at 1 hour. If HbS is present in any amount, the normocytic erythrocytes will begin sickling within 30 minutes and the majority of erythrocytes will be obviously sickled within 1 hour. Two other abnormal hemoglobins are less soluble than HbA: These are HbC and HbD, and they may give a positive screening test result. The hemoglobin electrophoresis will identify the specific hemoglobin present.

Hemoglobin electrophoresis is the separation, by electrical current, of the hemoglobins for identification and quantitation. Similar to the protein electrophoresis described in Chapter 6, hemoglobin electrophoresis (Hb EP) utilizes the different charges of the globin chains to separate the various Hb in a reproducible manner for identification and quantitation.

A hemolysate is prepared from whole blood (EDTA, heparin, or citrate) used fresh or after storage at 4° C. The hemolysate is applied to the electrophoresis medium (cellulose acetate, agarose gel, citrate agar gel, or starch gel) and allowed to migrate under electrical current (electrophorese) (Fig. 10–9). The medium is then stained or marked to allow identification and measurement of hemoglobin bands. There are more than 400 hemoglobins, many of which are so similar in globin chain structure that they will migrate together in a specific pH and medium. This is the reason why there are variations in electrophoresis techniques. The cellulose acetate medium is electrophoresed at a pH of 8.6 versus the citrate agar medium, which is electrophoresed at an acid pH of 6.8 in order to change the separation pattern of the hemoglobins in the specimen.

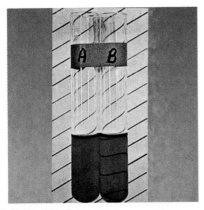

FIGURE 10–8

Sickle cell solubility screening test. The specimen containing HbS labeled A is cloudy, and the printed lines cannot be seen through the solution. The normal soluble HbA specimen labeled B is clear, and the printed lines are clearly seen.

Step 1. Application of hemolysate

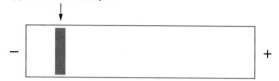

Step 2. Electrophoresis of hemoglobin on a strip of cellulose acetate connecting two buffer baths (pH of 8.4)

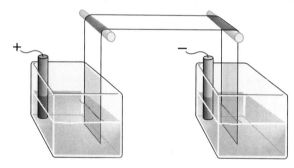

Step 3. Stained hemoglobin bands

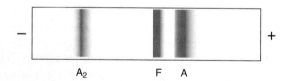

Step 4. Interpretation of results compared with a known control specimen

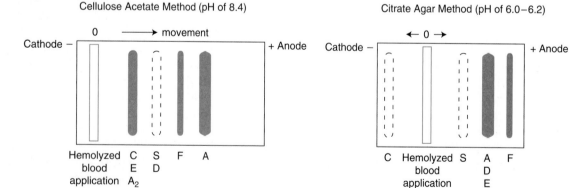

FIGURE 10–9

Hb electrophoresis procedure for identification of Hb present in the specimen. Solid bands are examples of normal hemoglobins; open bands are examples of abnormal hemoglobins. Citrate agar, at an acid pH, is used to separate HbS from HbD.

Hb electrophoresis is done to facilitate identification of a decreased, increased, or abnormal hemoglobin in the patient's erythrocytes.

HbF, in fetal cells, is discovered by the **resistance of HbF to acid elution and alkali denaturation.** The **presence of fetal cells, containing HbF, in the mother's circulation** aids in diagnosis and treatment of **hemolytic disease of the newborn (HDN).** During **pregnancy,** the **maternal blood** and fetal blood should never come into contact with one another. All substances move through membranes to and from the mother. If a pregnant woman experiences bleeding of the fetal blood into her blood stream, there is a potential for an **immune response.** If the fetal cells carry strong antigens from the father (e.g., RhD), which the mother does not have, these antigens will be recognized as foreign invaders and **antibodies will be produced against these fetal cells.** The antibody (anti-Rh D) produced will then pass the placenta into the fetal circulation and destroy the baby's cells. The resultant hemolytic disease of the newborn (HDN) will produce anemia, mental retardation, or stillbirth. In order to try to avoid such an outcome, the blood bank (immunohematology) area of the laboratory must know **how many of the fetal cells entered the mother.** This information will facilitate **administration of the correct amount of Rh immune globulin (RhIg) to prevent a primary immune response in the mother,** resulting in the production of anti-D antibodies directed against the baby's anti-D erythrocyte antigens. The hemoglobin electrophoresis is not adequate for this fetal hemoglobin quantitation due to the small quantity of HbF. Agglutination tests are available and are used more often to identify fetal cells in the mother's circulation. These tests are described later in this section. The agglutination tests are performed in the blood bank area of the laboratory. If the alkali denaturization test is done, the blood bank, hematology area, and chemistry area work together for the benefit of the mother and the fetus.

The **acid elution test** utilizes the fact that whereas **HbF is resistant to acid elution,** the mother's **HbA is not** and will be destroyed. All hemoglobin is precipitated when a peripheral blood smear is made and fixed in alcohol for staining. Treatment of the smears with an acid-phosphate buffer (pH of 3.3) will elute all precipitated hemoglobin except HbF. This results in only cells containing HbF staining red with the eosin stain component of the Wright-Giemsa stain. The remaining cells are ghost cells without hemoglobin. Known normal and abnormal (cord cells and adult cells) control blood smears should be stained and evaluated in the same manner as the duplicate patient slides.

The **alkali denaturation** test can also be used for the detection of **resistant hemoglobin F** present in the red blood cells of the fetus in the mother's blood for diagnosis of hemolytic disease of the newborn (HDN). This determination of fetal hemoglobin in the mother's blood is necessary for effective treatment of HDN by administration of Rh immune globulin (RhIg). A hemolysate of the mother's blood is read by the cyanmethemoglobin method in a spectrophotometer for total Hb level of both the fetal HbF and the mother's Hb. A second hemolysate of the mother's blood is incubated at 20° C with potassium hydroxide (KOH; pH of 12.7) for 2 minutes. The reaction is stopped; and the specimen is filtered and read in duplicate with known normal and known abnormal controls. The mother's Hb would have denatured and the solution would contain only the HbF available for the cyanmethemoglobin procedure. The calculation is as follows:

$$\frac{\text{Optical density of HbF}}{\text{Optical density of total Hb}}$$
$$\times \text{ fetal Hb dilution} \times 100 = \% \text{ HbF}$$

The manual Hb procedure used here may be done in the chemistry department where spectrophotometric methodology is readily available.

There are more practical tests available to aid in **diagnosis of Rh D HDN,** such as **slide agglutination tests** to detect fetal cells in the mother's blood. These tests agglutinate the Rh D positive fetal cells, while the mother's Rh D negative cells would remain free in suspension. If the quantity of fetal cells entering the mother can be determined, the correct amount of Rh immune globulin (RhIg) can be administered. RhIg is an antibody directed against the Rh D antigen on the baby's cells to destroy these cells in the mother's circulation before the mother develops a primary immune response with production of antibodies against the fetal red blood cells in subsequent pregnancies, which would move into the fetal circulation and be detrimental.

Iron, which is a key component of hemoglobin, is also used for the muscular oxygen transport by the myoglobin protein and is required for the proper function of a few body tissue enzymes. Iron is not synthesized in the body; therefore, iron levels are dependent on dietary intake and body metabolism (Fig. 10–10). The iron stores and iron in various capacities of transportation can be measured to assess the overall picture of the body's store of iron. Tests available for evaluation of the iron level are the serum iron, total iron-binding capacity, percent saturation, and ferritin. These tests are performed in the chemistry area of the laboratory and, combined with the hematology results, provide a more complete picture of the patient to the physician for diagnosis and treatment.

Serum ferritin is a soluble storage form of iron that is proportional to the iron stored throughout the body tissues. Serum ferritin is a sensitive indicator of iron deficiency and anemia of chronic disease discussed in Chapter 9. In **chronic disorders** such as inflammation, infection, malignancy, and viral hepatitis, serum **ferritin is elevated** and may mislead a laboratory investigation. If an individual is chronically ill and deficient in iron, the serum ferritin level may be normal. The serum ferritin test requires a very small amount of serum (20 to 110 μl) and is performed in the chemistry or a special area of the laboratory using techniques such as radioimmunoassay (RIA) and enzyme immunoassay (EIA). **Serum ferritin reference values are 20 to 200 ng/ml.**

Serum iron is the traditional colorimetric measurement used to determine the iron

available in the serum for use in erythropoiesis. Iron is lost through renal excretion if not bound to a transport protein such as transferrin. In order to measure serum iron, it must be disassociated from the carrier protein by exposure to strong acids. Serum iron is not as closely related to the body's stores as is the ferritin level. Diet, hemolysis, and other body parameters (e.g., sleep) can alter the serum iron for relatively short periods of time. Serum iron is low in iron deficiency anemia as well as anemia of chronic disease in which there are adequate iron stores. The reference values for serum iron are 75 to 175 μg/dl.

Total iron-binding capacity (TIBC) is a measure of the carrier protein **transferrin,** which is not bound to iron. For this reason, the TIBC values are inversely proportional to the iron level. If iron is decreased, the unbound transferrin or iron-binding capacity of transferrin is increased. Reference values for TIBC are 300 to 360 μg/dl and decrease with age. By age 70, the average value is 250 μg/dl.

Serum transferrin can now be measured by enzyme immunoassay and correlates very well with TIBC. Transferrin is a late acute phase reactant (APR) that will **rise late in inflammation.** This variation in proteins, due to an unrelated cause, **must be considered** when interpreting data.

Transferrin saturation (% saturation) is calculated from serum iron and TIBC values.

$$\frac{\text{Serum iron}}{\text{TIBC}} \times \% \text{ saturation}$$

This is a more accurate evaluation of iron than serum iron alone; however, this evaluation is not as accurate as that of serum ferritin. Reference values for iron saturation of transferrin are 20 to 55%.

Hemoglobin breakdown results in components other than iron being recycled, metabolized, or lost from the body. The following tests will provide key information for an accurate diagnosis and treatment of erythrocyte disorders (Fig. 10–11; see also Fig. 9–15).

Haptoglobin levels assist in the diagnosis of intravascular hemolysis. If cells are lysed within the vasculature, the free hemoglobin is rescued from loss through the kidneys primar-

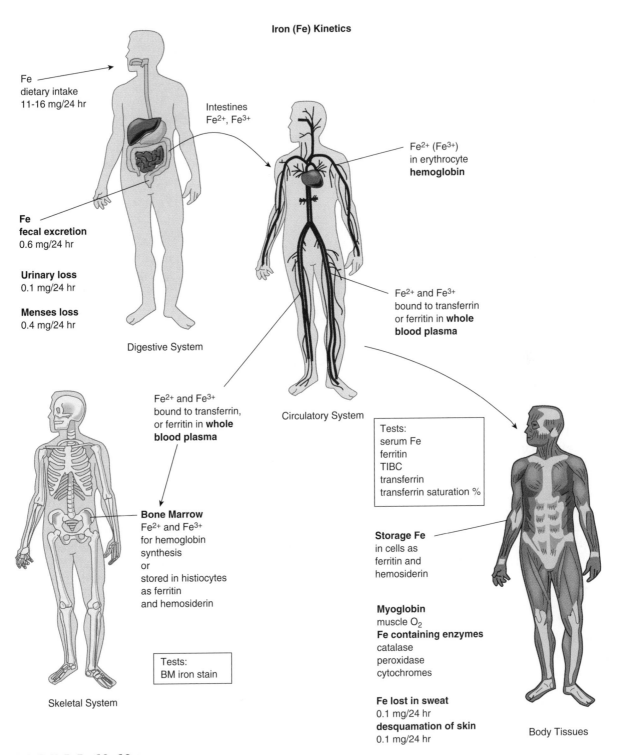

Iron (Fe) Kinetics

Fe
dietary intake
11-16 mg/24 hr

Intestines
Fe^{2+}, Fe^{3+}

Fe^{2+} (Fe^{3+})
in erythrocyte
hemoglobin

**Fe
fecal excretion**
0.6 mg/24 hr

Urinary loss
0.1 mg/24 hr

Menses loss
0.4 mg/24 hr

Fe^{2+} and Fe^{3+}
bound to transferrin
or ferritin in **whole
blood plasma**

Digestive System

Fe^{2+} and Fe^{3+}
bound to transferrin,
or ferritin in **whole
blood plasma**

Circulatory System

Tests:
serum Fe
ferritin
TIBC
transferrin
transferrin saturation %

Bone Marrow
Fe^{2+} and Fe^{3+}
for hemoglobin
synthesis
or
stored in histiocytes
as ferritin
and hemosiderin

Storage Fe
in cells as
ferritin and
hemosiderin

Myoglobin
muscle O_2
Fe containing enzymes
catalase
peroxidase
cytochromes

Tests:
BM iron stain

Fe lost in sweat
0.1 mg/24 hr
desquamation of skin
0.1 mg/24 hr

Skeletal System

Body Tissues

F I G U R E   10–10
Iron (Fe) kinetics and testing.

Hemoglobin Breakdown

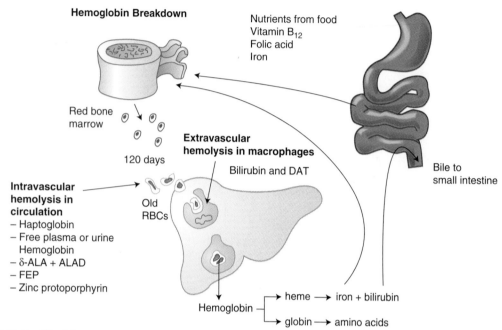

FIGURE 10–11
Hemoglobin breakdown and testing.

ily by the protein haptoglobin and, to a lesser extent, by hemopexin and albumin. The amount of haptoglobin that is not bound to free Hb is measured and is, therefore, **inversely proportional to the amount of free Hb.** If free hemoglobin is increased, haptoglobin will be decreased and vice versa. Haptoglobin is an acute-phase reactant (APR) that **increases in inflammation** and distorts the relationship with free Hb. Reference values for haptoglobin are **26 to 185 mg/dl,** and this test is performed in the chemistry area of the laboratory.

Free plasma or urine hemoglobin is seen in **hemolytic disorders** in which the rate of intravascular hemolysis exceeds the carrier protein's (e.g., haptoglobin) ability to bind with the hemoglobin for recycling in the body rather than be lost through the kidney. Excess free Hb passes readily through the kidney into the urine **(hemoglobinuria)** and is detected as part of a routine urinalysis. Hemosiderin (storage form of iron) may also be present in the urine **(hemosiderinuria)** due to excess iron from hemoglobin breakdown. Free Hb at high levels will be evident by red

plasma. Hb or hemosiderin in excess will result in a **red to brown urine.**

Bilirubin is a product of **hemoglobin breakdown.** The plasma will look yellow, and excessive bilirubin is toxic to tissues of the central nervous system. Bilirubin is **detoxified in the liver** for excretion as urobilinogen; therefore, liver failure (i.e., newborns with undeveloped liver enzymes) as well as hemolysis will result in high levels of bilirubin in the blood. Bilirubin is a **chemistry test** that relates directly to hemolytic anemia. Bilirubin can be tested and reported in several forms—total, conjugated, and unconjugated. The reference values for total bilirubin are 0.3 to 1.1 mg/dl.

Direct antiglobulin test (DAT) is a diagnostic test for **autoimmune hemolytic anemias (AIHA)** such as paroxysmal cold hemoglobinuria **(PCH) and alloimmune hemolytic anemias** such as hemolytic disease of the newborn **(HDN)** and hemolytic transfusion reactions **(HTR).** The specimen of choice is whole blood suspended in EDTA anticoagulant. The DAT is performed in the **blood bank area** of the laboratory and demonstrates the presence of **antibodies and complement components directed against erythrocyte antigens** that opsonize or coat the cell. Erythrocytes are not coated with antibodies unless there is an abnormality of some kind; therefore, DAT results should be negative. A **positive DAT** result indicates that the erythrocytes are opsonized, which will result in their destruction by macrophages (i.e., **extravascular hemolysis**).

Delta-aminolevulinic acid (δ-ALA) synthetase and δ-aminolevulinic acid dehydratase (ALAD) levels in urine are tests to aid in the diagnosis and treatment of heme synthesis abnormalities (e.g., porphyria or lead poisoning) and in the event of excessive intravascular hemolysis. δ-ALA reference values are 1.3 to 7 mg/dl per 24-hour urine.

Free erythrocyte protoporphyrin (FEP) and these tests are performed in the chemistry area of the laboratory. Reference values are less than 35 mg/dl FEP. This test provides additional information concerning intravascular hemolysis.

Zinc protoporphyrin is elevated and, therefore, is useful as a diagnostic screening test in inorganic lead poisoning. The zinc protoporphyrin assay is a fluorimetric procedure that is performed in the chemistry area of the laboratory. This test, along with the urine ALA and free erythrocyte protoporphyrin level, provides information to the primary care provider regarding the diagnosis of lead poisoning. Zinc protoporphyrin reference values are 10 to 38 μg/dl packed cells.

Erythropoietin levels (EPO) are measured by radioimmunoassay (RIA) and enzyme immunoassay (EIA) in chemistry or a special area of the laboratory. Reference levels for EPO are 5 to 36 mU/ml.

Glucose-6-phosphate dehydrogenase (G-6-PD) levels are done to determine if hemolytic anemia is due to unstable hemoglobin. The unstable Hb is unable to carry O_2 and forms Heinz bodies leading to extravascular hemolysis. The specimen required is whole blood (WB) suspended in EDTA or heparin anticoagulant. This chemistry test has reference values of 10 to 14 U/g of Hb.

Erythrocyte folate concentrations are more reliable than are the serum folate levels. The specimen of choice is whole blood suspended in EDTA anticoagulant. An aliquot of the specimen is hemolysed to free the folate from the erythrocyte for testing. This test is performed in the chemistry department of most laboratories, and the normal reference range is 166 to 640 μg/l.

Shilling urinary excretion test is one method **for testing B_{12} absorption.** In order to first saturate body binding sites, 1000 μg of nonradioactive B_{12} is injected intramuscularly. The patient is simultaneously given 0.5 to 2 μg of radioisotope-labeled B_{12} orally. Urine specimens are collected 24 to 72 hours after ingestion and **assayed for radioactivity.** If the patient is absorbing the oral vitamin B_{12}, the radioisotope will be excreted in the urine as a by-product of vitamin B_{12} metabolism. This test is performed in a special area of chemistry or a separate radionuclide area of the clinical laboratory.

Vitamin B_{12} levels, serum folate levels, and lead levels can be determined to provide valuable information for the diagnosis and treatment of deficiencies. The specimen of choice for **vitamin B_{12}** and **folate** is **clear, fresh serum** after the patient has been **fasting. Lead** testing requires **whole blood in a metal-free container and suspended in EDTA** anticoagulant. These tests are done in the chemistry area of the laboratory. **Reference** values for **B_{12} are 200 to 835 pg/ml** for an adult, up to 1300 pg/ml for a newborn, and as low as 110 pg/ml for an individual over 60 years of age. **Serum folate reference** levels are **3 to 20 ng/ml. Lead** levels should not be **above 25 μg/dl**; greater than 100 μg/dl is toxic.

The **osmotic fragility test** indicates erythrocyte fragility to lysis. To maintain viable cells in vivo (in the body) or in vitro (outside the body), the cells must be suspended in a solution with an osmotic concentration relatively equal to their interior osmotic concentration. **Erythrocytes have a large surface:volume ratio that allows them to deliver oxygen more efficiently,** maintain flexibility to travel in small or obstructed areas of the body, and expand **without lysis** when the osmotic concentrations of the body are not isotonic (equal to 0.85% NaCl). **Normal healthy erythrocytes** can tolerate a broad range of osmotic concentrations **(0.85 to 0.55% and less)** due to their ability to expand or collapse as the environment changes (Fig. 10–12). If erythrocytes are osmotically fragile, they will swell and lyse, before normal healthy erythrocytes, in low osmotic (hypotonic) solutions. The osmotic fragility of the erythrocytes is increased in disorders such as **hereditary spherocytic anemia.** The already spherical cells have lost the ability to expand under osmotic pressure and will begin to **lyse significantly in a hypotonic solution** that is **less than 0.65%** (111.2 mmol/l). Large flat cells, such as target cells, have the ability to take in more water than normal, resulting in a decreased osmotic fragility. The osmotic fragility test is available as a kit with a series of osmotic concentrations (0.75 to 0.2% or 128.3 to 34.2 mmol/l NaCl) already dis-

pensed, and the laboratory practitioner needs only to add the patient's blood. The specimens are mixed and examined for hemolysis after 30 minutes at room temperature (25° C) and again after 24 hours at 37° C. The results are recorded. To measure the amount of hemolysis, the **specimens can be visibly compared** as cloudy versus clear, or they are centrifuged and an aliquot of the supernatant is **read spectrophotometrically.** The value for each NaCl concentration is then plotted and interpreted in relation to the reference curve. This test is time consuming and is not often requested.

The **sugar water test, sucrose hemolysis test, and the acidified serum test (Ham's test)** are associated with the diagnosis of **paroxysmal nocturnal hemoglobinuria (PNH).** These tests are available to investigate rare hemolytic anemias but are no longer practical to perform in most cases. PNH demonstrates hemoglobin in the urine right

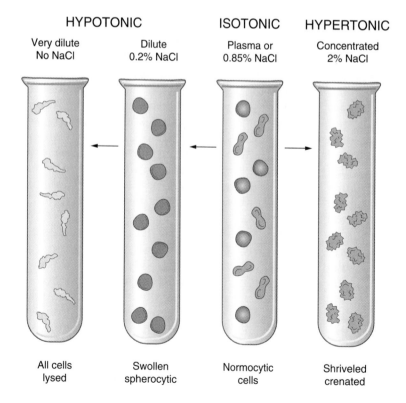

HYPOTONIC

Very dilute No NaCl	Dilute 0.2% NaCl

ISOTONIC

Plasma or 0.85% NaCl

HYPERTONIC

Concentrated 2% NaCl

All cells lysed

Swollen spherocytic

Normocytic cells

Shriveled crenated

FIGURE 10–12
Erythrocyte membrane shape changes associated with the osmotic environment.

after sleep in 25% of patients. **Hemosiderin-uria** (hemosiderin in the urine) is seen in most patients with PNH. This disease is an acquired sensitivity to complement activity, resulting in hemolysis that is enhanced by altering the pH or osmotic concentration. PNH, which is seen mostly in young adults, develops into a **chronic intravascular hemolytic anemia.**

Serum lactate dehydrogenase isoenzymes, LD-1 and LD-2, are **elevated** in vitamin B_{12} deficiency (pernicious anemia, [PA]) due to **increased hemolysis.** The isoenzyme LD pattern seen in hemolysis is similar to that seen in a **myocardial infarction** (MI, heart attack). The total LD activity can be up to $50\times$ normal in B_{12} deficiency hemolysis and returns to normal following successful treatment. The specimen of choice is fresh, clear serum, although heparinized plasma may also be used. The LD is made up of five fractions (LD-1 to LD-5) measured in the chemistry area of the laboratory. **LD** is also **elevated** in a variety of other disorders, such as **liver injury** and **muscle injury** or **inflammation.** All of these involve **cell damage.** LD reference values are different for each fraction, depending on the method used. In a healthy individual, a cellulose acetate electrophoresis of LD isoenzymes would reveal a total **serum LD of 100 to 190 U/l in which LD-1 makes up 18 to 33% and LD-2 makes up 28 to 40%.**

The **erythrocyte sedimentation rate (ESR)** is an inexpensive test to discover and monitor a significant elevation in serum proteins associated with disease. The specimen of choice is **whole blood** suspended in **EDTA or Na citrate anticoagulant.** Each manufacturer requires a specific type of specimen that provides the most accurate ESR test results in its system. This test is not testing erythrocytes and has little relevance to the erythrocytes themselves. The knowledge of the rouleaux phenomenon (see Fig. 5–12) (the stacking of red cells like coins in high-protein solutions, which results in increased sedimentation) is used to crudely **evaluate whole blood protein concentrations.** The more

plasma protein present, the more rapidly rouleaux phenomena will occur and the more elevated the sedimentation rate will be. The types of serum protein that are most often the cause of an elevated ESR are **antibodies** produced in autoimmune disorders such as rheumatoid arthritis (RA) or **inflammatory proteins,** which are produced in diseases such as Crohn's disease. An alternative test to detect inflammation is the C-reactive protein (CRP) test. The level of C-reactive protein is elevated in inflammatory conditions and can be detected using a latex agglutination technique. The CRP test is usually performed in the clinical immunology or serology area of the laboratory.

The ESR methodology requires forcing the **blood** up **into a 150-mm** long, narrow, **calibrated tube,** setting the filled tube **in a level rack at room temperature,** and observing how far the blood settles in **1 hour** (Fig. 10–13*B*). The tubes and other equipment necessary are readily available and disposable. This test can never be done for an emergency (STAT) rapid order. If the erythrocytes demonstrate any **anisocytosis** or **poikilocytosis** (abnormal sizes or shapes), rouleaux phenomena may not occur; thus, an **erroneously decreased** sedimentation rate will be observed and reported and will jeopardize the diagnosis and treatment of the patient. **Corrections** also need to be made for the ESR value if

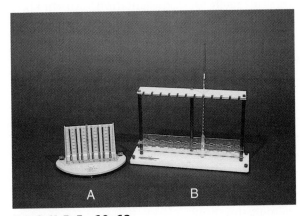

FIGURE 10–13
A. Westergren and *B.* Wintrobe erythrocyte sedimentation rate (ESR) equipment.

there is a decreased or increased erythrocyte count, as seen in **anemia** and **polycythemia.** Reference values for the Westergren method for children (0 to 10 mm/hr), for adult **women (0 to 20 mm/hr),** and adult men **(0 to 15 mm/hr)** increase by 5 to 10 mm/hr in persons older than 50 years of age.

The classical, but outdated, ESR procedure is the **Wintrobe method,** which requires filling a narrow, 10-mm, glass tube **(Wintrobe tube)** with a long Pasteur pipette, placing the filled tube in a **level rack** at room temperature, and observing for the **sedimentation of the cells over 1 hour** (see Fig. 10–13*A*). The placing of the blood in the Wintrobe tube with the long Pasteur pipette makes it difficult to fill the tube accurately and avoid air bubbles. The Wintrobe technique is now used primarily for **centrifuging** the blood in the Wintrobe tube to **concentrate the white blood** cells (in the **buffy coat**) for more accurate analysis of low white blood cell counts. The Wintrobe reference values are: 0 to 13 mm/hr for children; 0 to 20 mm/hr for adult women; and 0 to 9 mm/hr for adult men.

There are several Westergren **sedimentation rate test systems** available. The **differences** between them include the **specimen** anticoagulant, the **tube** used, how the tube is filled, and the **accuracy** of reading the result. It is very important to mix the specimen well before testing, have no air bubbles in the tube, and place the tube in a level vertical rack for sedimentation. Air bubbles will slow sedimentation and break up the column of cells. Sedimentation will be increased if the tube is held at an angle.

A more rapid centrifugal method for ESR, called the zeta sedimentation rate (ZSR) method, was developed, which provided rapid (approximately 15 minutes) results that were not altered by anemia. Reference values for ZSR were 41 to 54%. This method was not successful due to the requirement of a special centrifuge called a zetafuge, which was not easily repaired and quality assurance protocols were in question.

Red blood cell survival in the healthy individual is 120 days. If **hemolytic anemia** is present, this survival rate will be shortened

and may need to be confirmed by survival studies. An aliquot of the individual's erythrocytes in whole blood is **tagged with radioactive chromium (^{51}Cr).** These cells are injected back into the individual, and the survival of these erythroctyes (hence the radioactivity) is measured by drawing blood every 1 to 2 days for 2 weeks and counting the amount of ^{51}Cr that remains. When one half of the radioactivity is gone, the value is reported. The reference range for healthy individuals is **25 to 32 days,** keeping in mind that this is reduced from the expected 60 days due to the bound radioisotope that initiates the early destruction of some of the cells. In hemolytic anemia, the value will be less than 25 days.

Red blood cell mass is measured to **differentiate a physiologic polycythemia from an absolute or true polycythemia.** The red blood cell mass test is similar to the red blood cell survival presented previously; however, there is only one subsequent blood collection to determine the dilution of the original aliquot. The red blood cell mass can be determined by **calculating the dilution of the radioisotope-labeled red blood cells** within the total number of red blood cells. Other radioisotopes that are used instead of radioactive chromium (^{51}Cr) are technetium (^{99m}Tc) and phosphorus (^{32}P). Reference values for red blood cell mass are **20 to 30 ml/kg for women and 25 to 35 ml/kg for men.**

Plasma volume is used to **differentiate a transient shift of fluid producing a relative polycythemia versus a true decrease in plasma,** which is seen in **dehydration, shock, Addison's disease, and absolute polycythemia. Increased plasma volume is seen in starvation, splenomegaly, aldosteronism, and Cushing's syndrome.** The principle involves injecting **radioactive albumin ^{121}I** (a usual plasma protein) into an individual and drawing blood 20 minutes after injection to determine **how much the radioisotope was diluted.** This is similar to the red blood cell mass test previously explained. Reference values for plasma volume are related to gender and size. **Short, fat men and women** average **29 mg/kg and 27 mg/kg,** respectively. **Tall, thin men and women** average **46 mg/kg and 41 mg/kg.**

   Blood volume is represented by the **sum of the red blood cell mass and plasma volume.** This is also called the **whole body hematocrit.** The whole body hematocrit (blood volume) is lower than the venous hematocrit presented as part of the complete blood count.

STUDY QUESTIONS

Choose the best answer for the following:

1. A clot tube (red top) is delivered to the laboratory for diagnostic tests to support anemia. The blood component(s) obtained from this for hematology associated testing is (are):
   A. Clear, fresh serum
   B. Clear, fresh plasma
   C. Clotted blood
   D. Whole blood

2. The most likely test to perform using the specimen in question 1, which would rule out a common anemia, is the:
   A. Complete blood count (CBC)
   B. Hemoglobin and hematocrit
   C. Ferritin test
   D. Peripheral blood smear evaluation

An acceptable specimen for a CBC was analyzed. The results were:

RBC	Hb	Hct	MCV	MCHC	RDW
3×10^6 /ul	8.9 g/dl	28%	93.8 fl	32.9 g/dl	18%

3. Are there any reasons to question the validity of these results?
   A. Yes
   B. No

4a. If you chose "no" for question 3, choose the correct morphology based on the indices:
   A. Normocytic, normochromic
   B. Microcytic, hypochromic
   C. Macrocytic, normochromic
   D. Target cells are present.

4b. If you chose "yes" for question 3, what results need to be validated?
   A. The erythrocyte count is too low.
   B. The Hb and Hct do not correlate.
   C. The MCV does not reflect the RDW.
   D. The MCHC does not reflect the Hb.

5. An inclusion seen in erythrocytes when lead poisoning is suspected is:
   A. Basophilic stippling
   B. Siderotic granules
   C. Heinz bodies
   D. Polychromasia

6. Cells seen in association with most hemoglobinopathies are:
   A. Sickled cells
   B. Target cells
   C. Microcytic cells
   D. Spherocytes

7. The test done to confirm a positive result on a sickle cell screening test is:
   A. The reticulocyte count
   B. The peripheral blood smear morphology
   C. Genetic karyotyping
   D. Hb electrophoresis

Match the following mechanism of disease with the best test for diagnosis:

8. Increased destruction of erythrocytes   A. A reticulocyte count

9. Decreased production of erythrocytes   B. Direct antiglobulin test (DAT)

10. Abnormal synthesis of erythrocytes   C. Hb electrophoresis, ferritin level

Fill in the missing words:

11. _____ are used to determine the accuracy of the CBC test results.

12. _____ is determined by running each sample in triplicate to demonstrate the ability to obtain a similar acceptable result each time that the test is run.

13–15. Explain the impedance methodology of counting cells that is used by Coulter.

PART IV

Hemostasis

O U T L I N E

Origin, Maturation, and Morphology of Thrombocytes

Physiology and Function of Thrombocytes and Vasculature

Normal Responses and Diseases of Thrombocytes and Vasculature

Study Questions

Thrombocytes (Platelets) and Vasculature (Blood Vessels)

O B J E C T I V E S

Upon completion of this chapter the student should be able to:

1. Recognize a diagram or picture of a thrombocyte and be able to make a comparison to white blood cells.

2. Explain the life span, origin, and parent cell of the thrombocyte.

3. List the functional stages of the thrombocyte in the order in which these stages occur.

4. Explain the interaction between the thrombocyte and the coagulation pathways.

5. Apply knowledge of thrombocyte physiology to explain the effects of ingestion of aspirin and von Willebrand's disease.

6. Describe the testing for thrombocytes and the interpretation of the data.

7. Contrast and compare idiopathic thrombocytopenic purpura (ITP), thrombotic thrombocytopenic purpura (TTP), and disseminated intravascular coagulation (DIC).

Thrombocytes, also called **platelets,** differ significantly from erythrocytes and leukocytes. There is only **one population** of thrombocytes. The erythrocyte spends a lengthy life within the vasculature, whereas the thrombocyte has a shorter **life span** and **functions** both in and out of the vasculature (as does the leukocyte). The thrombocyte's **function is to initiate hemostasis,** which is a much different function than that of the five diverse white blood cells' function of defense against infection. The thrombocyte and the erythrocyte function **without a nucleus when they are mature,** whereas the leukocyte maintains (and in some cases utilizes) the nucleus throughout the life of the cell. The thrombocyte **requires cytoplasmic granules** to function (as do the granulocytic and monocytic leukocytes), whereas the lymphocytic leukocyte and erythrocyte do not. One unique aspect of the thrombocyte is its origin from the cytoplasm, rather than from maturation of a parent cell.

ORIGIN, MATURATION, AND MORPHOLOGY OF THROMBOCYTES

All of the blood cells originate from the pluripotent stem cell **(PSC),** which is under the influence of hematopoietic regulatory proteins **(cytokines).** The PSC becomes the hematopoietic stem cell **(HSC),** also known as the colony-forming unit–spleen **(CFU–S).** The HSC then differentiates into the colony-forming unit–granulocyte, erythrocyte, monocyte, megakaryocyte **(CFU–GEMM).** Growth factors specifically for the thrombocyte (megakaryocyte) cell line, such as **megakaryocyte colony-stimulating factor–mega (mega–CSF)** and a **thrombopoietin-like factor (TPO),** stimulate the CFU–GEMM to become the **colony-forming unit–megakaryocyte (CFU–mega, megakaryoblast),** which differentiates into the **promegakaryocyte,** the **megakaryocyte,** and then into the metamegakaryocyte, which loses fragments of the

mature cytoplasm and forms the **mature thrombocyte.** Normally, only the mature thrombocyte is found in the peripheral blood and in the tissues. The immature cells are found only in the bone marrow (Fig. 11–1). In megakaryocytic leukemia (FAB M7), immature megakaryocytes may circulate in the peripheral blood.

The **megakaryocyte is the largest cell in the bone marrow,** with abundant cytoplasm and a multi-lobed nucleus that is polyploid (i.e., has an increased DNA content). The megakaryocyte (Fig. 11–2) makes up only 1% of the nucleated bone marrow cells, because one parent cell can produce many mature thrombocytes. Unlike the other cell maturation schemes, the megakaryocytic cell line becomes larger as it matures until only the cytoplasmic fragments leave the bone marrow as the mature product (thrombocytes) (Fig. 11–3).

Formed elements of the blood were discussed earlier. The thrombocyte is about **2 to 4 μm** in diameter and up to 10 femtoliters (fl) in volume compared with the erythrocyte, which is 6 to 8 μm and 80 to 95 fl. Similar to the erythrocyte cell line, **larger thrombocytes** are a sign of **premature** release from the bone marrow under stress. The normal reference range is **150 to 400 $\times$ 10^9/l** or an approximate average of 8 to 20 per high-power field (40$\times$) in the random monolayer area of a peripheral blood smear. These cytoplasmic fragments of the parent megakaryocyte in the bone marrow appear with Wright-Giemsa stain to have a **gray-blue cytoplasm** and **purple functional granules** with **no nucleus** (see Fig. 11–3). There are two kinds of functional granules of interest in the thrombocyte as well as in the mitochondria, lysosomes, and other cytoplasmic organelles normally found in cells (Fig. 11–4). The lighter-staining granules are **alpha granules,** which contain several proteins including fibrinogen, von Willebrand's protein, and platelet factor 4 (PF4), which neutralizes the action of heparin, thus encouraging coagulation. Dense core granules (dense bodies) contain proteins and energy molecules such as adenosine diphosphate **(ADP)** and adenosine triphosphate **(ATP),** which are necessary

Hematopoietic Chart
of Cell Differentiation.

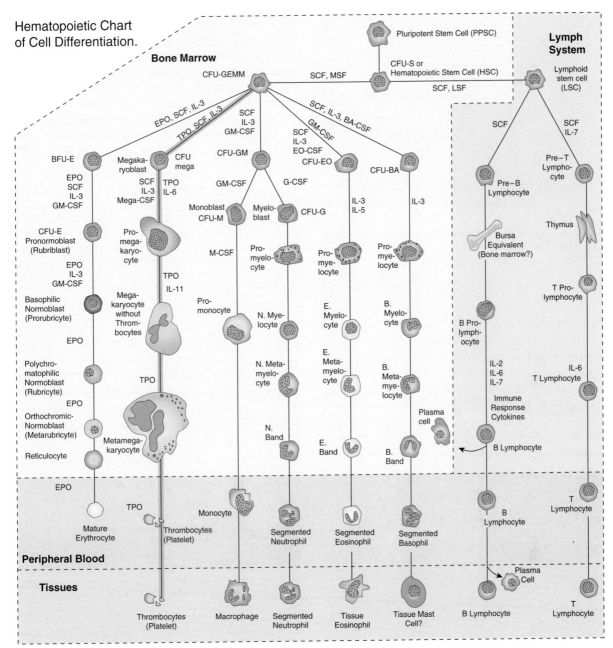

FIGURE 11-1
Hematopoietic chart with the thrombocyte (platelet) production highlighted.

for thrombocytes binding to each other (a process that is called aggregation).

Blood flows through **arteries, veins, arterioles, venules, and capillaries**, making up the circulatory **vasculature**, to deliver oxygen to all parts of the body. Two essential factors are required to maintain the blood within the vessels **(vascular integrity)** by resistance to vessel disruption: (1) **functional, circulating thrombocytes** to

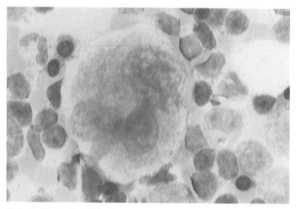

F I G U R E 11–2
A megakaryocyte, found only in the bone marrow. Note the size and nuclear pleomorphism.

sure without breaks in the endothelial lining. Blood leaking from the vasculature under the pressure of a tourniquet would produce small hemorrhagic spots called **petechiae.** The vasculature experiences small breaks and tears daily as a natural part of the processes of life. These normal weaknesses in the blood vessels are closed before enough blood escapes to produce petechiae, which are not normally seen.

These routine and expected disruptions of the blood vessel wall are minor and are quickly plugged by activated platelets (usually before any blood leakage is obvious). For this reason, vascular integrity cannot be evaluated unless an adequate number of functional thrombocytes are present in the blood vessel for the normal vascular integrity.

initially plug small tears, and (2) adequate connective tissue such as **collagen** and **hyaluronic acid** production to hold together the endothelial cells that line the vasculature. Connective tissue function is compromised by a lack of ascorbic acid (vitamin C) or long-term administration of corticosteroids. **Vascular integrity** is obvious every time that a **tourniquet is applied** and the blood vessels manage to contain the blood under this pres-

The endothelial surface of the lumen of the blood vessel (the tubular cavity) is smooth and constant. Any **alteration in the endothelial surface** may activate platelets and coagulation pathways with resulting **thrombus (clot) formation.** Examples of this would include cuts, cholesterol (lipid) plaque build-up or rupture, and artificial material such as heart valves and grafts.

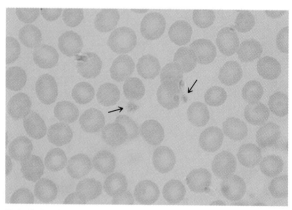

F I G U R E 11–3
Two normal-size platelets in the 100× microscopic field among normal-size erythrocytes. Note that there is some debris on the photograph. Don't mistake debris for platelets.

Do It Now — Thrombocyte Origin, Maturation, and Morphology

1. Make a chart with drawings of the relative sizes of formed elements in the peripheral blood. Start with the largest element, and end with the smallest element. Write the size and volume next to each drawing.
2. Together with other classmates, contrast and compare the origin, maturation, morphology, life span, and reference values of thrombocytes, erythrocytes, lymphocytes, granulocytes, and monocytes.
3. Discuss with other students or the instructor why there are four times as many granulocytic cells as there are erythroid cells and why there are only a few megakaryocytes in the bone marrow smear.

Thrombocyte (platelet) structure

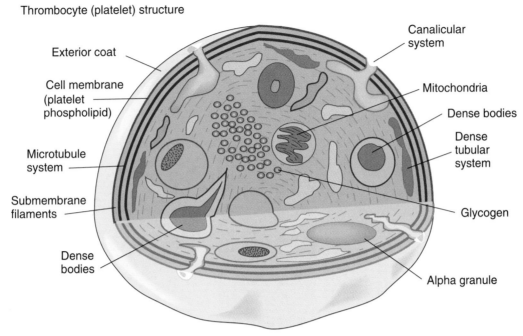

FIGURE 11–4
Platelet structure.

PHYSIOLOGY AND FUNCTION OF THROMBOCYTES AND VASCULATURE

The **thrombocyte** is a key component in the **initiation and conclusion of hemostasis.** The activated thrombocyte physically **forms a plug** at the site of injury along with other thrombocytes and this, as well as coagulation, is dependent on platelet-secreted proteins, energy molecules, Ca^{2+}, and platelet factors (Fig. 11–5). The **platelet-produced protein regulators** stimulate the **vasculature (blood vessels) to constrict** when injured, **activate other thrombocytes and coagulation factors,** and **finally contract or rearrange the thrombus** (clot) that is formed for adequate arrest of blood flow. Seven **factors** are associated with thrombocytes **(PF1–7).** Platelet factor 4 (PF4) neutralizes heparin, and PF3 is a platelet phospholipid

(PPL) that is necessary for adequate platelet function and coagulation. A major use of PF3 is in the production of **thromboxane A_2,** a potent platelet-**aggregating agent** and **vasoconstrictor.** Ingestion of **aspirin inhibits** the production of thromboxane A_2, which interferes with platelet function.

The functional stages of the thrombocyte include **shape change** and **adhesion** to nonthrombocyte surfaces in response to vascular **(blood vessel) injury, thus exposing the subendothelial surface.** Thrombocytes are also activated by any **artificial surface contact** or the plasma coagulation protein **thrombin.** The adherence of thrombocytes to an unnatural surface is **dependent on the von Willebrand factor (vWF)** from the platelet and also the plasma vWF associated with coagulation factor VIII (VIII : vWF). Following thrombocyte adhesion, **primary aggregation** of thrombocytes occurs. This initial plug is formed by thrombocytes attaching

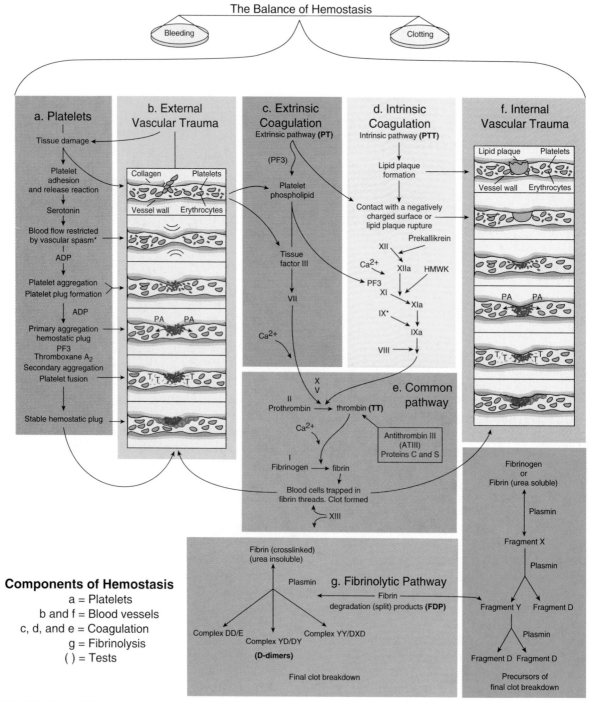

FIGURE 11–5

Hemostasis, including all components. The thrombocyte and vascular activity are shown in *A*, *B* and *F*.

reversibly to each other. **Release of thrombocyte granule contents** follows both adhesion and primary aggregation. Some of the energy molecules and chemicals released are **ADP** (to provide energy for platelet function), **serotonin** (to constrict blood vessels), and **platelet factor 4** (PF4 to neutralize heparin). **Secondary aggregation** results from increased levels of ADP, resulting from primary aggregation and granule release. This irreversible joining of thrombocytes to each other results in **PF3** (platelet membrane phospholipid), which is made available as a surface for the formation of fibrin by the coagulation pathways. The contraction **(rearrangement and compaction)** of the **final clot** depends on the contractile protein **thrombasthenin,** which is associated with thrombocyte membrane glycoproteins (IIa and IIIb). A genetic **absence** of glycoproteins IIa and IIIb (Glanzmann's thrombasthenia) will not allow binding of fibrinogen for conversion to fibrin, and **clot retraction cannot occur.**

NORMAL RESPONSES AND DISEASES OF THROMBOCYTES AND VASCULATURE

In the previous section of this chapter, the normal function of the vasculature was presented. Blood vessels are responsive to vaso-constrictors, which narrow the lumen to restrict blood flow, and vasodilators, which increase the size of the lumen and encourage a greater blood flow. **Disorders of vascularity** produce **petechiae** (very small hemorrhagic spots), **ecchymoses** (bruises and hemorrhagic spots larger than petechiae), and **purpura,** which is extensive hemorrhage into skin, mucous membranes, and organs. Petechiae are seen when a weak blood vessel is placed under pressure, such as when a tourniquet is applied. The tourniquet test is explained in Chapter 13. **Petechiae, ecchymoses,** and **purpura** may be the result of the following:

1. Direct **endothelial damage** (vascular trauma) from physical or chemical causes; lipid plaque formation; microbes such as rickettsia, bacterial toxins, antibody-mediated injury, drug reactions, insect bites, or activation of the plasma protein complement (see Fig. 11–5*F*).
2. **Hereditary telangiectasia,** an inherited decrease of vascular integrity
3. **Secondary** consequences of **another disease,** such as diabetes, which alters the vascular framework
4. **Decreased mechanical strength** of vessels as a result of scurvy (vitamin C deficiency) or amyloidosis
5. Development of **microthrombi** as in disseminated intravascular coagulation (DIC), which consume the thrombocytes
6. **Vascular malignancies,** such as Kaposi's sarcoma and vascular tumors

When a **small blood vessel** is injured, the vessel walls constrict to reduce blood flow. This process is called **vasoconstriction** (see Fig. 11–5*B* and *F*). This is a short-lived reflex action of the muscle. Vasoconstriction is then maintained as needed by the release of **serotonin** by activated thrombocytes. The **thrombocytes adhere** to the damaged vessel, **aggregate** with other platelets, and **release their granular content** to form an initial plug to stop the bleeding. This platelet plug of the blood vessel **provides the phospholipid surface** on which the final blood

Thrombocyte and Vascular Diseases and Disorders

Disorder	Etiology	Tests/Comments
Loss of vascular integrity:		
Endothelial damage	Trauma to the blood vessel	Petechiae, ecchymoses, and purpura
Hereditary telangiectasia	Genetic	Tourniquet test positive
2° to another disease	Diabetes	Poor circulation and nutrition
Decreased mechanical strength	Scurvy (vitamin C deficiency) or amyloidosis	Less connective tissue holding endothelial cells together
Microthrombi present	Disseminated intravascular coagulation (DIC)	Consuming thrombocytes Not a vascular problem False-positive result on a tourniquet test
Vascular malignancies	Kaposi's sarcoma and vascular tumors	
Thrombocytopenia:		
Inaccurate specimen or blood smear preparation	Poor technique Satellitism syndrome	$<100 \times 10^9/l$ thrombocytes Always examine the specimen. Carefully review the results.
Decreased thrombocyte production	Aplasia Bone marrow infiltration Vitamin B_{12} deficiency	Thrombocyte count Bone marrow examination Vitamin assay
Increased consumption or destruction	TTP, DIC, ITP, drug-induced immune response	Antibodies and complement
Abnormal distribution and dilution	Splenomegaly Liver cirrhosis Massive transfusion	Sequestration Alters body fluid distribution Dilution of thrombocytes in the blood
Thrombocytosis:		
Reactive thrombocytosis	Hemorrhage, trauma, postsurgery, malignancy, chronic infections, chronic iron deficiency, connective tissue disease (e.g., rheumatoid arthritis)	$>450 \times 10^9/l$ thrombocytes
Myeloproliferative diseases	Chronic myelocytic leukemia Polycythemia vera	CML $>1000 \times 10^9/l$ thrombocytes
Acute megakaryocytic leukemia (FAB M7)	Genetic tendency, leukemia virus, and initiating event (toxin exposure)	Cytochemical stains
Essential thrombocythemia	Uncontrolled megakaryocyte and platelet production	
Abnormal distribution	Post splenectomy	Two thirds of thrombocytes are sequestered in the spleen.
Thrombocyte dysfunction:		
	Genetic disorders	von Willebrand's disease Glanzmann's thrombasthenia Bernard-Soulier syndrome Gray platelet syndrome
	Acquired	Aspirin ingestion Hyperglobulinemia Myeloproliferative disorders Uremia and chemical toxicity Bleeding time test, adhesion tests, aggregation tests, factor assays

CML = chronic myelocytic leukemia; ITP = idiopathic thrombocytopenic purpura; TTP = thrombotic thrombocytopenic purpura.

coagulation takes place. The coagulation factors are activated and result in the **formation of fibrin** strands that engulf cells and platelets to **form the final blood clot** (Fig. 11–6), which holds the blood vessel intact for the injury to heal. Once the injury has healed, the **fibrinolytic pathway** of the hemostatic scheme **dissolves the clot** to allow blood to flow freely through the blood vessel. Not all bleeding can be controlled by the body. When an artery or vein is damaged extensively, beyond the ability of the thrombocytes and coagulation pathways, surgical intervention may be required in order to stop the bleeding.

As long as the blood is moving through the smooth surfaces of the circulatory system, all is well. If the **blood flow** becomes **sluggish,** there are **increased opportunities for clotting** to occur. This scenario is seen most often in individuals who are bed-ridden, experiencing post surgery inactivity, and possible activation of the coagulation system by the surgical procedure itself. For this reason walking is encouraged after surgery, and support stockings are used.

Clotting that appears to be spontaneous may occur **in response to tissue damage** due to an undiagnosed malignancy **(cancer).** This involves the coagulation system more than the platelets.

Atherosclerotic plaques develop at sites of altered blood flow, such as areas of arterial branching. Lipid or cholesterol plaque formation, on the walls of the blood vessels, decreases the flow of blood and encourages clotting. The lipids are measured in the **chemistry area** of the clinical laboratory, as **high-density lipoprotein (HDL),** which is antiplaque forming, and **low-density lipoprotein (LDL),** which is a known contributor to **plaque formation.** Research has shown that consumption of a moderate amount of red wine every day increases the level of HDL, thus reducing the risk of cardiovascular disease. If a plaque ruptures, a rough surface is exposed, which activates platelets and coagulation factors to **encourage and enhance clot formation** (see Fig. 11–5F).

The routine complete blood count (CBC) will reveal a **quantitative** thrombocyte disorder. A decrease in the number of thrombocytes is called **thrombocytopenia** and is defined as **< 100 × 10⁹/l thrombocytes.** Thrombocytopenia results in spontaneous clinical bleeding, which is seen as petechiae (small purple hemorrhagic spots), ecchymoses (purple hemorrhagic bruises that are larger than petechiae), or purpura (diffuse bleeding in large purple to brown areas) in the patient's mucous membranes and skin.

Thrombocytopenia may be the result of:

1. An **inaccurate specimen** leading to **erroneously low thrombocyte counts.** If the **specimen is not mixed well** upon collection, platelets may have already aggregated, resulting in several platelets being counted as one large platelet and thus decreasing the number available for the counting procedure. If the patient has **satellitism syndrome,** the platelets in the specimen adhere to the neutrophil membrane when exposed to EDTA anticoagulant. **The thrombocytes attached to the neutrophil** will not be counted and, therefore, an erroneous count results. This syndrome, however, can be **seen on the peripheral** blood smear. Redrawing the specimen into an **Na citrate (blue top) tube** instead of an EDTA tube will **maintain free flowing platelets,** inhibiting the satellitism seen with an EDTA specimen.

The **peripheral blood smear** must be

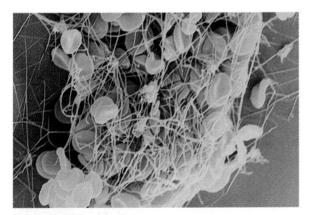

FIGURE 11–6
A scanning electron microscope photograph of a blood clot (also called a thrombus or a red clot), magnified 125,000 times. Note the cells trapped within the fibrin strands.

adequately made after mixing the specimen thoroughly to prepare a **random distribution of cells and platelets.** Any evaluations should be performed only in the randomly distributed **monolayer of a Wright-Giemsa–stained slide.**

2. **Decreased thrombocyte production** (hypoproliferation) or ineffective megakaryocytopoiesis in the bone marrow may be acquired or hereditary. Diseases associated with this are **aplasia** (inability of the bone marrow to produce any blood components), **infiltration of the bone marrow** by abnormal cell growth (i.e., myelofibrosis and leukemia), and **vitamin B$_{12}$ deficiency,** which prevents adequate DNA synthesis for normal and adequate cell production.

3. **Increased consumption** due to utilization in the clotting process may be another cause. Diseases associated with consumption are **thrombotic thrombocytopenic purpura (TTP)** and **disseminated intravascular coagulation (DIC).**

Thrombotic thrombocytopenic purpura (TTP) involves the development of clots, which are made up mostly of platelets and, therefore, are called "white clots." The white clots consume the thrombocytes, resulting in **thrombocytopenia,** and also block the erythrocytes from traveling freely throughout the blood vessels. The result of the erythrocytes forcing their way through the clots is the presence of **schistocytes,** which are torn pieces of erythrocytes (Fig. 11–7). All coagulation tests are normal.

Disseminated intravascular coagulation (DIC) occurs secondary to another disease process taking place in the body. Some initiating circumstance such as the tissue destruction associated with obstetric complications, surgery, or toxic substances, such as the bacterial cell wall lipopolysaccharide (LPS) from infection, results in small clots being formed throughout the body. The massive development of the clots consumes the thrombocytes and the coagulation factors. DIC is diagnosed clinically by **thrombocytopenia, prolonged coagulation testing,** and the **presence of fibrin degradation products (FDPs),** indicating massive clotting and fibri-

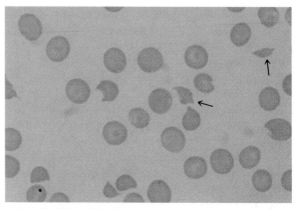

F I G U R E 11–7
Schistocytes due to the erythrocytes tearing on the fibrin strands from the clots in thrombotic thrombocytopenic purpura (TTP).

nolysis. Schistocytes may also be seen (see Fig. 11–7).

4. **Immune destruction** by macrophage phagocytosis occurs due to opsonization (coating with immunoglobulin or complement). Diseases resulting in the production of these detrimental antibodies are **idiopathic thrombocytopenic purpura (ITP)** and **drug-induced immune response or complement destruction.**

Idiopathic thrombocytopenic purpura (ITP) is a misnomer. It is now known that this destruction of thrombocytes is not idiopathic (unknown pathology). The **thrombocytes are opsonized** (coated with antibodies and complement), which marks them for destruction by the macrophages found primarily in the spleen. **No clots are formed; the thrombocytes are decreased due to phagocytosis by the macrophages.** ITP can be seen **following a viral infection,** in which case it is usually **transient.** Primary ITP is an **autoimmune disorder** and can be treated only by use of immunosuppressants such as steroids or by the removal of the spleen, which is the primary destructive organ.

A thrombocytopenia similar to ITP is **drug-induced immune response or complement destruction.** The thrombocytes are altered by the drug administered for another illness, and an antibody is formed against them. These antibodies and complement opsonize the thrombocytes, which makes them appetizing to the macrophages for phagocytosis. Once the drug is stopped, the thrombocyte count should return to the patient's pre-therapy range.

5. **Abnormal thrombocyte distribution** throughout the body, which is observed when the spleen is enlarged **(splenomegaly),** results in the pooling or **sequestration** of thrombocytes.

6. **Dilution of thrombocytes** in the body may be due to **cirrhosis of the liver,** which alters fluid distribution, or **massive transfusion** of packed red blood cells, which adds volume to the blood and contains no thrombocytes, resulting in a dilution of the patient's own thrombocytes.

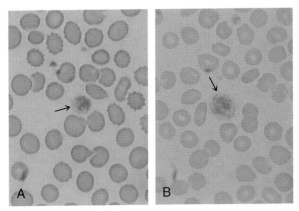

FIGURE 11–8

A and *B*, giant platelets. Platelets must be one half the size of the nucleus of an erythrocyte or small lymphocyte nucleus to be classified as giant platelets. A few giant platelets are normal. An increase in giant platelets is often the bone marrow response to bleeding.

An increase in thrombocytes found in the peripheral blood ($>450 \times 10^9$/l) is a **thrombocytosis.** Thrombocytosis may be the result of:

1. **Reactive thrombocytosis** is a normal healthy response to blood loss. The bone marrow responds to the need for thrombocytes by releasing the most mature available thrombocytes from the bone marrow and also increasing production (thrombopoiesis). Incidences utilizing thrombocytes appropriately are **hemorrhage, trauma, postsurgery, malignancy, chronic infections, chronic iron deficiency, and connective tissue disease (e.g., rheumatoid arthritis).** The reactive thrombocytosis may result in the premature release of thrombocytes (some of which will be larger in size) to meet the need. In this normal response, the count is rarely over 1000×10^9/l. If a thrombocyte is approximately one half the size (or larger) of a normal-sized erythrocyte or the nucleus of a small lymphocyte, it is noted as a "giant platelet" (Fig. 11–8*A* and *B*). There is often an inverse relationship between the size of the platelet and the platelet count. When giant platelets are seen, the count may be low. Every laboratory has its own criteria; however, observance of more than three giant platelets throughout the blood smear evaluation and differentiation

of white blood cells is usually reported as a significant finding.

2. **Myeloproliferative diseases,** such as **chronic myeloid (myelocytic) leukemia (CML)** and **polycythemia vera,** involve bone marrow proliferation of early cells of all cell lines. Excessive proliferation of leukocytes, erythrocytes, and thrombocytes is evidence of an abnormal proliferation or a malignancy. The **thrombocyte count is often greater than 1000×10^9/l.**

3. **Acute megakaryocytic leukemia (FAB M7)** is a very rare leukemia. The leukemic cells are identified by electron microscope visibility or by flow cytometry identification of platelet peroxidase and platelet membrane glycoproteins by immunocytochemical methods (Table 11–1).

4. **Essential thrombocythemia** results from **uncontrolled megakaryocyte and platelet production.** This is also considered to be a myeloproliferative disorder and involves uncontrolled proliferation of thrombocytes.

5. **Abnormal distribution** of thrombocytes throughout the body can produce an increase in circulating thrombocytes. The best example of this is post splenectomy. One third of the mature peripheral blood thrombocytes are normally sequestered in the spleen. If

TABLE 11–1 FRENCH-AMERICAN-BRITISH (FAB) CLASS OF ACUTE MYELOID/LYMPHOID LEUKEMIAS

FAB Class	Cells Observed	Unique Criteria	Cytochemistry/CD*	%†
M1(AML)	> 90% **myeloblasts** with minimal maturation (Pros)	Occasional Auer rods	Myeloperoxidase (**MP**), Sudan black B (SBB), NASDC	20
M2(AML)	< 90% Myeloblasts **>10% More mature**	**Auer rods**	Myeloperoxidase, Sudan black B, NASDC	30
M3(APL)	Predominantly **promyelocytes**	Often causes disseminated intravascular coagulation (DIC)	Myeloperoxidase, Sudan black B, NASDC	10
M4(AMML)	**Myeloblasts** and **monoblasts** with stages of both	Occasional Auer rods	> 20% MP, SBB, NASDC > 20% Nonspecific esterase (NSE)	12
M4eo	Same as M4 except with **eosinophilia**	Some with large **basophilic granules**	Same as M4 eos may be PAS	4
M5a(AMoL) Poorly differentiated	**>80% Monoblasts** promonocytes and monocytes	Later stages are poorly granulated and vacuolated	**NSE (fluoride inhibitor)**	5
M5b(AMoL) Differentiated	**<80% Monoblasts** promonocytes and monocytes		Same as 5a	6
M6(AEL)	**>50% Erythroblasts** also myeloblasts and monoblasts	50% Dysplastic megaloblastic	Periodic acid-Schiff (PAS) stain	6
M7(AMegL)	**>30% Megakaryoblasts**		Platelet peroxidase by EM; platelet glycoprotein by immunocytochemistry	1
L1(ALL)	Small lymph cells	2 to 10 year olds	PAS/CD 10,19, 24	71
L2(ATL)	Large irregular cells	Adult T cells associated with HTLV-I	PAS/CD 10	27
L3(ALL)	Large uniform cell	Burkitt's type	PS/CD 10	2

* Cluster differentiation markers for flow cytometry identification of cells.
† Represents the percentage of acute myeloid leukemias (M) or acute lymphoid (L) leukemias.

the spleen is removed, the **platelets that would reside in the spleen now go into the circulation, thus elevating the cell count.**

Qualitative platelet disorders are much less common than are quantitative disorders. Tests to **evaluate thrombocyte function** include the **bleeding time test, clot retraction, glass bead adhesion test, aggregation testing** using various activators (e.g., collagen, ADP, ristocetin), and factor assays. These tests are presented in more detail in Chapter 13. **Abnormal thrombocyte function** (dysfunction) can be hereditary or acquired. **Hereditary disorders** include:

1. **Platelet-type von Willebrand's disease,** an autosomal dominant disease **decreasing platelet adhesion** with resultant mild bleeding. The platelet count may be normal or low. This will **prolong the bleeding time test** and **decrease the aggregation response to ristocetin.**

2. **Thrombasthenia** (Glanzmann's disease) is a **failure of primary aggregation** due to a deficiency of membrane glycoproteins (gp) IIb and IIIa. Thrombocytes that lack these proteins are unable to bind fibrinogen for conversion to fibrin. **Abnormal clot retraction** is a diagnostic test.

3. Platelets in **Bernard-Soulier syndrome**

are larger than normal and lack **membrane glycoprotein (gp) Ib.** The absence of gp Ib does not allow effective binding to von Willebrand's factor, resulting in **defective adhesion and aggregation** with ristocetin.

4. **Storage pool disease (gray platelet syndrome)** demonstrates large platelets with an absence of alpha or dense granules. There is **defective secondary aggregation** due to a lack of stored ADP.

Abnormal thrombocyte function can also be acquired. Disorders of **acquired platelet dysfunction** include:

1. **Aspirin ingestion** is the most common cause. The aspirin, as well as other drugs, such as sulfinpyrazone and indomethacin, inhibit thromboxane A_2 synthesis and result in **deficient aggregation** (with adrenaline and ADP) and release of factors.

2. **Hyperglobulinemia** is associated with excessive protein produced in diseases such as multiple myeloma or Waldenström's macroglobulinemia, which **interferes with adhesion, aggregation, and release of factors.**

3. **Myeloproliferative disorders** resulting in intrinsic abnormalities of platelet function are seen with thrombocythemia and other myeloproliferative disorders.

4. **Uremia** secondary to renal (kidney) failure is associated with various functional thrombocyte abnormalities. The production of **thromboxane A_2 is decreased,** resulting in poor aggregation.

5. Chemical toxicity due to **heparin** (administered in a high concentration), **alcohol, radiographic contrast agents,** and **dextrans inhibits platelet aggregation and factor release.**

Do It Now — Normal Responses and Diseases of Thrombocytes and Vasculature

1. Using index cards, draw the various platelet responses and abnormalities, including the tests involved. You may want to begin with a chalk board or a white board to explore all the options before you record the diagram on your permanent card. Present the diagrams in the fashion that facilitates your learning of the material. Be creative.
2. Write your theory of why elderly individuals present with purpura and petechiae more commonly than do younger individuals. Relate this phenomenon to your knowledge of hematopoiesis, vascular and thrombocyte physiology, and function.

FAST FACTS

Thrombocyte General Information

Origin: Bone marrow
Maturation: Megakaryoblast—medium to large, with a large round nucleus containing nucleoli and light blue cytoplasm. The morphology is similar to that of the myeloblast of leukocytes. The micromegakaryocytic leukemic cell resembles a large lymphocyte to the inexperienced eye.
Promegakaryocyte—larger than the blast, multilobed nucleus, gray cytoplasm with purple granules.
Megakaryocyte—larger than the promegakaryocyte with a multilobed nucleus and an increased amount of DNA (polyploid). The cytoplasm is gray with purple granules, especially around the periphery of the cell where the mature thrombocytes are developing.
Mature thrombocyte—2 to 4 μm in diameter, 9 fl volume, anucleate disk, gray irregular cytoplasmic fragment with purple granules.
Function: Respond to a break in the vasculature (blood vessels) by **adhering** to the site, **releasing regulatory factors** such as phospholipid (PF3), which provides a surface for coagulation pathway reactions to enhance the formation of a thrombus (clot), **aggregating** to form an initial plug and secondary retraction to prevent blood from escaping from the injured blood vessel.
Major regulatory factors: GM-CSF, Mega-CSF, and thrombopoietin (TPO)
Reference ranges: Count = 150-400 $\times$ 10^{12}/mm^3 or 150-400 $\times$ 10^9/l
Size = 2 to 4 μm diameter, 9 fl mean platelet volume (MPV)

STUDY QUESTIONS

Choose the Best Answer.

1. The life span of a platelet is:
   A. 8–10 hours
   B. 8–10 days
   C. 120 days
   D. Years

2. A positive result on a tourniquet test is used for diagnosis of and indicates:
   A. Dysfunctional thrombocytes
   B. Thrombocytopenia
   C. Impaired vascular integrity
   D. Increased consumption of thrombocytes

3. Apply knowledge of thrombocyte physiology to choose the correct effects of aspirin ingestion on hemostasis.
   A. Thrombocytes are unable to release granule content.
   B. The vasculature cannot constrict if the patient has ingested aspirin.
   C. Thrombocytes are unable to produce thromboxane A$_2$, which is necessary for proper aggregation.
   D. Aspirin does not allow the binding of fibrinogen to the PF3 for conversion to fibrin.

True or False:

4. The thrombocyte develops from the megakaryocyte in the bone marrow and loses its nucleus before entering the peripheral blood in a manner similar to the erythrocyte.

5. A prolonged bleeding time test indicates a problem with platelet function, provided that adequate platelets are present.

6. The functional stages of the thrombocyte in the order in which they occur are: change of shape, primary aggregation, factor release, secondary aggregation, and adhesion.

7–8. List at least **two ways** in which the platelets and the coagulation pathways are interdependent.

For the Following Questions, Use as Many Parameters as Possible.

9–14. Contrast and compare the thrombocyte, erythrocyte, and lymphocyte.

15–20. Contrast and compare idiopathic thrombocytopenic purpura (ITP), thrombotic thrombocytopenic purpura (TTP), and disseminated intravascular coagulation (DIC).

CHAPTER 12

OUTLINE

Coagulation and Fibrinolytic Proteins and Pathways

Appropriate Coagulation and Fibrinolysis

Inappropriate Coagulation and Fibrinolysis

Study Questions

Blood Coagulation and Fibrinolysis

O B J E C T I V E S

Upon completion of this chapter the student should be able to:

1. Diagram and explain hemostasis using a figure that includes all four components.

2. Explain the significance of coagulation and fibrinolytic factor synthesis, especially the vitamin K–dependent coagulation proteins.

3. Discuss the viability and function of the coagulation and fibrinolytic proteins.

4. Apply knowledge of hemostasis physiology when given a clinical scenario to analyze the situation.

5. Correlate the appropriate testing for blood coagulation and hemostasis with disease.

6. Explain the following conditions and associated diseases: hypercoagulation, hypocoagulation, and combination diseases.

7. Contrast and compare heparin and warfarin (Coumadin) therapy and monitoring.

Blood coagulation involves the biologic **generation of thrombin,** which **converts soluble plasma fibrinogen to insoluble fibrin strands.** Fibrin enmeshes the platelet aggregates at the sites of vascular injury and converts the unstable primary platelet plug into a firm, definitive, and stable hemostatic plug called a **thrombus** (blood clot) (Fig. 12–1). Due to the presence of large numbers of erythrocytes in a normal thrombus, it may be referred to as a **red clot,** as opposed to the **white clot** discussed in Chapter 11 involving mostly platelets. If a piece of the thrombus breaks off and moves through the body to another site, this piece is called a **thromboembolus** or **embolus.**

There are approximately **13 original glycoprotein coagulation factors, numbered I to XIII and a total of 17 factors.** There is **no factor IV;** this is Ca^{2+}, and there is also **no factor VI,** due to a duplication of naming the factors originally. Other proteins discovered after the first twelve are **proteins S, C, prekallikrein, high-molecular-weight kininogen, and antithrombin III (Table 12–1).** All except fibrinogen are enzyme precursors or co-factors. Three fibrinolytic factors are listed with the coagulation factors in Table 12–1. These factors of fibrinolysis are activated simultaneously with the coagulation factors to keep the clotting and dissolution of clots in a dynamic balance.

Coagulation takes place on various surfaces within the body. Surface-mediated reactions occur on exposed **collagen, platelet phospholipid (PPL, PF3), and tissue factor (III). Calcium ions (Ca^{2+})** are also a requirement for the formation of a clot. This mechanism is used to anticoagulate blood for testing. Many of the anticoagulants (EDTA, citrate) available are Ca^{2+} binding chemicals.

The process of blood coagulation and fibrinolysis has been separated into four pathways in order to simplify the complex interactions. These do not exist separately in the body. Although one pathway may be more active than another, the processes described here are often occurring simultaneously (Fig. 12–2).

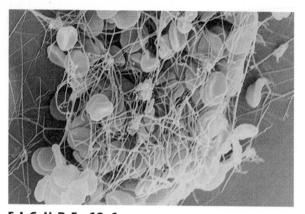

FIGURE 12–1
A scanning electron microscope photograph of a blood clot. The fibrin strands enmesh the erythrocytes.

COAGULATION AND FIBRINOLYTIC PROTEINS AND PATHWAYS

The specimen of choice to assess the coagulation pathways is a **full and well-mixed Na citrate blue-stoppered tube maintained on ice and tested within 2 hours.** The initial specimen for evaluation must be drawn before any treatment or therapy has been administered. This is discussed more in Chapter 13.

The **intrinsic coagulation pathway** involves initiating factors that are activated within the vasculature by **contact with rough or irregular surfaces (ruptured cholesterol plaques) as well as collagen and other negatively charged subendothelial connective tissue. Fletcher factor (prekallikrein), Fitzgerald factor (high-molecular-weight kininogen, HMWK), and factors XI and XII interact with calcium (Ca^{2+}) on a phospholipid (PF3) surface to activate factor IX. Factor IX$_a$ reacts with factor VIII, PF3, and calcium ions (Ca^{2+})** to activate primarily factor X of the common pathway (see Fig. 12–2d and e). Factor VIII is most commonly associated with **hemophilia A,** which is a genetic deficiency of the **VIII.** Factor VIII is also associated with **von Willebrand's (VIII:vWF)** factor, which is required for normal thrombocyte adhesion. If the VIII:vWF form of factor

TABLE 12-1   COAGULATION/FIBRINOLYTIC PROTEINS

Designation/Name		Comments	Active Form
I	Fibrinogen	Large protein, 200 to 400 mg/dl, consumed in clotting	Fibrin subunit
II	Prothrombin	*Vitamin K dependent*	Serine protease
III	Tissue thromboplastin receptor/co-factor	Not present in PB, released by tissue disruption	
IV	Old name for Ca^{2+}		
V	Labile factor	Proaccelerin, consumed	Co-factor
VI	Not used	Activated factor V (V_a)	
VII	Stable factor	Proconvertin, *vitamin K dependent*	Serine protease
VIII	Antihemophiliac factor (AHF)	Antihemophiliac globulin (AHG) consumed	Co-factor
IX	Christmas factor	Plasma thromboplastin component (PTC) Antihemophiliac factor B	Serine protease
X	Stuart-Prower factor	*Vitamin K dependent*	Serine protease
XI	Plasma thromboplastin antecedent	Antihemophiliac factor C (PTA)	Serine protease
XII	Hageman factor	Contact factor	Serine protease
XIII	Fibrin-stabilizing factor (FSF)	Polymerizes fibrin	Transglutaminase
•	Prekallikrein	Fletcher factor, contact factor	Serine protease
•	High-molecular-weight kininogen	Fitzgerald factor or HMWK	Co-factor
•	Protein C	X_a inhibitor, *vitamin K dependent*	Serine protease
•	Protein S	enhances protein C, *vitamin K dependent*	Cofactor
•	Antithrombin III Plasminogen	ATIII/heparin co-factor Converted to plasmin	Breaks down fibrin and fibrinogen
•	Plasminogen activator	Tissue plasminogen activator (tPA), urokinase, streptokinase, staphylokinase, thrombin, kallikrein, XI, XII_a	
•	Plasminogen inhibitors	α_2-Plasmin inhibitor, tissue plasminogen activator inhibitor	

VIII is deficient, the compromised platelet function may result in bleeding. This pathway is the most **sensitive to intravenous (IV) heparin therapy** given to patients to prevent cardiac (heart) and circulatory thrombosis. The **partial thromboplastin time (PTT) test measures the intrinsic system and therefore also monitors the effectiveness of heparin therapy.**

The **extrinsic coagulation pathway** is activated by the **exposure to tissue thromboplastin (factor III).** Tissue thromboplastin, normally extrinsic to the blood, is derived from phospholipoproteins and organelle membranes from disrupted tissue cells. PF3 is not necessary in this system because **factor III supplies its own phospholipid (PPL)** surface for coagulation. **Factor VII** binds to the

factor III and becomes activated. Along with ionized calcium, factor VII is a potent activator of the common pathway (factor X) (see Fig. 12-2c and e). Evidence suggests that tissue factor pathway inhibitor (TFPI), a naturally occurring proteinase, keeps the VIIa/tissue factor complex in check. The **prothrombin time (PT) test measures the extrinsic system, which is primarily factor VII. Factor VII is the most sensitive factor to oral warfarin (Coumadin) anticoagulant therapy** due to its short half-life resulting in a high rate of synthesis by the liver. The **PT test** is the most useful to monitor the effectiveness of **oral warfarin (Coumadin) treatment.**

The **common coagulation pathway** is utilized by both the intrinsic and extrinsic

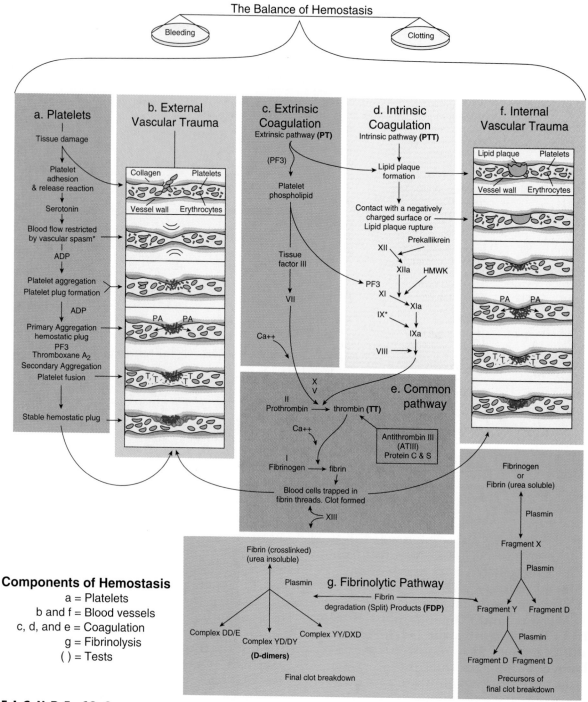

FIGURE 12–2
Hemostasis showing the interrelationship of the vasculature, platelets, coagulation, and fibrinolysis.

pathways to accomplish the common goal of converting fibrinogen to fibrin. **Factor X** in association with cofactor **factor V on the phospholipid (PPL) surface and Ca²⁺,** converts **prothrombin into thrombin,** which then converts **fibrinogen into fibrin** (see Fig. 12–2e). Fibrin monomers link spontaneously by hydrogen bonds to form loose, fibrin polymers. **Factor XIII** activated by thrombin and calcium **stabilizes the fibrin polymers** with the formation of covalent bond cross-links. Laboratory investigation of the common pathway would include the **thrombin time test (TT)** and the **fibrinogen assay.**

Not all coagulation factors are procoagulants. There is a direct inactivation of thrombin and other serine proteases by **circulating inhibitors.** This is necessary to avoid inappropriate thrombosis. **Antithrombin III (ATIII),** a circulating protein, is the most potent of these inhibitors. ATIII works with **heparin** anticoagulant to enhance (synergize) the inhibition of thrombin. There are also inhibitors of factors V and VIII. Thrombin binds to an endothelial cell surface receptor known as thrombomodulin. This complex then activates the vitamin K–dependent serine protease **protein C,** which when combined with protein S (see later), is able to destroy activated factors V and VIII. This prevents further production of thrombin. In addition, protein C enhances fibrinolysis by inactivation of plasminogen activator inhibitor I (PAI-I). The action of protein C is dependent on another vitamin K–dependent protein co-factor known as **protein S.** There is also a tissue factor pathway inhibitor (TFPI) that forms a complex with factors VII_a and X_a to limit the main in vivo pathway.

The **fibrinolytic pathway** removes fibrin clots, which are temporary structures that seal off a damaged area until healing can take place. **Plasminogen,** the precursor to plasmin, circulates in the plasma until an injury occurs. Plasminogen is then activated to plasmin by a variety of proteolytic "kinase" enzymes. Examples of these **plasminogen activators** are: **tissue plasminogen activator (tPA), urokinase, and streptokinase.** The fibrinolytic factor, **plasmin,** digests fibrin, fibrinogen, and factors V and VIII by hydrolysis to produce progressively smaller fragments, some of which act as anticoagulants and inhibit further thrombus formation (see Fig. 12–2g). **Tests to assess the fibrinolytic pathway are the fibrin split products (FSP) test, the D-dimer test, the euglobin lysis test (ELT), and fibrinogen levels.** As the

> ### Do It Now Coagulation Pathways
>
> 1. Draw the coagulation pathways together in as many different ways as you can. Figure 12–2 depicts this, but there are many other ways to show the same information. Be sure to include tests for each pathway. Perhaps you will discover a relationship between the tests, factors, or the pathways by picturing the process in different ways.
> 2. While you draw, think of how and where this process is occurring. Note any questions that you have as you explore this process.
> 3. Once you have several drawings, choose the one that you like best and explain it to a classmate or copy it onto an overhead and explain it to the class. Ask the questions generated in part 2.

injured tissue heals, the fibrinolytic process removes the fibrin. Macrophages phagocytize the debris from this process, which restores the blood vessel or site of coagulation back to the precoagulation state.

As with every system in the body there are also **fibrinolytic inhibitors. Alpha-2 plasmin inhibitor and tissue plasminogen activator inhibitor** are examples.

As individuals **grow older,** they demonstrate signs of **increased coagulation** (hypercoagulability). Higher levels of several coagulation factors and increased fibrinolysis have been demonstrated in individuals over 100 years old. Obviously, this observation is compatible with a long life and does not indicate risk of arterial or venous thrombosis.

APPROPRIATE COAGULATION AND FIBRINOLYSIS

Any **disruption of the blood flow, cell membranes, vascular tissue, or the presence of bacterial toxins and by-products, such as cell wall lipopolysaccharides (LPS), can stimulate thrombus formation.** Thrombus formation is a life-saving mechanism when a blood vessel has been cut and blood is leaking out. This mechanism is normal and desirable. If, on the other hand, the **thrombus does not form when**

Coagulation and Fibrinolytic Proteins and Pathways

Pathway	Factors	Notes and Tests
Intrinsic	Prekallikrein, high-molecular-weight kininogen, XII XI, IX, VIII:vWF, PF3, Ca²⁺, VIII:C	Contact initiation group **Partial thromboplastin time (PTT),** heparin therapy, hemophilia (VIII:C deficiency) Von Willebrand's disease (VIII:vWF) Cholesterol plaque rupture
Extrinsic	Tissue thromboplastin III VII, Ca²⁺	Cell injury, cut **Prothrombin time (PT) test** Warfarin (Coumadin) therapy; warfarin decreases VII synthesis in the liver
Common	V, X, PF3, Ca²⁺, prothrombin (II) Fibrinogen (I), XIII Proteins C and S Antithrombin III (ATIII)	Dysfibrinogenemia Hypofibrinogenemia or afibrinogenemia **Thrombin time test (TT)** **Fibrinogen assay**
Fibrinolytic	Plasminogen activators (kinases) Plasminogen Plasminogen inhibitors	tPA, streptokinase Fibrin split products test **D-dimer test**

needed or a **thrombus forms due to abnormal occurrences in the body** not involving a cut in the vessels, a life-threatening coagulation disorder develops.

As presented earlier in Figure 12–2, when injury occurs several incidents happen before the formation of fibrin. The **blood vessel** itself responds by a **reflex constriction,** and **platelets** begin to **change shape, adhere to the injured tissue, aggregate** to one another, and **release platelet factors** such as serotonin, which maintains the constricted blood vessel. Proteins from the damaged cells and activated platelets stimulate coagulation. **Thrombin transforms fibrinogen into the insoluble gel, fibrin,** the visible result of coagulation. Fibrin forms a loose covering over the injured area to reinforce the platelet plug and close off the wound. After a short time the platelets send out cytoplasmic processes that attach to the fibrin strands and pull the fibers closer together. This secondary aggregation of the platelets pulling the clot tighter is called **clot retraction.** Clot retraction as seen in the blood tube (in vitro) expresses the clear serum out of the clot for use in chemistry and blood bank testing.

Normal coagulation, as discussed, involves **fibrinogen,** which is normally present in a **high concentration** (200 to 400 mg/dl) in the plasma as a large (340,000 MW), soluble molecule. A high concentration of this large protein, fibrinogen, in plasma results in a **cloudy or hazy appearance.** Protein and other chemistry studies are more accurate if fibrinogen is not present since it masks the proteins of interest; therefore, **serum, which does not contain fibrinogen,** is the specimen of choice for chemistry testing. Serum is also the specimen of choice for the blood bank, due to the absence of an anticoagulant that may interfere with reactions rather than the absence of fibrinogen.

The escape of blood from the vasculature, resulting in the formation of a thrombus, can occur in veins, arteries, or capillaries and takes place externally or internally, such as when an organ ruptures. A large clot of blood outside a blood vessel is a **hematoma.** The hematoma is visible as a bruise and will be degraded by the fibrinolytic system within a few days. Placing direct pressure on the site of bleeding will allow coagulation to occur inside the blood vessel to stop the bleeding, rather than leakage outside of the vessel with clotting occurring both inside and outside the blood vessel. **Petechiae** are very small irregular spots of visible bleeding due to loss of **vascular integrity** (weakening of the endothelium). **Ecchymosis** is larger than the petechia and is a hemorrhagic bruise in the skin or mucous membranes. **Purpura** are areas of bleeding into the mucous membranes resulting in a purple area of the skin, which is often seen in elderly individuals. **Petechiae, ecchymosis, and purpura suggest vascular defects, thrombocyte defects, or decreased numbers of thrombocytes.**

INAPPROPRIATE COAGULATION AND FIBRINOLYSIS

If thrombus formation does not occur when there is a break in the blood vessel, the result is **hemorrhage** (blood loss). If a thrombus does develop in the absence of a blood loss, there is a **thrombotic coagulopathy** (abnormal coagulation) present.

   Hemorrhagic disorders occur if coagulation is necessary and is not possible. The inability to form a thrombus may be due to a factor deficiency or factor inhibitor. The deficiency can be genetic or acquired. Genetic bleeding disorders are not common; however, when seen, the most common genetic hemorrhagic disorder is **hemophilia A.** A patient with hemophilia A is genetically **deficient in factor VIII (antihemophiliac factor [AHF])** of the intrinsic coagulation pathway. Factor VIII exists in a stable complex with another glycoprotein, von Willebrand factor, which is necessary for normal thrombocyte adhesion. The hemophiliac individual will also have a prolonged bleeding time test (which measures platelet function) due to a lack of vWF with the factor VIII (VIII:vWF). This individual will bleed spontaneously into joints and mucous membranes, resulting in swollen, tender, arthritic joints and visible bruises. **He-**

mophilia A is diagnosed by a **prolonged partial thromboplastin time (PTT)** test that assesses the intrinsic factors. Once this test has been shown to be prolonged, the cause must then be determined. The **PTT test is prolonged due to factor deficiencies or circulating inhibitors** (anticoagulants). To determine which one of these is involved, the patient's abnormal citrated plasma is mixed with an equal volume of the normal control citrated plasma and this mixture is then used as the patient's unknown specimen. If the prolonged PTT was due to a factor deficiency, it will be **corrected by the 1:1 mixed specimen,** because all of the factors have been added. If the PTT is not corrected, this indicates that there is a circulating anticoagulant in the patient's blood that inhibited the normal control factors as well as the patient's factors. This PTT performed on a **mixed specimen (one-half patient specimen + one-half normal control serum) is called the circulating anticoagulant test.** Once a deficiency is established, further testing can be performed to identify the missing factor. Testing for hemostasis is presented in more detail in Chapter 13.

   Hereditary coagulation factor deficiencies in addition to hemophilia A (factor VIII) include hemophilia B (factor IX deficiency), factor XI, prekallikrein, high-molecular-weight kininogen (HMWK), and factors X, VII, V, and I (fibrinogen). **Factors may also be decreased, not totally absent, or present in adequate quantity but nonfunctional.** Hypofibrinogenemia and dysfibrinogenemia are examples. Hemorrhage is not associated with factor IX, prekallikrein, or high-molecular-weight kininogen deficiencies. Factor XI deficiency demonstrates minor bleeding. Deficiencies of factors X, VII, and V vary in severity of bleeding.

   Treatment for the genetic factor deficiencies involves replacement of the missing factor or the administration of drugs that stimulate production of the factor. **Factor VIII concentrates** and **cryoprecipitate** (factor VIII precipitated upon thawing of frozen plasma and pooled to concentrate) are administered on a regular basis by the patient in his or her home. If the patient is totally deficient in factor VIII, antibodies may develop against this product, which is foreign to the body. The antibodies produced will bind to factor VIII and render it nonfunctional. Alternatives such as the administration of factor VIII from another source (bovine, which is cow) or performing a plasmapheresis to remove the IgG antibodies from the hemophiliac's plasma have been somewhat successful. Complications of factor VIII replacement therapy have been the risk of contracting hepatitis B virus (HBV) and now the human immunodeficiency virus ([HIV], AIDS virus) from the donors. **Recombinant** (made in the laboratory) **factor VIII is now available** and will eliminate these human exposure risks. In cases of von Willebrand's disease, a drug can be given to increase production of factor VIII:vWF. The drug is 1-desmino-8-D-arginine vasopressin **(DDAVP).** This drug is a synthetic analog to vasopressin, which **stimulates the production of factor VIII:vWF** in the body and will result in a twofold to 10-fold rise in factor VIII titer after intravenous infusion.

Acquired hemorrhagic disorders include the development of inhibitors (antibodies), vitamin K deficiency, liver disease, intravascular coagulation (secondary to another disorder), systemic fibrinolysis, massive blood transfusion, renal failure, cancer, obstetric hemorrhage, lymphoid and myeloid proliferative disorders, and toxins.

Developing **inhibitors** to the coagulation factors is best seen in hemophilia A, in which the administration of a factor VIII not found normally in the body induces an immune response resulting in **antibodies produced against the coagulation factor** administered. These antibodies can be alloantibodies (antibodies whose targets are coagulation factors from another member of the same species) or on rare occasions autoantibodies (antibodies whose target is their own coagulation factors).

Antiphospholipid antibodies (APA), often referred to as **lupus anticoagulants,** constitute a very complex entity that actually blocks natural anticoagulants and fibrinolytic factors, resulting in thrombosis. Therefore this will be discussed later under thrombotic disorders.

Vitamin K deficiency and liver disease involve the same mechanism or etiology of abnormal coagulation and result in a bleeding tendency. Vitamin K is metabolized in the liver to produce functional coagulation factors. The **vitamin K–dependent factors synthesized in the liver are factors II, VII, IX, and X, and factor VII is the most sensitive to lack of vitamin K.** This sensitivity is due to the short half-life of factor VII, which requires constant synthesis to maintain an adequate plasma level. The oral anticoagulant administered to individuals with a clotting tendency, **warfarin (Coumadin), inhibits synthesis of vitamin K–dependent coagulation factors, thus clotting, by competing with the vitamin K in the liver.** Warfarin is a vitamin K antagonist and results in less of the vitamin K–dependent coagulation proteins being produced, thus reducing the risk of unnecessary clotting. Since factor VII is the most sensitive to this therapy and is part of the extrinsic coagulation pathway, the **prothrombin time (PT) test, which tests the extrinsic pathway, is the test used to monitor warfarin (Coumadin) therapy.** Keep in mind that intake of vitamin K depends on the diet. If the diet changes, altering the intake of vitamin K, warfarin therapy must also be altered, resulting in changes in the PT. The production of the coagulation factors that are synthesized in the liver is dependent on a functional liver. If the patient is suffering from liver damage, such as **alcoholic cirrhosis, hepatitis, or hepatocarcinoma (liver cancer), the PT will be prolonged** due to decreased production of the coagulation factors synthesized in the liver. If the primary problem is improved, the tendency to bleed will decrease.

Intravascular coagulation occurs secondary to another disorder. As discussed in Chapter 11, small clots of thrombocytes and fibrin **(white clots)** occur throughout the body in **thrombotic thrombocytopenic purpura (TTP).** The laboratory results indicate a **thrombocytopenia,** which will **prolong the bleeding time tests,** and **schistocytes** (torn, fragmented erythrocytes) seen on the peripheral blood smear due to passage through the fibrin strands that tear the cells. A secondary coagulation disorder that is seen more often is **disseminated intravascular coagulation (DIC),** which involves the production of small clots **(microthrombosis)** and the lysis of these clots throughout the body **(systemic fibrinolysis).** This massive clotting consumes the platelets and coagulation factors so that they are not available when normal coagulation is needed. The products of clot lysis act as anticoagulants, further decreasing the ability of the blood to clot when necessary. Massive bleeding will occur in this individual. **Treatment** includes administration of **heparin** to reduce the systemic clotting while administering **fresh frozen plasma (FFP)** to replace the consumed coagulation factors. Laboratory diagnosis includes a **decreased platelet count, prolongation of all coagulation tests, a decreased fibrinogen level, and a positive test result for fibrin split products (FSP) or D-dimers** from the lytic component. DIC is seen secondary to conditions such as obstetric complications, surgical procedures, sepsis (systemic infection), and malignancies.

Primary systemic fibrinolysis occurs when active forms of the fibrinolytic enzymes (factors) circulate in the blood. Plasmin destroys fibrinogen, factor V, and factor VIII, which does not allow adequate coagulation to occur. This is a rare disorder, and enzyme-linked immunosorbent assay (EIA) techniques are available to measure plasmin-α_2-antiplasmin complexes, in order to aid in the diagnosis. **Treatment** includes administration of inhibitors of fibrinolysis, such as **epsilon aminocaproic acid or tranexamic acid orally** or intravenously to control immediate bleeding. Blood volume loss is replaced by the administration of erythrocytes or whole blood (given as packed erythrocytes and fresh frozen plasma).

A **massive blood transfusion** is defined as the replacement of more than one total blood volume (e.g., 10 units of blood) in less than 24 hours. The bleeding tendency is the result of dilution of the coagulation factors or the development of DIC. The results for the **dilutional coagulopathy** are similar to those found in DIC, prolonged coagulation tests (PT and PTT), decreased fibrinogen, and

thrombocytopenia, except that the FSP or D-dimer test results are negative. Fresh frozen plasma (FFP) is given to replace diluted coagulation factors.

Renal failure (chronic or hemolytic uremic syndrome **[HUS]), cancer, obstetric hemorrhage, lymphoid and myeloid proliferative disorders, and toxins** all have the potential to interfere with platelet function and normal coagulation. The test results and treatment vary from one disorder to another. The treatment also varies from one disease to the next but should always include correction of the underlying primary cause.

Thrombotic disorders include **disseminated thrombosis** (e.g., TTP, DIC), **deep vein thrombosis** (DVT), **venous thromboembolic disease,** and **arterial thrombosis. Until 6 months of age,** a newborn is at risk for blood clotting due to **low levels of coagulation inhibitors and also fibrinolytic agents.** The factor balancing this tendency toward thrombosis is the **low level of the coagulation factors** produced in the liver, which is not yet functioning fully. **This risk of clotting is increased in premature or at-risk babies** in which artificial devices (e.g., indwelling lines) are inserted into the blood vessels. Newborns may be genetically deficient and require testing and treatment, if possible, to avoid hemorrhage (factor VIII) or thrombosis (protein C). Diagnosis of the infant or child is based on physical observation, platelet count, PT, APTT, TCT, FDP, contrast angiography (blood vessel studies), and imaging studies (e.g., ultrasound, sonography). The last two tests are performed in the radiology department.

Hypercoagulable states are hereditary or acquired. Acquired disorders are more common and include venous stasis (sluggish blood flow), endothelial injury, and circulating activated clotting factors. Less common are the hereditary disorders such as deficiency of factor XII, defects of natural anticoagulants, inadequate fibrinolysis, or circulating activated thrombocytes. Venous thromboembolism is a common clinical problem. **Deep vein thrombosis (DVT)** tends to develop in sluggish blood flow areas near a valve and increases in size filling the lumen and great lengths of the vein. In a normal individual, small clots are formed after situations such as surgery and are rapidly degraded by the fibrinolytic system. In individuals with clotting tendencies, the clotting exceeds the fibrinolytic degradation. If antithrombotic therapy is not administered, new clots will form on the surface of the original clot and the **risk of embolization (pieces breaking off)** increases. Pulmonary emboli (PE) (pieces of thrombi that block blood supply to the lungs) are usually the outcome of embolization, and this accounts for 5 to 10% of all hospital deaths. The diagnosis involves testing for **protein C, protein S, and ATIII deficiencies** in young patients as well as the **radiologic studies.** Monitoring of any anticoagulant therapy is the clinical laboratory's responsibility. Thrombolytic therapy is the treatment of choice in severe DVT and PE. Anticoagulation therapy by intravenous infusion of heparin or subcutaneous injection of low-molecular-weight heparin is started immediately. Oral warfarin (Coumadin) therapy is then established and continued from 3 months to the lifetime of the individual, depending on the risk of recurrence.

Deficiencies associated with thrombosis include **antithrombin III (ATIII, hereditary or acquired), protein C, and protein S, resulting in venous thromboembolism. Heparin therapy** is dependent on adequate levels of **functional ATIII.** Heparin is much less effective and may need to be administered in a higher dose to the ATIII-deficient patient. ATIII is measured in the chemistry department. **Protein C** can be measured by **immunologic antigen assay** and is performed in the chemistry department. This test is less sensitive than is the **functional assay** performed in the coagulation area of the hematology department. Keep in mind that the quantitative assays may indicate an adequate level with no indication of function. **Skin necrosis** (cell death) occurs in some protein C–

deficient individuals who are given warfarin anticoagulation therapy since protein C is also vitamin K–dependent. Individuals who are deficient in protein S may demonstrate necrotic tissue with or without warfarin therapy. **Management** of these deficiencies includes administration of **warfarin** and **fresh frozen plasma (FFP).** Warfarin prevents further clotting and must be monitored by the clinical laboratory, and the FFP replaces coagulation factors consumed by the clotting. Protein C concentrates are now available in the United States for treatment of protein C deficiency.

There are **thrombotic events** associated with **fibrinolytic defects, myeloproliferative disorders, paroxysmal nocturnal hemoglobinuria (PNH), cancer, atherosclerosis, vascular disorders, cardiac disease, cerebrovascular disease, and as a complication of pregnancy.** Treatment is determined by the cause of the thrombus. If the disorder involves deep vein thrombosis, cardiac disease, and so forth, anticoagulant therapy is the treatment of choice. Individuals who are deficient in certain factors can be treated with factor concentrates. Disseminated intravascular coagulation (DIC) is treated with a balance of fresh frozen plasma, to replace consumed factors, and heparin anticoagulant therapy.

Do It Now   **Abnormal Coagulation and Fibrinolysis**

1. Make a table in which the disorders are listed down the left side and the coagulation and fibrinolysis tests are listed across the top. Fill in the results that you would see for each one (e.g., prolonged, no change, positive, negative).
2. Take turns explaining one disorder and the associated testing to another classmate. Debate points that are not clearly understood.

Blood Coagulation and Fibrinolysis

Disorder	Diagnostic Tests	Comments
Hemorrhagic:		
Factor VIII deficiency	Prolonged PTT Corrected 1:1 mix	Hemophilia A, genetic Cryoprecipitate treatments
Deficiency in factor IX	Prolonged PTT Corrected 1:1 mix	Genetic hemophilia B
XI, XII, and prekallikrein	Prolonged PTT Corrected 1:1 mix	Factor assays to identify deficient factors
High-molecular-weight kininogen (HMWK)	Prolonged PTT	Factor assays to identify deficient factors
I, V, VII, X	Prolonged PT and PTT	Factor assays to identify deficient factors
Inhibitors: antibodies	Prolonged PTT	Antifactor VIII
Vitamin K deficiency	Prolonged PT	Warfarin (Coumadin) therapy
Liver disease	Prolonged PT and PTT	
Disseminated intravascular coagulation (DIC)	All coagulation tests are prolonged and abnormal Positive fibrin split products (FSP) Positive D-dimer tests	2° to another disorder Heparin and FFP treatment Thrombocytopenia
Systemic fibrinolysis	Positive FSP; decreased euglobin lysis time (ELT) Decreased α_2-plasmin α_2-antiplasmin complexes	
Massive blood transfusion	All coagulation tests are prolonged and abnormal Negative FDP	>10 units in 24-hour dilution of factors
Renal failure, cancer, obstetric hemorrhage, lymphoid/myeloid proliferation, toxins, and infections	Abnormal results vary with the disorder	
Thrombotic:		
Deep vein thrombosis (DVT)	Protein C and S levels low Antithrombin III level low	Antithrombotic therapy Pulmonary emboli (PE)
Antithrombin III (ATIII)	ATIII level in chemistry	Heparin co-factor
Protein C and S deficiency	Protein C and S levels	Warfarin (Coumadin) necrosis Warfarin/FFP/protein C concentration
Fibrinolytic defects	Euglobin lysis test (ELT) Positive FSP	

STUDY QUESTIONS

Choose the Best Answer for Each Question:

1. Hemostasis involves which of the following components:
   A. Hemorrhage, clotting, fibrinolysis
   B. Leukocytes, erythrocytes, thrombocytes
   C. Vasculature, thrombocytes, coagulation, fibrinolysin
   D. PT, PTT, FSP

2. Coagulation factor deficiencies can be due to:
   A. Decreased production
   B. Nonfunctional factor
   C. Increased consumption (use)
   D. All of the above

Choose the Best Answer for Each, and Match the Following:

3. Genetic coagulopathy
4. Vitamin K deficiency
5. Following obstetric complications
6. Liver disease
7. Bleeding after the administration of cryoprecipitate

A. Decreased production
B. Nonfunctional factor
C. Increased consumption (use)
D. Increased production

Choose the Best Answer for Each Question:

8. The drug _____ is a vitamin K analog that

9. _____ the production of

10. factor _____, and this response is measured by the

11. _____ coagulation test.
    A. Heparin
    B. Warfarin
    C. Increases
    D. Decreases
    E. VII
    F. VIII
    G. PTT
    H. PT

12. The successful function of the coagulation factors in the process of forming a clot is dependent on the presence of at least two necessary components, which are:
    A. Ca^{2+} and phospholipid
    B. Vitamin K and B_{12}
    C. Vasculature, thrombocytes, and coagulation
    D. Tissue factor and fibrin

The Following Patient Specimens for Coagulation Profiles are Received in the Laboratory. The Following Results Are Obtained:

13. The PT is normal, and the PTT is prolonged. The follow-up test that will provide some further information is the:
    A. Thrombin time test
    B. Circulating anticoagulant test ("mix")
    C. Fibrin split products
    D. D-dimer test

14. The appropriate test chosen in question 13 would determine which of the following diagnoses?
    A. Factor deficiency
    B. Coagulation inhibitors present
    C. Increased fibrinolysis
    D. Both a and b

Match the Following Conditions and Associated Treatments that Would Be Monitored for Success by the Laboratory:

15. Hypercoagulation

16. Hypocoagulation

17. Combination diseases

18. Heparin therapy

19. Warfarin (Coumadin) therapy

A. Factor replacement and FFP

B. Heparin or warfarin

C. Heparin and FFP

D. PTT

E. PT

O U T L I N E

Vascular Testing and Evaluation

Thrombocyte Testing and Evaluation

Coagulation Testing and Evaluation

Fibrinolysis Testing and Evaluation

Study Questions

Hemostasis Testing

OBJECTIVES

Upon completion of this chapter the student should be able to:

1. Describe the acceptable specimens for thrombocyte, coagulation, and fibrinolytic testing.

2. Explain the various hemostasis test methodologies.

3. Correlate the various hemostasis tests to one another and their significance in the diagnosis.

4. When given a testing scenario, analyze the data and information available to determine if there are reasons to question the validity of the results or to alter the way in which the results are reported.

5. Contrast and compare heparin therapy, warfarin (Coumadin) therapy, fibrinolytic therapy, and the relevant testing.

The **specimen of choice for thrombo-cyte testing is a fresh, clear, well-mixed (lavender top) ethylenediaminetetra-acetic acid (EDTA) specimen.** EDTA is the anticoagulant of choice for cellular testing because it **preserves cell function and morphology** better than do any of the other anticoagulants. For most accurate results the specimen should be kept at room temperature (not chilled), and the platelets should be counted within 2 hours because in time all cells begin to change. However, some individual cells become altered immediately after exposure to the anticoagulant. If a patient's cells are altered by EDTA, Na citrate can be used if testing is performed within a short period of time.

The **specimen** required for assessment of the **coagulation** pathways is a **full, clear, and well-mixed solution of sodium citrate (Na citrate, blue top) in an unopened tube (to maintain pH) that is stored on ice, and tested within 2 hours.** The Na citrate tube for coagulation testing must be full to achieve the correct ratio of blood to liquid sodium citrate. This is critical for accurate results. The ratio should be **9:1 or 4.5 ml blood:0.5 ml sodium citrate anticoagulant.** A patient with a hematocrit of more than 55% will require less anticoagulant.

If less than 4.5 ml of blood is drawn or the patient's hematocrit is higher than 55%, test results will be prolonged due to excess anticoagulant. The initial specimen for evaluation must be drawn before any treatment or therapy has been administered as a reference value for the treatment and further testing.

Some special tests to evaluate **fibrinolysis** include **fibrin degradation products (FDP), also called fibrin split products (FSP).** This test requires serum preparations *or* an alternative anticoagulant and additive, **thrombin with soy bean trypsin inhibitor (light blue top tube).** This additive inhibits further breakdown of the fibrinolytic products before testing. The fibrinolytic testing is discussed later in this chapter.

If the laboratory practitioner is not correlating results, fragmented or inaccurate information is provided to the clinical practitioner, which can hinder the efficiency of the health care and can be detrimental to the patient.

Our mission in the clinical laboratory is: (1) to provide test results that reflect the condition within the body (in vivo), not changes that took place once the blood was removed from the patient and was placed into a glass tube (in vitro), and (2) to correlate results from all test information (puzzle pieces) available to provide the primary health care provider with a clear and accurate picture of the patient's state of health.

VASCULAR TESTING AND EVALUATION

Disorders involving decreased vascular integrity are rare, and no sophisticated accurate tests are available to evaluate vascularity. Capillary fragility tests can be performed to aid in the diagnosis. An example of a vascular test procedure is the **tourniquet test.** Blood flow is obstructed by application of some form of tourniquet. Use of a **blood pressure cuff adjusted to a specific pressure** (usually at the midpoint between the systolic and diastolic pressures), and **observation for petechiae** are carried out for a specific period of time (e.g., 5 minutes) as stated in the established procedure protocol in the laboratory. The number of petechiae seen are recorded. Increased numbers of petechiae indicate an increased capillary fragility. Reference values are approximately up to five petechiae. A decreased number of thrombocytes will also result in petechiae.

A tourniquet test is performed in a crude fashion each time that a tourniquet is used for phlebotomy (blood collection). If petechiae are prominent during a phlebotomy procedure, this should be brought to the attention of the nurse or physician assigned to the patient.

THROMBOCYTE TESTING AND EVALUATION

Quantitative testing of thrombocytes is the most convenient value to obtain for an initial evaluation of bleeding due to platelets. The most common test performed in the hematology laboratory is the **complete blood count (CBC),** which is part of the routine examination upon the patient's admission to the hospital. Many hematology tests are performed simultaneously by one instrument, and the final CBC report contains information relevant to leukocytes, erythrocytes, and thrombocytes. Components of the CBC include a **platelet count with a histogram, platelet indices, reference ranges,** and **flags for out-of-range values** (Fig. 13–1). There is also a "delta check," which notes if a patient's value has changed significantly from the previous performance of that same test. This allows you to correct or verify the result before releasing the information. The typical reference value for a total thrombocyte count is 150 to 450 $\times$ 10^9/l. References are 3 to 15 fl for the mean platelet volume (MPV) index and a platelet distribution width (PDW) of less than 20%. Keep in mind that reference values are given for the adult in the general population. **Each laboratory must establish its own normal reference values,** owing to variations in instrumentation, procedures, and local populations, which may render a less accurate interpretation of the generic normal reference values because of the differences in the specific laboratory involved in the testing.

Several instruments (with a variety of methodologies) perform the complete blood count. Electronic impedance (voltage-pulse variation), laser light scatter, light absorbance, and staining characteristics are the various principles utilized by cell counting instruments. These instruments are explained in greater detail in Chapter 6 in reference to leukocyte testing.

Correlation Factors. Known values of control and standard specimens should be run regularly to **determine the accuracy and precision of the system.** Many of the results will appear within the normal reference range and, although they must still be re-viewed for appropriateness, can be verified and sent to the patient's chart without additional correlation. If there is a special mark or "flag" near a result to alert the laboratory practitioner to an abnormal value, other tests should be considered to support and validate this result. The platelet count should correlate with the platelet estimate from looking at a peripheral blood smear of the specimen.

Sources of Error. An appropriate blood specimen is essential to perform an accurate platelet count. If the specimen **clots,** is **physically damaged,** tested at a **temperature other than room temperature,** or the **tube is inappropriately filled,** the blood must be redrawn. If the problem only involves temperature, the specimen is brought to the correct temperature before testing. When a whole blood (WB) specimen is refrigerated, the white blood cells and platelets may stick together.

Abnormalities that will **alter** a **platelet histogram** and count are: (1) small **schistocytes** (fragmented red blood cells) and extremely **microcytic red blood cells,** which would be counted as platelets, thus giving an erroneously high count; (2) **large platelets,** which may be counted as erythrocytes resulting in an erroneously low platelet count; (3) the presence of **satellitism** (platelets coating the white blood cells), which would result in a low count of free platelets; and (4) a **poorly mixed specimen** providing a less than random count (this is less likely because the newer instruments rotate the blood before sampling).

A **manual platelet count** from an **unopette dilution** is the most reliable **manual method** (Fig. 13–2). Manual counts are not often done and are performed only if the cell count is too low for accuracy on the automated instruments or when establishing a new protocol or procedure and another method of verifying results is needed. Low platelet counts occur occasionally in patients with hypoplastic disorders, after chemotherapy or radiation treatments, with thrombotic thrombocytopenic purpura (TTP), idiopathic thrombocytopenic purpura (ITP), and disseminated intravascular coagulation (DIC).

The **hemocytometer** is used for **manual**

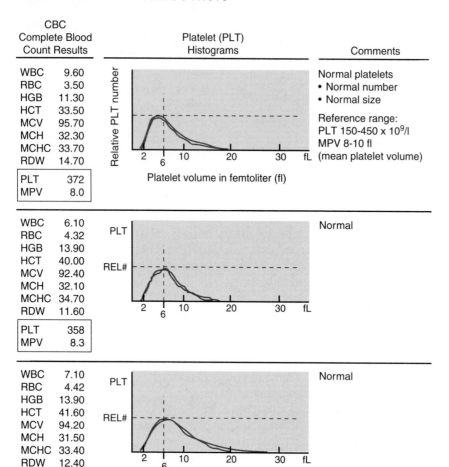

CBC Complete Blood Count Results	Platelet (PLT) Histograms	Comments

WBC 9.60
RBC 3.50
HGB 11.30
HCT 33.50
MCV 95.70
MCH 32.30
MCHC 33.70
RDW 14.70

PLT 372
MPV 8.0

Normal platelets
• Normal number
• Normal size

Reference range:
PLT 150-450 x 10⁹/l
MPV 8-10 fl
(mean platelet volume)

WBC 6.10
RBC 4.32
HGB 13.90
HCT 40.00
MCV 92.40
MCH 32.10
MCHC 34.70
RDW 11.60

PLT 358
MPV 8.3

Normal

WBC 7.10
RBC 4.42
HGB 13.90
HCT 41.60
MCV 94.20
MCH 31.50
MCHC 33.40
RDW 12.40

PLT 248
MPV 9.8

Normal

FIGURE 13–1
Complete blood count results with the platelet values and platelet histograms are highlighted. Note the histograms' reflection of the MPV by location of the peak and by the length of curve to the right. The height of the curve is less sensitive to the number of platelets.

cell counts of any specimen (refer to cell counts in Chapter 6). The variation in the procedure and calculation is dependent on the specimen used, the dilution of the specimen, and the area of the hemocytometer counting chamber grid in which cells are counted. The diluent characteristics are very important in any laboratory test situation. Particle counting, such as platelets, requires the diluent to maintain the platelets unaltered while destroying the red blood cells. The large number of red blood cells would obstruct the counting of platelets and, therefore, they must be removed. The center area of the hemocytometer is **engraved with squares to allow accurate counting** of the cells (Fig. 13–3). The Neubauer ruling on the central chamber area is 9 mm². The area is divided into smaller squares to facilitate counting. This procedure is explained in detail in Chapter 6, which refers to white blood cell counting. The modifications for the **platelet count** include: (1) the use of a different **diluent,** generically called a Rees-Eker fluid made of **ammonium oxalate;** (2) a higher dilution **(1:100);** (3) the **loaded chamber** must sit in a **moist dish for 10 minutes** to allow the platelets to settle down on the surface for accurate counting in one plane of focus; and (4) the **center 1-mm square** of the hemocytometer chamber is **counted** rather than the four corner squares counted for the white blood cell count (see Fig. 13–3). These changes can easily be inserted into the calculation to determine the number of platelets per cubic millimeter (mm³).

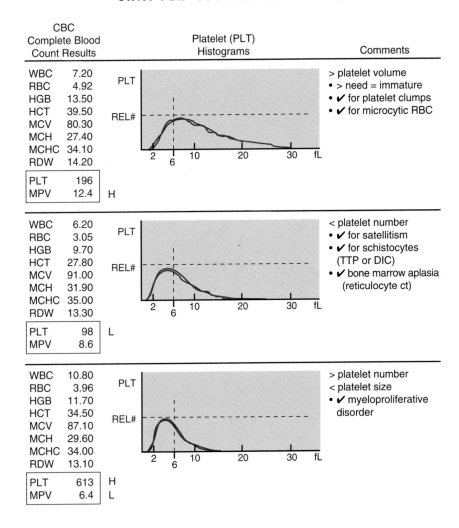

CBC Complete Blood Count Results		Platelet (PLT) Histograms	Comments
WBC 7.20 RBC 4.92 HGB 13.50 HCT 39.50 MCV 80.30 MCH 27.40 MCHC 34.10 RDW 14.20	PLT REL#		> platelet volume • > need = immature • ✔ for platelet clumps • ✔ for microcytic RBC
PLT 196 MPV 12.4	H		

WBC 6.20
RBC 3.05
HGB 9.70
HCT 27.80
MCV 91.00
MCH 31.90
MCHC 35.00
RDW 13.30
	PLT
	
	REL#
			< platelet number
			• ✔ for satellitism
			• ✔ for schistocytes
			  (TTP or DIC)
			• ✔ bone marrow aplasia
			  (reticulocyte ct)

PLT 98 MPV 8.6	L		
WBC 10.80 RBC 3.96 HGB 11.70 HCT 34.50 MCV 87.10 MCH 29.60 MCHC 34.00 RDW 13.10	PLT REL#		> platelet number < platelet size • ✔ myeloproliferative disorder
PLT 613 MPV 6.4	H L		

FIGURE 13–1
Continued

A manual hemocytometer count calculation and platelet count calculation follow:

$$\frac{\text{No. of white blood cells counted}}{\text{No. of 1-mm squares counted}} \times \text{dilution}$$
$$\times \text{ depth factor } 10* = \text{No. of cells/mm}^3$$

Adapting this formula to the platelet procedure would look like this:

$$\frac{\text{No. of platelets counted}}{1 \text{ (large square)}} \times 100$$
$$\times \text{ depth factor } 10 = \text{No. of platelets/mm}^3$$

* The hemocytometer chamber is only 0.1 mm deep; thus to report mm³, the depth must equal 1 mm; thus 0.1 × 10* = 1 × 1 × 1 mm² counted on the chamber.

In order to accurately count the platelets, it is important to let them settle to the surface of the counting grid and to utilize the fine focus constantly. Air bubbles and debris can mimic platelets; therefore, it is very important

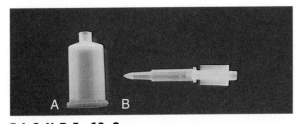

FIGURE 13–2
Unopette diluting reservoir (A) and micropipet (B) for manual platelet counts.

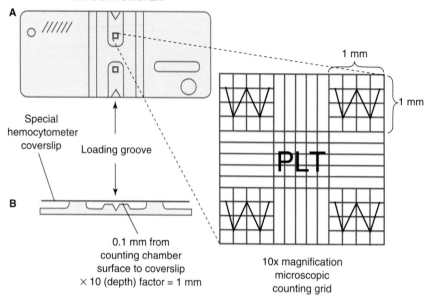

HEMOCYTOMETER

A

Special
hemocytometer
coverslip

Loading groove

B

0.1 mm from
counting chamber
surface to coverslip
× 10 (depth) factor = 1 mm

1 mm

1 mm

PLT

10x magnification
microscopic
counting grid

Two methods to calculate the cell count are as follows:

$$\frac{\text{No. of cells counted}}{\text{No. of 1 mm squares counted}} \times \text{dilution} \times \frac{\text{(depth factor)}}{10^*} = \text{No. of WBC/mm}^3 \text{ or /}\mu\text{l}$$

or

$$\text{Total cells counted} \times \text{dilution factor} \times \text{volume factor}^\dagger = \text{cells/}\mu\text{l or cell} \times 10^6\text{/l}$$

The hemocytometer chamber is only 0.1 mm deep, therefore to report mm³ the depth must equal 1 mm. Thus 0.1 × 10 = 1 mm × the 1 mm by 1 mm square counted on the chamber.
† If 10 mm³ × 0.1 mm (depth factor) = 1 μl.

FIGURE 13–3
The hemocytometer counting grid. Note the nine large 1-mm squares and the center one, which is the only square counted for platelets.

to look for a small particle that changes from black to white as the focus plane changes and that is moving slightly but does not change size throughout the focusing. Air bubbles and debris will change size and shape slightly throughout focusing and may not change from black to white. Begin counting in the upper left hand corner of the center 1-mm square and record, with a counter, the number of platelets seen. To avoid counting some cells more than once, which fall on a line, count only cells on the same two adjacent lines of each small square (Fig. 13–4).

Safety Precautions

1. Wear or use personal protective equipment (PPE) such as gloves, laboratory coats, and shields.
2. Never pipette by mouth. Use a suction apparatus to draw the specimen into the pipette.

Correlation Factors. The manual cell count should reflect the peripheral blood smear platelet estimate. The 1-mm center square is counted on each side of the chamber to check

CELL COUNTING PROTOCOL

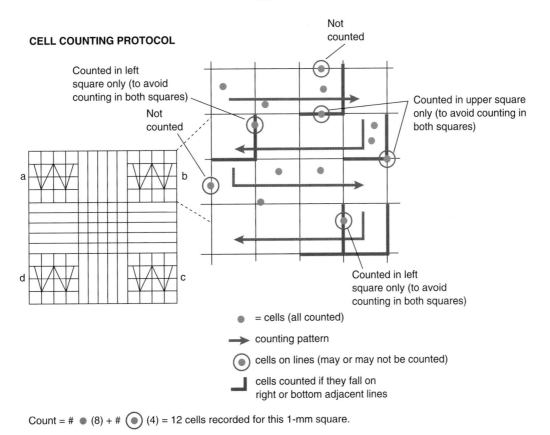

Count = # ● (8) + # ⊙ (4) = 12 cells recorded for this 1-mm square.

FIGURE 13–4

The protocol for counting cells to avoid missing cells or counting cells twice is shown. Cells on two adjacent lines within each small square are counted, and they are not counted if they lie on the two nondesignated lines.

precision of technique and randomness of distribution. The two counts should agree within 10% of each other. If a significant difference exists between the squares counted, an alternative large 1-mm square can be counted. This value would replace the original square that was not in agreement, or the hemocytometer can be cleaned and refilled with the same pipette after mixing and release of the first two drops.

Sources of Error. Error could be caused by: an incorrect or inadequate specimen; inadequate mixing of the specimen prior to sampling; incorrect dilution, diluting fluid, or calculation of the count; incorrect counting; counting some cells twice; or not counting all of the cells.

Microscopic Evaluation. An evaluation of the peripheral blood smear and a platelet esti-

mate can be done to support or rule out automated or manual count results. The estimate of the number of platelets is done by counting the platelets in at least five random fields in the good monolayer reading area of the peripheral blood smear. An **average of 8 to 20/100× field (oil immersion) is adequate** if the slide is truly a random representation of whole blood. If the five fields are very erratic and are not within a few platelets of each other, up to 10 additional fields should be counted. To ensure precision, a second smear should be examined and the results should agree within 10%. If a count is low, the blood smear evaluation may demonstrate **aggregation of platelets,** which in the automated instrument will appear as fewer large platelets. **Satellitism** could also be present, in which the platelets stick to the neutrophil membrane and are not counted individually. Inadequate mixing of the sample can also result in a decreased count. An important observation when evaluating the peripheral blood smear is the size and morphology of the platelets. **Large platelets are associated with a decreased count owing to increased demand.** If the platelets are too large, they may be counted on the automated instruments as red blood cells, which will erroneously decrease the platelet count and increase the red blood cell count. The morphology of the thrombocytes should be noted, also, for any variation from the gray cytoplasm with purple granules in the center.

Qualitative thrombocyte testing is recommended when the thrombocyte count is normal and there is still presence of bleeding (e.g., petechiae or purpura). Thrombocyte function is tested in general by the **bleeding time test.** As with most of the tests explained in this text, there are a variety of methods. The method that is most often used currently is the template bleeding time test, which is provided by several different companies. It is important that the specific equipment, procedure, or the laboratory's established protocol be followed. A generic sample of a procedure is presented here to provide some insight into how this test is performed.

The laboratory practitioner selects and **cleans a site** 2 inches below the elbow on the forearm. The area must be dry and clear of heavy hair growth, skin lesions, or eruptions. **Apply 40 mm Hg pressure** (with a blood pressure cuff) to the patient's arm. This provides a standardized capillary pressure for testing. **Two punctures are made** for duplication on the forearm using a lancet device (Fig. 13–5) that is 1 mm wide and 3 mm deep. A **stopwatch is started** with the first sign of blood. The **blood is blotted with filter paper** and care is taken not to touch the incision itself, which would enhance platelet function, but rather to touch only the drop of blood. When **blood is no longer absorbed onto the filter paper, the watch is stopped, the time is recorded,** and the blood pressure cuff is released. Reference values are usually **less than 10 minutes.** The bleeding time test is the **easiest and least expensive test to evaluate platelet function.** The disadvantage, however, is the subjective variation from one test to another due to practitioner bias; thus it is less accurate.

If proper platelet function is present, normal bleeding time, adhesion, and primary aggregation of the platelets will occur within 10 minutes to stop blood flow. Accurate interpretation of bleeding time test results is dependent on an adequate number of platelets present. **If the patient is thrombocytopenic, the bleeding time test will be prolonged** owing to a lack of platelets and not because of their dysfunction.

A second test to evaluate platelet function, which is easy and inexpensive, is the **clot retraction.** Fresh **whole blood** is collected without anticoagulant into a **graduated glass tube** (a conical centrifuge tube works well). Record the volume before clotting. Place the tube in a 37° C (body temperature) water bath or incubator **and observe for clot retraction at 1 hour, 2 hours, 4 hours, and 24 hours.** Clot retraction is indicated by the **clot** pulling away from the walls of the tube and **shrinking** as it **expresses the serum**

Do It Now **Vascular and Quantitative Thrombocyte Testing Exercise**

1. Write out the procedure for a manual platelet count using the unopette method. The basic unopette manual counting procedure is discussed in Chapter 6. The modifications for the platelet count are provided in this chapter.
2. Exchange the written procedure from question 1 with another classmate. As you read through each other's procedure, make note of the following:
   a. Are all the steps clearly explained?
   b. Which steps, if done incorrectly, could increase the platelet count, and how could this occur?
   c. Which steps, if done incorrectly, could decrease the platelet count, and how could this happen?
3. Discuss with another knowledgeable individual, or write out on your own, the controls necessary to ensure accuracy of the unopette manual platelet count value.

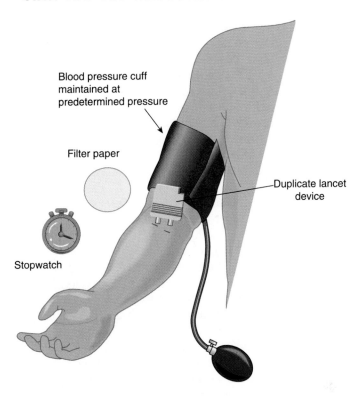

Blood pressure cuff
maintained at
predetermined pressure

Filter paper

Duplicate lancet
device

Stopwatch

FIGURE 13–5
The template method of the bleeding time test.
The lancet and forearm procedure is shown.

out. This process should begin within 1 hour and should be complete **within 24 hours.** Upon completion the **clot should be approximately half the original volume.** If the clot is observed to clot and dissolve again after 24 hours, a fibrinolytic abnormality is indicated. Additional information can be obtained if a wire or wooden stick is placed in the specimen initially, which allows removal of the clot upon completion to **observe the firmness or friability** (how easily it can be pulverized or crumbled) of the clot formed. The clot is removed and rolled across a paper towel or protective bench workpaper (behind a Plexiglas shield). If the clot is stable, very few, if any, cells will come off the clot and it will remain intact. If there is an abnormality in platelet retraction or the coagulation pathways, the clot may leave a significant number of cells behind in the tube and on the paper or it may fall apart. **A known healthy person's blood is set up for clot retraction and is recorded as a control.**

Special tests of platelet function that require special specimens, supplies, and equip-

ment are also available. Each manufacturer has an established procedure and protocol that must be followed for the equipment and supplies used. Most platelet testing requires a platelet-rich plasma (PRP) specimen. A **platelet-rich plasma** specimen is prepared by centrifuging an anticoagulated (**9:1 ratio of blood:anticoagulant of 3.8% sodium citrate**) specimen at **60 to 100 g for 10 minutes** to allow the separation of red blood cells and plasma with the platelets remaining in the plasma. Coagulation tests, which are explained later, require a **platelet-poor plasma (PPP)** specimen. PPP is prepared by centrifuging a 9:1 ratio (4.5:0.5 ml) of whole blood:anticoagulant of 3.8% sodium citrate at **2000 g for 10 minutes.** A modification to ensure a PPP is to draw off the supernatant after the PPP initial centrifugation and to spin this again to remove any residual platelets. A general explanation of platelet function tests is provided here.

Platelet adhesion can be evaluated by use of the **glass bead retention test.** The basic principle for this test is observing whether platelets exposed to the glass bead surfaces will be stimulated to adhere to the beads. A column of glass beads is the primary equipment used. A **PRP specimen is counted for platelet content, passed over the glass bead column,** collected as it comes out, and a **post-column platelet count is done.** If the platelets are functioning properly, **at least 70% of the platelets in the pre-test count should have been retained in the column.**

Aggregation studies of platelets are performed on platelet-rich plasma (PRP) as explained earlier. An aliquot of the **PRP is placed into an aggregometer** instrument, and the amount of light transmitted through the specimen is recorded. **An aggregating agent is added, and the change in light transmittance is recorded** and graphed. As aggregates form, the PRP becomes clear and the light transmission is increased. Aggregating agents used are **ADP, epinephrine, collagen, thrombin, ristocetin, and arachidonic acid.** All of these agents will induce aggregation in a healthy platelet. In specific diseases the platelets will demonstrate diminished or absent aggregation in response to a specific agent. An example of this is the diminished response associated with aspirin ingestion (Fig. 13–6). Recently **flow cytometry** laboratories have established procedures **to assess platelet aggregation** and **factor release** by flow cytometry. This methodology may provide a more accurate picture of the platelet abnormality or disease process; however, the equipment is expensive and a specially trained technician must test the specimen.

Platelet factor (PF) assays can also be performed, although the cost and expertise needed limit the procedure to primarily PF3 and PF4 and this is not often done. **PF3 assays** involve preparing a **series of dilutions** of the patient's PRP with the patient's platelet-poor plasma (PPP). The **clotting time** is then measured, demonstrating the availability of PF3. Platelet factor 4 **(PF4) is measured by radioimmunoassay** technique, which is performed in the chemistry area of the clinical laboratory and is explained in Chapter 6 in relation to measuring substances required for white blood cells.

COAGULATION TESTING AND EVALUATION

Tests routinely performed to evaluate the coagulation system are the **prothrombin time (PT) test** and the **activated partial thromboplastin time (APTT) test.** The PT reflects the function of the extrinsic pathway and warfarin (Coumadin) anticoagulant therapy involving primarily factor VII. The APTT demonstrates the functional intrinsic pathway and the effects of heparin therapy involving Fletcher and Fitzgerald factors, as well as factors XII, XI, IX, VIII, PF3, and Ca^{2+}. Most coagulopathies involve one of these two pathways. Less common is a disorder of the common pathway that would be detected by the **thrombin time (TT) test.** When any of these tests are prolonged, further testing such as the circulating anticoagulant test, factor substitution tests, factor assays, **fibrinogen**

Do It Now **Quantitative Testing and Evaluation of Thrombocytes Individually or in a Small Group**

1. Request two anticoagulated blood tubes from the instructor. From one tube prepare platelet-poor plasma (PPP), and from the other tube prepare platelet-rich plasma (PRP). Perform platelet counts (preferably manual) on each specimen to be sure that one is platelet rich and one is platelet poor. The patient's whole blood platelet count would be a good comparison for your preparations.

2. Request one clotted specimen from the instructor. Arrange the tubes prepared as in no. 1 next to the clotted specimen. Contrast and compare these three specimens in terms of: (a) name the various components in each tube, (b) estimate the liquid percentage of whole blood, (c) describe the appearance (color and clarity) of the fluid component, and (d) describe the testing associated with each specimen.

3. Exchange lists and begin reading each characteristic, followed by discussion or debate.

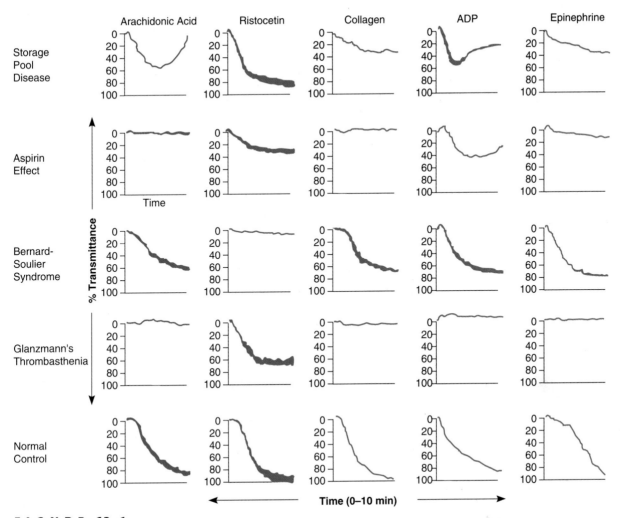

FIGURE 13-6
Platelet aggregation charts show the difference in the normal pattern and the abnormal patterns. This information is useful in the diagnosis of coagulation disorders, when the platelets are stimulated with a variety of aggregating agents.

levels, and factor immunoassays can be done to aid in the identification of the problem. The **fibrinogen degradation products (FDP) test** or the **D-dimer test** (fibrin products only) is the easiest and most common test performed in the clinical laboratory to assess the involvement of breakdown products of fibrinogen and fibrin in the coagulopathy under investigation. Specific FDPs act as circulating anticoagulants to inhibit clotting.

Be aware of the interpretation of the test results. Is the test measuring how much is present or the function of what is present? Factor assays performed in which clot formation is the indicator evaluate factor function. Immunoassays employ monoclonal antibodies to determine the quantity of a factor with no information regarding function.

Two methodologies are available for coagulation testing. The most common **coagulation methodology (optical clot detection)** is associated with instruments capable of performing several coagulation tests and several patient samples in duplicate. The original pre-test plasma is cloudy owing to the soluble fibrinogen present in the specimen. The

FAST FACTS

Vascular and Thrombocyte Information

Hemostasis Component	Tests to Evaluate	Diseases and Comments
Vasculature Platelet serotonin, epinephrine, and thromboxane A_2 constrict vessels Endothelial prostacyclin dilates	Tourniquet test (measures capillary integrity) >5 Petechiae = a positive test result Vitamin C levels	Hereditary telangiectasia Vitamin C deficiency (scurvy)
Thrombocytes 2–4 μm diameter 8–10 fl volume (MPV)	Automated count Manual count Peripheral blood smear schistocytes Normocytic and normochromic smear	150–450 × 10⁹/l reference <150 × 10⁹/l is thrombocytopenic <8 average/HPF results in hemorrhage TTP and DIC ITP and aplasia

DIC = differentiated intravascular coagulation; ITP = idiopathic thrombocytopenic purpura; HPF = high power field; MMV = mean platelet volume; TTP = thrombotic thrombocytopenic purpura.

cloudy plasma impedes the passage of light through the specimen, resulting in minimal light transmitted through the sample to the detector. When the **fibrinogen is converted to fibrin** as a clot forms, the **plasma clears, increasing the amount of light transmitted through the specimen to the detector.** The amount of time that it takes to form a fibrin clot is the reported value. The value on the instrument reflects the increase in light transmittance detected when the clot is formed, removing the fibrinogen and therefore clearing the specimen.

Sources of Error. The correct **specimen** (full, mixed, Na citrate tube) is essential. If the **9:1 blood:anticoagulant ratio** is not present, the test results are invalid. The **plasma** must be **fresh** (less than 4 hours old) and **clear** (no hemolysis, lipemia, or extreme icterus). If the specimen is hemolyzed, this may facilitate clotting that will result in an **abnormal specimen clotting within the normal reference interval in error.** A normal range result will then be released when the patient truly has impaired clotting ability. Since this methodology depends on accurate transmittance of light in relation to the clot, **any pre-existing alteration of the specimen** such as red color from hemolysis, white milky color from lipemia, or yellow color from bilirubin **may interfere with the accuracy of the value** obtained using the optical methodology.

A **second coagulation methodology** used as a back-up procedure or to perform special coagulation tests not adapted to the more sophisticated automation, involves **electromechanical probes.** Two electrodes are immersed in the test solution. One electrode stays stationary in the plasma test solution, while the other probe moves back and forth through the plasma. When a **clot forms** the electrical circuit is complete, **stopping the moving probe** and the timer. The time elapsed for the clot formation is recorded (Fig. 13–7).

Sources of Error. The correct **specimen** (full, mixed, Na citrate tube) is essential. If the 9:1 blood:anticoagulant ratio is not present, the test results are invalid. The plasma must be **fresh** (less than 4 hours old) and **clear** (no hemolysis, lipemia, or extreme icterus). If the specimen is **hemolyzed,** this may facilitate clotting, which will result in an abnormal specimen clotting within the normal reference interval in **error.** A normal range result will then be released when the patient has impaired clotting ability.

The **prothrombin time (PT) test** is most often ordered to monitor warfarin (Coumadin)

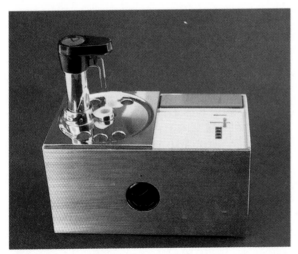

FIGURE 13-7
A fibrometer electromechanical coagulation instrument is useful in the performance of manual prothrombin time (PT), partial thromboplastin time (PTT), thrombin time (TT), fibrinogen, and factor substitution testing.

oral anticoagulant therapy. Warfarin competes with vitamin K in the liver, which is necessary for synthesis of the vitamin K–dependent coagulation factors. The factor most sensitive to vitamin K deficiency is factor VII of the extrinsic coagulation pathway. If factor VII is significantly decreased, the PT test will be prolonged. Due to the variation in PT reagent (tissue thromboplastin, factor III) from one company to another and from lot to lot, an international sensitivity index (ISI) has been established by the manufacturer for each lot of thromboplastin reagent produced. The ISI value is then used to calculate the international normalized ratio (INR) to generate consistent standardized results. The calculation is as follows:

INR =
the patient's PT value/mean reference value)^{ISI}

If the patient on **warfarin (Coumadin) therapy** has a PT value of 16 seconds, the control value is 12 seconds and the thromboplastin reagent has an ISI value of 2.0:

The PT ratio is $16/12 = (1.48)^{2.0\ ISI} = 2.19$ INR

The **PT** reference range is **11 to 13 seconds,** and the **INR** reference value is **less than 2.0.** The clinician administers warfarin to treat disorders such as deep vein thrombosis and strives to reach a therapeutic INR of 2.0 to 3.0. Patients with mechanical heart valves or more severe clotting problems may receive warfarin at a higher dose, bringing the INR between 3.0 and 4.5. The clinician is using the INR to effectively balance a level of oral anticoagulant, which is enough to inhibit clotting without placing the patient at risk for hemorrhage.

The procedure involves placing a small amount of **platelet-poor plasma (PPP)** from a sodium citrate specimen in a test well, adding the **tissue thromboplastin reagent** (factor III), and observing and recording the time required for a fibrin clot to develop.

A test measuring the **intrinsic coagulation pathway** is the **partial thromboplastin time (PTT) test.** The intrinsic system is the most sensitive to anticoagulation therapy with **heparin** and is, therefore, the test of choice to monitor heparin administration. The intrinsic system includes the contact factors (Fletcher, Fitzgerald, and XII) as well as factors VIII, IX, and XI. Most coagulation factor deficiencies and circulating anticoagulants involve these factors; therefore, an investigation and significant interpretation of an abnormal PTT are warranted. The standard reference value for the **PTT is less than 35 seconds,** and the specimen with values greater than this, with no history of anticoagulant therapy, is subjected to the circulating anticoagulant test (also called the "mix" test).

The PTT procedure involves placing a small amount of platelet-poor plasma (PPP) from a sodium citrate specimen in a test well, adding a cephaloplastin reagent (contact factors), incubating for 3 minutes to allow all of the many intrinsic pathway factors to become activated, then adding calcium chloride (CaCl), observing, and recording the time required for a fibrin clot to develop. The PT reagent thromboplastin contains the Ca^{2+} needed for clotting to occur, thus eliminating the need to add it later.

Sources of Error. The **correct specimen** (full, mixed, Na citrate tube), which is drawn at the proper time, is essential. The **time and the mode of administration** of the intravenous (IV) **heparin** must be documented. If a continuous IV pump administers the anticoagulant, drawing from the opposite arm of the IV is mandatory; however, timing is not critical. If heparin is administered in any other mode in which the level is erratic, the time and the amount of administration must be noted on the result sheet. If the **9:1 blood: anticoagulant** ratio is not present, the test results are invalid. The **plasma must be fresh (less than 4 hours old) and clear (no hemolysis, lipemia, or extreme icterus).** If the specimen is hemolyzed, this may facilitate clotting and will result in an abnormal specimen clotting within the normal reference interval in error. A normal result will then be reported when the patient has impaired clotting ability. The color of the plasma would not affect the electromechanical method, because there is no optical system involved in this methodology. Due to the manual nature of the electromechanical instrumentation, incubation and reaction times are critical and meticulous technique must be used to precisely duplicate and ensure accurate values.

The **circulating anticoagulant test** (or "1:1 **mix**") is done to determine if the prolonged APTT is due to a factor deficiency or to an unknown circulating anticoagulant in the patient's blood. This is done by mixing **equal volumes of prolonged patient plasma and the normal reference control plasma and performing an APTT on this "mix" solution.** If a **factor deficiency** was the cause of the prolonged result, the addition of all the factors present in the normal reference control plasma **should correct** the prolonged value. If the abnormal result was caused by an unknown **circulating anticoagulant,** such as fibrin degradation products from fibrinolysis, this will also inhibit the added factors in the normal reference plasma and the APTT will **remain abnormal.**

If a factor deficiency is indicated, the next test of choice is the **factor substitution test.** It would be cost prohibitive to purchase control plasmas, each containing a single factor to add back in one at a time, in order to determine which factor corrects the test. A more efficient alternative to single factor substitution involves the addition of either aged plasma or absorbed serum, each of which is artificially depleted of a variety of factors. **Aged serum (AS) contains only factors I, II, VII, IX, X, XI, and XII. Absorbed plasma (AP) contains factors I, V, VIII, XI, and XII.** Some coagulation factors are in both AS and AP, whereas others are unique to one reagent, thus allowing a process of elimination to aid in the determination of the deficient factor (Fig. 13–8). The **fibrinogen level** is the easiest and least expensive factor assay and will detect hypofibrinogenemia or afibrinogenemia. Factor immunoassays can also be done to aid in the identification of the problem.

The **Lee-White whole blood clotting time test** is a crude method of testing the **intrinsic pathway.** A sample of 4 ml of blood is drawn into a syringe. The last 3 ml are dispensed—1 ml into three small glass tubes numbered so that the freshest 1 ml is in tube 1 and the third milliliter is in tube 3. A stopwatch is started as soon as the blood is placed in the glass tubes. Tube 3 is tilted every 30 seconds until clotting occurs. If tube 2 has not clotted, tilt tube 2 every 30 seconds until this blood has clotted, then move to tube 1 and repeat the process. At the moment when tube 1 clots, the stopwatch is stopped and the whole blood clotting time is recorded. The reference value is **5 to 10 minutes.** This test is **not recommended** because of the lack of standardization from one test to another and owing to the excessive exposure of the person performing the test to the blood.

Additional tests, which are available but are seldom done, are the **prothrombin consumption test** (which tests the extrinsic pathway), the **thromboplastin generation time test** (tests factors VIII and IX of the intrinsic pathway), and the **protamine sulfate test** (neutralizes heparin in order to detect fibrin split products).

Patient scenario: The PTT was prolonged. A "mix" specimen of patient plasma and normal reference control plasma was combined in equal volumes (1:1) and mixed, and another PTT was performed. This circulating anticoagulant PTT is within the reference range, corrected by the addition of all of the factors in the control plasma, which suggests a factor deficiency and not a circulating anticoagulant. Aliquots of the patient's plasma are then "mixed" in equal volumes with either the absorbed plasma or the aged serum reagents. PTT tests are performed with these specimens, and the following results are possible.

AP*	AS†	Interpretation	Disease
Correction	No correction	Deficient factor is in AP. Only factors V and VIII are unique to AP	Hemophilia A (factor VIII deficiency)
No correction	Correction	Deficient factor is in AS. Only factors IV, VII, IX, X are unique to AS	Hemophilia B (factor IX deficiency)
Correction	Correction	Deficient in factor common to both AP and AS. Factors I, XI, and XII	Afibrinogenemia Hemophilia C (factor XI deficiency)
No correction	No correction	Circulating anticoagulant	
		Normal control "mix" would not have been corrected, thus no substitution studies	

* *Absorbed plasma (AP) contains only factors I, V, VIII, XI, and XII.*
† *Aged serum (AS) contains only factors I, II, VII, IX, X, XI, and XII.*

FIGURE 13–8
Coagulation factor substitution studies using aged serum (AS) and absorbed plasma (AP) for determination of which coagulation factor is deficient.

FIBRINOLYSIS TESTING AND EVALUATION

The most common test done to determine if inappropriate fibrinolysis is occurring is the **fibrinogen degradation products (FDP) test,** which is also called the **fibrin split products (FSP) test.** The specimen is serum or plasma from a special tube that inhibits further breakdown of these fibrinolytic products and must be used to obtain accurate results. This alternate additive is **thrombin with soy bean trypsin inhibitor (light blue top tube).** The test itself is a latex agglutination immunoassay for serum FDPs. Kits are available from various manufacturers and include the thrombin with soy bean trypsin inhibitor tube for the blood specimen, latex beads coated with antibody that will bind with D or E fibrin fragments, negative and positive control sera, and buffered saline. The serum from the **specimen is diluted** 1:5 and 1:2 in order to **detect** only **more than 2 μg/ml of FDPs.** One drop of the specimen is mixed with one drop of the well-mixed reagent in a ring on a clean glass agglutination slide. The slide is rotated and observed for agglutination for up to 2 minutes. The negative and positive control sera are run identically to the patient's unknowns and must yield expected results in order to report the patient's test results.

A more specific test for fibrin breakdown is the **D-dimer test.** D-dimer is the product of stabilized fibrin breakdown only. The FDP test also detects several fibrin associated fragments, some of which are not indicative of clot lysis. The specimen can be citrated or heparinized plasma, and the test is available as a latex ag-

1. Draw the coagulation pathways in your own creative, original format.
2. Add the various tests to the area of the diagram with which they are associated.

Request from your instructor (or find on your own with the instructor's help) a copy of the thrombin time, fibrinogen, prothrombin time, partial thromboplastin time, and fibrin degradation products test procedures. Contrast and compare the following aspects of the procedures:

1. Specimen collection and preparation for testing
2. Equipment and reagents used—what are they; how are they prepared; and why are they used?
3. What quality assurance or control measures are required to validate the test results?
4. What can interfere with or render the test results incorrect?

glutination methodology or an enzyme-linked immunosorbent assay (ELISA).

Additional fibrinolysis tests, which are available but are not often ordered, are the ethanol gelatin test, which detects fibrin monomers, and the euglobulin lysis test for excessive fibrinolytic activity. **Factor assays** can also be done **for plasminogen.**

Tests ordered to further investigate clotting tendencies are **protein C levels, protein S levels, and antithrombin III (ATIII) levels.** These are all natural inhibitors of coagulation, and the effectiveness of heparin therapy is dependent on ATIII, which is the heparin cofactor.

The hemostasis testing described in this chapter does not encompass every test or instrument available. A flow chart of the hemostasis tests from this chapter is presented in Figure 13–9. Coagulation and fibrinolysis are rapidly moving areas of medicine, and the

successful laboratory will have to keep up with the clinical practitioner's needs for patient diagnosis and management of disease. All tests and procedures must have controls; all have various sources of error, many of which are redundant. Correlation of results can never be emphasized enough. Isolated numbers mean nothing, but the relationship of those numbers to other tests and to the patients themselves will paint a picture from which the patient and health care providers can benefit.

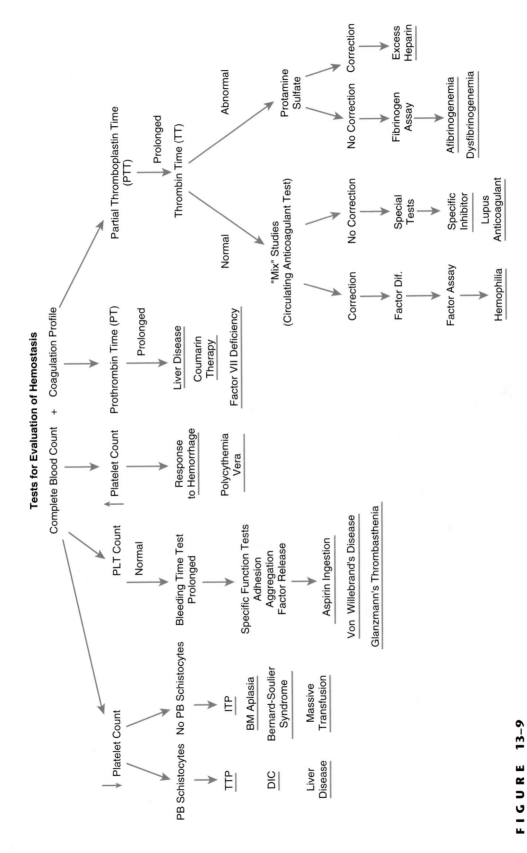

FIGURE 13-9

Flow chart of hemostasis testing. A logical approach to the diagnosis of hemostasis disorders.

Coagulation and Fibrinolysis Information

Pathway	Test	Comments
Extrinsic pathway	Prothrombin time (PT)	Warfarin (Coumadin) therapy 11–13 seconds, INR < 2.0
Intrinsic pathway	Partial thromboplastin time (PTT) Circulating anticoagulant test or "mix" test	Heparin therapy monitoring <35 seconds 1:1 "mix" of the patient's plasma to the normal control plasma Corrected PTT mix = factor deficiency Prolonged PTT mix = circulating antico-agulant
Common pathway	Thrombin time Fibrinogen level	17–25 seconds 200–400 mg/dl
Fibrinolytic pathway	Fibrinogen degradation products (FDP) test, also called the fibrin split products (FSP) test	Positive or negative latex agglutination for >2 μg/ml of fibrinogen or fibrin degra-dation products Specially diluted 1:5 and 1:20 to avoid a false positive result due to the normal ex-isting level

The specimen of choice for most coagulation testing is a full, well-mixed sodium citrate (Na citrate) blue top tube. The plasma should be placed at 4° C, and the test should be done within 4 hours owing to labile factors.

STUDY QUESTIONS

Match the Following Specimen Appropriate for Each Test Listed:

1. Prothrombin time (PT)

2. Platelet count

3. Fibrin degradation products (FDP)

4. Partial thromboplastin time (PTT)

5. Bleeding time

A. EDTA plasma

B. Na citrate plasma

C. Whole blood in vivo

D. Thrombin and soy bean trypsin

Choose the Best Answer to the Following Questions:

6. The test methodology most often used for coagulation testing is _____.
   A. Electromechanical
   B. Flow cytometry
   C. Photometric/optical
   D. Latex agglutination

7. The fibrometer is a back-up instrument for coagulation testing and uses _____ methodology.
   A. Electromechanical
   B. Flow cytometry
   C. Photometric/optical
   D. Latex agglutination

8. The D-dimer test utilizes this type of test methodology:
   A. Electromechanical
   B. Flow cytometry
   C. Colorimetric
   D. Latex agglutination

9. Before a bleeding time test can be interpreted the _____ test value must be known.
   A. Clotting time

   B. Platelet count

   C. D-dimer

   D. PTT

10. The bleeding time test evaluates:
    A. Platelet function

    B. Vascular integrity

    C. Intrinsic coagulation pathway

    D. All components of hemostasis

11. If the PTT is prolonged and hemophilia is suspected, what test is the first step to support a factor deficiency as the cause of the prolonged test?
    A. PT test

    B. TT test

    C. Circulating anticoagulant test

    D. PTT with a new specimen

12. The PTT, PT, and TT are all prolonged. These tests are repeated to rule out technical error. Correlation and interpretation of results should include:
    A. Report the results; this suggests a factor deficiency.

    B. Report the results with a request for a new specimen to repeat and verify the results.

    C. Do not report results; verify correct and acceptable specimen. If not, redraw.

    D. Do not report results; contact the supervisor.

13. As you are drawing blood from an elderly patient you notice the development of 15 petechiae on the arm just below the tourniquet. A test that should be done to help determine the cause of the small hemorrhages is:
    A. Bleeding time test

    B. Platelet count

    C. D-dimer test

    D. PTT

14. Explain your choice of answer for question 13.

15–20. Contrast and compare heparin therapy and warfarin (Coumadin) therapy and testing.

Body Fluids

The fluids analyzed in hematology are not easily obtained and arrive in the laboratory after patient stress and duress from specimen collection. Keep this in mind during analysis of the specimen, and handle these fluids carefully, using only the amount that is required. Try to complete the tests as soon as possible with the utmost precision and accuracy.

CHAPTER 14

OUTLINE

Cerebrospinal Fluid

Synovial Fluid (Joint)

Serous Fluids

Urine Analysis and Miscellaneous Body Fluids

Study Questions

Body Fluid Analysis

O B J E C T I V E S

Upon completion of this chapter the student should be able to:

1. Recognize or fill in on a diagram or picture of the human body, the source location for the various body fluids.

2. Describe the test procedure and methodology for analyzing body fluids and interpretation of the data.

3. Contrast and compare an exudate and a transudate in reference to location, origin, chemistry, cells, and associated disease.

Body fluids, which are examined and analyzed in the hematology area of many laboratories, include **cerebrospinal fluid (CSF), synovial fluid, seminal fluid, and serous fluids, such as pleural fluid, pericardial fluid, and peritoneal (ascites) fluid.** Except for seminal fluid, these fluids are almost cell free and are present in very small quantities in various areas of the body (Fig. 14–1). These fluids become specimens for clinical laboratory analysis only when clinical symptoms exist or when excess accumulation occurs, suggesting a pathologic condition. Body fluids are analyzed for **physical, microscopic, chemical, microbiologic, and sometimes immunologic (antigen) characteristics.** Seminal fluid is examined for the presence or absence of various cells and spermatozoa. Brief comments are presented on **urine, amniotic fluid, and wound aspirates.** These body fluids are not examined or analyzed in hematology.

CEREBROSPINAL FLUID

Cerebrospinal fluid (CSF) is a clear, watery, cell-free liquid that is present in the spinal column and surrounding the brain. Its

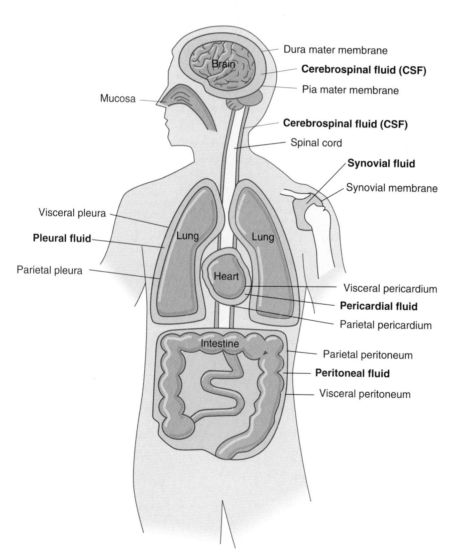

F I G U R E   14–1
The various body fluids, which are examined and evaluated in the clinical laboratory, are drawn from various parts of the body. (Modified from Applegate EJ: The Anatomy and Physiology Learning System. Philadelphia: WB Saunders, 1995, p 76.)

Dura mater membrane
Cerebrospinal fluid (CSF)
Brain
Pia mater membrane
Mucosa
Cerebrospinal fluid (CSF)
Spinal cord
Synovial fluid
Synovial membrane
Visceral pleura
Pleural fluid
Lung   Lung
Parietal pleura
Heart
Visceral pericardium
Pericardial fluid
Parietal pericardium
Intestine
Parietal peritoneum
Peritoneal fluid
Visceral peritoneum

Body Fluid Analysis General Information

Types of Body Fluids
Cerebrospinal fluid (CSF)
Serous fluids (pleural, peritoneal, and pericardial)
Synovial fluid
Seminal fluid

Body Fluid Characteristics
Physical appearance and volume
Microscopic evaluation for cells, crystals, or
    microorganisms
Chemical analysis for glucose and protein
Microbiologic analysis for infectious agents
Immunologic analysis for antigens or antibodies
    (not routine)

purpose is to cushion the central nervous system (CNS) and provide a medium for nutrients and removal of waste products. The brain is surrounded by three membranes called the **meninges,** which are **infected** in a highly fatal disease known as spinal **meningitis.** The spinal fluid exists between two of the membranes in the **subarachnoid space** and **spinal column.** The endothelium of the capillaries in the CNS is more selective than is the capillary endothelium in other parts of the body. The passage of substances between the blood and the CSF is restricted. This is called the **blood-brain barrier** and allows only low molecular weight proteins and certain antibiotics to pass into the CSF. The CSF is in a dynamic balance between production by the brain cells, circulation, and reabsorption into the blood. A 20-ml turnover occurs every hour with a total volume of 85 to 150 ml in the average adult. If an obstruction occurs, an accumulation of CSF and the development of hydrocephalus may result in brain damage, mental retardation, and death. To obtain spinal fluid, the patient is placed in a fetal position on a treatment table or in bed. The site is cleansed and anesthetized, and a needle is inserted between the third or fourth lumbar interspace (Fig. 14–2). A **maximum of 20 ml** can be taken from an adult if the spinal pres-

sure is normal. The preference is to remove less than 20 ml. After collection of the spinal fluid, the volume is recorded and the fluid is dispensed into at least three sterile tubes for distribution to areas of the clinical laboratory. **Testing** should take place as soon as possible after the CSF has been collected. The **first tube** is used for **chemical and immunologic testing** since these results will not be affected by cells introduced through blood vessel injury during the tap procedure. The **second tube** is sent to the **microbiology** department for testing, and the **third tube** is sent to the **hematology** department for cellular evaluation and cytology preparations. If only a small volume is collected, the health care provider (e.g., physician, nurse practitioner) must prioritize the tests ordered. Microbiologic analysis may be the most important test and must be done from an unopened sterile specimen. If only **one tube of CSF** is collected, the **microbiology** department should process the specimen **first** and then pass it on to the hematology and chemistry departments.

The **physical examination of the cerebrospinal fluid** includes the observation of volume, color, and viscosity. Normal CSF is **clear** and **colorless** and has the **viscosity of water.** A thin film or clot may form and is associated with the puncture from collection. Cloudy CSF indicates the presence of more than $200/\mu l$ white blood cells and more than $400/\mu l$ red blood cells. Microorganisms and protein can also appear cloudy in CSF. Yellow discoloration is described as **xanthochromic** and may be due to **protein greater than 150 mg/dl, the presence of hemoglobin, or products of hemoglobin breakdown.** The appearance of **gross amounts of whole blood** will be evident, and a **traumatic tap must be ruled out.** This is done by comparing the cell counts from each collection tube, which will vary greatly if a traumatic tap is the source of the cells. If this is a pathologic process in the CSF, the cell counts should be consistent. Another indication of subarachnoid hemorrhage is the appearance of phagocytes with ingested erythrocytes on microscopic examination.

Microscopic examination of CSF in-

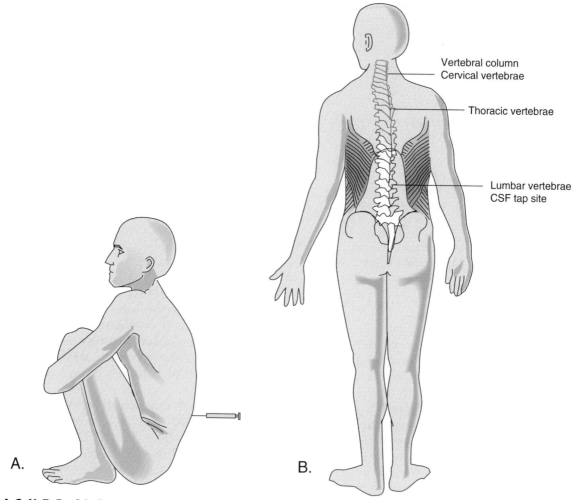

F I G U R E   14–2

A and *B,* Lumbar puncture for collection of cerebrospinal fluid (CSF). During this procedure, the patient must lie in the fetal position in order to extend and separate the vertebrae. A needle is inserted between the third or fourth lumbar interspace.

cludes a **total cell count** by the manual hemocytometer method of cell counting and a **cytocentrifugation slide differential.** The manual cell count and cytocentrifuge preparation are explained in Chapter 15. Reference values for **normal CSF are up to 5 mononuclear cells/µl for adults,** up to 10 mononuclear cells/µl for children aged 5 to puberty, up to 20 mononuclear cells/µl for children younger than 5 years of age, and up to 30 mononuclear cells/µl for neonates. Adult mononuclear cells in CSF are lymphocytes, whereas the neonate cells are primarily monocytes. The presence of increased numbers of

mononuclear cells is suggestive of a **viral infection,** whereas the presence of a significant number of **neutrophils** suggests a **bacterial infection.** These diseases are described as viral meningitis or bacterial meningitis and demonstrate white blood cells and sometimes microorganisms (Fig. 14–3). Cells shed from the CNS (**ependymal cells** or choroid plexus cells) can be seen occasionally in the CSF (Fig. 14–4). These cells are not significant and may be difficult to distinguish from malignant cells. Any unusual cells (e.g., tumor cells) or obvious microorganisms (e.g., *Cryptococcus*) should be reported (Fig. 14–5). Keep in mind

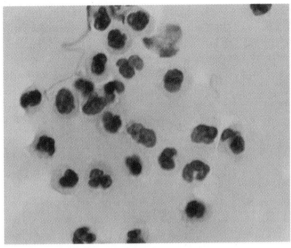

FIGURE 14–3
Meningitis (bacterial), as seen on a Wright-Giemsa–stained cytocentrifuge slide preparation of CSF. Note that the majority of white blood cells are segmented neutrophils, which are indicative of a bacterial infection. Primarily lymphocytes would be seen with a viral meningitis.

that **only a fresh CSF is valid and accurate.** Cells will become altered and lyse upon sitting.

Chemical analysis of CSF is also important in the diagnosis. The major chemistry tests performed are the tests for CSF **protein** (15 to 45 mg/dl) and CSF **glucose** (10 to 30 mg/dl). Additional tests that may assist in di-

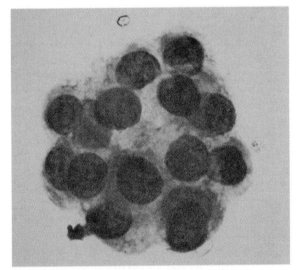

FIGURE 14–4
Ependymal cells are seen occasionally in normal cerebrospinal fluid (CSF). (From Henry JB: Clinical Diagnosis and Management, 18th ed. Philadelphia: WB Saunders, 1991, p 449.)

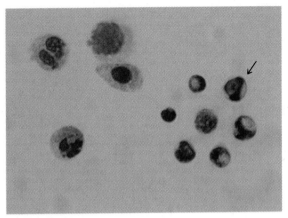

FIGURE 14–5
Cryptococcus microorganisms in a cerebrospinal fluid (CSF) cytospin preparation.

agnosis detect and measure specific **protein fractions** and **immunoglobulins** associated with disease states. **Elevated lactate levels** are seen in **CNS tissue hypoxia; enzymes** (aspartate aminotransferase [AST] and lactate dehydrogenase [LD]) rise in **cerebral infarction** (stroke); **glutamine** levels are useful in diagnosis of **encephalopathy** (degenerative brain disease); specific **amino acids** are associated with genetic **metabolic disorders;** and diagnosis of **CNS diseases** such as **multiple sclerosis** utilize the detection of certain **immunoglobulins** and their levels. Biogenic **amine levels** in the CSF provide treatment information for patients with **seizure disorders** and **Parkinson's disease.** The effectiveness of various drugs such as antibiotics and anticonvulsants depends on the maintenance of therapeutic CSF levels.

Microbiologic examination of CSF includes: a **Gram stain** for bacterial or fungal organisms, an **acid-fast stain** for *Mycobacterium tuberculosis* identification, concentrated CSF stained with **auramine-rhodamine** for identification of *Mycobacterium* species, and possibly (but not the best choice) the india ink stain for *Cryptococcus neoformans.* There are **latex agglutination** tests for *Cryptococcus* that are much more reliable than is the india ink preparation. **Immunologic assays** for microorganism antigens or antibodies to these antigens provide a rapid presumptive diagnosis for *Haemophilus influenzae, Neisseria menin-*

gitides, Streptococcus pneumoniae, and group B *Streptococcus.* CSF is **cultured to detect many pathogens,** some of which are difficult to recover. Isolation of viruses from CSF involves special media and techniques that are not readily available in every laboratory. **Lymphocyte subsets** that are present in the CSF can be identified by monoclonal antibodies to help in the investigation of **CNS inflammatory responses.**

Analysis of cerebrospinal fluid can provide information for early diagnosis of central nervous system disease and life-threatening central nervous system infections.

SYNOVIAL FLUID (JOINT)

Synovial fluid is the result of **ultrafiltration of plasma** across the synovial membrane and from **secretion by synoviocytes.** Synovial fluid is a viscous lubricant for the joints and has a unique composition. The **glucose** and **uric acid** concentrations are equivalent to blood plasma levels, while total protein and immunoglobulin values are one fourth to one half of those of blood plasma. Ideally, the **patient should have fasted for 4 to 6 hours** or overnight to allow a synovial fluid-plasma equilibrium to occur. A blood sample should be drawn at approximately the same time as the fluid for comparison of components. Testing of the fluid should be done as soon as possible. The **anticoagulant** of choice for synovial fluid is **sodium heparin at approximately 25 units/ml of fluid.** Approximately 5 to 10 ml is collected into a sterile tube containing sodium heparin for **microbiology tests.** A second tube for **microscopic examination** should contain 2 to 5 ml. The remaining synovial fluid should be placed in a plain empty tube for further studies, such as chemistry determination of uric acid content.

The **physical examination of synovial fluid** begins with documentation of the total volume collected. Due to the distribution of the total volume collected in a syringe into three different tubes, the total volume should be recorded at the patient's bedside at the time of aspiration. The **color and clarity** should be noted. Normal synovial fluid is **pale yellow or colorless and clear.** Turbidity of the synovial fluid can result from the presence of leukocytes, erythrocytes, synoviocytes, crystals, fat droplets, fibrin, and cellular debris. These can be identified microscopically. Synovial fluid is **viscous** due to the presence of the mucoprotein hyaluronate, a connective tissue component that holds membrane cells together.

The **microscopic examination** includes a **total cell count** by the manual hemocytometer method of cell counting, a **wet preparation,** and a **cytocentrifugation slide differential.** The total cell count can be done using a light microscope or a phase-contrast microscope to allow better visibility of the unstained cells. The wet preparation is best viewed with a **polarized microscope to identify crystals.** The manual cell count, wet preparation, and cytocentrifuge preparation are explained in Chapter 15. The **clear specimen** can be **manually counted undiluted for the total cell count.** If the **specimen is turbid,** however, a **dilution may be necessary. Dilutions** can be made with **normal saline** (0.85% NaCl) or with a hyaluronidase buffer solution. If saline is used, the viscosity will remain high and the cells will require more time to settle down on the chamber for counting. **Acetic acid should not be used** because this will result in mucin clot formation and the clumping of cells, thus making an accurate random cell count impossible. If the erythrocytes must be removed, a hypotonic saline solution (0.3%) can be used for dilution. Synovial fluid usually contains **less than 2000/μl erythrocytes** and **less than 200/μl leukocytes.** Leukocyte counts of higher than 2000/μl are significant, however, not specific. Infectious (bacterial) arthritis, gouty arthritis, and rheumatoid arthritis will all result in elevated leukocyte counts in synovial fluid.

The **synovial fluid wet preparation** is done primarily to discover and identify crystals that will aid in the diagnosis. **Monosodium urate (MSU) crystals** (1 to 30 μm in length) are indicative of gouty arthritis (Fig. 14–6). **Cholesterol crystals** are associated with chronic inflammatory conditions such as

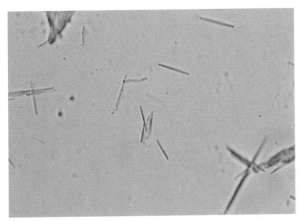

FIGURE 14-6
Monosodium urate (MSU) crystals seen in synovial fluid with gout.

rheumatoid arthritis (Fig. 14–7). **Calcium pyrophosphate dihydrate (CPPD) crystals** (1 to 20 μm) are seen in calcification of articular cartilages, degenerative arthritis, and arthritis associated with metabolic diseases such as hypothyroidism, hyperparathyroidism, and diabetes mellitus. MSU and cholesterol crystals are bright and easy to visualize compared with pyrophosphate dihydrate crystals. These crystals all have fairly characteristic shapes (Fig. 14–8). **Hydroxyapatite (HA) crystals** require electron microscopy in order to visualize them due to their small size and leukocyte intracellular location. HA crystals are associated with calcium deposit disorders. Crystalline **corticosteroid crystals** will be seen af-

ter intra-articular injection for treatment and should not be mistaken for a biologic crystal of significance for diagnosis (see Fig. 14–8). Consultation with the primary care provider concerning treatment would facilitate accurate identification and significance of crystals present.

A **synovial fluid cytocentrifugation slide differential**, stained with Wright-Giemsa, normally demonstrates approximately **60% monocytes and macrophages,** approximately 30% lymphocytes, and approximately **10% neutrophils. Synovial lining cells (synoviocytes)** may also be seen (Fig. 14–9). Greater than 80% neutrophils is associated with bacterial arthritis and urate gout. An increase in the lymphocyte percentage is seen in early stages of rheumatoid arthritis; the later stages demonstrate an increase in neutrophils.

Chemical examination of synovial fluid for diagnostic purposes is limited due to the viscosity of the specimen. The chemistry tests that can be performed on synovial fluid to provide useful information are glucose, total protein, uric acid, and lactate. The **synovial fluid glucose** must be accompanied by a blood specimen collected at the same time to determine the **plasma-synovial fluid glucose difference.** If the patient has been fasting, the plasma and synovial fluid glucoses should agree within 10 mg/dl. If there is more than 25 mg/dl less glucose in the synovial fluid than in the plasma, an inflammatory condition is indicated. If there is more than 40 mg/dl difference, sepsis (infection) is present. **Synovial fluid total protein** is normally about one third of the plasma value. An elevated value is due to membrane permeability changes and indicates an inflammatory condition. This is **not specific enough** to affect treatment and, therefore, is not usually done. Gout is most reliably diagnosed by elevated **plasma and synovial fluid uric acid levels;** however, frequently **microscopic examination for monosodium urate crystals** is used to determine the diagnosis. Although not of clinical utility yet, the **synovial fluid lactate level** is associated with several diseases. An elevated lactate level is associated with rheumatoid arthritis and

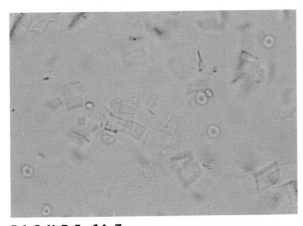

FIGURE 14-7
Cholesterol crystals as seen in body fluids.

Crystal	Morphology	Disease
Monosodium urate (MSU)		Gouty arthritis
Calcium pyrophosphate (CPPD)		Degenerative or metabolic arthritis
Cholesterol		Tuberculosis or rheumatoid arthritis
Corticosteroid		Drug injection for inflammation

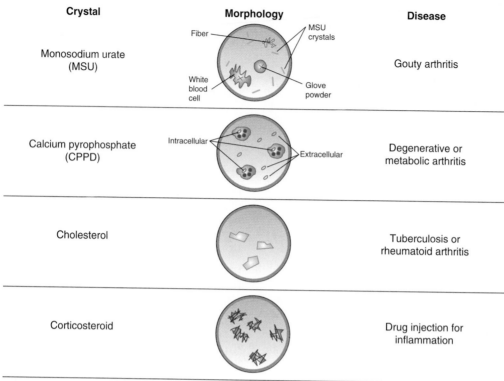

F I G U R E 14–8
Synovial fluid (SF) crystals most often seen in various diseases.

septic arthritis; however, gonococcal arthritis displays a normal lactate level.

Immunologic studies can also be done with synovial fluid to detect proteins associated with a primary disease and concomitant accumulation of synovial fluid in the joints. **Rheumatoid arthritis (RA)** antibodies and **lupus erythematosus (LE)** protein are examples of disease proteins in this category.

Microbiology studies of synovial fluid aid in the differential diagnosis of joint disease. A positive **Gram stain** suggests a bacterial disease. A Ziehl-Neelsen stain should be used for diagnosis if tuberculosis arthritis is suspected. The **synovial fluid culture** is positive in most cases of bacterial arthritis. **If diseases due to mycobacteria, fungi, and anaerobic organisms are suspected, special culture media and conditions must be considered. This is a key example of the need for communication and collaboration between the laboratory practitioner and the primary care clinician.** Without this interaction of health care providers, the suspected diagnosis and appropriate tests will not be considered and the efficiency and quality of patient care will be compromised.

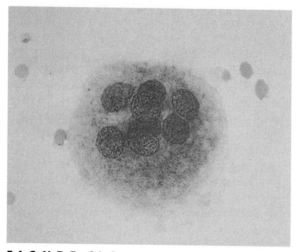

F I G U R E 14–9
Synoviocyte occasionally seen in normal synovial fluid (SF). (From McClatchey KD (ed): Clinical Laboratory Medicine. Baltimore, Williams & Wilkins, 1994, p 555.)

SEROUS FLUIDS

Serous fluids such as pleural fluid, pericardial fluid, and peritoneal (ascites) fluid exist **between two thin mesothelial-lined membranes** referred to as serous membranes. Serous membranes surround various body cavities (see Fig. 14–1). In a healthy individual, only a small amount of serous fluid is present between the serous membranes **to lubricate their surfaces for normal body movement of one membrane against the other.** Examples are lung expansion, heart contraction, and movement of the viscera in the abdomen. Excessive accumulation of these fluids accompanies the development of various diseases and is called an effusion. The various mechanisms for an accumulation of serous effusions are: **a decrease in osmotic pressure** (due to a decrease in plasma proteins); **an increase in hydrostatic pressure** (excess water in the blood and body tissues); an **increase in capillary permeability** (more water and solute movement); a **decrease in lymphatic reabsorption;** or an **obstruction** of lymph flow. All of these mechanisms involve tissue damage or an imbalance in fluid distribution.

Establishing whether a serous effusion is a transudate or exudate is an aid in the establishment of a diagnosis or a cause of fluid accumulation. Exudates and transudates are differentiated by their specific gravity, total protein, and cell content. In general, **exudates** have a higher **specific gravity (>1.015)** and a total protein of more than 3 g/dl, which should represent more than 50% of the serum total protein level. Exudates result from the decreased permeability of the capillaries and the decreased absorption of fluid by the lymphatic system. The **leukocyte count is higher than 1.0×10^9/l,** with increased **neutrophils or lymphocytes,** and the **erythrocyte count is higher than 100×10^9/l,** especially with a malignancy. Exudates appear cloudy or they may be bloody and clotted. **Transudates** are clear, colorless, and watery. The **specific gravity is less than 1.015,** and the total protein is less than 3 g/dl. The **leukocyte count is less than 100×10^9/l** with more than 50% mononu-

clear cells. Transudates result from a decrease in osmotic pressure and an increase in hydrostatic pressure. Fluid formation is a dynamic process involving the constant formation and reabsorption of the body fluid. Formation of fluids occurs via filtration of plasma through capillary endothelium, and fluid is reabsorbed by the capillaries and lymph system.

Serous fluid analysis includes a physical examination for volume, clarity, and color; **total cell count** to determine the increased presence of cells; **microscopic examination of cytocentrifuge slide** in order to differentiate mononuclear cells (usually lymphocytes) from neutrophils, which indicate a bacterial infection; **cytology examination** to identify any neoplastic cells present; **chemical examination** of total protein, lactate dehydrogenase, glucose, amylase, triglyceride, pH, and carcinoembryonic antigen (CEA); **and microbiologic examination** of stained slides and culture growth. All of these analytic tests are presented in more detail in Chapter 15.

In a healthy individual there is less than 15 ml of **pleural fluid** between two serous membranes in the **thoracic (chest) cavity.** In disease, however, more than 1000 ml may accumulate and must be removed to avoid shortness of breath, lung compression, and development of pneumonia. To remove the pleural fluid, the chest wall is punctured and the fluid is drained. This procedure is called a **thoracentesis.** In order to determine the cause of the pleural effusion, the fluid is sent to the laboratory for analysis. The analytic tests are presented in Chapter 15. A microscopic examination of a cytocentrifuge slide stained with Wright-Giemsa will routinely demonstrate **mesothelial cells** from the membrane lining, **monocytes, macrophages,** and **neutrophils** if there is an inflammatory process, or **lymphocytes** in response to tuberculosis, neoplasms, and systemic diseases (Fig. 14–10). If a neoplasm is suspected in the lung, suspicious neoplastic or cancerous cells may be seen (Fig. 14–11). Notice how these cells have **lost their contact inhibition** and appear to be "stuck together" with no defined margins. The cells have **large nuclei with nucleoli,** which may be

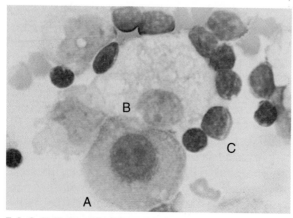

FIGURE 14-10

Pleural effusion showing a mesothelial cell (*A*), a macrophage (*B*), and lymphocytes (*C*). The lymphocytes are a cell population characteristically seen with a malignancy, such as this case of lung cancer, or tuberculosis. A bacterial infection would be indicated by neutrophils. Note how the cells are individual although they are close to each other. (Cells courtesy of Margaret Liffick.)

pleomorphic (abnormal cell structure), and are **dark blue,** indicating a high level of activity. Many pleural effusions result from congestive heart failure, which is a systemic disease; therefore, primarily lymphocytes should be seen.

Pericardial fluid is the lubricating fluid between the serous membranes **surrounding the heart** in the pericardial cavity. Approximately 10 to 50 ml of this clear, straw-colored ultrafiltrate of plasma is adequate to serve as a lubricant and to allow contraction and relax-

ation of the heart without pain due to friction between membranes. Any damage to the lining of the pericardial cavity is associated with **infection, malignancy** (neoplasm), or **metabolic damage from increased toxic waste products,** such as in kidney damage, resulting in a fluid increase and uremia from renal failure. This pericardial effusion exerts a mechanical interference on heart movement and function, which requires immediate aspiration. Microscopic examination of a cytocentrifuge slide stained with **Wright-Giemsa** will routinely demonstrate **mesothelial cells** from the membrane lining, **monocytes, macrophages,** and **neutrophils** if there is an inflammatory process, or **lymphocytes** in response to tuberculosis, neoplasms, and systemic diseases (see Fig. 14-10). If a neoplasm is suspected in the lung, suspicious **neoplastic or cancerous cells** may be seen (see Fig. 14-11). Notice how these cells appear to have **lost the contact inhibition** and are "stuck together" with no defined margins. The cells have **large nuclei with nucleoli** demonstrating **pleomorphism** (abnormal structure), and the cells are **dark blue,** indicating a high level of activity.

Peritoneal (ascitic) fluid bathes the abdominal membranes to allow visceral organ movement without friction pain. In healthy individuals less than 100 ml of clear, straw-colored fluid is found between the serous membranes of the abdomen. The presence of a peritoneal effusion (increased collection of fluid) is the result of increased hydrostatic pressure of systemic circulation (associated with congestive heart failure), decreased plasma osmotic pressure (hypoproteinemia), decreased lymphatic reabsorption (neoplastic blockage), and increased permeability of local capillaries (due to peritonitis). Microscopic examination of a cytocentrifuge slide stained with Wright-Giemsa will routinely demonstrate **mesothelial cells** from the membrane lining, **monocytes, macrophages,** and **neutrophils** if there is an inflammatory process, or **lymphocytes** in response to tuberculosis, neoplasms, and systemic diseases (see Fig. 14-10). If a **neoplasm** is suspected in the lung, suspicious neoplastic or cancerous cells may be seen (see Fig. 14-11). Notice how

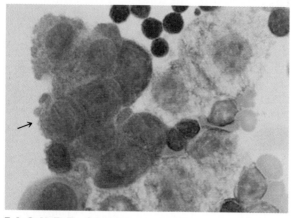

FIGURE 14-11

Pleural effusion demonstrating malignant adenocarcinoma cells originating from the lung. Notice the loss of contact inhibition that makes them look continuous. (Cells courtesy of Margaret Liffick.)

these cells appear to have **lost their contact inhibition** and appear to be "stuck together" with no defined margins, **large nuclei with nucleoli,** often demonstrating **pleomorphism** (abnormal morphology), and the **dark blue cytoplasm,** indicating a high level of activity. Many peritoneal effusions result from congestive heart failure, which is a systemic disease of abnormal hydrostatic pressure that forces movement of fluid from one area of the body to another. **Lymphocytes** are associated with neoplasms and diseases other than bacterial infection. If an infectious process was responsible for the effusion, segmented neutrophils would be present instead of the lymphocytes, such as those seen in Figure 14–10.

Seminal fluid or semen is produced by the prostate, the testes, the epididymis, the seminal vesicles, and a small amount by the bulbourethral gland. This viscous fluid is used to transport spermatozoa (sperm cells). Analysis of seminal fluid is done most often to evaluate infertility or to provide information concerning the lack of sperm present following a vasectomy to confirm the success of the procedure. A variation in the sperm concentration of seminal fluid warrants analysis of at least two specimens. Specimen collection for duplicate **specimens should be at least 7 days, but no more than 3 months, apart.** Sexual **abstinence for at least 48 hours** (and not more than 7 days) prior to collection allows a more accurate evaluation, and **this information should be recorded on the identification label.** The specimen is collected by the patient through masturbation (not involving a lubricant or condom) into a **clean sterile wide-mouthed container,** such as a sterile urine container, which has been **approved by the clinical laboratory.** Some containers are toxic to spermatozoa. The patient must be instructed in written form as well as verbally, and he must be provided with a quiet, comfortable, and private room near the laboratory. The collection process should be handled using the utmost sensitivity. Before collection, the container of seminal fluid and the **specimen following collection must be kept at room temperature** in order to avoid cold shock and to

enhance the quality of the evaluation of the spermatozoa mobility. A **white blood cell count of more than 1 × 10⁶/ml** of seminal fluid is indicative of an **inflammatory condition,** usually involving the seminal vesicle or the prostate.

The **seminal fluid evaluation** includes the **physical examination,** which includes recording the **color** (gray-white and opalescent), **volume** (2 to 5 ml), and **viscosity** after liquefaction (tested by dropping from a Pasteur pipette, which should demonstrate discrete droplets after 1 hour). **Microscopic examination of seminal fluid** includes an assessment of the **motility** by placing a drop of the specimen on a slide, adding a coverslip, and observing the percentage of sperm moving. Additional tests of seminal fluid include the total **spermatozoa count,** a determination of the percentage of spermatozoa with **normal morphology** (Figs. 14–12, 14–13, and 14–14), the **physical orientation,** the **viability** or survival, and the number of **leukocytes/ml in the specimen.** The last portion of the evaluation of the seminal fluid is the **chemical examination.** Critical to the survival of spermatozoa is the **pH,** which should be between 7.2 and 7.8. A pH of less than 7.2 can indicate abnormalities of the genital tract, and a pH higher than 7.8 suggests an infection. **Fructose** determinations assess the secretory function of the seminal vesicles where fructose is produced and secreted. A normal fructose value in seminal fluid is **13 μmol/specimen** or greater. Seminal fluid **acid phosphatase** activity provides information relative to the secretory function of the prostate gland. The expected level is **200 units/specimen or greater,** unlike other body fluids that contain insignificant activity. This knowledge is used to aid in the determination of vaginal intercourse during rape. If the victim has been raped, the vaginal fluid will contain abnormally high acid phosphatase activity from the presence of seminal fluid. Decreased **citric acid levels** (<52 μmol/specimen) are associated with prostate dysfunction. Citric acid, which is the primary anion in seminal fluid, is normally **52 μmol/specimen,** and can be quantitated spectrophotometrically. **Zinc** values are another indi-

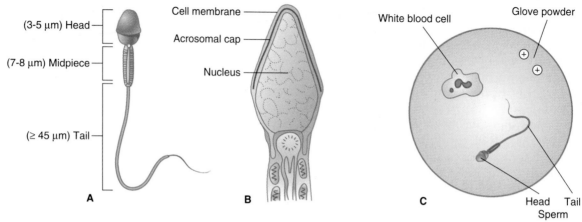

FIGURE 14-12

Normal spermatozoon morphology (*A* and *B*) and a microscopic field containing a leukocyte, a spermatozoon, and glove powder (*C*). Note the size and shape relationship to provide orientation for accurate identification. (Redrawn from Brunzel NE: Fundamentals of Urine and Body Fluid Analysis. Philadelphia: WB Saunders, 1994, p 340.)

cator of prostate function. Seminal fluid zinc concentrations are 2.4 μmol/specimen or greater if the prostate is healthy. Zinc can be measured spectrophotometrically or by atomic absorption spectroscopy techniques. All of these procedures are presented in more detail in Chapter 15.

URINE ANALYSIS AND MISCELLANEOUS BODY FLUIDS

Urine is a body fluid **produced by the kidneys** that is valuable for providing informa-

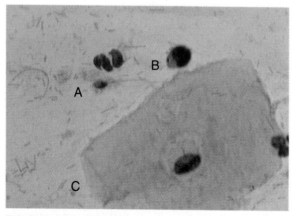

FIGURE 14-13

Seminal fluid spermatozoa (*A*) with leukocytes (*B*) and epithelial cells (*C*) for comparison of size.

tion for the patient's diagnosis and treatment. **Urine** or **blood** is **not considered as a "body fluid"** since the contents of the fluid may change and the presence of these fluids in large quantities is normal. The urine itself is the result of a body process for the purpose of **ridding the body of waste products** and **maintaining the osmotic concentration of the plasma.** The body fluids presented previously are drawn from the body and manually analyzed as a single individual specimen due to the short specimen viability, significance of results, and randomness of the need for testing. Urine and blood testing are done routinely using sophisticated instruments in groups of specimens or "batches." Entire books and courses are available to learn how to properly analyze urine and blood specimens.

Amniotic fluid is the fluid **within the uterus** that cushions the fetus throughout prenatal life. The formation and composition of amniotic fluid changes throughout the fetal development. Aspiration of this fluid, **amniocentesis,** is done to **assess diseases and detect chromosomal abnormalities** that are life threatening to the fetus, to the mother, or that have an impact on the quality of life. The hematology department does not usually test amniotic fluid. The **chemistry** department performs the most significant clinical laboratory testing of amniotic fluid by way of the

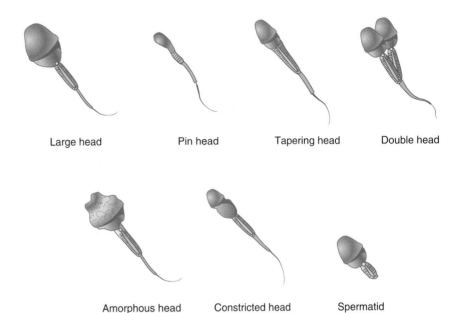

Large head   Pin head   Tapering head   Double head

Amorphous head   Constricted head   Spermatid

FIGURE 14–14
Abnormal spermatozoon mor-
phologies are recorded if seen.
(Redrawn from Brunzel NE: Fun-
damentals of Urine and Body
Fluid Analysis. Philadelphia: WB
Saunders, 1994, p 340.)

**lecithin/sphingomyelin (L/S) ratio and
the phosphotidylglycerol level.** These
tests aid the physician, or primary care provider, in evaluating and treating complicated
pregnancies **involving fetal lung development.** Other tests performed on amniotic
fluid are genetic, endocrine (hormonal) abnormalities, and infectious disease. Testing for genetic conditions by analyzing the chromosomes in the cells obtained from the amniotic
fluid is called **karyotyping.** Amniocentesis
introduces a small risk to both the mother
and the fetus and, therefore, is not done without a medical or genetic reason. The sex of the
fetus can be determined in the genetic analysis, but the risk far outweighs the desire to
know the sex of the fetus as a sole reason for
the procedure.

Wound aspirates drained from infectious
sites in the body are not analyzed in hematology. The fluid specimens are sent to the **microbiology** department where a **Gram stain**
is made to look for infectious organisms. Any
cells present are also reported, such as segmented neutrophils, which suggests a bacterial
infection; a "round cell" response of lymphocytes and monocyte/macrophages suggestive
of a chronic inflammatory response; epithelial
cells and sulfur granules, which may provide

Do It Now Body Fluids

1. Make a chart comparing the various body
   fluids. Be creative. List all the characteristics
   such as origin, location in body, analytical
   tests, and diseases.
2. Look at Figure 14–10. Draw the basic outline
   of the cells and nuclei, or trace the picture
   from the text. If you had never seen these
   cells before, how would you analyze and
   compare this cellular picture? Make a list
   contrasting and comparing the characteristics
   of the cells. Include the size, nucleus (shape,
   color, texture), and cytoplasm (amount,
   color, texture).
3. Once you have done this, try to find another
   example of a Wright-Giemsa–stained body
   fluid cytocentrifuge slide preparation in another book, or ask the instructor for different
   kodachrome slides or glass slide preparations.
   You can then perform the same analysis to
   determine what cells are present. Check your
   conclusions with other classmates or with
   your instructor.

information about the specimen's environmental source and the organism involved. The specimen is placed in both **aerobic** (with O_2 and CO_2) and **anaerobic** (without O_2) cultures as well as in a **thioglycollate broth** to encourage growth if only a few organisms are present and nothing grows in the cultures. All of these specimens are **incubated at 35 to 37° C** to simulate body temperature and to encourage rapid growth of any organisms present. **After 48 hours the broth is subcultured.** If any **organisms** are grown and **identified,** an **antibiotic sensitivity test is done** to determine which antibiotic will best destroy the invading organism. This antibiotic sensitivity information is then given to the physician or primary care practitioner so that he or she can prescribe the most effective drug therapy for the patient.

The "Do It Now" activity on page 295 is an exercise in perspective. It applies to **any** microscopic specimen. Don't look at a specimen and jump to a conclusion. **Analyze all the facts** using your knowledge of the cell, microorganism, or crystal characteristics **to draw a logical and valid conclusion.** One cell cannot be identified by itself. Only in relation to the other cells and to the patient can an accurate analysis and report be generated.

Study Questions

Match the Following:

1. Abdominal cavity of the body

2. Heart cavity of the body

3. Lung cavity of the body

4. Central nervous system

5. Male reproductive tract

6. Bone joints

A. Pleural fluid

B. Cerebrospinal fluid (CSF)

C. Peritoneal fluid

D. Synovial fluid

E. Pericardial fluid

F. Seminal fluid

Choose the Best Answer:

7. Methods to differentiate a traumatic CSF tap from a subarachnoid hemorrhage resulting in erythrocytes in the spinal fluid are:
   A. A count of more than $100 \times 10^9/l$ erythrocytes indicates a traumatic tap.

   B. A count of less than $2000/\mu l$ erythrocytes and less than $200/\mu l$ leukocytes indicates a hemorrhage.

   C. A consistent cell count in three tubes delivered to the laboratory and the presence of erythrophagocytosis on microscopic examination indicate a hemorrhage.

   D. A variable erythrocyte cell count and consistent leukocyte count in all three tubes indicate a traumatic tap.

8. Malignant cells in any body fluid have similar characteristics such as:
   A. Large cells with a large nucleus and very little cytoplasm

   B. Large cells with nucleoli and indistinct borders, which are on top of each other

   C. Small cells resembling resting lymphocytes, which appear very round

   D. Cells can be any size with a small nucleus and abundant dark blue cytoplasm.

9–10. Compare and contrast an exudate and a transudate in reference to location, origin, chemistry, cells, and associated disease.

11–12. The cerebrospinal fluid (CSF) is examined to determine if an abnormal process is in progress. Describe what is found upon microscopic examination in normal healthy CSF and what would be found if viral meningitis was in progress.

O U T L I N E

Physical Characteristics of the Body Fluid

Body Fluid Cell Counts

Microscopic and Cytologic Evaluation of Body
Fluids

Chemical Analysis of Body Fluids

Microbiologic and Immunologic Tests of
Body Fluids

Study Questions

Body Fluid Testing

O B J E C T I V E S

Upon completion of this chapter the student will be able to:

1. Describe the acceptable specimen and treatment of that specimen for each body fluid being tested.

2. List the components of testing for each body fluid.

3. Correlate the various body fluid tests and their significance.

4. When given a testing scenario, determine if there are reasons to question the validity of results.

5. State the various reasons for development of body fluid effusions.

Proper **identification** of the body fluid specimen, as with any specimen for testing, is a priority. Owing to the unique collection of body fluids in a variety of situations by a variety of health care providers, the information must be clear and must include the patient's **name, identification number, fluid collected, time, and date of collection.** The **specimen** for body fluid testing varies from a small amount of cerebrospinal fluid (CSF) (6 ml or less) to larger quantities of serous fluid (up to 50 ml). Fluid is **freshly drawn or collected into a sterile container,** does not require maintenance at a lower temperature, and may not require an anticoagulant to prevent clotting. Some body fluids, such as serous fluids, may require ethylenediaminetetraacetic acid (EDTA) for cell counts and heparin for pH determination. Synovial fluid may clot and require the addition of an enzyme such as hyaluronidase to digest the clot for random sampling to occur. All of the body fluid specimens, except seminal fluid, should be collected into at least three different tubes for distribution in the laboratory with minimal contamination.

If the body fluid specimen appears red, indicating the presence of red blood cells, an assessment of the source of the erythrocytes present may be significant. In the case of cerebrospinal fluid, it is important to determine if the erythrocytes present are a result of a traumatic CSF tap or the result of a subarachnoid brain hemorrhage. Only with this information can an evaluation of the CSF be accurately performed. **All body fluid specimens should be tested at room temperature immediately upon their arrival in the laboratory.**

The abnormal content or accumulation of body fluids is secondary to a disease in progress. The purpose of testing body fluids is to diagnose, determine treatment, and follow treatment for the primary disease process. Body fluids are not easily obtained without the patient incurring pain and discomfort; therefore, the clinical laboratory analysis of body fluids is not routine and must be performed accurately on a single specimen.

PHYSICAL CHARACTERISTICS OF THE BODY FLUID

The first component of evaluation is an assessment of the physical appearance of any body fluid. This begins with observations of the specimen by the laboratory practitioner upon receipt of the specimen in the hematology department.

The **volume** is measured by reading a value off of a calibrated tube containing the specimen, or the specimen may be transferred to a graduated cylinder and the volume is then recorded.

The **color** is observed and recorded. As stated earlier, a red color may indicate recent bleeding, which could be due to a traumatic aspiration (tap) of the fluid or may be due to primary bleeding into the fluid, such as seen in a subarachnoid hemorrhage into the CSF. Identification of the source of the erythrocytes is very important. This is done by comparing the cell counts from each collection tube, which will vary greatly if a traumatic tap is the cause. If this is a pathologic process in the CSF, the count should be consistent. An indication of subarachnoid hemorrhage is the appearance of phagocytes with ingested erythrocytes on microscopic examination. This process would not have time to occur in the time between traumatic spinal fluid tap and the laboratory analysis.

The **turbidity** of any specimen can be determined by attempting to read newsprint through the specimen and then grading the clarity or turbidity on a scale of 0 (clear) to 4+ (newsprint not readable). Standard criteria must be written and used for this procedure. An example would be to always use a specific size of tube and to hold it at a specific distance from the newspaper. Turbidity is a result of increased cellularity or the presence of microorganisms or lipids.

Viscosity is evaluated by pulling the specimen up into a Pasteur pipette and observing the formation of droplets as the fluid is expelled. Again, a standard written test protocol must be available in order to ensure a precise and accurate evaluation. Increased viscosity will be evident by the formation of a string

(>2 cm in length) from the pipette tip instead of the formation of discrete droplets. If any clot formation occurs, this must be noted and reported.

BODY FLUID CELL COUNTS

The **hemocytometer method** is used for manual cell counts as well as for sperm counts on seminal fluid. The variation in the calculation is dependent on the specimen, the procedure (dilution), and the size of the squares on the hemocytometer grid in which the cells are counted. A hemocytometer is a thick glass slide with a central area 0.1 mm lower than the sides. A special thick glass coverslip, ground to a perfect plane, unlike ordinary coverslips that have uneven surfaces, rests on the higher sides of the central counting area, and the diluted specimen is delivered under this coverslip. The center area of the hemocytometer is engraved with squares to allow accurate counting of the cells. The Neubauer ruling on the central counting area is 9 mm^2. This area is divided into smaller squares to facilitate counting (Fig. 15–1).

SAFETY PRECAUTIONS IN THE LABORATORY

1. Wear or use personal protective equipment such as gloves and shields.
2. Never pipette by mouth; use a micropipette or a suction apparatus to draw a specimen into a pipette.

DILUTION METHOD FOR MANUAL BODY FLUID COUNTS

1. Obtain the recently collected body fluid specimen maintained at room temperature.
2. Owing to the **low number of cells** seen in most body fluids, no dilution may be necessary. Mix the specimen, then insert a Pasteur pipette and allow it to fill by capillary action. Place a gloved finger over the top of the pipette; remove the pipette from the specimen; touch the tip to the loading

---

groove of the hemocytometer; and slowly release the finger to fill the chamber slowly and smoothly. Fill both sides of the hemocytometer. Overfilling (flooding) or underfilling the chamber will result in erroneous counts. Always remix the specimen before refilling the chamber if counts don't agree and must be repeated. Repeat as in the following sperm count procedure. If the specimen has a **high cell count**, which is determined by looking at the specimen microscopically and finding the cells too numerous to count (TNTC), the specimen must be diluted. Dilute the sample with a micropipette into an isotonic diluent. A unopette may also be used (see Figs. 6–6 and 6–7).

3. Once the chamber is filled, place it in a humidifying chamber (e.g., a moist petri dish) for 3 to 5 minutes to allow the cells to settle down on the counting surface all in one plane of focus. If the specimen on the hemocytometer chamber begins to evaporate, the count will not be accurate.

DILUTION METHOD FOR MANUAL SPERM COUNTS

1. Obtain the recently collected sperm specimen, which is maintained at room temperature.
2. Dilute the sample by preparing a premeasured amount of isotonic diluent, then add a specific amount of the sperm specimen using a calibrated micropipette to produce a 1:20 dilution.
3. The hemocytometer and the coverslip should be washed with a mild, dilute, liquid detergent followed by distilled water and alcohol. Dry them with a soft lint-free cloth such as cheesecloth to avoid scratching the surface of the chamber or leaving particles on the counting surface. Water droplets will resemble cells.
4. Mix the specimen and load it onto a clean hemocytometer by touching the end of the delivery pipette to the groove on the side of the hemocytometer. (See Figs. 6–4 and 6–5.) Fill both sides of the hemocytometer at a slow steady pace. Overfilling (flooding) or underfilling the chamber will result

Box continued on following page

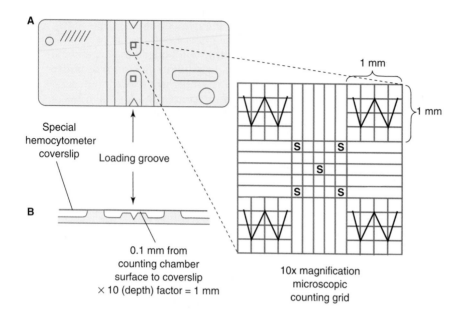

1 mm

1 mm

Special
hemocytometer
coverslip   Loading groove

A

B

0.1 mm from
counting chamber
surface to coverslip
× 10 (depth) factor = 1 mm

10x magnification
microscopic
counting grid

Two methods to calculate the cell count are as follows:

$$\frac{\text{No. of cells counted}}{\text{No. of 1 mm sq. counted}} \times \text{dilution} \times \underset{10^*}{\overset{\text{(depth factor)}}{}} = \text{No. of WBCs/mm}^3 \text{ or } /\mu l$$

or

Total cells counted × dilution factor × volume factor† = cells/μl or cells × 10^6/l

*The hemocytometer chamber is only 0.1 mm deep, so to report mm³ the depth must
  equal 1 mm; thus 0.1 × 10* = 1 mm × the 1 mm by 1 mm square counted on the chamber.
†If 10 mm³ × 0.1 mm (depth factor) = 1 μl.

FIGURE 15–1

A, Top view of the improved
Neubauer Hemocytometer
Counting Chamber. Note that
there are nine large 1 × 1-mm
squares. The four large corner
squares are used for counting
white blood cells (W). The five
small squares within the center
1-mm square are used for counting high-concentration cells,
such as red blood cells and spermatozoa (s). *B*, Side view of a
hemocytometer.

in erroneous counts. Always remix the dilution before refilling the chamber if
counts don't agree and must be repeated.
5. Once the chamber is filled, place it in a
humidifying chamber (e.g., a moist petri
dish) for 3 to 5 minutes to allow the sperm
to settle down on the counting surface all
in one plane of focus. If the specimen on
the hemocytometer chamber begins to
evaporate the count will not be accurate.
6. Count the number of spermatozoa in the
five small squares within the center 1-mm
square on the hemocytometer counting
grid (see Fig. 15-1). Each of these small
squares is equal to ¹⁄₂₅ of 1 mm. Be sure to
insert this number into the calculation for
the area counted. The large number of
sperm present allows an acceptably accurate count when only five small squares

are counted instead of a full 1-mm square
necessary if the count is less than 1 mil-
lion.

HEMOCYTOMETER CELL COUNTING

1. With the light off, place the loaded hemocytometer on the microscope stage.
2. Center one of the two chambers under
   the shortest (5× or 10×) objective.
3. Turn the light on, and limit the light exposure to avoid evaporation of the specimen.
4. **Looking from the side,** move the lowest (shortest) objective and the hemocytometer as close to each other as possible.

This is important to prevent the objective from breaking the chamber.

5. While looking through the oculars, **move** the objective and the specimen **away** from each other until the counting grid comes into focus (see Fig. 15–1).

6. Center the middle 1-mm square (which contains 25 smaller squares).

7. Rotate the microscope objectives to the 10× objective. At this point there may appear to be no cells on the chamber due to an excess amount of condensed light.

8. Lower the condenser and adjust the light to provide maximum contrast in order to enhance the visibility of the unstained cells.

9. Begin in the upper left hand corner of the small upper left hand corner square of the center 1-mm square and record, on a counter, the number of spermatozoa. It is important not to count cells on a line twice, thus the cells on two adjacent lines are counted. Any two adjacent lines can be used, but be consistent throughout the count (Fig. 15–2).

10. Progress back and forth, as shown in Figure 15–2, across the small square until all the spermatozoa in the entire square (15-1s) have been counted. The visibility of the sperm is dependent on the contrast of the light. The condenser should be slightly lowered, and the fine focus must be used for maximum visibility (Fig. 15–3).

11. Record your results on an answer sheet.

12. Move over to the next small corner square of the center large square and repeat steps 9 to 11 until the five small corner squares and at least one small center square of the 1-mm center square have been counted.

13. If one of the squares has an inconsistent count, it may be discarded and another square can be counted instead. If the count is low, more squares may be included in the count. Follow the laboratory's written procedure.

14. Upon completion of one of the chambers, move immediately across to the other chamber and repeat steps 9 to 12. Remember that excessive exposure to the light will evaporate the specimen and alter the results.

15. The chamber must be decontaminated by placing the hemocytometer into a small container, such as a petri dish, flooding it with a disinfectant, allowing it to sit for at least 5 minutes, then rinsing it with 70% alcohol. Now the hemocytometer can be cleaned as described earlier.

16. Calculate the cell count:

$$\frac{\text{No. of cells counted}}{\text{No. of 1-mm squares counted}} \times \text{dilution} \times \frac{\text{(depth factor)}}{10*}$$

$$= \text{No. of WBC/mm}^3 \text{ or } /\mu l$$

* The hemocytometer chamber is only 0.1-mm deep, therefore to report mm³, the depth must equal 1 mm, thus $0.1 \times 10* = 1 \text{ mm} \times 1 \text{ mm} \times 1 \text{ mm} = 1 \text{ mm}^3$ counted on the chamber.

Sperm Count Reference Values. The values are 20 to 250×10^6 sperm/ml of the specimen.

Sources of Error. Error may be caused by an incorrect or inadequate specimen; inadequate mixing of the specimen prior to sampling; incorrect dilution, diluting fluid, or calculation of the count; incorrect counting; counting some cells twice or some not at all; counting dirt or water droplets as cells; or not allowing the cells to settle resulting in missing some cells in another plane of focus.

A Makler counting chamber, which is designed specifically for semen analysis, is another method available for determining sperm concentration. Another method is available for determining sperm concentration, motility, and morphology from the wet preparation.

MICROSCOPIC AND CYTOLOGIC EVALUATION OF BODY FLUIDS

Seminal fluid is the only body fluid that requires a **wet preparation** analysis in addition to the prepared glass slide. After complete liquefaction, approximately **10 to 20 μl** of the **well-mixed specimen** is placed **on a slide under a coverslip.** The specific volume and coverslip size should be included in the laboratory's written procedure. Two slides

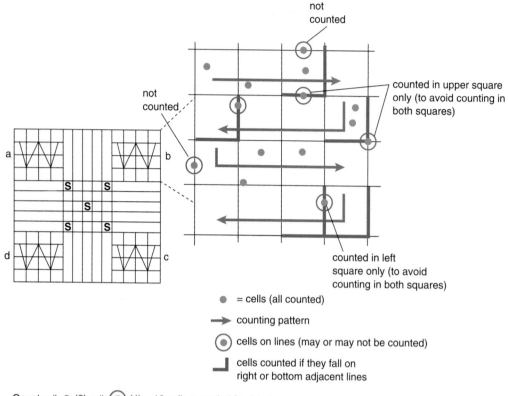

not
counted

not
counted

counted in upper square
only (to avoid counting in
both squares)

a

b

counted in left
square only (to avoid
counting in both squares)

d

c

● = cells (all counted)

→ counting pattern

⊙ cells on lines (may or may not be counted)

⌐ cells counted if they fall on
right or bottom adjacent lines

Count = # ● (8) + # ⊙ (4) = 12 cells recorded for this 1mm square.

F I G U R E 15–2
The protocol for counting cells to avoid missing cells or counting cells twice is shown. Cells on two adjacent lines within each small square are counted; however, they are not counted in the small square if they are on the two nondesignated lines. White blood cell counts are done on the large corner 1-mm squares. Sperm counts are done on five of the small squares within the center 1-mm square.

should be prepared to ensure precision. Allow these slides to settle for about 1 minute at 37° C or, if that is not possible, at room temperature (22° C ± 2°) before making an evaluation. As with any microscopic preparation, the first priority is to **scan the specimen** to determine if there is a random distribution of cells or movement to provide an accurate evaluation. Once the acceptability of the slide has been established, the **sperm motility** is graded from **0 (no movement) to 4+ (active movement)**. There are variations, such as an evaluation of one microscopic field under 200× or 6 to 10 fields under 400× magnification. The specific criteria will be written in the procedure manual of the laboratory. Up to **1 hour following collection, at least**

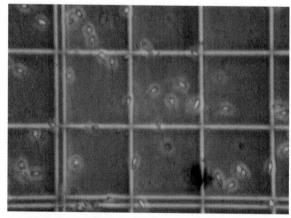

F I G U R E 15–3
Spermatozoa are shown on part of a small square within the 1-mm center square of the hemocytometer counting chamber grid. (From Ringsrud KM, Linne JJ: Urinalysis and Body Fluids. Boston: CV Mosby, 1995, p 212.)

50% of the sperm should be moving in a moderate to strong forward pattern.

In order to identify any variation from the normal **spermatozoa morphology,** a seminal fluid smear, or squash preparation, is made on a glass slide (refer to Chapter 1 for procedures). Similar to the preparation of a blood smear, a drop of fresh seminal fluid is placed at one end of a glass slide. Using the edge of a second glass slide, the drop is spread with a pushing motion across the length of the slide. An alternative slide preparation technique is the squash method in which a drop of seminal fluid is placed one third of the way from the end of the slide and a second slide is pressed (squashed) down on top to spread the drop out. The slides are then pulled across each other to spread the drop the length of both slides. This **seminal fluid slide preparation is allowed to dry and a stain such as Wright-Giemsa** is applied. Compare the differences in size, shape, and color among the cells within the microscopic field to maintain an accurate perspective for identification of cells (Fig. 15–4). The cells that are seen in Figure 15–4 are an epithelial cell (C), segmented neutrophils (B), and sperm (A). The normal morphology of a spermatozoa is a single, rounded head, a short narrow midpiece, and a long, thin, tapering tail (Fig. 15–5). A relative perspective of size, shape, and color based on objects present within the field is essential for accurate microscopic evaluation (see Figs. 15–4 [A, B, and C] and 15–5 [C]). Several morphologic variations are possible, many of which will affect fertility (Fig. 15–6).

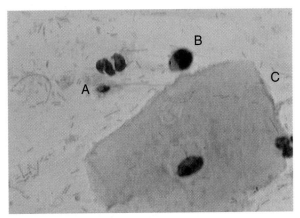

FIGURE 15–4
Seminal fluid spermatozoa (A) with leukocytes (B) and an epithelial cell (C) for comparison of size.

Keeping a perspective when performing microscopic examinations is essential for a precise and accurate evaluation. A single object is not always meaningful until compared with other objects present on the slide of known size and color or contrast. An example is a comparison of red blood cells, white blood cells, microorganisms, or sperm cells. This avoids reporting glove powder, debris, or incorrect identification of cells.

Body fluid specimens, other than semen, may need to be concentrated in order to accu-rately evaluate the small number of cells present. A **cytocentrifuge** (Fig. 15–7) is used to concentrate the cells or organisms in the body fluid onto a small area of a glass slide. The **glass slide** (Fig. 15–8A) and a **special filter paper** with a central hole are attached to a funnel and placed **in the cytocentrifuge holder** (see Figs. 15–8B and C and 15–9). A **specific amount** of the **well-mixed specimen,** as stated in the laboratory procedure, is placed into the funnel portion of the cytocentrifuge slide holder. The machine is closed, locked, and started. The cytocentrifuge **spins the sample for 5 to 10 minutes at 200 to 1000 rpm.** This forces the cells down **into a central 6-mm circle** on the slide at the hole in the filter paper, and the fluid is absorbed by the filter paper. This slide can then be **stained with Wright-Giemsa** or any other stains of interest. The stained cells on the cytocentrifuge slide can be differentiated and reported. The major cells of interest are **lymphocytes, which are associated with viral or malignant processes; neutrophils, which are associated with bacterial infections; and cancerous cells.**

The **sample of body fluid sent to the cytology** department will be concentrated and embedded in a block of paraffin. The sample will then be cut very thin, fixed on a glass slide, and stained for cell examination. Cyto-

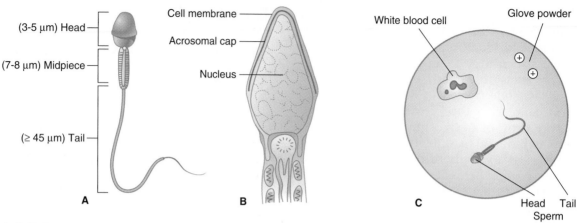

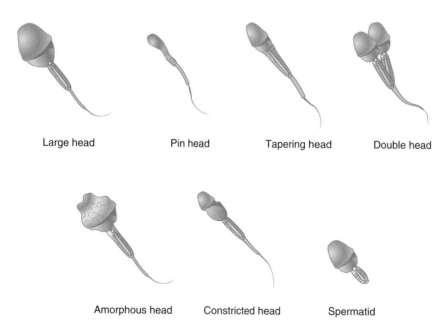

FIGURE 15-5

Normal spermatozoa morphology and a microscopic field containing a leukocyte, a spermatozoa, and glove powder. Note the size and shape relationship to provide orientation for accurate identification. (Redrawn from Brunzel NE: Fundamentals of Urine and Body Fluid Analysis. Philadelphia: WB Saunders, 1994, p 340.)

centrifuge smears are also sent to the cytology department, where the smears will be stained with a variety of stains **in order to identify any suspicious cells such as cancer cells.** The cytology examinations are performed by a cytologist and possibly a pathologist.

CHEMICAL ANALYSIS OF BODY FLUIDS

The chemistry tests performed on the various body fluids include: **total protein, glucose, uric acid, triglyceride, pH, citric acid,**

Large head

Pin head

Tapering head

Double head

FIGURE 15-6

Abnormal spermatozoa morphologies. (Redrawn from Brunzel NE: Fundamentals of Urine and Body Fluid Analysis. Philadelphia: WB Saunders, 1994, p 340.)

Amorphous head

Constricted head

Spermatid

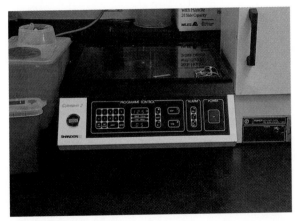

FIGURE 15-7
A cytocentrifuge is used with the apparatus seen in Figures 15–8 and 15–9 to concentrate cells found in body fluids.

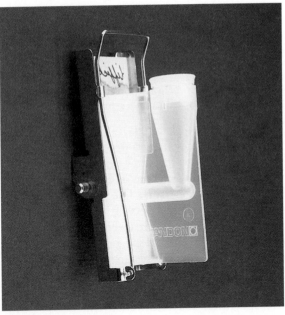

FIGURE 15-9
A cytocentrifuge holder with the glass slide and filter paper (attached to the funnel) containing the patient's specimen. This is placed in the cytocentrifuge, and the cells in the specimen are concentrated onto the slide for microscopic examination.

zinc, glutamine, amino acids, biogenic amines, enzymes such as aspartate aminotransferase (AST), lactate dehydrogenase (LD), amylase, and acid phosphatase. The tumor marker carcinoembryonic antigen (CEA) may also be part of the body fluid chemistry work-up. Most of these tests are performed in the chemistry area of the clinical laboratory. Some tests may be too expensive or too seldom ordered to be offered at one specific laboratory and will be

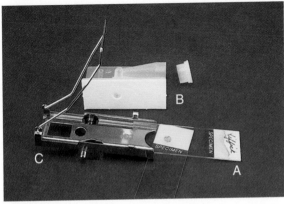

FIGURE 15-8
A cytocentrifuge holder (C) with filter paper (B), glass slide (A), and stained cytospin slide. These are used to concentrate cells in body fluids for the purpose of microscopic examination.

sent to a larger laboratory or a reference laboratory.

MICROBIOLOGIC AND IMMUNOLOGIC TESTS OF BODY FLUIDS

Cytocentrifuge slide preparations (explained under microscopic examination earlier) of the specimen are stained with a variety of microbiologic stains, which may vary depending on the organisms suspected. The most frequently used microbiology stain is the **Gram stain,** which will aid in identification of gram-negative and gram-positive microorganisms such as *Streptococcus pneumonia, Staphylococcus aureus, Neisseria meningitides,* and *Haemophilus influenzae.* A second commonly used stain is the **acid-fast stain,** which aids in identification of *Mycobacterium tuberculosis.* A slide with **no**

visible organisms does not rule out an infection.

If the specimen collection, handling, and processing or the technical competence of the microbiologic microscopist is substandard or compromised, inaccurate results will be generated.

In order to confirm a microorganism seen on the slide or to discover one that is not seen on the slide, a **culture** is set up using **the body fluid specimen.** The sample should be concentrated before inoculation of the growth media plates, and **both aerobic and anaerobic cultures** should be performed. The organisms are allowed to grow for at least 24 hours, delaying effective treatment. Microorganisms are not easily grown, and the quality of the specimen may influence the results, thus erroneously negative growth may occur in some cases. Once an organism is grown, further testing such as **biochemical or sensitivity testing may be required for confirmation of the microorganism found and treatment.**

Immunologic tests or assays are also available for some microorganism antigens and the antibodies produced against them. **Bacterial antigen detection tests** are in use to detect both **bacterial and fungal pathogens** that can cause various types of meningitis. The techniques used range from **agglutination, radioimmunoassay (RIA),**

and counterimmunoelectrophoresis and involve the use of antibodies directed against the microbial antigen of interest. If a reaction is detected, the corresponding microbe is presumed to be present. Due to the variation in specificity and sensitivity of these tests, the **Gram stain and cultures remain the standard diagnostic tests.** The immunologic assays are performed in other areas of the laboratory outside of the hematology department and are discussed in more detail in Chapter 6.

Do It Now Body Fluids

1. Draw a microscopic field demonstrating red blood cells, white blood cells, ependymal cells, synoviocytes, sperm, and glove powder. Take time to draw the size and structures as accurately as possible.

2. Obtain a blood specimen from the instructor. Make a 1:2 dilution with saline. Mix the dilution well; place one drop on a glass slide; and cover it with a coverslip. Examine this drop under the microscope. Scan first on low power (10×). Note if the distribution of the cells is random. Adjust the condenser and iris diaphragm to obtain the best contrast of this unstained specimen in order to demonstrate cell characteristics. Now move to the high-power objective (40×), and again adjust the light until the best visibility is found. Compare the cell sizes and characteristics.

Body Fluid Testing

Body Fluid	Source	Tests	Comments
Cerebrospinal fluid (CSF)	Spinal column	Physical examination: volume, color, clarity	Meningitis, CNS disease Hemorrhage 0–5 WBC/0 RBC reference
		Microscopic examination: Mononuclear cells	Lymphocytes
		Neutrophils	Bacterial infection
		Chemistry: protein, glucose	
		Immunology assays: antigens or antibodies	Microorganisms
		Microbiology	Stain and culture
Synovial fluid (SF)	Bone joints	Physical examination: volume, clarity, color	Infections, gout, rheumatoid arthritis
		Cell count	<200 WBC/μl reference
		Microscopic examination:	<2000 RBC/μl reference
		Mononuclear cells	Cytocentrifuge preparation
		Neutrophils	Lymphocytes
		Synoviocytes	Bacterial infection
Serous fluids	Between serous membranes	Same basic testing for all body fluids	Physician may vary tests done
Pleural fluid	Lung cavity	Physical examination: volume, color, clarity	<10,000 RBC/μl reference
		Microscopic examination: Mononuclear cells	<1000 WBC/μl reference lymphocytes
		Neutrophils	Bacterial infection
		Mesothelial cells	
		Cytology examination	Neoplastic cells
		Chemistry: total protein, glucose, lactate dehydrogenase, amylase, triglyceride, pH Carcinoembryonic antigen (CEA)	
		Microbiology stain and culture	
Pericardial fluid	Heart cavity	Same tests	Congestive heart failure (CHF)
Peritoneal fluid (ascites)	Abdominal cavity	Same tests	Change in pressure/permeability of vasculature, neoplasm, or infection
Seminal fluid (semen)	Male reproductive organs	Physical examination, volume, viscosity, appearance	
		Microscopic examination: $20–250 \times 10^6$/ml reference	Infertility studies
		Motility, viability total number of sperm and WBC morphology	Vasectomy confirm
		Chemistry values: pH, fructose, citric acid, acid phosphatase, zinc	Genital organ dysfunction

STUDY QUESTIONS

Choose the Best Answer:

1. Describe the acceptable cerebrospinal fluid (CSF) specimen and proper treatment prior to testing.
   A. 2 ml in a sterile plastic urine cup at room temperature

   B. 1 ml in a sealed glass tube at room temperature

   C. 2 ml in a sealed glass tube at 4° C

   D. at least 4 ml in an EDTA tube at 4° C

2–5. List the testing profile for each body fluid.

CSF	Serous Fluids	Synovial Fluids	Seminal Fluid

Correlate the Various Cells Found in Body Fluid and Their Significance.

6. Malignancy

7. Bacterial spinal meningitis

8. Tuberculosis

9. Traumatic aspiration

10. Viral spinal meningitis

A. Lymphocytes present

B. Erythrocytes present

C. Segmented neutrophils present

D. Very few, if any, cells present

Clinical Laboratory Practice

Interrelationships and the future of the clinical laboratory are intimately entwined. **As clinical pathways are developed,** health care providers must work together to use each expertise maximally. Each individual must understand his or her contribution to the entire facility in which he or she practices. This relationship between the various health care providers within a facility is becoming more apparent as the organizational structures change. An example is the grouping of previously independent ancillary services such as radiology, laboratory, respiratory therapy, and pharmacy under one manager. Patient testing is now taking place at the point of care (POC), which may be at the bedside, at the physician's office, or in a clinic. This new testing environment **requires interaction** with other health care professionals. **Physicians, pharmacists, laboratory practitioners, and nurses** are beginning to work together, and **dietitians** now feel the need to add a laboratory practitioner to the nutritional support team. These are opportunities for use of the expertise unique to each person on the team and this challenge must be met with enthusiasm and a positive proactive (not reactive) attitude. The personal rewards are evident in a team that shares mutual respect for each member and for his or her knowledge. As symphony director Boris Brott explains with parallels between a symphony orchestra and an organization, such as a health care system, **we must all "play together"** to achieve the goal of accurate and efficient health care.

CHAPTER 16

OUTLINE

Correlation of Clinical Laboratory Results

Validation of Fact Versus Fiction

Documentation, Verification, and Dissemination

Important Considerations of Clinical Hematology and Clinical Laboratory Practice

Study Questions

Correlation, Validation, Verification, and Considerations

OBJECTIVES

Upon completion of this chapter the student will be able to:

1. Diagram and explain the interrelationship of the clinical laboratory with other health care areas, the patient, and the community.

2. Discuss and debate the future of clinical laboratory practice, emphasizing hematology.

3. List the components of clinical laboratory practice.

4. Explain the rationale for insisting on an acceptable specimen and proper treatment of that specimen for clinical laboratory testing.

5. Correlate the various tests and their significance.

6. When given a testing scenario, determine if there are reasons to question the validity of the results.

7. Contrast and compare the various methods of verification, documentation, and dissemination of clinical laboratory information and results.

8. Recognize and discuss the considerations necessary to provide accurate and meaningful laboratory data to other members of the health care team.

CORRELATION OF CLINICAL LABORATORY RESULTS

The sum of the parts exceeds that of the whole. Each individual performing each laboratory test is a crucial part of the whole process. The ability to **correlate clinical laboratory results** begins with the knowledge of the **components of acceptable clinical laboratory testing** and depends on the **professional and positive attitude** of each person in the process. This begins with the physician's request, which is processed by the nurse, collected by the nurse or phlebotomist, transported to the laboratory, and analyzed by a laboratory practitioner. The results are verified, documented, and recorded in the patient's chart, then a nurse or physician interprets the data to help determine diagnosis, prognosis, or treatment. Every step in this entire process is critical, and the entire health care team must work together to strive for valid and accurate results. This means **getting out of the laboratory** and **communicating with the nurses and other health care providers** who are part of the process of patient care.

The first component of clinical laboratory testing includes the requisition, the patient, and the specimen. Each patient is unique and, therefore, cannot be approached routinely. This is sometimes called the **preanalytic component** of clinical laboratory practice. Once a specimen has been collected and accepted into the laboratory, the **analytic component** begins and the various requested tests are performed. The final component of clinical laboratory practice is the **postanalytic phase,** which involves responding to the results. Other references may describe the laboratory testing components using a variety of terms such as the input, process, and output. Each of these components undergoes continuous monitoring, evaluation, and improvement as part of the institution's **quality assurance** program, which may lead to a **false sense of security** in the absence of test correlation. Correlation of clinical laboratory components and results is crucial to the accuracy of health care and cost reduction. Although the quality assurance measures in your laboratory have been performed and demonstrate an accurate system in control, there may be unusual circumstances associated with a specific patient or testing event. There will always be a human entry of data or review of results at some point, which must involve the correlation of several patient values.

Tying it all together, **correlation**, mandates viewing the patient in terms of status; all tests performed; the critical pathways; and patient outcome assessment. Each part of the process is one piece of the puzzle, and if the pieces don't fit the patient may be incorrectly diagnosed and treated.

The values generated in a clinical laboratory or any laboratory diagnostic setting are meaningless unless the validation, verification, documentation, and dissemination of results all provide some insight to the physician or other primary health care provider into the in vivo state of the patient's blood.

VALIDATION OF FACT VERSUS FICTION

The primary health care provider who is using the clinical laboratory information to make health care decisions has no way of knowing of any errors in the process. These individuals depend on the **laboratory practitioner to provide accurate (factual) and timely (quick) dissemination of valid information** for the care of the patient. Results generated without validation are "fiction" with no relevance to the status of the patient but rather reflect an error or oversight in preanalytic (patient preparation, specimen collection, transport, and storage) or analytic (analysis of the specimen) components of clinical laboratory science. The clinical laboratory personnel, from the phlebotomist to the laboratory manager, have the responsibility of providing the best quality and most meaningful data for efficient patient health care.

Test result reporting in relation to standards, reference values, and so forth is addressed in Chapter 1 as part of the quality assurance information. The process of determining the validity of a result involves the ability to look at a value and say, **"given the value from test X, the value for test Y should support this information."** If this known relationship does not exist, one of the test results is erroneous and must be investigated before it is released from the laboratory. Specific tests with direct correlations to determine validity are:

1. $3 \times Hb = Hct$ value. A Hb of 12 g/dl would be accompanied by a Hct of approximately 36%. If the results do not relate in this way, either the Hb or Hct test result is incorrect. This must be investigated and corrected before the information is released. The specimen may be re-run; other results may be correlated; and the laboratory protocol for working up this discrepancy will be completed.

2. MCV should be abnormal if the RDW is abnormal. If one value is normal and the other is abnormal, one of the results is in error. A peripheral blood smear may need to be prepared to provide more information for the investigation of this inconsistent result.

3. If a specimen is known to be hemolyzed, icteric, lipemic, drawn from an alternative site, or any other alteration from routine, this should be noted with the result and documentation of the results include the corrections for the interfering circumstance.

These are examples of **correlation of data to validate results.** The following case provides an example of the need to correlate results:

An elderly man was admitted to the hospital because of diarrhea, blood in the urine, and possible seizures. The preliminary diagnosis was possible septicemia (bacterial infection). Blood was drawn for a complete blood count (CBC), chemistry profile, coagulation testing, and microbiology testing. Upon spinning the blood down to obtain serum from the red top tube for chemistry testing and plasma from the blue top tube for coagulation tests, severe hemolysis was noted. A second set of speci-

mens was drawn and the appearance of significant hemolysis was determined to result from the in vivo condition of the blood and not a result of the phlebotomy technique.

Finding no other alternative, the hemolyzed specimen was used to obtain the following results:

WBC $62.0 \times 10^9/l$ $(5.0–10.0 \times 10^9/l)$
RBC $2.45 \times 10^{12}/l$ $(4.0–5.0 \times 10^{12}/l)$
HGB   9.3 g/dl (12–16 g/dl)
HCT   23% (36–48%)
MCV   93 fl (85–95 fl)
RDW   15.1% (11–14%)
MCHC   41% (33–36%)
PLT $135 \times 10^9/l$ $(150–400 \times 10^9/l)$
PT   12.8 sec (11–13 sec)
APTT   21.6 sec (21–30 sec)
Fibrinogen   420 mg/dl (200–400 mg/dl)
FDP pos = >40 μg/ml (neg = <10 g/ml)
BUN   89 mg/dl (5–17 mg/dl)
Creatinine   8.3 mg/dl (0.2–0.59 mg/dl)

In this example, the physician or primary care provider would not know that these values are inconsistent and erroneous. The hemoglobin and hematocrit do not correlate due to the small red blood cells counted as large platelets, resulting in a lower than true red blood cell count, which in turn contributes to a Hct that is lower than its true value. The fibrinogen appears normal, when in fact the fibrinogen level is very low and the color from the hemolytic serum erroneously raised the value. The PT and APTT appear normal, when in fact they are erroneous. If the plasma was not hemolyzed, initiating coagulation and in-

Do It Now Correlation and Validation

1. Ask your instructor for some anonymous hematology results. Review these results in terms of correlation, validation, verification, and any additional considerations.
2. Mark any results that do not correlate.
3. Note any questions that you have concerning the tests listed or other tests or patient information that might be helpful in correlating and validating results.
4. Discuss this information with other classmates. Ask the instructor to clarify information.

terfering with the optical result, both the PT and APTT would be prolonged. The platelet count is normal, when in fact, the platelets are decreased and the extremely microcytic cells and schistocytes are counted as large platelets. This patient most likely had septicemia (bacterial systemic infection), which was not detectable but induced secondary complications such as disseminated intravascular coagulation (DIC). DIC then exacerbated a hemolytic uremic syndrome (HUS) and kidney failure. This is an example of what appear to individuals outside of the laboratory to be facts, but in reality these values are fiction. The astute, motivated laboratory practitioner must correlate and validate these results before they are verified, documented, and disseminated.

DOCUMENTATION, VERIFICATION, AND DISSEMINATION

Documentation (i.e., recording of information) occurs most often from the instrument to the laboratory computer and then to the nursing unit computer where the information can be placed in the patient's chart. Documentation **must always include the date, time, reference values, and any circumstances, or names of individuals, relevant to the test results.** Back-up mechanisms must be in place to record and disseminate information in case of computer failure.

Verification of results is the process of **checking the clinical laboratory data for error** (e.g., clerical, lack of validation, abnormal flags) and correcting these errors before final release of information. The most common cause of clinical laboratory error is **clerical error** due to the tendency of humans to transpose figures, misidentify patients or specimens, and record results on the wrong patient due to the multitude of thoughts and interruptions that distract from the laboratory practitioner's ability to focus on the current task. The use of computers has decreased the incidence of clerical error, but the computer does not know the patient or have any way of knowing if the specimen was collected and transported correctly. This may result in the generation of incorrect results if the results obtained fit the criteria in the computer logic and, therefore, appear acceptable when interfering factors have rendered inaccurate data. The ability to see the **"bigger picture"** of where a specific laboratory value fits in, and its relationship to the patient, **increases the laboratory practitioner's ability to focus** without distractions and **decreases the dissemination of erroneous results.** If the results are not directly recorded into a computer system, these results must be appropriately entered into the **laboratory information systems (LIS)** and verified before they are released from the laboratory. If the results are directly recorded, by the instrument into the computer system, they must demonstrate verification, which may involve the addition of the laboratory practitioner's initials or some mark added to the result in order for this information to be disseminated from the laboratory to the patient chart for health care use.

Dissemination of information, **from the laboratory to the patient care area or physician,** must be **timely** and **accurate.** The health care providers depend on the accuracy of laboratory results in order to treat the patient. Results must reach the patient care area in a reasonable amount of time to allow an efficient diagnosis and administration of treatment. The information must be readily accessible, easily understood, and presented in a manner that can be interpreted by nonlabora-

---

Do It Now Documentation, Verification, and Dissemination

1. Choose a clinical laboratory facility and arrange a visit to see and discuss how the laboratory information is documented, verified, and disseminated.
2. Write a brief report that includes the problem areas and the advantages of the system.

tory personnel. Laboratory results are of no use if they are inaccurate or misinterpreted.

IMPORTANT CONSIDERATIONS OF CLINICAL HEMATOLOGY AND CLINICAL LABORATORY PRACTICE

The **orientation and attitude** of each individual in the clinical hematology laboratory, the entire laboratory (Fig. 16–1), the entire hospital (Fig. 16–2), and even the community has an **impact on the practice of clinical laboratory science** and health care. Every test performed in the clinical laboratory and every patient with whom the laboratory personnel interact **influences the entire community outside of the hospital.** If the **laboratory personnel** as well as various **health care providers worked more closely together for the good of the patient** (Fig. 16–3), the practice of medicine and the efficiency and **quality of health care would increase and costs would decrease.** An example of this would be the **collaboration of the physician, the nurse, the pharmacist, and the hematology**

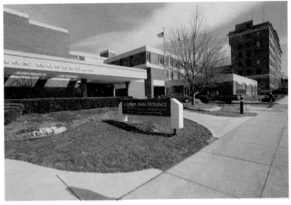

FIGURE 16–2
The entire hospital, as well as the community outside, have an impact on each other, and a more complete global perspective is necessary for the success of health care.

clinical laboratory scientist to ensure the proper anticoagulant therapy for a patient with a complicated clotting disorder (Fig. 16–4). The **physician** orders an anticoagulant such as heparin or coumadin as part of the patient's treatment and also orders tests, such as the APTT or PT, to monitor this treatment. The **nurse,** along with a **unit assistant or secretary,** processes and disseminates these orders. The **pharmacist** fills the order and provides the anticoagulant drug, which the nurse administers as the physician ordered. The **laboratory practitioners** collect the blood specimens and perform the tests to monitor the effectiveness of the treatment.

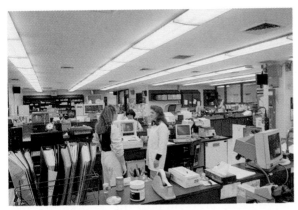

FIGURE 16–1
The clinical laboratory is a single entity. The various specialty areas must not function independently, but rather they must work together with all areas of patient testing to provide quality laboratory data. A pathologist (laboratory physician) works with a laboratory practitioner in hematology, while a chemistry practitioner enters data into a computer in the background.

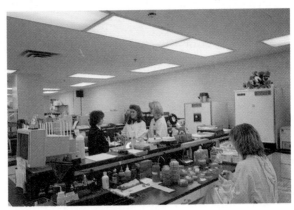

FIGURE 16–3
Laboratory personnel working together for the best diagnosis and treatment of the patients.

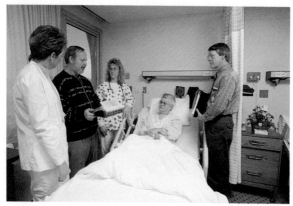

FIGURE 16–4
From left to right: The clinical laboratory scientist from hematology, the physician, the nurse, and the pharmacist work together to resolve problems for the good of the patient.

The APTT or PT test results will determine the next step in treatment to ensure the patient's recovery and release from the hospital.

The best prevention against errors and mistakes in the clinical laboratory is a **well-edu**-**cate laboratory practitioner,** who has a **professional attitude** and is **self-motivated.** Professional attitude and personal motivation include actively pursuing continuing education; maintaining professional involvement; disseminating knowledge to others (communication); having the ability and desire to stop, think, and transfer knowledge; readily accepting challenges; and adopting an attitude of "continuing to strive for the gold standard in clinical laboratory science" without complaints even if your facility never quite reaches that goal. If the application of the hematology from this textbook is viewed as part of an important profession, which it is, the laboratory practitioner will love what he or she does and will enjoy the profession and life! The **laboratory practitioner will benefit** from this change **in attitude,** but most important, the **patient will benefit from a caring "patient-oriented" clinical laboratory experience.**

STUDY QUESTIONS

1. Diagram and explain the interrelationship of the clinical laboratory with other health care areas, the patient, and the community.

2. Discuss and debate the future of clinical laboratory practice, emphasizing hematology.

3. List and define the components of clinical laboratory practice.

4. Explain the rationale for insisting on an acceptable specimen and proper treatment of that specimen for clinical laboratory testing.

5. In your own words, define the concept of correlation of clinical laboratory test results.

6. When given a testing scenario, what results would you look at to support the validity of the hematology results?

7. Contrast and compare the various methods of verification, documentation, and dissemination of clinical laboratory information and results.

8. List as many ways as you can think of to provide accurate and meaningful laboratory data to other members of the health care team.

Bibliography

Abbas AK, Lichtman AH, Pober JS: Cellular and Molecular Immunology. Philadelphia: WB Saunders, 1991

Adamson JW: The relationship of erythropoietin and iron metabolism to red blood cell production in humans. Semin Oncol 2(21):9–15, 1994

Applegate EJ: The Anatomy and Physiology Learning System. Philadelphia: WB Saunders, 1995

Arkin CF: Quality control and standardization in the hematology laboratory. *In* Bick RL (ed): Hematology, Clinical and Laboratory Practice. Boston: CV Mosby, 1993, pp 17–33

Bauer C: Introduction: The physiology of oxygen sensing and erythropoietin formation. Ann N Y Acad Sci 718:70–71, 1994

Becan-McBride K: Textbook of Clinical Laboratory Supervision. Englewood Cliffs, NJ: Appleton-Century-Crofts, 1982, pp 1–28

Bick RL (ed): Hematology Clinical and Laboratory Practice. Boston: CV Mosby, 1993

Bozzini CE, Alippi RM, Barcelo AC, et al: The biology of stress erythropoiesis and erythropoietin production. Ann N Y Acad Sci 718:83–93, 1994

Brandt JT: Measurement of factor VIII. Arch Pathol Lab Med 117:48–51, 1993

Brown AS, Martin JF: The megakaryocyte platelet system and vascular disease. Eur J Clin Invest 25(Suppl 1):9–15, 1994

Broze GJ: Tissue factor pathway inhibitor and the revised theory of coagulation. Annu Rev Med 46:103–112, 1995

Brunzel NA: Fundamentals of Urine and Body Fluid Analysis. Philadelphia: WB Saunders, 1994

Burtis CA, Ashwood ER: Tietz Fundamentals of Clinical Chemistry. Philadelphia: WB Saunders, 1996

Campbell JM, Campbell JB: Laboratory Mathematics, Medical and Biological Applications. Boston: CV Mosby, 1990

Carpenter MA, Kendall RG, O'Brien AE, et al: Reduced erythropoietin response to anaemia in elderly patients with normocytic anaemia. Eur J Haematol 49:119–121, 1992

Cembrowski GS, Carey RN: Quality control in the 1990s. Lab Med 20(6):375–376, 1989

Chernecky CC, Krech RL, Berger BJ: Laboratory Tests and Diagnostic Procedures. Philadelphia: WB Saunders, 1993

Cioffi WG, Burleson DG, Pruitt BA Jr: Leukocyte responses to injury. Arch Surg 128:1260–1267, 1993

Cline MJ: The molecular basis of leukemia. N Engl J Med 330(5):328–336, 1994

Cohen JJ: Apoptosis: The physiologic pathway of cell death. Hosp Pract 28(12):25–33, 1993

Cordell JL: A guide to developing clinical pathways. MLO 27(4):35–39, 1995

Cotes PM: Anomalies in circulation erythropoietin levels. Ann N Y Acad Sci 718:103–109, 1994

Davis BG, Bishop ML, Mass D: Clinical Laboratory Science: Strategies for Practice. Philadelphia: JB Lippincott, 1989

Dorland's Pocket Medical Dictionary. Philadelphia: WB Saunders, 1989

Epstein FH, Agmon Y, Brezis M: Physiology of renal hypoxia. Ann N Y Acad Sci 718:72–81, 1994

Ersboll J, et al: Comparison of the working formulation of non-Hodgkin's lymphoma with the Rappaport, Kiel, and Lukes and Collins classifications. Cancer 55:2442, 1985

Funk PE, Kincade PW, Witte PL: Native associations of early hematopoietic stem cells and stromal cells isolated in bone marrow cell aggregates. Blood 83(2):361–369, 1994

Gabrilove JL: Introduction and overview of hematopoietic growth factors. Semin Hematol 26(2):1–4, 1989

Garza D, Becan-McBride K: Phlebotomy Handbook. E. Norwalk, CT: Appleton & Lange, 1989

Gore MJ: Educator's corner, education and training for physician office laboratory personnel. Clin Lab Sci 8(4):204–205, 1995

Guterl GO: Lab managers accept POC testing trend—with reservations. Advance for Med Lab Prof 7(16):10, 11, 23, 1995

Hajjar DP, Nicholson AC: Atherosclerosis. Am Scientist 83:460–467, 1995

Harris PJ: Hematopoietic endocrinology: Role of autoantibodies to soluble mediators in hematopoiesis. Medical Hypothesis 41:61–62, 1993

Harruff RC: Pathology Facts. Philadelphia: JB Lippincott, 1994

Hathaway WE, Goodnight SH Jr: Disorders of Hemostasis and Thrombosis. New York: McGraw-Hill, 1993

Henry JB (ed): Clinical Diagnosis and Management by Laboratory Methods. Philadelphia: WB Saunders, 1991

Holmsen H: Significance of testing platelet functions in vitro. Eur J Clin Invest 24(Suppl 1):3–8, 1994

Horning SJ: Treatment approaches to the low-grade lymphomas. Blood 83(4):881–884, 1994

Hoyer JD: Laboratory medicine and pathology, leukocyte differential. Mayo Clin Proc 68:1027–1028, 1993

Issaragrisil S, Visuthisakchai S, Suvatte V, et al: Brief report: Transplantation of cord-blood stem cells into a patient with severe thalassemia. N Engl J Med 332(6):367–369, 1994

Jahn M: How to thrive—not just survive—with managed care. MLO 27(2):54–58, 1995

Karselis TC: The Pocket Guide to Clinical Laboratory Instrumentation. Philadelphia: FA Davis, 1994

Kaufman JL: Reply to hypercoagulable states as an evolving risk for spontaneous venous and arterial thrombosis. J Am Coll Surgeons 179:508–509, 1994

Kuby J: Immunology. New York: WH Freeman, 1994

Kuznetsov AI, Ivanov AL, Idelson LI, et al: Mechanisms of thrombocytopenia in patients with lymphoproliferative diseases. Eur J Haematol 49:113–118, 1992

Lee GR, Bithell TC, Foerster J, et al: Wintrobe's Clinical Hematology. Philadelphia: Lea & Febiger, 1993

Locht H, Lindstrom FD, Herder A: Large vessel occlusion, cerebral infarction and thrombocytopenia in the "primary" antiphospholipid syndrome: Response to anticoagulation. Clin Exp Rheumatol 9:169–172, 1991

Mari D, Mannucci PM, Coppola B, et al: Hypercoagulability in centenarians: The paradox of successful aging. Blood 85(11):3144–3149, 1995

Mauch PM: Controversies in the management of early stage Hodgkin's disease. Blood 83(2):318–329, 1994

Mayani H, Guilbert LJ, Janouska-Wieczorek A: Biology of the hematopoietic microenvironment. Eur J Haematol 49:225–233, 1992

McClatchey KD: Clinical Laboratory Medicine. Baltimore: Williams & Wilkins, 1994

Miller SM: Chemical safety: Dangers and risk control. Clin Lab Sci 5(6):338–342, 1992

Monroe DM, Roberts HR, Hoffman M: Platelet procoagulant complex assembly in a tissue factor-initiated system. Br J Haematol 88:364–371, 1994

National Safety Council: Bloodborne Pathogens. Jones and Bartlett, 1993

NCCLS: Methods of Erythrocyte Sedimentation Rate (ESR) Test, 3rd ed. NCCLS document H2-A3. Wayne, PA, NCCLS, 1993

Noe G, Schrezenheier H, Rich IN, Dubanek B: Circulating erythropoietin levels in pathophysiological conditions. Ann N Y Acad Sci 718:94–102, 1994

Otto CN: Safety in health care: Prevention of bloodborne diseases. Clin Lab Sci 5(6):343–345, 1992

Pantel K, Nakeff A: The role of lymphoid cells in hematopoietic regulation. Exp Hem 21:738–742, 1993

Parrott-Boyle M: Hazardous chemical waste disposal management. Clin Lab Sci 5(6):346–348, 1992

Pendergraph GE: Handbook of Phlebotomy. Philadelphia: Lea & Febiger, 1992

Peterson SN, Lapetina EG: Platelet activation and inhibition. Ann N Y Acad Sci 18(714):53–63, 1994

Powars DR: Questions and answers: Sickle cell disease in non-black persons. JAMA 271(23):1885, 1994

Purtillo R: Ethical Dimensions in Health Professions. Philadelphia: WB Saunders, 1993

Ratnoff OD, Forbes CD: Disorders of Hemostasis. Philadelphia: WB Saunders, 1991

Reid CDL: Annotation: In vitro studies of normal and pathological erythropoiesis. Br J Haematol 82:483–487, 1992

Rescitzky P, Haran-Ghera N: Influence of hematopoietic growth factor on leukemic cells. Exp Hematol 22:1, 1994

Rettmer RL: The laboratorian: A key player on the nutrition support team. Am Clin Lab 27(2):19–20, 1992

Rich IN, Lappin RJ (eds): Molecular, cellular, and developmental biology of erythropoietin and erythropoiesis. Ann N Y Acad Sci Vol. 718, 1994

Ringsrud KM, Linne JJ: Urinalysis and Body Fluids: A Color Text and Atlas. Boston: Mosby–Year-Book, 1995

Roby PV, Kenny MA, Garza D: The laboratory outside the laboratory: Our role in point of care testing. Clin Lab Sci 6(4):18–19, 1993

Rouault TA: Heredity hemochromatosis. JAMA 269(24):3152–3154, 1993

Rozman M, Masat T, Feliu E, Rozman C: Dyserythropoiesis in iron-deficiency anemia: Ultrastructural reassessment. Am J Hematol 41:147–150, 1992

Saven A, Piro I: Newer purine analogues for the treatment of hairy-cell leukemia. N Engl J Med 330(10):691–697, 1994

Sacher RA, McPherson RA: Widmann's Clinical Interpretation of Laboratory Tests. Philadelphia: FA Davis, 1991

Schafer AI: Hypercoagulable states: Molecular genetics to clinical practice. Lancet 344:1739–1742, 1994

Schlossman SF, Boumsell L, Gilks W, et al: CD antigens 1993. Blood 83(4):879–880, 1994

Schoeff LE, Williams RH: Principles of Laboratory Instruments. Boston: CV Mosby, 1993

Schumann GB: Clinical utility of body fluid analysis: An overview. Clin Lab Sci 7(1):28–31, 1994

Slack SM, Cui Y, Turitto VT: The effects of flow on blood coagulation and thrombosis. Thromb Haemostas 70(1):129–134, 1993

Smith MA, Knoght SM, Maddison PJ, Smith JG: Effect of the blunted response to erythropoietin and of interleukin 1 production by marrow macrophages. Ann Rheum Dis 51(5):753–757, 1992

Smith SV, Forman DT: Laboratory analysis of cerebrospinal fluid. Clin Lab Sci 7(1):32–38, 1994

Sohn D-S, Kim K-Y, Lee W-B, Kim D-C: Eosinophilic granulopoiesis in human fetal liver. Anat Rec 235:453–460, 1993

Springer TA: Traffic signals for lymphocyte recirculation and leukocyte emigration: The multistep paradigm. Cell 76:301–314, 1994

Stamatoyannopoulos G, Nienhuis AW, Majerus PW, Varmus H: The Molecular Basis of Blood Diseases. Philadelphia: WB Saunders, 1994

Statland BE: Vitamins and minerals: Passing fads or keys to health? Med Lab Obs 25(12):21–28, 1993

Stewart CE, Koepke JA: Basic Quality Assurance Practices for Clinical Laboratories. Philadelphia: JB Lippincott, 1987

Stites DP, Terr AI: Basic and Clinical Immunology. E. Norwalk, CT: Appleton & Lange, 1991

Straetmans N: Cell adhesion molecules and their role in hematopoiesis and in hematological diseases. Aust N Z J Med 23:504–512, 1993

Sweetenham JW: Mutated genes in myeloid leukemias. Exp Hematol 22:5–6, 1994

Tavassoli M: Embryonic origin of hematopoietic stem cells. Exp Hematol 22:7, 1994

Testa U, Pelosi E, Gabbianelli M, et al: Cascade transactivation of growth factor receptors in early human hematopoiesis. Blood 81(6):1442–1456, 1993

Theriot BL: Clinical Laboratory Science Review. Jeffersonville, LA: Creative Educators, 1995

Tietz NW (ed): Clinical Guide to Laboratory Tests. Philadelphia: WB Saunders, 1995

Timonen TTT, Kauma H: Therapeutic effect of heme arginate in myelodysplastic syndromes. Eur J Haematol 49:234–238, 1992

Tizard IR: Immunology. Philadelphia: Saunders College Publishing, 1995

Traycoff CM, Abboud MR, Laver J, et al: Evaluation of the in vitro behavior of phenotypically defined populations of umbilical cord blood hematopoietic progenitor cells. Exp J Hematol 22:215–222, 1994

U.S. Department of Health and Human Services: Biosafety in Microbiological and Biomedical Laboratories. HHS Publication No. (CDC) 93-8395. Atlanta, GA: U.S. Government Printing Office, 1993

Wallach J: Interpretation of Diagnostic Tests. Boston: Little Brown, 1992

Ward KM, Lehmann CA, Leiken AM: Clinical Laboratory Instrumentation and Automation: Principles, Applications, and Selection. Philadelphia: WB Saunders, 1994

Weinberg RS, He L, Alter BP: Erythropoiesis is distinct at each stage of ontogeny. Pediatr Res 2(31):170–174, 1992

Westgard JO, Quam EF, Barry PL: Establishing and evaluating QC acceptability criteria. MLO 26(2):22–26, 1994

Wilson JD, Braunwald E, Isselbacher KJ, et al (eds): Harrison's Principles of Internal Medicine. New York: McGraw-Hill, 1991

Winter J: Hematology: Hemoglobin E and beta-thalassemia: A case study report. Clin Lab Sci 7(1):19–20, 1994

World Health Organization (WHO) Laboratory Manual for the Examination of Human Semen and Semen-Cervical Mucous Interaction, 3rd ed. Cambridge University Press, NY, 1992, pp 5–6.

Xu L, Stahl SK, Dave HPG, et al: Correction of the enzyme deficiency in hematopoietic cells of Gaucher patients using a clinically acceptable retroviral supernatant transduction protocol. Exp Hematol 22:223–230, 1994

Young NS, Alter BP: Aplastic Anemia Acquired and Inherited. Philadelphia: WB Saunders, 1994

Comprehensive Glossary: A Shortcut to Knowledge!

ADP (adenosine 5'-pyrophosphate) is a nucleotide produced from adenosine triphosphate (ATP) to provide energy for cellular metabolism, such as platelet aggregation. For this reason ADP is one of the aggregating agents used as a reagent to test platelet aggregation. Refer to Chapter 13.

APCs (antigen-presenting cells) describe one of the functions of the macrophage cells throughout the body. The macrophage cells are not only the most efficient phagocytes of the body defense system but they also have the ability to process the phagocytized antigen and present this antigen to the CD4 lymphocyte for an efficient and effective initiation of a primary immune response. Refer to Chapters 4 and 5 as well as to Figures 4–4 and 5–4.

Abetalipoproteinemia is a hereditary deficiency of beta lipoproteins, which are part of the erythrocyte membrane. This lack of beta lipoprotein results in the development of acanthocytes, which are erythrocytes with irregular spicules off of the membrane. It is important to be able to tell the difference between acanthocytes and echinocytes, which are crenated erythrocytes. Crenated erythrocytes have more rounded protrusions in a more regular pattern. Individuals with abetalipoproteinemia also have decreased cholesterol, malabsorption, and other problems attributed to this condition. Refer to Chapters 7 and 9.

Absolute values refer to the true value and are not a reflection of the relationship of the component of interest to other blood components. The absolute value is an accurate value, whereas the relative value may appear erroneously normal or abnormal due to a change in one of the other components. For example, the percentage of lymphocytes in the peripheral blood multiplied by the total white blood cell count is equal to the absolute lymphocyte count (% lymphocytes × total white blood cell count = absolute lymphocyte count) versus the percentage of lymphocytes rela-

tive to the other cells in the specimen. If other cells are increased, the number of lymphocytes may appear to be decreased in proportion to the others, when in fact the absolute number of lymphocytes has not changed.

Absorbed plasma (AP) is a plasma reagent with some of the coagulation factors removed for the purpose of investigating an abnormal coagulation test result. AP is used when a coagulation test, such as the partial thromboplastin time (PTT) or the thrombin time (TT), is prolonged to determine the cause of the abnormal result. The AP is prepared by absorbing normal plasma with barium sulfate ($BaSO_4$), which removes some of the coagulation factors, leaving factors I, V, VIII, XI, and XII. An example of use is AP mixed in equal volumes with the patient's prolonged plasma, and the abnormal test or tests are repeated with this mixed specimen. If the testing now yields normal results, the laboratory practitioner knows that one of the factors in AP was deficient in the patient's specimen. This is one form of factor substitution assay and is used in conjunction with the aged serum (AS) reagent. Refer to Chapters 12 and 13.

Acanthocytes are abnormally shaped erythrocytes with pointed irregular spicules of the cell membrane. Acanthocytes are seen in association with abetalipoproteinemia, which is a hereditary deficiency of beta lipoprotein (a component of the erythrocyte membrane). This lack of the beta lipoprotein results in the development of acanthocytes. It is important to be able to tell the difference between acanthocytes and echinocytes, which are crenated erythrocytes. Crenated erythrocytes have more rounded protrusions in a more regular pattern. Refer to Chapters 7 to 9.

Accuracy is the closeness of the test result value to the true value of the component being measured as it exists in the patient. Samples with known values, such as standards purchased from the manufacturer of the instrument, are used to assess the accuracy of a test procedure or instrument. If the standard is tested exactly as the patient's specimen and the results are consistent with the known value of the standard (i.e., are accurate), then the patient's value, derived from the same procedure, is also accepted as being accurate. A test performance may render the same value in multiple determinations, but if that value is not correct, it is still useless for the patient's diagnosis or treatment.

Acid elution test demonstrates the presence of hemoglobin F in fetal cells within the mother's circulation. Normally the fetal blood and maternal blood never come into contact. All nutrients, waste products, and so forth are passed through membranes between the mother and the fetus. Occasionally, blood vessels are broken and bleeding occurs during pregnancy or at birth, and the baby's blood enters the mother's circulatory system. If hemolytic disease of the newborn (HDN) is suspected, the physician needs to know how much of the fetal blood is in the mother; thus a prophylactic treatment of immunoglobulin can be administered to the mother. This test is presented in more detail in Chapter 10. HDN is presented in Chapter 9 and fetal hemoglobin in Chapter 8.

Acid-fast stain is a microbiologic stain used on sputum smears to identify *Mycobacterium tuberculosis*.

Acidified serum test is used to diagnose paroxysmal nocturnal hemoglobinuria (PNH), a hemolytic anemia. This test is presented in detail in Chapter 10. PNH is presented in Chapter 9.

Acquired refers to an illness developed throughout life versus an inherited disease that is genetically determined from birth.

Acute refers to a condition with severe symptoms and a short course.

Acute erythroleukemia (FAB M6, AEL) is the proliferation of malignant erythrocytes and requires aggressive treatment. AEL demonstrates more than 50% erythroid dysplasia in the bone marrow with megaloblastic normoblasts containing diffuse blocks of cytoplasmic glycogen, which is visible with periodic acid-Schiff (PAS) stain. PAS staining can be used to differentiate AEL from other erythroproliferative (polycythemia) and myeloproliferative (myelodysplasia) disorders. Refer to Chapter 9 and Table 9–2.

Acute leukemias are the excessive proliferation of a malignant bone marrow cell. Acute leukemias are very aggressive; the onset is rapid; the prognosis is poor; and mostly immature cells (blasts) are seen in the bone marrow and peripheral blood. The acute leukemias are classified by the French, American, and British (FAB) system due to the morphologic similarities of the early undifferentiated cells involved. The FAB classification of acute leukemias allows consistent diagnosis

and treatment throughout the world and provides more information for better diagnosis and treatment. Identification of the cell line involved is done by using cytochemical stains and detecting specific membrane proteins with fluorescent monoclonal antibodies and flow cytometry. The use of the flow cytometry methodology is required for accurate cell identification. The white blood cell count varies from low to high. Due to the excessive proliferation of leukemic cells and the cytotoxic effect of treatment, a life-threatening decrease in neutrophils and thrombocytes predisposes the patient to infections and bleeding. These patients often die of pneumonia. These individuals may benefit from receiving white blood cells and thrombocyte transfusions. Growth factors (e.g., G-CSF) are commercially available to stimulate production of new healthy neutrophils, and thrombocyte growth factor is in development. The FAB classification is presented in Table 3–1.

Acute lymphocytic leukemia (ALL) is an abnormal proliferation of lymphocytic cells in the bone marrow. ALL has been classified by the French, American, and British (FAB) cooperative hematology group (see Table 3–1) into three categories—L1, L2, and L3—for consistency of diagnosis and treatment. The ALL classified as FAB L1 is the most common malignancy in children younger than 5 years of age. The leukemic blasts (see Fig. 5–7) have the membrane markers (immunophenotype) of pre-B cells and are common ALL antigen (CALLA/CD10) negative. Genetic translocations are common, especially t(4;11), 11q23-25, and 9p21-22. The peripheral blood may show a normocytic, normochromic anemia. In the past this leukemia was fatal. Currently more than 50% of the patients with this diagnosis are considered to be cured after treatment. This emphasizes the importance of accurate and early identification of cells in the laboratory. FAB L2 leukemia is found most often in adults; thus it is also called adult T-cell leukemia (ATL) and is associated with human T-cell lymphotrophic virus-1 (HTLV-1). The cells seen are small and homogeneous (the same appearance) and have a high N:C ratio (see Fig. 5–8). The FAB L3 acute lymphoblastic leukemia is the leukemic phase of Burkitt's lymphoma. The cells in this leukemia are large and uniform and have prominent nucleoli and deeply basophilic cytoplasm with vacuoles (see Fig. 5–9). These leukemic cells are determined to be mature B cells and are often common ALL antigen (CALLA/CD10) positive; some express IgM on the membrane. Other membrane protein markers that identify these cells are Ia/HLA-DR, CD19, CD20, and CD24. The most common chromosomal translocations associated with L3 are t(8;14)(q24;q32). Epstein-Barr virus (EBV) is associated with this leukemia. Refer to Chapters 5 and 6.

Acute megakaryocytic leukemia (FAB M7) is a very rare leukemia involving malignant proliferation of the early thrombocytic cell, the megakaryoblast. The leukemic cells are identified by the electron microscope, visibility of platelet peroxidase, and platelet membrane glycoproteins by immunocytochemical methods or flow cytometry. This leukemia is presented in Chapter 11 and Table 11–1.

Acute monocytic leukemia (AMoL, FAB M5) is the abnormal proliferation of malignant monocytic cells. AMoL accounts for less than 5% of acute nonlymphocytic leukemias. M5A presents in younger individuals and is poorly differentiated, with 80% monoblasts seen in the bone marrow. The M5B (well differentiated) demonstrates less than 80% blasts in the bone marrow and more promonocytes and monocytes, which are more differentiated cells and are not seen in M5A. For this reason cytochemical stains and membrane proteins recognized by the use of fluorescent monoclonal antibodies and flow cytometry are required for accurate cell identification to confirm M5A. Cytochemical staining, which differentiates the monocytic cells from the myelocytic cells, is the fluoride-inhibited esterase stain. Refer to Chapter 4, Figure 4–5, and Tables 4–1 and 4–2.

Acute myelogenous leukemia (FAB M1 and M2 AML), also called acute granulocytic leukemia (AGL), is an abnormal proliferation of malignant granulocytic cells. FAB classification M1 and M2 can occur in the first few months of life or in the mid to late years of life. There are two classifications of AML, depending on the cells seen. The first type of AML is classified as M1 (AML without maturation) by the FAB classification (see Table 3–1). The predominant cell is the myeloblast, which makes up at least 90% of the nonerythroid bone marrow cells and is seen in the peripheral blood (see Fig. 3–15). Some AML myeloblasts have cytoplasmic inclusions, called Auer rods, which are made of fused azurophilic peroxidase and ASD chloroacetate esterase positive granules. The similarity of blast cells makes cell line identification difficult; however, if Auer rods are seen, the cells are considered myeloblasts. The cytochemical stains used to diagnose AML are myeloperoxidase (MPO), Sudan black B (SBB), and ASD chloroacetate esterase (CAE) (see Fig. 3–16 and Table 3–2). The AML classified as M2 (AML with maturation) demonstrates only 30 to 89% of bone marrow cells as myeloblasts; more than 10% of the nonerythroid cells are promyelocytes, myelocytes, metamyelocytes, bands, and mature neutrophils (see Fig. 3–17). Due to the presence of primarily immature cells and few mature PMNs in AML, there is no concern that this is a normal leukemoid reaction or chronic myelogenous leukemia (CML). Refer to Chapters 3 and 5.

Acute myelomonocytic leukemia (FAB M4, AMML) is an abnormal proliferation of malignant bone marrow blast cells with characteristics of both granulocytic and monocytic cells that are thought to be derived from the CFU-GM cell and diagnosed by the presence of a peripheral blood monocytosis of more than $5 \times 10^9/l$, with 20 to 80% of the bone marrow nonerythroid cells monocytic. M4E is acute myelomonocytic leukemia with an accompanying eosinophilia. Refer to Chapters 3 and 5 and Tables 3–1, and 3–2.

Acute promyelocytic leukemia (APL, FAB M3) is an abnormal proliferation of malignant promyelocytes originating in the bone marrow. Characteristic of M3 are hypergranular promyelocytes dominating the bone marrow (see Fig. 3–18). A common complication of this leukemia is the development of disseminated intravascular coagulation (DIC), which is a blood clotting disorder. Refer to Chapters 3 and 5 and Tables 3–1 and 3–2.

Aerobic cultures involve the microbiologic growth of organisms in an atmospheric oxygen (O_2) or carbon dioxide (CO_2) environment that is adequate for most organisms to grow. The microorganisms are grown in culture to provide the physician with identification and treatment information. This is in contrast with anaerobic cultures, which are grown without oxygen.

Aged serum (AS) is a serum reagent with some of the coagulation factors removed for the purpose of investigating an abnormal coagulation test result. AS is used when a coagulation test time, such as the partial thromboplastin time (PTT) or the thrombin time (TT), is prolonged in order to determine the cause of the abnormal result. The AS is obtained from a clotted specimen; therefore, it does not contain the factors consumed in clotting as well as any labile factors that degrade over time. AS contains only factors XII, XI, IX, VII, X, II, and I. AS is mixed in equal volumes with the prolonged patient plasma, and the test, which was prolonged, is repeated with this mixed specimen. If the previously prolonged test is now corrected, the laboratory practitioner knows that one of the factors in AS was deficient in the patient's specimen. This is one form of factor substitution assay and is used in conjunction with the aged serum (AS) reagent. Refer to Chapters 12 and 13.

Agnogenic means of unknown origin.

Agranulocytosis is a marked decrease in the number of granulocytes.

Alder-Reilly anomaly is an inherited disorder in which all of the leukocytes demonstrate large irregular azurophilic granules in the cytoplasm. These dense azurophilic granulations resembling toxic granulation are present with no association to infection (see Fig. 3–22).

Alkali denaturation test demonstrates the presence of hemoglobin F in fetal cells within the mother's circulation. Normally the fetal blood and maternal blood never have contact. All nutrients, waste products, and so forth are passed through membranes between the mother and the fetus. Occasionally blood vessels are broken and bleeding occurs during pregnancy or at birth, and the baby's blood enters the mother's circulatory system. If hemolytic disease of the newborn (HDN) is suspected, the physician needs to know how much of the fetal blood is in the mother, so that a prophylactic treatment of immunoglobulin can be administered to the mother. Refer to Chapters 8 to 10.

Alkaline phosphatase (LAP) score, also called the neutrophil alkaline phosphatase (NAP) score, is done when the neutrophil (also called a polymorphonuclear cell or PMN) count is elevated to examine the amount of digestive enzyme in the cells. If the process occurring is a normal healthy response to infection (a leukemoid reaction), the LAP score should be high, demonstrating the cell's attempt to increase digestive enzymes and destroy the bacteria. If the LAP score is low, this demonstrates an increase in cells for no biologically normal reason, because they are not functioning properly and are merely proliferating to the detriment of the patient, as seen in chronic myelogenous leukemia (CML). LAP is also elevated in the erythrocyte disorder polycythemia. The score can range from 0 to 400, and a normal score is higher than 125. This test is discussed in more detail in Chapters 3 and 6.

Alloimmune hemolytic anemia is the result of the production of immune response antibodies in one individual against the antigens on the erythrocytes of another individual. This occurs in hemolytic transfusion reactions (HTR) when one person has an immune response to another person's cells, which have been introduced to their blood system, and hemolytic disease of the newborn (HDN) when the mother develops antibodies (has an immune response) to the fetal erythrocyte antigens. Any time that antibodies are produced, the cell or substance that they bind to is marked for destruction (opsonized) by the phagocytic cells of the body; therefore, in the case of erythrocytes, anemia develops.

Alpha-aminolevulinic acid (ALA) is a precursor of heme in the hemoglobin molecule. ALA is a precursor of the porphyrin of the hemoglobin molecule produced from succinyl coenzyme A and glycine in the mitochondria of the developing erythrocyte. In order to investigate abnormalities of hemoglobin synthesis, the level of ALA can be measured in a urine specimen collected over 24 hours. This test is discussed in more detail in Chapters 9 and 10.

Anaerobic cultures are microbiologic growth of microorganisms in an atmosphere depleted of oxygen (O_2) to provide the physician with diagnostic and treatment information. Some organisms (e.g., *Clostridia*), which are found in deep wounds of the body, thrive in this environment and do not grow well with oxygen present. Organisms that grow well with oxygen exposure are grown in aerobic cultures.

Anemia is a decreased number of erythrocytes ($<3 \times 10^{12}/l$) or a decreased amount of hemoglobin (<10 g/dl) present in the peripheral blood erythrocytes. This results in a decrease in oxygen distributed to the body tissue (hypoxia), which in turn should stimulate the kidney to produce (synthesize) the glycoprotein hormone erythropoietin (EPO), which in turn stimulates the release of reticulocytes and increases erythropoiesis. Causes of anemia may be lack of bone marrow production (hypoplasia or aplasia), abnormal production (dyserythropoiesis), or increased rate of destruction (hemolysis) after release from the bone marrow. Erythrocytes lacking the normal quantity of hemoglobin will appear pale through the light microscope and are described as hypochromic (less color). This decreased hemoglobin content will also be evident by a decreased mean corpuscular hemoglobin (MCH) and mean corpuscular hemoglobin concentration (MCHC). Refer to Chapters 9 and 10.

Anemia of chronic disease (ACD) is the anemia that is most commonly seen in the geriatric patient and accompanies the progression of a chronic disease (e.g., infections, rheumatoid arthritis, and cancers). ACD is characterized by shortened red blood cell survival and insufficient bone marrow response to erythropoietin (EPO). Tests show a decreased total iron-binding capacity (TIBC) of transferrin, decreased percentage of iron saturation, and increased free erythrocyte protoporphyrin (FEP) and serum ferritin reflecting increased iron in the macrophages (reticuloendothelial cells), which is not released as needed. The erythrocytes appear normochromic and normocytic. Refer to Chapters 9 and 10.

Anemia of pregnancy in the third trimester, a characteristic retention and shift of body fluids, increases the plasma and causes the blood composition to appear anemic. Refer to Chapter 9.

Anisocytosis refers to a variation in the size of erythrocytes that were formerly called corpuscles. The possible variations producing anisocytosis are macrocytic cells (>95 fl. MCV, which is the mean corpuscular volume) and microcytic cells (<80 fl. MCV). A normal blood specimen is normocytic (80 to 95 fl. MCV). Another index is the red blood cell distribution width (RDW), which provides the percentage of cells outside the normal size range, or in other words, provides insight into the uniformity of the erythrocyte population. The reference range is approximately 11 to 14.5%. Refer to Chapters 9 and 10.

Anomaly refers to a marked deviation (e.g., in the leukocytes) from the normal, especially as a result of congenital or hereditary defects. The hematologic anomalies are Alder-Reilly anomaly, Chédiak-Higashi anomaly, and Pelger-Huët anomaly. All of these have either nuclear or cytoplasmic abnormalities. Refer to Chapter 3.

Anoxia is the absence of oxygen supply to the body tissues despite adequate blood flow. This occurs when anemia is present or when a blood clot has blocked a vessel. Hypoxia is a reduced oxygen supply to the tissues.

Antigen, also called immunogen, is any substance capable of inducing a specific immune response (production of antibodies, also called immunoglobulins) and then reacting with these antibodies. Antigens are phagocytized by macrophages and a processed part of the antigen is presented to T lymphocytes, which then pass it on to a B lymphocyte, which produces the antibodies that will specifically bind to that antigenic determinate.

Antigen-presenting cells (APCs) are the macrophage cells throughout the body. The macrophage cells are not only the most efficient phagocytes of the body defense system but they also have the ability to process the phagocytized antigen and present this antigen to the CD4 lymphocyte for an efficient and effective initiation of a primary immune response. Refer to Figures 4–4 and 5–4.

Antiphospholipid antibodies (APA), often referred to as lupus anticoagulants, are abnormal plasma proteins that bind to the thrombocyte phospholipid (PF3) and interfere with normal blood clotting. When the partial thromboplastin time (PTT) test is prolonged and mixing normal plasma (containing all the coagulation factors) with the patient plasma does not correct the PTT, a circulating anticoagulant such as this is present. If this mixed specimen does correct the PTT, a factor deficiency is suspected instead. The APA is an autoantibody and is seen more commonly in the geriatric patient. Refer to Chapters 11 and 13.

Aperture is an opening or orifice. In hematology instrumentation, the aperture refers to the opening through which cells pass one at a time and are counted by the electrical impedance instruments. Refer to Chapters 6, 10, and 13.

Aplasia literally means without formation. This refers to the loss of cellular development in the bone marrow. It can be due to infiltration of the bone marrow by malignant tissue such as myelofibrosis or cancer cells. Damage to the bone marrow by toxic drugs, such as the antibiotic chloramphenicol, or radiation will cause aplasia. Refer to Chapters 3 to 6.

Aplastic anemia is a decreased number of erythrocytes due to lack of bone marrow production. Hereditary aplasias are Diamond-Blackfan syndrome and Fanconi's anemia. Acquired aplastic anemia can be due to toxic antibiotics (e.g.,

chloramphenicol), toxic chemicals (e.g., benzene), certain viruses (e.g., B19 parvovirus), or radiation. The hemoglobin and hematocrit will be decreased with normocytic and normochromic erythrocytes. The reticulocyte count will be normal to decreased. The reticulocyte is the best indicator of bone marrow function. Refer to Chapter 5.

Arachidonic acid is an essential fatty acid that is a source of prostaglandins (PG 9 hydroxy fatty acids with a variety of physiologic effects in the body) and is used as a reagent to stimulate platelet aggregation for testing in the laboratory. Refer to Chapter 13.

Arneth count is done to determine if a significant number of hypersegmented neutrophils are present in a specimen. Normal neutrophils have three to five lobes when mature; more than five lobes is considered hypersegmented. Hypersegmented neutrophils are associated with DNA synthesis disorders such as a vitamin B_{12} deficiency. This test is discussed in more detail in Chapter 6.

Aspirin is acetylsalicylic acid, which is an analgesic (relieves pain), antipyretic (reduces fever), and antirheumatic (relieves joint pain from rheumatoid arthritis and similar chronic diseases). One complication of aspirin ingestion is deficient thrombocyte aggregation and possible bleeding. Refer to Chapter 12.

Atherosclerotic plaques are lipid accumulations in the arteries associated with a group of diseases referred to as arteriosclerosis. These plaques appear as pearly white areas within an artery and cause the inner surface to bulge into the lumen. These plaques consist of cholesterol, lipids, cell debris, smooth muscle cells, and collagen, and in the older person they may also contain calcium. These plaques slow down the blood flow, which encourages clot formation. When these plaques rupture, the rough surface initiates clot development. Refer to Chapter 12.

Auramine-rhodamine is a microbiologic stain used for identification of the *Mycobacterium* species of microorganisms in a patient's specimen to facilitate the patient's diagnosis and treatment.

Autoimmune hemolytic anemia (AIHA) develops when antibodies produced are capable of binding to the individual's own erythrocytic cells (opsonization), which marks them for destruction by the phagocytic cells of the body (extravascular hemolysis). This can occur when the erythrocytes are altered by viruses or contain antigens similar to viral antigens. The direct antiglobulin test (DAT) is a diagnostic test performed in the blood bank or immunohematology area of the laboratory. When the macrophage digests the opsonized erythrocyte, one product is yellow bilirubin, which is detoxified by the liver and excreted in the urine and feces. Refer to Chapter 9.

Azurophilic granules are present in various granular cells, and they appear red after staining with the metachromatic basic dye. Azurophilic aggregates may be found occasionally in large lymphocytes and mistaken for granules. Lymphocytes are agranular, and the presence of the azurophilic aggregates is insignificant.

BFU-E (burst-forming unit–erythroid) is the earliest cell committed to the erythrocyte cell line for development. This is called a burst-forming unit rather than a colony-forming unit (CFU) due to the unique growth characteristic of seeming to "burst" all over the agarose gel culture plate. This cell originates from the CFU-GEMM and develops into the CFU-E, which is the erythroblast also called the pronormoblast. Refer to Chapter 7 and the hematopoietic chart in Figure 7–3.

B lymphocyte is a mature cell developed from the lymphocytic stem cell (LSC) in the bursa equivalent area of the body (believed to be the bone marrow) and is responsible for humoral immunity (HI), which is the production of antibodies (Ab), also called immunoglobulins (Ig), in an immune response. This cell, when stimulated, becomes a plasma cell and is the most efficient antibody-producing cell of the body. Approximately 20% of the peripheral blood lymphocytes are B cells, which cannot be morphologically distinguished from T lymphocytes. Antibodies (Ig) present in the cytoplasm and on the B lymphocyte membrane can be used to identify this cell. Plasma cells are seen primarily in the bone marrow and body tissues. Plasma cells make up less than 5% of the nucleated bone marrow cells. Refer to Chapter 5.

B lymphocyte memory cells are cells that are produced in the primary immune response and are able to remember the antigen. These long-lived cells will be sensitized to the specific foreign antigen that they were produced against, thus allowing an immediate and more intense immune response (secondary) if the same antigen enters the body in the future. This is the mechanism by which a vaccine protects against disease. Refer to Chapter 5.

Bacterial products, such as cell wall lipopolysaccharides (LPS) or secreted toxins, stimulate an immune response and inflammatory reactions in the body.

Band cells, also called stab cells, are slightly immature granulocytic cells that have not segmented yet. The nucleus is sausage shaped, and the cytoplasm is mature enough to be functional. These cells are released from the bone marrow when there is an increased demand for neutrophils and all of the mature neutrophils in the bone marrow have been released. These cells are associated with a leukemoid reaction. A few bands are seen routinely, and each laboratory has its own criteria for distinguishing bands from segmented neutrophils. It is important that everyone in the laboratory be familiar with the established criteria for the laboratory. If a new instrument is implemented in the laboratory, the band criteria must be established and the medical staff must know the significance of the count. Patients may not have changed status, although more bands may be reported due to a change in the method of testing or criteria used. Refer to Chapter 3, Figures 3–2 and 3–7.

Basophilic normoblast is an immature form of the erythrocyte that is only found in the bone marrow. This cell originates from the pronormoblast (erythroblast, CFU-E) and develops into the polychromatophilic normoblast. Refer to Chapter 7, Figures 7–3 and 7–5.

Basophils are the smallest, least common granulocytes and are derived from the CFU-Ba. Basophils mediate type I hypersensitivity reactions as seen with allergies and asthma. When the antibody IgE is produced in response to an allergen, it binds to the basophil and results in the release of the granule contents, such as histamine. Clinical symptoms such as watery eyes, runny nose, and sneezing are produced. Refer to Chapter 3 and Figure 3–10.

Beer's law is a combination of several calculations done to describe the colorimetric test methodology used in the clinical laboratory to measure substances such as hemoglobin. The law states: The absorbency (ABS) of a colored solution is equal to the product of the concentration of the color-producing substance (C) multiplied by the depth of the solution through which the light must travel (L) multiplied by a constant (K). When written as an equation, this becomes: $ABS = C \times L \times K$. In other words, the amount of color developed in the test procedure is proportional to the amount of substance being tested. Standard lines or curves are often used to apply this law. An example is a method to determine hemoglobin (or any spectrophotometric color determination) concentration using Beer's law with the calculated K value by measuring a known standard using the same methodology and instrumentation that will be used for the patient unknown. A known standard is read and the concentration is divided by the ABS, which gives the K value.

$$\frac{\text{Standard concentration}}{\text{Absorbency}} = \text{K value}$$

The patient's unknown hemoglobin concentration is then determined by taking the ABS of the unknown multiplied by the K value.

ABS of unknown test specimen
$$\times \text{ K value} = \text{Hb in g/dl}$$

Benign refers to a condition that is not life threatening.

Bernard-Soulier syndrome is a genetic abnormality in the thrombocyte membrane glycoprotein (gp) Ib, resulting in defective adhesion and aggregation. Refer to Chapter 11.

Bilirubin is a yellow pigmented toxic product of hemoglobin breakdown that is usually eliminated by the liver. An increase in bilirubin demonstrates a yellow (jaundiced) plasma, skin, and membrane color. This indicates an increase in erythrocyte breakdown (hemolysis) or liver failure; or, if observed in a newborn infant, the enzymes that degrade bilirubin in the liver are not yet developed and the infant is placed under a light to break down the bilirubin until the liver enzymes can. Bilirubin is a product of and indicator for extravascular hemolysis as seen in autoimmune and alloimmune hemolytic anemias. The reference value for bilirubin is 0.3–1.1 mg/dl. Refer to Chapters 9 and 10.

Bleeding time test is a crude method of assessing thrombocyte function. In order to accurately interpret this test, the thrombocyte count must be in the normal range. This procedure is provided in detail in Chapter 13.

Blood gases can be measured in arterial or venous blood, keeping in mind that the reference values are different, so that the source of the specimen is important. The arterial blood gas is usually drawn and often analyzed by the respiratory therapy department. Venous blood gases may be drawn and analyzed by the clinical chemistry department of the laboratory. The specimen should be kept sealed and on ice until tested. The parameters determining the blood gases are a standard pH of 7.4 in acid-base balance, the partial pressure of oxygen (PO_2), the partial pressure of carbon dioxide (PCO_2), carbonic acid (H_2CO_3), and bicarbonate (HCO_3^-). The acid-base balance of blood is affected by the respiratory and metabolic state of the individual, the ratio of $Na^+:K^+$, and Cl^- levels. Refer to Chapter 8.

Blood volume of an average adult is approximately 6 liters. There are circumstances in which there appears to be too much or too little blood volume. By measuring the plasma volume and the red blood cell mass, the total blood volume can be accurately determined. This information may be used to diagnose disorders such as polycythemia. Refer to Chapter 10.

Body fluids typically refer to fluids other than blood or urine, such as cerebrospinal fluid (CSF), synovial fluid, pleural fluid, and peritoneal fluid (ascites). These fluids are normally present in a rather small fixed volume for lubrication purposes and contain very few cells. In a state of disease, the volume increases and various cells or crystals may be present. Seminal fluid is also used for analysis of the sperm count, morphology, and motility. Refer to Chapters 14 and 15.

Body substance isolation (BSI) involves a more comprehensive approach than do universal precautions, which require protective measures to be used during exposure to *all* body specimens (not just fluids).

Bone marrow produces blood from the seventh month of gestation and continues to do so throughout life (see Fig. 2–2). Blood cell formation in the bone marrow is called medullary hematopoiesis, and the cells produced are listed in Figure 2–3.

Bone marrow microenvironment consists of stromal cells (fibroblasts, macrophages, endothelial cells, adipocytes/fat cells) in which the blood cells are influenced to become specific cells when needed by the body. Refer to Chapter 2 and Figure 2–1.

Boyden chamber is a device used to test the chemotaxis of neutrophils. In lazy leukocyte syndrome, the neutrophils do not respond appropriately to chemotactant substances, which should draw them to a site of possible bacterial infection. This is a rare disorder, and this test is rarely done. Refer to Chapters 3 and 6.

Buffy coat is the layer of white blood cells and platelets that forms between the erythrocytes and the plasma of centrifuged whole blood. The buffy coat makes up approximately 1% of whole blood volume. If the leukocyte count is extremely elevated, the buffy coat will be visibly increased. If the leukocyte count is very low, the cells may need to be concentrated. In this case a buffy coat preparation is done for leukocyte evaluation. The procedure for preparing a buffy coat is discussed in more detail in Chapter 6.

Bursa equivalent (bone marrow?) is the site of B lymphocyte development in the human body. Birds have a bursa of Fabricius in which their B lymphocytes become competent to produce antibody. Although humans have competent B lymphocytes, no bursa of fabricius has been found in humans. Perhaps the bone marrow is the equivalent site for development.

CBC or complete blood count consists of the erythrocyte count, leukocyte count, thrombocyte count, hemoglobin, hematocrit, red blood cell and platelet indices, reference ranges and flags for out-of-range values, histograms, and scattergrams providing additional information about the size and population of cells present in the counts. An automated differential of the leukocytes is provided. The specimen of choice for this procedure is an EDTA (purple top) tube containing blood. More details are provided in Chapters 6, 10, and 13.

CD4 (cluster differentiation marker 4) lymphocyte, also called the T helper (T_h) cell, orchestrates an immune response by receiving the processed antigen (immunogen) information from the monocyte/macrophage, which stimulates the CD4 cell to proliferate, produce cytokines to stimulate other immune response cells, and pass the information on to the B lymphocyte for the production of antibodies (immunoglobulins) to facilitate destruction of the foreign invader. This cell is counterbalanced by the CD8 cell, which is the T suppressor cell, to limit and control the immune response initiated by the CD4 cell. The virus that causes acquired immunodeficiency syndrome (AIDS) (human immunodeficiency virus [HIV]) resides in the CD4 cell, resulting in the inability to initiate an immune response to invading substances such as bacteria or cancer cells. Refer to Chapter 5.

CD8 (cluster differentiation marker 8) lymphocyte is also called the T suppressor (T_s or cytotoxic (T_c or CTL) cell. The T_s lymphocyte limits the immune response initiated by the T helper (T_h) lymphocyte to achieve the goal of eliminating the foreign invader without complications due to excess antibody. The T_c cell is activated by interaction with an HLA class I (also called MHC) antigen to physically destroy abnormal cells. When the T_c is involved in the delayed reaction of organ rejection, this cell is referred to as a T-delayed type of hypersensitivity (T_{DTH}) lymphocyte. Refer to Chapter 5.

CFU-E (colony-forming unit–erythroid) is an early erythroid cell called an erythroblast or a pronormoblast. Refer to Chapters 2 and 7.

Cancer is a malignant (life-threatening) uncontrolled growth of cells. The cause of cancer is unknown, although research has indicated the association of three factors: (1) the genetic sensitivity or tendency to develop a cancer; (2) exposure to the cancer-causing virus; and (3) an initiating event such as exposure to radiation or excessive caffeine, which is instrumental in changing normal genes with cancerous potential (proto-oncogenes) to malignant cancer-enhancing genes (oncogenes). These oncogenes become transformed to stimulate cancerous growth or are inactivated to turn off a protein product that suppresses cancer.

Carboxyhemoglobin (HbCO) is hemoglobin (Hb) combined with carbon monoxide (CO) instead of oxygen. The CO binds with 200 times greater affinity than O_2, blocking the ability of the Hb to carry O_2 to the tissue. Anoxia results, with a rapidly fatal outcome. Refer to Chapter 8.

Cell adhesion molecules (CAMs) are specific cell surface proteins found on the stromal cells of the bone marrow that direct and stimulate the growth and development of the hematopoietic cells. Specific CAMs within the microenvironment of the bone marrow are necessary for normal cell migration and development. Refer to Chapter 2.

Cerebrospinal fluid (CSF) is the fluid from the spinal column that cushions the brain; CSF is sterile and cell free. Part of the central nervous system (CNS), which is called the meninges, can become infected in a rapidly fatal disease known

as spinal meningitis. For this reason, rapid and accurate examination and analysis of the CSF is essential. Normal CSF is clear, colorless, and cell free and has the viscosity of water. Refer to Chapter 14.

Chédiak-Higashi anomaly is an autosomal recessive inherited abnormality that is lethal. The leukocytes show large, irregular, neutral-colored granules in the cytoplasm. Many other defects, such as infiltration of organs with histiocytes, are associated with this disorder. Refer to Chapter 3.

Chemotaxis is the response of neutrophilic granulocytes to chemical stimulants by migrating to the area of the body where they are needed. A Boyden chamber is a device used to test the chemotaxis of neutrophils. In lazy leukocyte syndrome, the neutrophils do not respond appropriately to chemotactant substances, which should draw them to a site of possible bacterial infection. This disorder is rare, and this test is rarely done.

Chronic refers to a condition with very few symptoms and a long duration. Chronic leukemias are often discovered in geriatric individuals while they are being treated for a totally unrelated disorder.

Chronic granulocytic leukemia. See Chronic myelogenous leukemia. Refer to Chapter 3.

Chronic granulomatous disease (CGD) is the inability of the neutrophilic granules to release their contents. A test for neutrophil function to assess the ability of the neutrophils to degranulate is the nitroblue tetrazolium reduction test (NBT), which is discussed more in Chapters 3 and 6.

Chronic lymphocytic leukemia (CLL) is most common in persons older than 60 years of age. Small lymphocytes of B-cell origin are elevated and dominate the bone marrow and blood. The presence of broken or deteriorated cells, called basket cells or smudge cells, is characteristic of the fragile cells present. Lymphosarcoma cell leukemia (LSL), a rare CLL, demonstrates genetic alterations that correlate with prognosis (survival). A lymphoma differs from a leukemia in the primary site of neoplastic cells. Refer to Chapter 5.

Chronic myelogenous leukemia (CML), also called chronic myelocytic leukemia or chronic granulocytic leukemia (CGL), is a disease that has a slow onset with proliferation of mature neutrophilic leukocytes. This disease is found most often in geriatric patients by accident when another problem is being investigated. An elevated leukocyte count of primarily mature neutrophils must be evaluated to distinguish a normal healthy leukemoid reaction from chronic myelogenous leukemia. A chromosomal abnormality has been associated with this disease in diagnosis and prognosis. The t(9;22) translocation, also called the Philadelphia (Ph′) chromosome, has been found in most cases of CML. Refer to Chapter 3.

Chronic myelomonocytic leukemia (CMML) is

one classification of the myelodysplastic syndrome seen in individuals older than 50 years of age. CMML presents with monocytosis and anemia. The myelodysplastic information is presented in Table 3–3.

Circulating anticoagulant test, or "mix" test, is done if the partial thromboplastin time (PTT) test is prolonged. The prolonged specimen is mixed with an equal volume of the normal control plasma, and this mixed specimen is used to repeat the PTT. If the prolonged PTT was due to a factor deficiency, it will be corrected by the "mixed" specimen because all of the factors have been added. If the PTT is not corrected, this indicates that there is circulating anticoagulant in the patient's blood that inhibited the normal control factors as well as the patient's factors. This PTT, which was performed on a mixed specimen (half of the patient's specimen + half of the normal control serum), is called the circulating anticoagulant test. Refer to Chapters 12 and 13.

Circulating inhibitors include the naturally occurring coagulation inhibition factors such as antithrombin III (ATIII), heparin, protein C, and protein S. The circulating inhibitors that are developed throughout life are the antiphospholipid antibodies (APA) and other autoantibodies or excessive proteins produced in diseases such as multiple myeloma. Refer to Chapters 12 and 13.

Circulatory system includes the heart and blood vessels (vasculature made up of arteries, veins, arterioles, venules, and capillaries). The heart pumps the blood through the body carrying oxygen from the lungs to the body tissue. Healthy blood vessels are said to have vascular integrity.

Clinical Laboratory Improvement Act (CLIA) is legislation aimed at ensuring quality testing in all laboratory practice settings. This was developed to protect individuals from inadequate testing in small clinics, physician office laboratories (POLs), malls, supermarkets, and so forth where testing such as cholesterol screens are being performed with no way to ensure the qualifications of the individual performing the test and quality of the testing performed.

Clinical laboratory scientist (CLS), formerly called a medical technologist (MT), is a laboratory practitioner who has completed an accredited bachelor's degree program and has demonstrated competency by passing a national certification examination.

Clinical laboratory technician (CLT), formerly called a medical laboratory technician (MLT), is a laboratory practitioner who has completed an associate's degree program and has demonstrated professional competency by passing a national certification examination.

Clinical pathways are the expected flow of individual health care interventions, such as clinical testing, used to progress in a meaningful direction toward the most efficient and useful out-

come for the prevention, diagnosis, and treatment of disease. Refer to Chapter 16.

Clot retraction is a crude test to evaluate platelet function. The whole blood specimen is placed into a tube marked with graduations for measurement. The volume is recorded, and the tube is placed in a 37° C water bath and the retraction of the clot is observed. This test is discussed in Chapters 11 and 13.

Clots (thrombi) (singular, thrombus) are platelets and fibrin strands that hold erythrocytes and leukocytes together to stop blood flow. This is blood coagulation. If thrombi form at a break in the blood vessel, they can be beneficial by stopping the loss of blood from the body. If thrombi form within the blood vessels and block the flow of blood to the body tissue, as seen in a stroke or heart attack, the tissue deprived of oxygen will necrose (die), which is life threatening. If a piece of the thrombus breaks off and travels to the lung where it blocks flow to the lung tissue, this is also life threatening and is called a thromboembolism. Refer to Chapters 11 and 12.

Cluster differentiation (CD) markers are proteins on the surface of many blood cells and can be used with the flow cytometry methodology to identify specific cells. As cells differentiate and mature, their CD markers change, providing information about the cell's stage of development.

Coagulation of blood is the biologic generation of thrombin in the blood plasma, which converts soluble plasma fibrinogen to insoluble fibrin strands, forming a thrombus or red clot of the erythrocytes, leukocytes, and thrombocytes. The fluid portion is serum that is clear and does not contain coagulation factors consumed in the clot, such as fibrinogen. A white clot consists primarily of leukocytes and thrombocytes. A thromboembolus is a piece of a clot that has broken off and moved to another part of the body where it blocks blood flow. An example is a pulmonary embolus, which is a piece of a blood clot blocking blood flow to the lungs. Coagulation involves the coagulation factors and thrombocytes, and it requires calcium ions (Ca^{2+}) and phospholipids (PF3). Some anticoagulants work by binding to the Ca^{2+}, rendering it unavailable for coagulation to occur. Refer to Chapters 11 to 13.

Coagulation factors consist of approximately 17 glycoprotein coagulation factors, numbered I to XIII (no IV or VI), and proteins S, C, prekallikrein, high molecular weight kininogen, and antithrombin III (see Table 12–1). Additional components necessary for coagulation to occur are a phospholipid surface such as exposed collagen, platelet phospholipid (PPL, PF3), or tissue factor (III). Calcium ions (Ca^{2+}) are also essential for coagulation to occur.

Coagulation testing is done to diagnose and treat coagulation problems. Most of these tests require a full, clear, and well-mixed sodium citrate (Na citrate; blue top) tube unopened (to maintain pH), stored on ice, and tested within 2 hours. Often the tube is opened and the plasma is transferred to another tube, covered, and placed on ice until it is tested. The blue top tube must be full, because the test procedures are based on a full tube of blood with a 9:1 ratio of blood to anticoagulant or 4.5 ml blood: 0.5 ml sodium citrate anticoagulant. If there is less blood in the tube, there will be excess anticoagulant, which will prolong the test results erroneously. Refer to Chapter 13.

Coefficient of variation (CV) is a value that expresses the relativity (to the mean) of the standard deviation. Calculated as $CV = SD - \bar{X}$. The CV is a measure of the relationship between two statistical variables, which are most commonly expressed as their covariance divided by the standard deviation of each; in other words, CV is a statistic to determine how variable the results are. How widely are they distributed from one another? Refer to Chapter 1.

Cold agglutinins are antibodies that, when combined with their corresponding antigens at relatively low temperatures such as 0° to 25° C, cause the antigen elements to adhere to each other in clumps. The most common cold agglutinin tested for in hematology is associated with *Mycoplasma pneumoniae* (atypical or walking pneumonia). This cold agglutinin agglutinates erythrocytes and causes erroneous blood counting results. When this test is ordered, the specimen should be kept at body temperature (37° C) until testing is done. If the specimen is allowed to cool before testing, the cold agglutinin will have bound to the cells and the serum removed to test for cold agglutinins will not contain any antibody. This test is usually performed in the blood bank (immunohematology) area of the laboratory. Refer to Chapters 9 and 10.

Collagen is the protein fibers of connective tissue that holds the cells of the skin, tendons, cartilage, and other connective tissue together. Collagen is also used as a platelet-aggregating reagent in laboratory testing and may be a target for the rheumatoid factor. Refer to Chapter 13.

College of American Pathologists (CAP) is an organization that provides proficiency testing to monitor the quality of the tests performed in the laboratory.

Colony-forming unit–eosinophil (CFU-Eo) cell is derived from the CFU-GEMM cell and differentiates into an eosinophilic granulocyte. If the CFU-GEMM responds to IL-5 and as of yet unknown eosinophil CSFs, it will become the colony-forming unit–eosinophil (CFU-Eo). Refer to Chapter 3.

Colony-forming unit–granulocyte, erythroid, monocyte, and megakaryocyte (CFU-GEMM) is the early myeloid cell that is derived from the hematopoietic stem cell (HSC) and is destined to become a granulocyte, an erythrocyte, a monocyte, or a megakaryocyte (platelet precursor) depending on the protein stimulation by plasma factors produced by the body in response to the need. Refer to Chapters 2 and 3.

Colony-forming unit–granulocyte or monocyte (CFU-GM) cell is derived from the CFU-GEMM cell and can be directed by specific growth factors to differentiate into the CFU-G, which becomes a neutrophilic granulocyte, or the CFU-M, which becomes a monocyte. Refer to Chapters 2 to 4.

Colony-forming unit–megakaryocyte (CFU-mega) is derived from the CFU-GEMM and is also called a megakaryoblast, which will develop into a promegakaryocyte and then a megakaryocyte and will eventually produce thrombocytes (platelets [PLT]). Platelets are cytoplasmic fragments of the megakaryocyte that are a component of blood coagulation. Platelets form the initial plug of an injured blood vessel to contain blood flow. These cellular elements are discussed in detail in Chapter 11.

Colony-forming unit–x (CFU-x) refers to the early cells of a cell line (x) that is noted after the dash. An example is the CFU-M, which is the earliest definitive monocytic cell. These cells are called colony-forming units because they can be grown in tissue culture and form colonies of progeny cells. For this reason they may also be called progenitor cells. Refer to Chapter 2.

Colony-stimulating factor (x-CSF) refers to a growth factor whose target cell (x) is abbreviated before the dash. These proteins, also called myeloid growth factors, are produced by various cells of the body that stimulate and influence the development of the hematopoietic cells. An example is the G-CSF, which stimulates the production of granulocytes. Refer to Chapter 2.

Colony-stimulating factors (CSF) are growth-regulatory proteins produced by cells in the body to specifically stimulate one blood cell line. The protein factors present and their concentrations determine the direction of development of the early cells. Refer to Chapter 2.

Common coagulation pathway is part of both the extrinsic and intrinsic coagulation pathways. In this pathway, factor X, in association with a cofactor, factor V, on the phospholipid (PPL, PF3) surface with Ca^{2+}, converts prothrombin into thrombin, which then converts fibrinogen into fibrin (see Fig. 12–2C). Fibrin monomers link spontaneously by hydrogen bonds to form loose fibrin polymers, trapping the erythrocytes, leukocytes, and thrombocytes to form a blood clot. Factor XIII, which is activated by thrombin and calcium, stabilizes the fibrin polymers. Tests to evaluate this part of the coagulation pathways for assessment of hemostasis are the thrombin time (TT) test and the fibrinogen assay. Refer to Chapters 12 and 13.

Complete blood count (CBC) consists of the erythrocyte count, leukocyte count, thrombocyte count, hemoglobin, hematocrit, red blood cell and platelet indices, reference ranges and flags for out-of-range values, histograms and scattergrams providing additional information about the size and population of cells present in the counts, and an automated differential of the leukocytes. The specimen of choice for this procedure is an EDTA (purple top) tube containing blood. More details are provided in Chapter 6.

Continuous quality improvement (CQI) is the constant monitoring and improvement of the quality of laboratory practice and data, generated by the laboratory, which is practiced in most clinical laboratories. Refer to Chapter 16.

Correlations to determine validity mean that the values produced in the laboratory have no true value or meaning unless there is some mechanism for determining the validity of the results. This is accomplished by comparing various test results throughout the laboratory, ensuring consistent repetition of test results for precision, testing standards, and controls with known values to verify accuracy, and by monitoring the quality control and clerical errors within the laboratory. The values produced within the laboratory must undergo correlation to determine their validity before they are generated for dissemination to the health care provider responsible for the diagnosis and treatment of the patient. Refer to Chapters 6, 10, 13, 15, and 16.

Coumadin (warfarin) is the trade name for a preparation of warfarin, which is used as an oral anticoagulant for patients with a tendency for thrombosis. The test to monitor the effectiveness of this drug is the prothrombin time (PT) test. Information required for interpretation of PT test results are the time and mode of administration of the drug. Refer to Chapters 12 and 13.

Covariance is the expected value of the product of the deviations of corresponding values of two random variables from their respective means; in other words, a calculation to determine if the values fall within an expected range from the mean for acceptable results. Refer to Chapter 1.

Crenated erythrocytes have lost their biconcave shape and become shriveled up like a raisin. Placing erythrocytes in a hypertonic solution will cause the phenomenon of osmosis to occur, due to the movement of water out of the cell.

Cytocentrifuge is an instrument used to concentrate a small number of cells in a solution for the purpose of microscopic evaluation and cytochemical staining. The carriers in the cytocentrifuge are filled with a holder containing a glass slide, a special filter paper containing a central hole for the cells to pass through onto the slide, and a funnel containing a specific amount of the well-mixed specimen, as stated in the procedure. Refer to Chapter 15.

Cytochemical stains such as myeloperoxidase (MPO), Sudan black B (SBB), and ASD chloroacetate esterase (CAE) can be used to aid in the identification of cells and in the diagnosis of leukemia (see Table 3–2 and Fig. 3–16).

Cytokines are proteins secreted by cells that regulate other cells. Cytokines produced by lymphocytes are called lymphokines; those produced by monocytes are called monokines. These proteins can be stimulating, growth promoting, or inhibitory. Examples of lymphokines are interleukin-2 (IL-2), colony-stimulating factors (CSFs), interferon (IFN), which is antiviral, and monokines such as IL-1. Others include interleukin-3 (IL-3), interleukin-4 (IL-4), interleukin-9 (IL-9), interleukin-11 (IL-11), and tumor necrosis factor (TNF).

Cytology examinations are performed by a registered cytologist and confirmed by a pathologist to identify any inflammatory cells, questionable cells, or neoplastic cells present in a body specimen such as a tissue biopsy.

Cytomegalovirus (CMV) infection is similar to mononucleosis. The symptoms and blood picture are the same, but the mononucleosis test result is negative. Large reactive lymphocytes make up 90% of the peripheral blood leukocytes. The mode of transmission is multiple blood transfusions or from exchange of saliva as seen with mononucleosis. A definitive diagnosis is made by isolating the CMV by microbiologic techniques from blood or urine or by a rise in CMV antibody titer. The CMV isolation is done in the microbiology department or is sent to a reference laboratory. A titer of CMV antibodies produced in the patient is more useful if done several times over a period of days. The titer is significant only if a rise or a fall is seen. There are chronic cases of CMV, which is one of the chronic fatigue syndromes. Refer to Chapter 5.

Cytotoxic cell (T_c) is identified by the CD8 membrane protein and is also called the cytotoxic T lymphocyte (T_c or CTL) or the suppressor T lymphocyte (T_s). The T_c cell is activated by interaction with an HLA class I (also called MHC) antigen to physically destroy abnormal cells. The T_s lymphocyte limits the immune response initiated by the T_h lymphocyte to achieve the goal of eliminating the foreign invader without complications due to excess antibody. Refer to Chapter 5.

DDAVP (1-desamino-8-D-arginine vasopressin) is a synthetic analog to vasopressin, which stimulates the production of coagulation factor VIII in the body and will result in a two- to tenfold rise in factor VIII titer after intravenous infusion. DDAVP may be useful in treatment of an individual with liver damage or disease or in an individual who is deficient in factor VIII. Refer to Chapter 12.

Deep vein thrombosis (DVT) is the development of blood clots in the deep veins of the body, usually in the legs. This is characterized by leg pain and swelling. If a portion of the clot breaks loose, it may travel to the lungs and cut off the blood supply, resulting in shortness of breath and possibly death. This traveling blood clot is called a thromboembolus. Individuals with a tendency toward clotting are often placed on heparin therapy while they are hospitalized and given oral coumadin therapy for home anticoagulation to prevent the formation of clots. Refer to Chapter 12.

Delta check is a quality assurance check and balance included in some of the computerized hematology instrumentation. Through correlation of more than one test result, release of erroneous test values can be avoided. If a count in the morning is 4000/mm^3 and that same patient has a 12,000/mm^3 (>10% change) count on a later specimen, a delta check would be noted. The laboratory practitioner would address the delta check by repeating the test and by investigating any changes in the patient in order to resolve the discrepancy and ensure accurate results. The most common cause of a laboratory error is clerical error with release of erroneous values, owing to incorrect transcription or lack of correlation, even when a test has been performed correctly.

Deoxyhemoglobin is hemoglobin that is not combined with oxygen. Deoxyhemoglobin is produced in the body tissues when the hemoglobin carrying oxygen (oxyhemoglobin) from the lungs releases that oxygen to the tissues as needed. This deoxyhemoglobin then returns to the lungs to pick up more oxygen. Refer to Chapter 8.

Diamond-Blackfan syndrome is a hereditary inability of the bone marrow to produce hematopoietic cells, resulting in aplastic anemia. Refer to Chapter 9.

Differentiation is the development of undifferentiated parent cells into the functional mature cells. This is evident by the appearance of functional cell organelles such as granules and surface antigens at different stages of development. Direction and speed of differentiation are determined by the protein factors that interact with the pluripotent stem cell (PSC). Refer to Chapter 2.

Disseminated intravascular coagulation (DIC) is a coagulation disorder (coagulopathy) that occurs secondary to another problem within the body. DIC is triggered by destruction of cells, which occurs in cancer and surgery and in association with pregnancy and childbirth (obstetrics). The cell's destruction activates thrombocytes and the coagulation pathways, resulting in small clots at various locations in the body. Tests reveal thrombocytopenia, prolonged coagulation testing due to consumption of the factors in the clots, and the presence of fibrin degradation products (FDPs) from the continuous attempt by the body to dissolve the clots. Treatment involves the administration of intravenous heparin to inhibit clotting, while simultaneously administering fresh frozen plasma (FFP) to replenish the coagulation factors that have all been consumed in the clotting process. The only true treatment is to attempt to eliminate the primary problem, such as by removing the necrotic fetus or the cancer. These individuals are at risk of bleeding to death despite the fact that they are continuously clotting. Refer to Chapter 12.

Documentation and dissemination of laboratory results from the health care provider at the patient "point of care" must always include the date, time, reference values, and any circumstances, or individuals, relevant to the test results. The accurate (factual) and timely (quick) dissemination of valid information is crucial for efficient and cost-effective health care. If the documentation is not valid, it is "fiction" with no relevance to the status of the patient; and if the information is not received within an adequate time frame, the patient is in jeopardy of becoming worse or expiring due to lack of appropriate treatment.

Döhle bodies are patches of rough endoplasmic reticulum (RER) that are made of RNA and are seen in the cytoplasm of the neutrophils in response to a bacterial infection. The neutrophilic response is called a leukemoid reaction, which is characterized by an increase in band cells and mature neutrophils, both of which demonstrate cytoplasmic vacuolation, Döhle bodies, and toxic granulation. Refer to Chapter 3.

Dyserythropoiesis is abnormal or bad formation of erythroid cells in the bone marrow. An example of dyserythropoiesis is the production of large megaloblastic (undergoing asynchronous maturation) erythrocytes due to lack of adequate vitamin B_{12}. Refer to Chapter 9.

Dysplasia is an abnormality of cell development resulting in pathology and alteration in size, shape, and organization of adult cells. Dyserythropoiesis is an example of dysplasia. When cells taken from body tissue, such as in a biopsy, look abnormal but do not yet fit the characteristics of a specific cancer, they are described as dysplastic cells or are said to demonstrate dysplasia.

Ecchymosis is a small hemorrhagic spot (larger than petechia) on the skin or mucous membrane, forming a nonelevated, rounded or irregular, blue or purple patch. This is the result of blood seeping under the skin due to thrombocytopenia (decreased platelets) or a loss of vascular integrity, both of which are common in the geriatric population.

EDTA (ethylenediaminetetraacetic acid) is an anticoagulant found in the purple top vacuum tubes used for phlebotomy. The tube must be at least one-third full of blood and well mixed to prevent clotting. Mixing is done by inverting the filled tube completely six to eight times. Never shake a blood tube, or the blood cells may be damaged. If testing cannot be done immediately, refrigerate the specimen at 4° C until it is needed. If the liquid portion of the blood in the EDTA tube appears dark yellow (icteric), milky (lipemic), or red (hemolyzed), this will interfere with accurate testing and must be corrected for. EDTA is the anticoagulant of choice for cell counting and evaluations because EDTA preserves the cell function and morphology better than do any of the other anticoagulants. If a patient's cells are altered by EDTA, such as is seen in the satellitism phenomenon, sodium citrate (Na citrate) anticoagulant can be used if the blood is tested within a few hours of collection. EDTA chelates the Ca^{2+} ions in the blood, which are necessary for coagulation to occur.

Elderly anemia is anemia of individuals older than 65 years of age. Another term for the elderly is geriatric. As the aging process progresses, the active red bone marrow decreases, thus slowing the hematopoiesis that is occurring. Other factors that may add to the decrease in bone marrow cell production are less production of erythropoietin (EPO) by the kidney, less responsiveness by the bone marrow cells to the stimulation by EPO and other growth factors, and changes in diet and metabolism, which is the source of the vitamins, minerals, and other factors necessary for production of new blood cells. This concept is still in debate. It is possible that all elderly naturally slow down their erythropoiesis due to less need from the body; a mild anemia in an individual older than 65 years of age should not be investigated or treated. However, many believe that any anemia should be investigated and treated. There are currently no established reference values for the geriatric population because there is a question as to whether you can find enough geriatric individuals who are healthy, who take no drugs, and who are not ill in order to establish normal values. Refer to Chapter 9.

Electroimmunodiffusion (EID) is the diffusion of antigens and antibodies accelerated by the application of an electrical current. This is a modification of basic immunodiffusion and is discussed further in Chapter 6.

Electrolyte solution contains ions that are capable of conducting electricity. The electrolytes found in the body are sodium (Na^+), potassium (K^+), chloride (Cl^-), and bicarbonate (HCO_3^-). These ions and the blood pH (7.4) are important for proper functioning of the body, especially the electrical circuitry of the heart. Abnormal body metabolism or respiratory problems that affect the proper levels of these ions will alter the pH, resulting in a metabolic acidosis or alkalosis or a respiratory acidosis or alkalosis.

Electromechanical probe for clot detection is the older and back-up methodology of the fibrometer coagulation instrument. The reaction cup containing the patient's plasma and the reagents is placed under two electromechanical probes. One probe is stationary and the other probe moves back and forth at a steady rate. When the fibrin strands begin to form between the probes, the electrical circuit is complete and the moving probe and the timer stop. The number on the timer registers the seconds that it took for fibrin to form, hence the clotting time. Tests such as the prothrombin time (PT), partial thromboplastin time (PTT), thrombin time (TT), fibrinogen, circulating anticoagulant test (mix), and factor assays can be performed with this instrument. Only two specimens can be tested simultaneously by this instrument. Refer to Chapter 13.

Electronic impedance is the methodology used for some particle counters such as the Coulter instruments. A glass tube with a small hole (aperture) and two electrodes, one on the inside of the tube and one on the outside of the tube, pulls an electrolyte solution through the aperture as the current flows through also. Each particle or cell that passes through the aperture will momentarily increase the resistance (i.e., interrupt) of the electrical flow between the electrodes generating a pulse, which can be counted, measured, and displayed on a screen. The size of the particle passing through the aperture is proportional to the amount of resistance; therefore; the size of the particles or cells can be collected by the instrument. Refer to Chapters 6, 10, and 13.

Electrophoresis is a test methodology used to identify the presence or absence of proteins and, if present, to evaluate the quantity of proteins. Many protein elements in blood can be electrophoresed for identification or quantitation purposes. Examples are hemoglobin electrophoresis and protein electrophoresis; enzymes such as LD (from the breakdown of cells in the heart muscle, skeletal muscle, liver tissue, and erythrocytes) and CK (from heart muscle damage) can also be analyzed by this methodology. Examples of some of the variables that must be changed to separate different components are the media used, the pH, the current, the ionic strength of the solution, the temperature, and the length of time that the electrical current is applied. High-resolution agarose media is currently the best choice. Protein electrophoresis is pertinent to protein (immunoglobulin) terminology. The protein electrophoresis separates the proteins by their ability to move through a medium in which an electrical current is flowing. The proteins are primarily separated by net charge, but size and shape have some effect. Most immunoglobulins migrate in the gamma region of protein electrophoresis; another term for immunoglobulins or antibodies is gammaglobulins. Other regions of migration are the albumin, α_1, α_2, and β regions. Protein electrophoresis is discussed further in Chapter 6. The hemoglobin electrophoresis separates the various hemoglobins for identification and quantification. Hemoglobin electrophoresis is discussed further in Chapter 10. The electrophoresis procedure is done in the chemistry department of the laboratory.

Embden-Meyerhof pathway of glucose metabolism produces 90% of the energy required by the erythrocyte. Adenosine triphosphate (ATP) is produced by a series of enzymatic reactions in the anaerobic (without oxygen) conversion of glucose to lactic acid. This metabolic pathway generates 2,3-diphosphoglycerate (2,3-DPG) for adequate hemoglobin oxygen affinity. The methemoglobin reductase helps to maintain hemoglobin in a functional state, and it provides energy to maintain the membrane flexibility, shape, and sodium-potassium pump mechanism. If there is interference with this glycolytic pathway, the erythrocyte will lyse prematurely. Refer to Chapter 7.

Endosmosis is the inward passage of fluid through a membrane of a cell or cavity.

Endothelial damage is due to trauma, secondary to another disease, decreased mechanical strength, or surface change such as that seen in the formation of atherosclerotic (lipid) plaques. Endothelial damage triggers the thrombocytes and coagulation pathways to initiate clotting. Refer to Chapters 11 and 12.

Enzyme immunoassay (EIA) is used for the detection of antibodies developed in response to infectious agents or, less often, the infectious agents themselves. EIA is well adapted for automation and instrumentation and is one of the most sensitive assays (most accurate results for detection). The use of known antigens and antibodies to detect the corresponding element in the patient's specimen can be done by an indirect or competitive binding protocol. This test is discussed further in Chapter 6. An example of a test using EIA methodology involves antibody titers.

Eosin stain is an acid that stains the basic components of the cells, such as cytoplasmic granules, hemoglobin, and organelles, an orange color. This is one component of the routine Wright-Giemsa (polychrome) stain that is used to examine peripheral blood smears.

Eosinophilic granuloma is one of the original rare histiocytosis X proliferative histiocyte disorders. These diseases demonstrate a "foamy" cell in bone granulomas and are often found in young children, who have a very short survival span.

Epinephrine is an adrenal gland hormone used as a reagent to test platelet aggregation.

Epitope is the configuration at the antigen-binding site of an immunoglobulin or antibody that is specific for one antigenic determinant.

Epstein-Barr virus (EBV) is the causative agent for infectious mononucleosis and Burkitt's lymphoma. Refer to Chapter 5.

Erythrocyte indices are calculations that are correlated with the cell morphologies to aid in the diagnosis of disease. The mean corpuscular volume (MCV) is 80 to 95 fl. The mean corpuscular hemoglobin (MCH) is 26 to 34 g/dl. The mean corpuscular hemoglobin concentration (MCHC) is 32 to 36%. The red cell distribution width (RDW) is 11.5 to 14.5%. Refer to Chapters 9 and 10.

Erythrocytes (red blood cells) are biconcave disk-shaped cells making up approximately 54% of whole blood. These cells originate in the bone marrow from the burst-forming unit–erythroid (BFU-E) as nucleated cells and lose their nucleus when they mature. Their function is to carry oxygen (O_2) from the lungs to the body tissue, maintain functional hemoglobin and cell shape, aid in the maintenance of blood gases (PO_2, PCO_2, H_2CO_3, HCO_3^-), and act as a buffer for the acid-base balance (Cl^-, Na^+, K^+) of the blood to maintain a blood pH of approximately 7.4. The Embden-Meyerhof glycolytic pathway and the hexose monophosphate shunt provide the energy to function properly. Refer to Chapter 7.

Erythroleukemia, acute (FAB M6) (AEL) demonstrates more than 50% erythroid dysplasia in the bone marrow. Megaloblastic normoblasts with diffuse blocks of cytoplasmic glycogen, when stained with periodic acid-Schiff (PAS) stain, will differentiate AEL from polycythemia. Differentiation from myelodysplastic syndrome can be done with monoclonal antibodies and flow cytometry. The old name for this disorder is DiGuglielmo's disease. Refer to Chapter 9.

Erythropoietin (EPO) is a glycoprotein hormone that is produced primarily by the kidney in response to low O_2 in the body. This protein stimulates red blood cell production in the bone marrow. Refer to Chapters 7 to 9.

Essential thrombocythemia (ET) involves uncontrolled megakaryocyte and platelet production. Refer to Chapter 11.

Ethylenediaminetetraacetic acid (EDTA) is an anticoagulant found in the purple-top vacuum tubes used for phlebotomy. The tube must be at least one-third full of blood and well mixed to prevent clotting. Mixing is done by inverting the filled tube completely six to eight times. Never shake a blood tube, or the blood cells may be damaged. If testing cannot be done immediately, refrigerate the specimen at 4° C until it is needed. If the liquid portion of the blood in the EDTA tube appears dark yellow (icteric), milky (lipemic), or red (hemolyzed), this will interfere with accurate testing and must be corrected for. EDTA is the choice anticoagulant for cell counting and evaluations because the EDTA preserves the cell function and morphology better than do any of the other anticoagulants. If a patient's cells are altered by EDTA, such as is seen in the satellitism phenomenon, sodium citrate (Na citrate) anticoagulant can be used if the blood is tested within a few hours of collection. EDTA chelates the Ca^{2+} ions in the blood plasma, which are necessary for coagulation to take place.

Etiology is the study of the cause of disease, and the term is used interchangeably with "cause of the disease."

Euchromatin is the light, loose, active chromatin with nucleoli that indicates the cell is engaged in mitosis and transition. The cytoplasm will be rich with RNA (blue) if a lot of protein synthesis is occurring. Euchromatin and dark blue cytoplasm are characteristic of reactive lymphocytes and immature cells.

Extramedullary hematopoiesis refers to blood cell production outside of the bone marrow. Within the mesenchyme (cells of the mesodermic developmental layer) of the embryonic yolk sac, in the fetal liver, and after birth production of lymphocytes in the lymph system—all are considered to involve extramedullary hematopoiesis.

Extravascular hemolysis occurs when antibodies or other immune proteins bind to erythrocytic cells (opsonization), which marks them for destruction by the phagocytic cells (macrophages) of the body. The direct antiglobulin test (DAT) is a diagnostic test performed in the blood bank or immunohematology area of the laboratory. When the macrophage digests the opsonized erythrocyte, one product is yellow bilirubin, which is detoxified by the liver and excreted in the urine and feces. An example of a cause for extravascular hemolysis is autoimmune hemolytic anemia (AIHA). Refer to Chapter 9.

Extrinsic coagulation pathway is initiated by tissue factor III, which then activates coagulation factor VII, which is most sensitive to anticoagulation therapy with coumadin. The test for the extrinsic coagulation pathway and Coumadin therapy is the prothrombin time (PT) test. Refer to Chapter 12 and Figure 12–12D.

Exudates are one type of abnormal fluid accumulation in the body due to inflammation associated with infection or malignancy. An exudate has a higher specific gravity (>1.015) than does a transudate, a total protein of more then 3 g/dl, a leukocyte count of more than $1.0 \times 10^9/l$ with increased neutrophils, and an erythrocyte count of more than $100 \times 10^9/l$, especially with a malignancy. Exudates appear cloudy and may be bloody and clotted. Refer to Chapters 14 and 15.

FAB classification of acute leukemias was established by the French, American, and British (FAB) cooperative hematology group to standardize the diagnosis and treatment of acute leukemias. Due to the similarities of many of the cells in acute leukemia, it is difficult to accurately and consistently diagnose, treat, and share clinical and research information. The FAB classification of acute leukemias appears in Table 3–1.

Fabry's disease is a lipid storage disease caused by a genetic lack of ceramide trihihexosedase or α-galactosidase enzymes that are necessary for lipid catabolism.

Fanconi's anemia is a hereditary inability of the bone marrow to produce blood cells, resulting in aplastic anemia.

Ferritin is the iron-apoferritin complex, which is one of the storage forms of iron in the body. Apoferritin is the protein without the iron molecule. The serum ferritin level is the best indicator of the body's iron stores to diagnose disorders such as iron deficiency anemia. The reference range for serum ferritin is 20 to 200 ng/ml. Refer to Chapters 7 to 10.

Fibrin is an insoluble protein that holds the blood clot together. Fibrin is produced from plasma fibrinogen by the action of thrombin. Refer to Chapter 12.

Fibrinogen is coagulation factor I of the common coagulation pathway. The fibrinogen protein is a substrate for thrombin, which converts the soluble plasma fibrinogen to insoluble fibrin to complete the coagulation pathways and form a blood clot. The normal fibrinogen level of plasma is 200 to 400 mg/dl. Refer to Chapters 12 and 13.

Fibrinolysis testing requires a special anticoagulant containing thrombin with soy bean trypsin inhibitor (light blue–top tube) for the fibrin degradation products (FDP), also called fibrin split products (FSP) or the D-dimer test. Additional tests used to assess fibrinolytic activity are the euglobulin clot lysis test and observation of the clot retraction over 24 hours. Refer to Chapters 12 and 13.

Fibrinolytic pathway is activated by the initiation of clotting to dissolve the clot when it is no longer needed and also to degrade fibrinogen to prevent excessive clotting from occurring. The plasma protein plasminogen is acted upon by plasminogen activators such as tissue plasminogen activator (tPA), urokinase, and streptokinase to form plasmin. Plasmin is responsible for degrading both fibrinogen and fibrin. Refer to Chapters 12 and 13.

Flow cytometry is used to evaluate cell membrane markers, nuclear chromatin, and cytoplasmic components. Monoclonal antibodies with a fluorescent marker are incubated with the patient's cells, and if the corresponding membrane protein is present, the antibody will bind and the fluorescence will be detected as the cells go through the flow cytometer. This technique is used to identify leukemic cells, cancer cells, and CD4 and CD8 lymphocytes in order to assess immune abnormalities such as AIDS. Cell membrane proteins are the most commonly used definitive markers to identify cells. The flow cytometer has also been adapted to assess platelet aggregation and factor release. Some flow cytometers are more specifically called fluorescence-activated cell sorters (FACS). See Figure 6–17.

Fluorescence-activated cell sorter (FACS) is another name for a flow cytometer. Cells of interest are marked with fluorescent monoclonal antibodies, and the flow cytometer will then recognize these cells and sort them as programmed. This allows the collection of specific cells for research or clinical purposes. See Figure 6–17.

Folate is a coenzyme that promotes one-carbon transfer and is present in natural foods. The reference range for folate is 6 to 21 μg/l. Erythrocyte folate concentrations are 166 to 640 μg/l. Folic acid is a vitamin of the B group that is involved in the synthesis of amino acids and DNA. A folic acid deficiency is seen most often in pregnant women and in the elderly. Folic acid deficiency has the same presentation as vitamin B_{12} deficiency. The erythrocytes are megaloblastic and macrocytic. Refer to Chapter 9.

Free erythrocyte protoporphyrin (FEP) is protoporphyrin without iron and is, therefore, not incorporated into the hemoglobin molecule. The FEP level is the most sensitive early indicator of iron deficiency anemia. FEP is also elevated in chronic disease and lead poisoning. Reference values vary depending on the laboratory and the method, but a typical range is 15 to 18 μg/l of erythrocytes. The FEP is discussed more in Chapters 8 to 10.

Free plasma or urine hemoglobin is hemoglobin that is outside of the erythrocyte but is still intact as a molecule. It gives the plasma or urine a red color. This free hemoglobin molecule binds to carrier molecules such as haptoglobin in order to reach a macrophage for recycling of components in lieu of loss through the kidneys.

Fresh frozen plasma (FFP) is prepared from the plasma drawn off of a unit of whole blood immediately after collection. The plasma is frozen within 6 hours and kept at $-20°$ C until it is needed. The unit of FFP is then thawed at 37° C for 30 minutes before administration. FFP contains the coagulation proteins as well as other essential plasma proteins and is used to replenish the coagulation factors for hemostatic defects, such as disseminated intravascular coagulation (DIC) and to maintain fluid in burn patients.

Gaucher's disease is the most common of the lipid storage diseases and is caused by a genetic lack of β-glucocerebrosidase enzyme necessary for lipid catabolism. Gaucher's cells, with a fibrillar cytoplasm, can be found in the bone marrow and spleen for diagnosis. The build-up of lipids in the cells of the body is detrimental and may be fatal. Refer to Chapter 4.

Genetic abnormality (anomaly) of the leukocytes. The anomalies are characterized by a change in morphology that may or may not affect the function of the cell. In leukocytes, for example, Alder-Reilly anomaly has azurophilic cytoplasmic inclusions; Chédiak-Higashi anomaly has prominent lysosomal granules in the cytoplasm; May-Hegglin anomaly has blue patches (Döhle bodies) in the cell's cytoplasm; and Pelger-Huët anomaly has neutrophils that do not segment beyond two lobes. Refer to Chapter 3.

Genetic alteration occurs when normal genes with cancerous potential (proto-oncogenes) are transformed to malignant genes (oncogenes), or when a gene whose protein product normally suppresses cancer is inactivated. An example of a specific genetic alteration associated with disease is the transposition of chromosome 9 to 22, called the Philadelphia chromosome (Ph'), seen in patients with chronic myelogenous leukemia (CML). Refer to Chapter 3.

Geriatric anemia (anemia of aging) is found in individuals who are older than 65 years of age. As the aging process progresses, the active red bone marrow decreases and the process of hematopoiesis is slowed down. Other factors that may add to the decrease in bone marrow cell production are less production of erythropoietin (EPO) by the kidney, less responsiveness by the bone marrow cells to the stimulation by EPO and other growth factors, and changes in diet and metabolism, which is the source of the vitamins, minerals, and other factors necessary for production of new blood cells. This concept is still in debate. It is possible that all elderly naturally slow down their erythropoiesis due to less need from the body; therefore, mild anemia in an individual older than 65 years of age should not be investigated or treated. However, many believe that any anemia should be investigated and treated. There are currently no established reference values for the geriatric population because there is a question as to whether you can find enough healthy geriatric individuals who do not take drugs and who have no illnesses to establish normal values. This is not the same as the anemia of chronic disease that is often seen in the elderly. Refer to Chapter 9.

Gloves are a safety option that should be worn at all times as part of the personal protective equipment (PPE) used in the clinical laboratory and when collecting specimens. These should be changed often, and you should never touch a "clean" area or piece of equipment until the gloves have been removed and the hands have been washed. This procedure is to protect you as well as the patient against contamination and infection.

Glucose-6-phosphate dehydrogenase (G-6-PD) deficiency anemia is due to a genetic lack of G-6-PD, which is a significant enzyme in the hexose monophosphate shunt (HMS) of aerobic glycolysis in the erythrocyte. G-6-PD is responsible for reducing glutathione (GSH), which in turn maintains the hemoglobin iron in the reduced and functional ferrous state (Fe^{2+}). Due to various oxidative reactions in the blood, the hemoglobin is oxidized to the ferric (Fe^{3+}) state, which is not capable of carrying oxygen. The erythrocytes are normochromic and normocytic, and with use of a special stain, Heinz bodies, inclusions of denatured hemoglobin, are visible. The Heinz bodies mark the cells for early destruction, thus decreasing the number of erythrocytes available. Refer to Chapters 7 and 10.

Gower 2 and 1 hemoglobins are early hemoglobins produced in the fetus. Refer to Chapter 8.

Gram's stain is done to detect bacterial or fungal organisms on slides of body specimens. The organisms retaining the dark blue stain are gram-positive. The organisms decolorized by alcohol following the Gram's stain are then stained with an orange safranin counterstain and are described as gram-negative. The gram-negative organisms have a more complex cell wall composition than do the gram-positive organisms. This is a preliminary screen of the specimen prior to culturing for the purpose of isolating and definitively identifying any microorganism present. Throughout the culture and identification process, a series of Gram's stains is done to ensure the presence of the same microorganism and to contribute to the identification.

Granulopoiesis is the production of granulocytes. This involves the production of mature granulocytic cells from the CFU-G, CFU-EO, and CFU-BA (all of which are also called myeloblasts) in the bone marrow, which differentiates into the promyelocyte, then the myelocyte, then the metamyelocyte, and then the band cell before becoming the mature neutrophil, eosinophil, or basophil. Refer to Chapter 3.

Gray platelet syndrome or thrombocyte storage pool disease is a rare disease characterized by defective secondary aggregation due to the lack of granules and their contents. Refer to Chapter 11.

Growth factors include colony-stimulating factors (CSFs) and interleukins (ILs). The CSFs are preceded by a cell line designation such as G-CSF for granulocyte growth factors or M-CSF for monocyte growth factors. The ILs are followed by a number that is the order in which they were characterized and has become associated with their function. These proteins are produced by various cells of the body that stimulate and influence the development of the hematopoietic cells. Examples are proteins such as stem cell factor (SCF, also known as *kit* ligand and the Steel factor), which is essential for normal bone marrow hematopoiesis, interleukin-1 (IL-1) to enhance monocyte phagocytosis, and interleukin-3 (IL-3), which is a hematopoietic growth factor.

HAV is hepatitis A virus that is transmitted by the fecal-oral route (poor sanitation and hygiene) and is most common in contaminated food. The incubation time for HAV is 15 to 45 days after exposure, and elevated liver enzymes (aspartate aminotransferase [AST] and lactate dehydrogenase [LD]) precede symptoms. There is no chronic carrier state. Refer to Chapter 5.

HBV is hepatitis B virus, which causes serum hepatitis. HBV is transmitted by body fluids through sexual contact or parenterally (e.g., needles used for drugs). Liver enzymes (aspartate aminotransferase [AST] and lactate dehydrogenase [LD]) are elevated, and jaundice may be evident. Chronic carriers will harbor this virus for a lifetime with a higher risk of liver cancer (hepatocarcinoma). Refer to Chapter 5.

HCV is hepatitis C virus, which produces a serum hepatitis. HCV was previously called non-A, non-B hepatitis and has similar characteristics to HBV. HCV is transmitted by body fluids through sexual contact or parenterally (e.g., needles used for drugs). Liver enzymes are elevated (aspartate aminotransferase [AST] and lactate dehydrogenase [LD]), and jaundice may be evident. Chronic carriers will harbor this virus for a lifetime with a higher risk of liver cancer (hepatocarcinoma). Refer to Chapter 5.

Hairy cell leukemia (HCL) is a rare disease involving a B cell subtype, with the characteristic lymphocytes demonstrating hair-like projections off the cytoplasm, hence the name. HCL is seen in individuals older than 50 years of age. Symptoms include splenomegaly (enlarged spleen). The development of this disease has been associated with irradiation and the human T-cell lymphotrophic virus-II (HTLV-II). These malignant cells are confirmed by the tartrate-resistant acid phosphatase (TRAP) cytochemical stain. Refer to Chapter 5.

Ham's test (acidified serum test) is used to aid in the diagnosis of paroxysmal nocturnal hemoglobinuria (PNH), a hemolytic anemia presented in Chapter 9. This test is presented in more detail in Chapter 10.

Hand-Schüller-Christian syndrome is one of the original histiocytosis X proliferative histiocyte disorders. These diseases demonstrate "foamy" cell bone granulomas and are often found in young children, who have a very short survival. Refer to Chapter 4.

Haptoglobin is a carrier protein in the plasma that binds with free plasma hemoglobin released from erythrocytes in the blood stream due to intravascular hemolysis. If the free hemoglobin level exceeds the ability of plasma protein binding, it will be lost through the kidney to the urine, where free hemoglobin can be detected. Haptoglobin carries the hemoglobin to the macrophages for processing and recycling of the components to produce new erythrocytes in the bone marrow. Haptoglobin levels measure the protein that is not bound to free hemoglobin; thus the test results are inversely proportional to the amount of free hemoglobin. If there is an increase in free hemoglobin, there will be a decrease in haptoglobin available to measure. Note that haptoglobin will be increased in inflammatory disease. Refer to Chapter 8.

Hashimoto-Pritzker syndrome was originally one of the histiocytosis X proliferative histiocyte disorders. These diseases demonstrate a "foamy" cell in bone granulomas and are often found in young children, who have a very short survival. Refer to Chapter 4.

Health care providers include physicians, physician assistants, nurse practitioners, pharmacists, laboratorians, and nurses as well as any other persons involved in patient care. The health care providers must work closely together for the good of the patient and the practice of medicine. Efficiency and quality of health care would increase and costs would decrease. The health care provider who takes direct care of the patient is called the primary care provider. Refer to Chapter 16.

Hematocrit determinations provide information relative to the percentage of red blood cells in whole blood. These determinations are calculated by the automated instruments from the erythrocyte number and cell size. Manual testing involves centrifugation of a sample of whole blood, which is then measured for the percentage of erythrocytes. Hematocrits are reported as a percentage or a decimal in liters/liter (l/l) (i.e., 36% or 0.36 l/l). The automated instruments in use today do not use centrifugation. These instruments count the cells and measure their size, which allows the calculation of the hematocrit. The average adult body contains approximately 6 liters (6.36 quarts) of blood. This life-giving fluid is made up of approximately 45% formed elements (red blood cells, white blood cells, and platelets) and 55% plasma. The plasma consists of 90% water and 10% of various proteins, vitamins, nutrients, ions, and solutes. The hematocrit is correlated with the hemoglobin value, which should be one third of the hematocrit value. Refer to Chapters 1, 2, and 10.

Hematology is literally the study of blood, but more specifically it involves the determination of the number of formed elements, the correct morphology and function of the formed elements, the amount of coagulation proteins, and the correct function of coagulation proteins. Hematologic disease is due to: (1) not enough of a formed element or coagulation protein; (2) too much of a formed element; or (3) adequate amount of the formed element or coagulation protein but with abnormal function.

Hematoma is a blood tumor formed from the collection of clotted blood beneath the skin.

Hematopoiesis is the production of blood cells. This process occurs primarily in the bone marrow, which is called medullary hematopoiesis as opposed to production of blood cells outside of the bone marrow (e.g., production of lympho-

cytes in the lymph system and fetal hematopoiesis in the liver). Hematopoiesis outside of the bone marrow is called extramedullary hematopoiesis. Refer to Chapter 2.

Hematopoietic stem cell (HSC) is the first cell in the bone marrow that is committed to become a blood cell. This early hematopoietic progenitor cell has the potential to become any of the blood cells. The protein factors (cytokines) influence the pluripotent stem cell to become the HSC and then direct this cell to become the specific cell that is needed by the body. Refer to Chapter 2.

Hemochromatosis is a disorder of iron metabolism with excess deposition of iron in the tissues. This deposit of iron in the skin, liver, and other organs of the body results in a brown skin pigmentation, hepatic (liver) cirrhosis, and other illnesses. Treatment includes administration of drugs that chelate (bind) iron. The removal of a unit of blood periodically may also help to remove some of the iron.

Hemocytometer is an instrument used for manual counting of blood cells or any particles that cannot be accurately counted by automated instrumentation. This device is a thick glass slide with engraved measurements on the surface to allow cells or particles of any kind, suspended in a solution and placed on the hemocytometer, to be counted through a light microscope. This instrument is commonly used for counting cells in body fluids such as cerebrospinal fluid. Refer to Chapters 1 and 6.

Hemoglobin (Hb) is the oxygen transport protein within the erythrocyte that gives the blood its red color. Hb binds to O_2 in the lungs, carries it to the body tissues, and releases the O_2 to areas of the body that are deficient in oxygen. If adequate hemoglobin is not produced (iron deficiency), abnormal hemoglobin is produced (sickle cell hemoglobin), or erythrocytes are lost (hemorrhage), not enough oxygen will reach the body tissues and anemia will develop and can be life threatening. Adult hemoglobin is 96 to 98% Hb A (also referred to as Hb A_1), 0.5 to 0.8% Hb F, and 1.5 to 3.2% Hb A_2. Hb A_{1c} is the best test for monitoring a diabetic. Refer to Chapter 8.

Hb A (Hb A_1) is the major adult hemoglobin in the erythrocytes. The reference range for Hb A is 96 to 98%, and Hb A_2 and F make up the other 2 to 4%. There are subgroups of Hb A_1 designated Hb A_{1a}, Hb A_{1b}, and Hb A_{1c}. HbA_{1c} is glycosylated (contains sugars) and is the most sensitive to glucose levels in the body. For this reason Hb A_{1c} is the best test to monitor diabetic patients. A serum glucose determination is subject to the patient's recent diet, exercise, and fluid intake. The glycosylated Hb reflects an average level of glucose in the body over several days. This is a special test that is usually performed in the chemistry department. Refer to Chapter 8.

Hb A_{1c} monitoring of a diabetic is the most

sensitive test for glucose levels in the body. For this reason Hb A_{1c} is the best test to monitor diabetic patients. Hb A_{1c} is glycosylated (contains sugars) and reflects the body's glucose metabolism. A serum glucose determination is subject to the patient's recent diet, exercise, and fluid intake. The glycosylated Hb reflects an average level of glucose in the body over several days. This is a special test that is usually performed in the chemistry department. Refer to Chapter 8.

Hb A_2 or hemoglobin A_2 is a minor component of adult Hb. The normal reference range is 1.5 to 3.2% of adult hemoglobin. An elevation in Hb A_2 is associated with an anemia called thalassemia. Refer to Chapters 8 and 9.

Heinz bodies are erythrocyte inclusions of denatured hemoglobin that are only visible when stained with a special stain. The erythrocytes appear normochromic and normocytic, and anemia is present. The enzyme glucose-6-phosphate dehydrogenase (G-6-PD) is essential for the function of Hb. Individuals with a genetic G-6-PD deficiency are unable to maintain their Hb iron in the reduced state (Fe^{2+}) once it is oxidized (Fe^{3+}) by normal body metabolism. The individual has oxidized iron incapable of carrying oxygen and unstable hemoglobin forming Heinz bodies, which mark the cells for early destruction, thus decreasing the number of erythrocytes available. Refer to Chapters 7 to 10.

Hemoglobin C (Hb C) is an abnormal Hb that becomes insoluble in the erythrocytes and forms dark red crystals that distort the erythrocyte morphology. Refer to Chapters 8 and 9.

Hemoglobin electrophoresis is a test methodology used to identify the presence or absence of specific hemoglobins and, if present, to evaluate the quantity. The net charge of each hemoglobin determines how far it will migrate from the point of application. Of the adult hemoglobins A_2 is the slowest, followed by F; and A is the fastest. These hemoglobins are easily seen as bands of protein in the media. There are two types of hemoglobin electrophoresis—the acetate media method at a pH of 8.6 and the agarose gel method that requires a lower pH of 6.0. The hemoglobins migrate differently in the agarose at the lower pH, which may clear up a question by separating two hemoglobins that migrated together in the acetate procedure. This methodology is used to confirm the presence of any abnormal hemoglobin. Refer to Chapter 10.

Hemoglobin F (Hb F) is the primary fetal Hb, and a small percentage (0.5 to 0.8% Hb F) continues to be produced as part of the adult Hb. If an adult persistence of hemoglobin F occurs, anemia develops. Hb F has a higher O_2 affinity than does Hb A and will not release the O_2 to the body tissues, which results in anoxia, or lack of oxygen. Hb F is identified and quantitated by hemoglobin electrophoresis in the adult. If hemolytic disease of the newborn is suspected in a pregnant woman, the quantity of Hb F in fetal red blood cells that have mistakenly entered the mother's blood stream must be determined. This is too small an amount to quantitate by Hb electrophoresis. Tests to measure fetal-maternal bleeding are agglutination tests, acid elution tests, and alkali denaturization tests. These tests are performed in the blood bank or immunohematology area of the laboratory. Refer to Chapters 8 to 10.

Hemoglobinopathies are genetic abnormal hemoglobin disorders such as sickle cell anemia and thalassemia. The abnormal hemoglobins are suspected if an individual has a normocytic, normochromic anemia with the presence of occasional target cells. Some hemoglobinopathies have screening tests, such as the sickle cell screening test, but confirmation is done by hemoglobin electrophoresis. Refer to Chapters 9 and 10.

Hemolysis is the destruction of erythrocytes, resulting in free hemoglobin or bilirubin in the blood plasma and possibly also in the urine.

Hemolytic anemias are the result of destruction (lysis) of the erythrocytes after their release from the bone marrow. This hemolysis can occur due to change in shape, inclusions, or antibodies, or complement attached to the cell membrane. The cells can lyse within the blood stream, which is a process called intravascular hemolysis, or outside the blood stream in the macrophage cells of the body, which is a process called extravascular hemolysis. This is discussed further in Chapter 9.

Hemolytic disease of the newborn (HDN) develops when the mother produces antibodies (has an immune response) to the fetal erythrocyte antigens. Any time antibodies are produced, the cell or substance that they bind to is marked for destruction by the phagocytic cells of the body; thus, in the case of erythrocytes, anemia develops. Normally the fetal blood and maternal blood never make contact with each other. All nutrients, waste products, and so forth are passed through membranes between the mother and the fetus. Occasionally blood vessels are broken and bleeding occurs during pregnancy or at birth, and the baby's blood enters the mother's circulatory system. If hemolytic disease of the newborn is suspected, the physician needs to know how much of the fetal blood is in the mother; a prophylactic treatment of immunoglobulin can be administered to the mother. Refer to Chapters 9 and 10.

Hemorrhage is blood loss from the blood vessels, often resulting in anemia if the loss of erythrocytes is great enough.

Hemosiderin is an insoluble form of storage iron in the tissues that is visible microscopically with or without iron stain. Refer to Chapters 8 to 10.

Hemostasis is the arrest of bleeding out of the vasculature through vasoconstriction, thrombocyte initiation of the clot, and formation of a fibrin clot. Included in the practical application of hemostasis is the need to limit blood clotting and dissolve the formed clots in order to achieve a hemostatic balance. There are naturally occurring inhibitors of clotting (e.g., antithrombin III), and the fibrinolytic system is activated when clotting occurs to aid in limiting the clotting and dissolving the formed clot when the area has healed. This is not to be confused with homeostasis, which is the physiologic balance of the entire body of which hemostasis is one aspect. Refer to Chapters 11 to 13.

Heparin is an acidic mucopolysaccharide that is present in many body tissues. Heparin is used as an anticoagulant and is found in the green-stoppered vacuum tube of blood collection; it is also administered to patients suffering from coagulation disorders (coagulopathies). Heparin inhibits platelet aggregation and platelet factor release and is an antithrombin that binds in the body with antithrombin III (ATIII) to neutralize thrombin and inhibit the activation of prothrombin. The mechanism of anticoagulation for heparin takes place in the blood stream, directly affecting the coagulation factors; thus this drug is given intravenously. Heparin monitoring is best done by use of the partial thromboplastin time (PTT) test for evaluation of the intrinsic system. The reference range for the PTT is approximately 11 to 13 seconds. Important information necessary for proper collection of the PTT blood specimen and interpretation of results includes the time of administration and the mode of administration. If problems develop in testing, it may be necessary to also know the lot number and company that is supplying the heparin. Heparin activity varies from one company to the next and from one lot number to the next. Refer to Chapters 12 and 13.

Hepatitis is literally inflammation of the liver caused by alcohol and other toxic drugs, viral infection, or heat damage. The liver enzymes (aspartate aminotransferase [AST] and lactate dehydrogenase [LD]) will be elevated, and the individual may appear jaundiced (yellow). Several viruses are associated with hepatitis. The most common viruses are hepatitis A virus (HAV), hepatitis B virus (HBV), and hepatitis C virus (HCV). Hepatitis can be fatal. Refer to Chapter 5.

Heterochromatin is the tightly coiled, dark staining, and inactive chromatin seen in most mature cells, such as in the segmented neutrophil.

Hexose monophosphate shunt (HMPS) is the aerobic glycolytic pathway present in the mature erythrocyte. This pathway provides 10% of the cell's energy and is the major mechanism for maintaining hemoglobin iron in the ferrous (Fe^{2+}) state, which is capable of transporting oxygen. The glucose-6-phosphate dehydrogenase enzyme reduces glutathione (GSH), which in turn reduces the oxidized ferric (Fe^{3+}) back to the functional ferrous state. Refer to Chapters 7 to 10.

High-resolution agarose electrophoresis is a modification of the protein electrophoresis using agarose as the media instead of acetate.

Histiocytes are the bone marrow macrophage cells, which are also called antigen-presenting cells (APCs). The macrophage cells are not only the most efficient phagocytes of the body defense system, but they also have the ability to process and present antigen to the CD4 lymphocyte for an efficient and effective initiation of a primary immune response. In addition to the two functions stated earlier, the body's macrophages also store iron (Fe) for use within the body as needed. This is especially important in the bone marrow, where iron is critical for the production of hemoglobin. Refer to Chapter 4.

Histiocytosis X was labeled as such due to a lack of knowledge of the proliferative histiocyte disorders. The more recent classifications are: Langerhans cell histiocytosis, Hand-Schüller-Christian syndrome, Letterer-Siwe disease, eosinophilic granuloma, Hashimoto-Pritzker syndrome, self-healing histiocytosis, and pure cutaneous histiocytosis. These diseases demonstrate a "foamy" cell in bone granulomas and are often found in young children, who have a very short survival. Refer to Chapter 4.

Histograms are graphs produced by the automated cell counting instruments for leukocytes, erythrocytes, and platelets by plotting numbers on the x axis and size on the y axis. This depicts an alteration in cell number and size and indicates the abnormal specimen to be examined, thus eliminating the need to view each specimen manually. Refer to Chapters 6, 10, and 13 for examples.

Hodgkin's lymphoma is a malignant proliferation of cells in the lymph system that are most often seen in the 15 to 35 age group. The diagnostic cell is the Reed-Sternberg cell in the lymph node biopsy. This cell is large and multilobed (see Fig. 5–15). Peripheral blood specimens show normal leukocytes and a normocytic, normochromic anemia. The leukocyte count is variable and may range from a reduced to an increased number. Refer to Chapter 5.

Homeostasis is the tendency of an organism such as the human body to maintain stability in the normal body physiology. This is done by maintaining the structures, the temperatures, and all the elements within the body to achieve a healthy balance of life. All aspects of clinical laboratory science involve evaluating and measuring this balance.

Hormones are chemical substances that are produced in the body and have a specific regulatory effect on the activity of certain cells or on a certain organ or organs. An example is erythropoietin (EPO), which is produced in the kidneys in response to low oxygen in the body and stimulates the bone marrow to produce and release more erythrocytes into the blood stream.

Humoral immunity (HI) occurs when B lymphocytes and plasma cells are stimulated to produce immunoglobulins (antibodies). This terminology is derived from the original designation of proteins that protect against disease as "humors." Refer to Chapter 5.

Hydrogen peroxide is a bactericidal product of neutrophilic granulocyte phagocytosis and digestion. Following digestion, the neutrophil undergoes destruction and dies. Refer to Chapter 3.

Hypergammaglobulinemia involves increased gammaglobulins in the blood. This excess of proteins, which is often seen in the geriatric patient and in individuals with autoimmune disorders, interferes with thrombocyte adhesion, aggregation, and release of factors. Excessive production of one protein inhibits the production of others, so that normal, healthy immune responses are not possible and infections are easily established. Refer to Chapter 5.

Hypersegmented neutrophil is a neutrophil with more than five lobes, indicating a nuclear maturation abnormality such as that seen with vitamin B_{12} deficiency. This is also called a "shift to the right," indicating that older cells are not leaving the blood stream as soon as expected. Refer to Chapter 3.

Hypersensitivity reactions such as the type I seen with allergies, hay fever, and bronchial asthma are due to cytokine mediators released from basophils following stimulation by IgE antibody. This action in turn activates eosinophils to release their granule contents. Refer to Chapter 3.

Hypertonic refers to solutions that contain less water and more solute. The cells in this solution will lose water through the membrane into the diluent (osmosis), resulting in a shriveling effect called crenation. Any alteration of the cells in vitro (out of the body) will interfere with accurate testing and interpretation of test results.

Hypochromic literally means very little, or less, color. This term refers to erythrocytes that stain red with the Wright-Giemsa stain. The amount of color in the erythrocytes is directly related to the amount of hemoglobin in the cell. A hypochromic erythrocyte would be very pale and would be expected to contain less hemoglobin.

Hypoplastic anemia is a decreased production of bone marrow cells due to the lack of a component or the presence of an inhibitor. Refer to Chapter 9.

Hyposegmented neutrophil is a neutrophil with fewer than three lobes, indicating a less mature cell that is called a band cell. The presence of immature cells is described as a "shift to the left" towards immaturity. This is seen in severe bacterial infections when the bone marrow is releasing neutrophils early to meet the needs of the body to fight the infection. The Pelger-Huët leukocyte anomaly is a genetic hyposegmentation of the neutrophils that mimics the band cell. Refer to Chapter 3.

Hypotonic refers to a solution that contains more water and less solute. Water will pass into the cell and will try to equalize or dilute the concentration within the cell to equal the exterior environment. This action will cause the cell to become swollen (spherocytic) and burst.

Hypoxia is the condition of decreased oxygen in the body's tissues despite an adequate blood supply to the tissues. This condition will stimulate the increased production of erythropoietin (EPO) by the kidney, which in turn will stimulate the bone marrow to produce more erythrocytes and to release any erythrocytes stored.

Icterus is another name for yellow jaundice due to an increased level of bilirubin in the blood. Bilirubin is a breakdown product of hemoglobin, and the liver is responsible for detoxifying the bilirubin. Kernicterus is a high level of bilirubin that results in severe neural symptoms. This condition occurs primarily in newborns who are unable to detoxify and eliminate the bilirubin due to underdeveloped liver enzymes. In the adult, icterus is due to excessive breakdown of erythrocytes or liver damage.

Idiopathic thrombocytopenic purpura (ITP) was called idiopathic when the cause was unknown. We now know that the thrombocytes are opsonized by autoimmune antibodies (a chronic problem) or antibodies directed against viral antigen that cross-react with the platelet antigens (a transient condition following viral infection). No clots are formed; the thrombocytes are decreased due to phagocytosis by the macrophages. Refer to Chapter 11.

Immunoassay is a test methodology used to identify the presence or absence of proteins, such as antigens or antibodies, as well as quantitation of the proteins present. Immunoassays are performed in the chemistry department and involve a radioactive (radioimmunodiffusion [RIA]) or chromogenic enzymatic (enzyme immunoassay [EIA]) indicator for detection of the antigen or antibody of interest.

Immunodiffusion is a test methodology used to identify the presence or absence of proteins, such as antigens and antibodies, as well as to quantitate the proteins present. The indicator here is the visible precipitation observed if the corresponding antigen and antibody are present in acceptable concentrations. If the diffusion occurs in a circle (radially), this is called radial immunodiffusion (RID) and the diameter of the circle can be compared with standards to determine the concentration.

Immunoelectrophoresis (IEP) is a modification of immunodiffusion by first electrophoresing the serum proteins through a gel medium and then allowing the antibody (known reagent) to diffuse into the media and precipitate with the corresponding antigen (patient's serum is unknown) that has been electrophoresed. Refer to Chapter 6.

Immunogen, also called an antigen, is a protein on the surface of a foreign substance that stimulates an immune response and that will react with the products (antibodies) of that immune response.

Immunoglobulin (Ig), also called antibody (Ab), is protein produced by B lymphocytes and plasma cells in response to a specific immunogen or antigen. This process is called humoral immunity (HI). The Ig structure is four polypeptide chains held together by disulfide bonds. There are two heavy chains, which determine the class of Ig, and two light chains, which consist of only one of two types, kappa or lambda, combined with the antigen (immunogen)-binding end of the heavy chain to produce a configuration unique to the antigen that the antibody was produced against. This configuration is specific for one antigenic determinant called an epitope. There are five classes of Ig, each demonstrating a variety of characteristics and functions. The classes are IgA for alpha heavy chain; IgG for gamma heavy chain; IgM for mu heavy chain; IgD for delta heavy chain; and IgE for epsilon heavy chain. The class provides the basic size and characteristics, but each antibody produced is unique for one antigen only; therefore, within each class there are many different immunoglobulins.

Immunoglobulin alpha (IgA) is the second most abundant class of antibody in the serum; however, IgA is mostly found in the body fluids as a first line of defense against invasions of the body. The endothelial cells add the secretory unit to the IgA molecule to allow it to be secreted with the body fluids. IgA often exists as a dimer, which is two molecules connected by a J chain. Plasma concentrations of IgA are 6% or 0.4 to 2.2 mg/ml. The structure of IgA is two heavy alpha chains bound by disulfide (—S—S—) bonds to two light polypeptide chains.

Immunoglobulin delta (IgD) is in very low concentration in human plasma (1% or 0.03 mg/ml), and its function is not clear. The structure is two delta heavy polypeptide chains bound by disulfide bonds (—S—S—) to two light polypeptide chains.

Immunoglobulin E (IgE) is associated with hypersensitivity reaction such as allergies and is responsible for the degranulation of basophils and mast cells. IgE makes up only 0.002% or 17 to 450 ng/ml of plasma immunoglobulin. The structure of IgE is two epsilon heavy polypeptide chains bound by disulfide bonds (—S—S—) to two light polypeptide chains.

Immunoglobulin G (IgG) is the most abundant in the human blood plasma (80%, 8 to 16 mg/ml) and is also the most important antibody for fighting off infection. IgG exists as a monomer or as a single unit molecule consisting of two heavy gamma polypeptide chains bound by disulfide (—S—S—) bonds to two light polypeptide chains. There are four subclasses of IgG with slightly different characteristics. IgG$_4$ is the only one that binds and partially activates (to the C3 component) the plasma protein complement. This partial activation of complement results in opsonization of the cell carrying the corresponding immunogen, which will mark it for extravascular hemolysis by macrophages in the body. IgG also has the ability to bind with receptors on the placental cells, allowing it to pass into the fetus. This is advantageous for fighting infection in the fetus but may be detrimental if the antibodies involved are a result of hemolytic disease of the newborn (HDN) in which the IgG antibodies that can pass into the fetus are directed against the fetal cells and result in their destruction. IgG functions well at body temperature (37° C) and may be less reactive if testing is performed at or below room temperature (25° C).

Immunoglobulin M (IgM) is the second most important for immune defense and the third highest level in human plasma (13%, 1.2 to 4 mg/ml). IgM exists as a pentamer that consists of five single molecules (monomers) attached together by a J chain. This makes a large molecule; therefore, IgM is described as a macroglobulin. One characteristic of IgM is its ability to readily bind and activate a plasma protein (complement) responsible for cell lysis, thus causing hemolysis of erythrocytes carrying the corresponding immunogen on the cell surface. The large size of the IgM allows it to bind immunogen particles together easily in the absence of complement to form a visible agglutination. IgM functions well at room temperature and does not always require high concentrations and incubation for testing.

Immunoprecipitin tests, such as the turbidimetric immunoprecipitin assay, are used to quantitate protein by light detection. The greater the amount of antigen-antibody complexes, the more light is absorbed. Nephelometric immunoprecipitin assays are similar to the turbidimetric assays in that the greater the antigen-antibody reaction, the more of the unknown protein is present, thus producing more light scatter to indicate and quantitate the protein of interest. Refer to Chapter 6.

India ink stain can be used in microbiology to stain body fluids for *Cryptococcus neoformans*. A better technique to detect *Cryptococcus* is latex agglutination.

Indices are values that will indicate sizes, shapes,

and content of cells to facilitate an accurate assessment. This mathematical correlation with the cell morphology is used to ensure accurate results and provide additional information to the health care provider. Refer to Chapters 1, 9, and 10.

Infectious lymphocytosis occurs mainly in young children. It is contagious and has a 12- to 21-day incubation period. Refer to Chapter 5.

Infectious mononucleosis is an acute self-limiting (days to weeks) infection of Epstein-Barr virus (EBV), which is a herpes virus. The EBV is passed by exchange of saliva, which occurs during kissing; thus, the alternate name for this is the "kissing disease." It is most common in the 17- to 25-year-old age group. Symptoms include sore throat, lymphadenopathy, and splenomegaly. The white blood cell count is usually elevated from 12 to 25 $\times$ 10^9/l, but it can reach as high as 80 $\times$ 10^9/l with 60 to 90% lymphocytes with over 20% reactive. The responding cell is a lymphocyte (see Fig. 5–3), not a monocyte. Abnormally elevated liver enzyme levels (aspartate aminotransferase [AST] and lactate dehydrogenase [LD]) are seen in most cases due to liver infection, and occasionally a normocytic, normochromic hemolytic anemia is seen. Cytomegalovirus (CMV) infection is similar to mononucleosis. The symptoms and blood picture are the same with a negative result on a mononucleosis test. Large reactive lymphocytes will make up 90% of the peripheral blood leukocytes. The mode of transmission is multiple blood transfusions or from an exchange of saliva, as seen with mononucleosis. A definitive diagnosis is made by isolating the CMV in the microbiology laboratory, from blood or urine or by a rise in CMV antibody titer. The CMV isolation is done in the microbiology department or is sent to a reference laboratory. A titer is more useful if done several times over a period of days. The titer is significant only if a rise or a fall is seen. Chronic cases of CMV can cause chronic fatigue. Refer to Chapter 5.

Inflammatory response is a protective vascular and exudative tissue response to injury or destruction of tissue. The inflammatory response may also attract various leukocytes and may initiate coagulation. Symptoms are pain, heat, swelling, redness, and loss of function.

Inherited refers to characteristics or qualities that are transmitted from parents to offspring through the genetic material and are passed down from one generation to the next.

Initiating event includes exposure to toxic drugs such as benzene, caffeine, and saccharin or to radiation, which may damage the genetic material in an organism and result in a greater chance of developing a malignancy or cancer.

Interferon (IFN) is a cytokine that is produced by monocytes, lymphocytes, and other cells and that acts as an antiviral protein. Refer to Chapter 5.

Interleukin (IL) is a protein produced by one leukocyte that stimulates or has an effect on another leukocyte. Examples are: IL-1, which is produced by monocytes and enhances other monocytes; IL-2, which is produced by the T lymphocyte (CD4 cell) that activates other lymphocytes; and many others produced by the CD4 lymphocyte and other leukocytes.

Intravascular hemolysis is the destruction of erythrocytes in the blood stream, thus releasing free hemoglobin into the plasma. This can be caused by abnormal cells, such as spherocytes, which are very fragile and lyse easily; activation of complement to C8 by the IgM antibody; or mechanical destruction from artificial body parts (e.g., heart valves) and getting torn passing through blood clots. The free plasma hemoglobin makes the plasma red and, if not bound to the carrier protein haptoglobin, it will pass through the kidney and make the urine red.

Intrinsic coagulation pathway has unknown initiators, but one we know is contact with rough or irregular surfaces (ruptured cholesterol plaques) as well as collagen and other negatively charged subendothelial connective tissue. Fletcher factor (prekallikrein), Fitzgerald factor (high molecular weight kininogen [HMWK]), and factors XII and XI interact with calcium (Ca^{2+}) on a phospholipid (PF3) surface to activate factor IX. Factor IX$_a$ reacts with factor VIII, PF3, and calcium ions (Ca^{2+}) to activate primarily factor X of the common pathway (see Fig. 12–2A). Factor VIII is associated with von Willebrand's factor (VIII:vWF), which is required for normal thrombocyte adhesion. This pathway is the most sensitive to heparin therapy given to patients intravenously, and the best test to monitor this pathway is the partial thromboplastin time (PTT) test. The PTT requires platelet-poor plasma (PPP) from a sodium citrate tube (blue top), and the reference values are <35 seconds. Refer to Chapters 12 and 13.

In vitro refers to a specimen in a container outside of the body. In order to be relevant to the health of the individual or the disease process, the laboratory values must reflect the in vivo values and not the in vitro changes, which have no bearing on the state of the individual specimen being tested.

In vivo means in the body. A test performed in vivo involves injecting a substance into the patient and performing the test inside the patient's body. All testing is done to determine the status within the patient's body, which is the in vivo environment. The laboratory must guard against changes that take place once the patient's specimen is taken from the body and placed in a glass or plastic container.

Iron (Fe) is an essential component of hemoglobin with the oxygen binding directly to the ferrous (Fe^{2+}) iron. When cells break down and the iron is released, it becomes bound to the transferrin carrier protein for recycling in new cells rather than being lost through the kidneys. Storage forms of iron are ferritin and hemosiderin. Ferritin levels are the best indicators of iron deficiency. Hemosiderin can be seen in the cells with a light microscope, with or without stain. Iron in the ferric state (Fe^{3+}) cannot transport oxygen and must be reduced or anemia will develop. Refer to Chapter 8.

Iron deficiency anemia results from decreased intake or utilization of dietary iron. The iron-deficient erythrocytes are microcytic (small) and hypochromic (pale) due to the inability to make hemoglobin molecules without iron. The ferritin, serum iron, and percent saturation are low, whereas the total iron binding capacity (TIBC) is elevated. A bone marrow smear with cells stained with the vital iron stain (Prussian blue) would show a lack of storage iron in the cytoplasm of the histiocytes. Of these tests, the amount of ferritin is the best indicator of storage iron. Refer to Chapters 9 and 10.

Iron stain (Prussian blue) is a vital stain that means the cells are stained while they are still alive before the smear is made. This stain makes the iron granules in the bone marrow histiocytes more visible with light microscopy.

Isopropyl alcohol at a concentration of 70% is the cleanser of choice for routine phlebotomy. Special tests such as blood alcohol levels and blood cultures require an alternative cleansing protocol.

Killer lymphocyte (K cell) is programmed to destroy any cell that is coated with antibody, so it is called an antibody-dependent cytotoxic cell (ADCC). Antibodies are produced by the B cells and plasma cells in response to invading substances such as bacteria and virally infected cells of the body. The antibody then coats the cell, which marks (opsonizes) it for destruction by the K cells and macrophage cells of the body. Refer to Chapter 5.

Kupffer cells, the liver macrophages, are also called antigen-presenting cells (APCs). The macrophage cells are not only the most efficient phagocytic cells of the body defense, but they also have the ability to process and present antigen to the CD4 lymphocyte for an efficient and effective initiation of an immune response. In addition to these two functions, the body macrophages also store iron (Fe) for use within the body when needed. Refer to Chapter 4.

LD (LDH or lactic dehydrogenase) is a group of isoenzymes found in various cells of the body and in the plasma. When cells are damaged, LDH is released and can be measured to indicate which cells are damaged and how much damage has occurred. The isoenzymes are LD-1 through LD-5 (also called LDH_1 through LDH_5) are in cardiac (heart) cells, renal (kidney) cells, and erythrocytes. Excessive erythrocyte death releases LD; thus, an increase in LD is associated with hemol-

ysis. Hemolysis that is associated with an increase in LD may be considered part of the diagnosis in vitamin B_{12} and folate deficiencies.

Laboratory information systems (LIS) are a vital (computer) link to the patient and the health care provider. Most instruments are computerized and provide a natural link to the point of care, not to mention the development of rural health clinics and physician office laboratories (POLs) that need rapid and accurate information at a distance via computers within the laboratory information systems.

Lactate dehydrogenase (LD or LDH) is a group of isoenzymes found in various cells of the body and in the plasma. When cells are damaged, LDH is released and can be measured to indicate which cells are damaged and how much damage has occurred. The isoenzymes are LD-1 through LD-5 (also called LDH_1 through LDH_5). These isoenzymes are found in cardiac (heart) cells, renal (kidney) cells, and erythrocytes. Excessive erythrocyte death releases LD; thus, an increase in LD is associated with hemolysis. The hemolysis-associated increase in LD may be considered part of the diagnosis in vitamin B_{12} and folate deficiencies.

Langerhans cells are skin macrophages and are also called antigen-presenting cells (APCs). The macrophage cells are not only the most phagocytic cells of the body defense but also have the ability to process and present antigen to the CD4 lymphocyte for an efficient and effective initiation of an immune response. In addition to the two functions stated earlier, the macrophages also store iron (Fe) for use within the body as needed. Refer to Chapter 4.

Langerhans cell histiocytosis is one of the original histiocytosis X proliferative histiocyte disorders. These diseases demonstrate a "foamy" cell in bone granulomas and are often found in young children, who have a very short survival. Refer to Chapter 4.

LAP score is the leukocyte alkaline phosphatase (LAP) stain applied to a peripheral blood smear, after which the neutrophils are scored for the amount of LAP present. Another name is the neutrophil alkaline phosphatase (NAP) score. The purpose of this test is to determine if a high neutrophil count is due to a normal healthy response to bacterial infection (a leukemoid reaction) or due to the proliferation of leukemic cells as seen in chronic myelogenous leukemia (CML). The score ranges from 0 to 400. A high score indicates a normal response to bacterial infection, whereas a low score indicates leukemic cells. Refer to Chapters 3 and 6.

Laser light scattering is used in several laboratory instruments to characterize a cell or solution. The cell or solution is exposed to laser light, and a detector measures the pattern of scattering or the amount of scatter. Cells with various nuclei and cytoplasmic granules will have their own characteristic light scatter pattern. This is used in the complete blood counting (CBC) instruments to classify and identify the leukocytes for the automated differential. This concept is also used by flow cytometers to analyze chromosomes and thrombocytes.

Latex agglutination tests use latex particles coated with either an antigen or antibody that corresponds with the complementary antigen or antibody of interest in the patient specimen. Examples of latex agglutination are for *Cryptococcus* in cerebrospinal fluid (CSF) and for fibrin split products in plasma.

Lazy leukocyte syndrome demonstrates poor response to chemotactic factors resulting in a lack of migration to the site of inflammation or injury. Refer to Chapter 3.

Lead poisoning is an inhibitor of heme synthesis resulting in anemia. The lead interferes with heme synthesis by inhibiting the enzymes necessary to produce heme. A classic hallmark of lead poisoning is the appearance of basophilic stippling in some of the erythrocytes. Basophilic stippling is small dark blue dots throughout the erythrocyte that are associated with any heme synthesis disorder. The basophilic stippling may be so faint that it is not visible without adjustment of the fine focus on the light microscope. Refer to Chapters 8 and 9. See Figure 9–14.

Lee-White clotting time test is an outdated test performed at the patient's bedside to evaluate the intrinsic coagulation pathway. This test is discussed further in Chapter 13.

Left shift refers to the presence of immature cells in the peripheral blood. This is most often seen in the neutrophil's response to a bacterial infection (leukemoid reaction) with the appearance of the band cells, which are immature neutrophils prematurely released from the bone marrow to meet the body's need for neutrophils. A few bands are seen routinely, and each laboratory has its own criteria for distinguishing band cells from segmented neutrophils. It is important that everyone in the laboratory be familiar with the established criteria for the laboratory. If a new instrument is implemented in the laboratory, the band criteria must be established and the medical staff must know the significance of the count. Patients may not have changed status, although more bands may be reported due to a change in the method of testing or criteria used. Refer to Chapters 3 and 6.

Letterer-Siwe disease is one of the original histiocytosis X proliferative histiocyte disorders. These diseases demonstrate a "foamy" cell in bone granulomas and are often found in young children, who have a very short survival. Refer to Chapter 4.

Leukemia literally means white blood due to the excessive amount of white blood cells present in leukemia. Leukemia is a progressive malignant proliferation of one of the bone marrow cells. This is analogous to cancer. Leukemia can have an acute, rapid onset of early cells and a poor prognosis or a chronic, slow onset of mature cells with a better prognosis. The malignant leukemic cell proliferates uncontrolled and infiltrates the organs of the body, beginning with the bone marrow, and disrupts function. The quality and quantity of life for the leukemic patient depends on an accurate identification of the leukemic cell. Some leukemias can be cured if there is correct identification of the cell followed by early diagnosis and treatment.

Leukemic phase of lymphoma refers to the advanced stages of lymphoma when it has progressed beyond the lymph system and is invading the body via the bone marrow. A lymphoma differs from a leukemia in the primary site of neoplastic cells.

Leukemoid reaction is a visible response to bacterial infection that includes an increase in segmented neutrophils, which demonstrate an increase in leukocyte alkaline phosphatase (LAP) granules. These granules are visible under light microscopy and are called toxic granulation. In addition, phagocytic vacuoles and patches of cytoplasmic RNA called Döhle bodies are present in the cytoplasm of the responding cells. There is also an increase in slightly immature hyposegmented neutrophils (band cells), which is called a "left shift." The opposite is a "right shift," which reflects the appearance of hypersegmented neutrophils, demonstrating abnormal DNA synthesis (vitamin B_{12} deficiency) over mature or old cells. Refer to Chapters 3 and 6.

Leukocyte alkaline phosphatase score (LAP score) is the leukocyte alkaline phosphatase stain applied to a peripheral blood smear, and then the neutrophils are scored for the amount of LAP present. Another name is the neutrophil alkaline phosphatase (NAP) score. The purpose of this test is to determine if a high neutrophil count is due to a normal healthy response to bacterial infection (a leukemoid reaction) or due to the proliferation of leukemic cells as seen in chronic myelogenous leukemia (CML). The score ranges from 0 to 400. A high score indicates a normal response to bacterial infection, whereas a low score indicates leukemic cells. Refer to Chapters 3 and 6.

Leukocytes (white blood cells) are nucleated cells responsible for defending the body from invasion from microorganisms and other foreign substances. There are three categories of leukocytes: granulocytes, monocytes, and lymphocytes. Each of these cells has a unique and separate function. The normal total leukocyte count is approximately 5 to 10 × 10⁹/l; however, each laboratory must establish its own reference range with its procedure, equipment, personnel, and local population. Of the total leukocytes, approximately

60% are neutrophilic granulocytes, 30% are lymphocytes, and the remaining 10% are monocytes, eosinophilic granulocytes, and basophilic granulocytes.

Leukopoiesis is the production of leukocytes. This primarily refers to the production of granulocytes in the bone marrow versus the production of lymphocytes in the lymph system (lymphopoiesis).

Levey-Jennings quality control graph is used to plot laboratory quality control results. The numerical result is plotted on the vertical axis, and the time is plotted on the horizontal axis. Within the chart, the solid center line represents the mean value and the broken lines represent the standard deviations (SD) from the mean. Changes in QC testing, indicating errors or problems, can be determined by reviewing these graphs. Refer to Chapter 1.

Light absorbence is used to measure color development or a change in association with the concentration of a substance of interest. An example is the hemoglobin procedure in which the hemoglobin is combined with a color reagent and the amount of color developed is proportional to the amount of hemoglobin present. A light is passed through the colored hemoglobin solution, and the difference in the light detected on the other side of a control solution without hemoglobin compared with the change in light due to the hemoglobin color absorbing some of the light is used to determine the hemoglobin concentration.

Lipemia is an excess of lipids in the blood plasma. This occurs after ingestion of a meal that is high in fats and lipids. Until the body can metabolize the lipids, they appear white and milky. An individual with hyperlipemia has a milky appearance of the veins and arteries, which can be seen in the retinal area of the eyes. This is one reason it is best to fast before getting blood drawn for testing because the lipemic serum is not suitable for testing.

Lipid storage diseases are caused by a genetic lack of an enzyme necessary for lipid catabolism. Each of the following diseases is attributed to the deficiency of an enzyme necessary for the normal metabolism of the corresponding lipid substrate. The first indication of a lipid storage disease may be pancytopenia and hepatosplenomegaly. Diseases in this classification are Gaucher's, Tay-Sachs, Sandhoff's, Niemann-Pick, sea-blue histiocytosis, and Fabry's diseases. Refer to Chapter 4.

Lipopolysaccharide (LPS) is a molecule in which lipids and polysaccharides are linked. LPS is found in the cell wall of certain bacteria. This bacterial by-product acts as a chemotactant to draw defending cells (e.g., neutrophils and monocytes) to the area of bacterial invasion as well as stimulating lymphocytes to proliferate in an immune response.

Liver (hepatic) is an essential body organ that is responsible for blood cell production in the fetus, protein synthesis, and degradation of toxins such as bilirubin from birth to death. Blood cell formation by the liver (extramedullary hematopoiesis) during fetal development is the primary source of cells until the bone marrow takes over. Medullary hematopoiesis surpasses the liver's production of the blood cells by the time of birth. The liver maintains the ability to begin producing blood cells again if necessary in extreme cases such as bone marrow failure. The adult liver is responsible for the detoxification of bilirubin (a breakdown product of hemolysis) and other toxic body substances. Instances of increased bilirubin resulting in a yellow jaundice are seen in newborns, due to the undeveloped liver enzymes; alcoholic cirrhosis, due to liver damage from the toxic effects of alcohol; hepatitis, liver inflammation due to viruses; or liver failure due to cancer, called hepatocarcinoma.

Lupus anticoagulants (LA), which are more accurately called antiphospholipid antibodies (APA), are abnormal plasma proteins that act as circulating anticoagulants by binding to the thrombocyte phospholipid (PF3) interfering with normal blood clotting. When the partial thromboplastin time (PTT) test is prolonged and mixing normal plasma (containing all the coagulation factors) with the patient's plasma does not correct the PTT, a circulating anticoagulant such as this is present. If this mixed specimen does correct the PTT, a factor deficiency is suspected instead. The APA is an autoantibody that is seen more commonly in the geriatric patient and is not usually associated with lupus erythematosus. Refer to Chapters 11 to 13.

Lupus erythematosus (LE) is an autoimmune disease characterized by the production of an antibody-like protein called the LE factor. This protein binds with various body substances, and these antigen-antibody complexes deposit in various organs of the body. This disease occurs most often in women aged 20 to 40 years old. The first sign is usually a butterfly rash over the nose and cheeks of the face, and the terminal sign is kidney (renal) failure due to deposits of these immune complexes in the kidneys. A latex agglutination method is available for screening. This test must be confirmed by use of a fluorescent antinuclear antibody (FANA) test. The lupus erythematosus preparation (LE prep) was done in the past and is discussed in Chapter 6.

Lymphocytes are agranular and produced outside of the bone marrow (extramedullary hematopoiesis) in the lymph system of the body. There is a wide variety of lymphocytes, the most common of which are the T lymphocytes and B lymphocytes. Other lymphocytes described include the K lymphocyte, the NK lymphocyte, the large granular lymphocyte (LGL), and the lymphokine-activated killer (LAK) cells, which, when activated by

IL-2, lyse fresh tumor target cells that are resistant to NK cell lysis. Some lymphocytes are classified as "null" cells because they demonstrate neither T nor B markers.

Lymphopoiesis is influenced by the regulatory proteins called interleukins, followed by a number designation to identify the specific protein (e.g., IL-1, IL-3). Lymphocytes produce many of the regulatory proteins such as interleukins as well as being regulated by some of these proteins. Reference values for blood lymphocytes are 1.5 to $4 \times 10^9/l$, and T cells account for 80% and B cells account for 20% of this value. Within the T cell population, the normal ratio for CD4 (T_h):CD8 (T_s) is $2:1$. Refer to Chapter 5.

The most common reasons for reactive lymphocytosis are viral diseases such as mononucleosis, cytomegalovirus infection, and infectious lymphocytosis. These conditions are followed closely by hepatitis, influenza, mycoplasma pneumonia, mumps, measles, rubella, varicella, and other viral infections. A few bacterial and protozoan infections also produce lymphocytosis. These infections are pertussis (whooping cough), tuberculosis, cat-scratch fever, toxoplasmosis, and malaria. The most common reasons for malignant lymphocytosis are acute lymphoblastic leukemia (ALL), chronic lymphocytic leukemia (CLL), leukemic phase of lymphoma, and Waldenström's macroglobulinemia.

Lymphocytopenia is a decrease in lymphocytes that may be due to an increase in another blood cell, genetic impairment, malignancy with cancerous cells invading the lymph tissue, adrenocortico-steroids, chemotherapy, or radiation. It is very important to distinguish a relative lymphocytopenia from an absolute lymphocytopenia. If any other white blood cell is increased in number, this may result in a relative decrease in lymphocytes in which the lymphocytes appear decreased in reference to the other cells. Refer to Chapter 5.

Lymphocytosis is an increase in lymphocytes, which is the result of a decrease in the other white blood cells, a normal response to viral infection (called a reactive lymphocytosis), or due to an abnormal proliferation of lymphocytes called a malignant lymphocytosis. The most common reasons for malignant lymphocytosis are acute lymphoblastic leukemia (ALL), chronic lymphocytic leukemia (CLL), leukemic phase of lymphoma, and Waldenström's macroglobulinemia. It is very important to distinguish a relative lymphocytosis from an absolute lymphocytosis. If any other type of white blood cell is decreased in number, this may result in a relative increase in lymphocytes so that the lymphocytes appear elevated in reference to the other cells. Refer to Chapter 5.

Lymphoid stem cell (LSC, 10 to 20 μm) is the result of influence on the pluripotent stem cells

(PSC) by lymphoid growth factors such as IL-7 and SCF. The PSC under lymphocytic growth factor stimulation will proliferate and differentiate into a lymphoid cell, which is found primarily in the lymphatic system of the body instead of the bone marrow. This lymphoid progenitor cell is committed to the lymphoid hematopoietic cell line. The LSC will migrate either to the thymus gland to become a T lymphocyte (6 to 10 μm) or to the bursa equivalent (bone marrow?) to become a B lymphocyte (6 to 10 μm), or the LSC may become a killer lymphocyte (K) or a natural killer (NK) lymphocyte. The lymphoid cells are considered to be a product of extramedullary (outside of the bone marrow) hematopoiesis. Refer to Chapter 5.

Lymphoma refers to a malignant lymphocyte cell proliferation in the lymph tissue. As the disease progresses, the lymphoma cells will travel to the blood and bone marrow, which is called the leukemic phase of lymphoma. A lymphoma differs from a leukemia in the primary site of neoplastic cell origin. These are both treated with chemotherapy and radiation. Successful treatment depends on accurate identification of the malignant cell and early diagnosis and treatment. Refer to Chapter 5.

Lymphopoiesis is the production of lymphocytes primarily in the lymph system. Refer to Chapter 5.

MCH (mean corpuscular hemoglobin) is the average hemoglobin per erythrocytic cell. The normal reference range is 26 to 32 picograms (pg). This calculation provides an indication of hemoglobin present but does not take into consideration the size of the cells. The MCHC includes cell size in the calculation and is more accurate and useful. Refer to Chapters 1 and 10 for the formulas and application.

MCHC (mean corpuscular hemoglobin concentration) is the average concentration of hemoblobin per erythrocyte. The normal reference range is 32 to 36%. Less then 32% would correlate with hypochromic erythrocytes, 32 to 36% would be normochromic, and greater than 36% would require the cell to alter its shape and be spherocytic. Refer to Chapters 1 and 10 for the formulas and application.

MCV (mean cell volume) is the average erythrocyte volume in a specimen. The normal reference range is 80 to 95 femtoliters (fl). An average of less than 80 fl would correlate with the presence of microcytes, 80 to 95 fl with normocytes, and greater than 95 fl with macrocytes. Refer to Chapters 1 and 10 for the formulas and application.

MPV (mean platelet volume) is a calculated index to provide the average size of the platelets in a specimen. The normal reference range for MPV is approximately 7 to 10 fl. MPVs above 10 fl indicate a release of immature platelets in response to use of all the mature platelets due to clotting in the body, an anomaly, or other disorder.

Macrocytic describes a large erythrocyte. Macrocytes have a mean corpuscular volume (MCV) greater than 95 fl. This can be a normal bone marrow response to anemia by releasing as many erythrocytes as possible, including less mature cells that are larger, or this can be the result of abnormal maturation as seen in vitamin B_{12} deficiency and liver disease.

Macrophage describes the large phagocytic cells of the body that have different names depending on where they are located. In the bone marrow, they are histiocytes; liver cells are Kupffer cells; the brain macrophages are microglial cells; osteoclasts are bone macrophage cells; Langerhans cells are skin macrophages; and the monocyte is the peripheral blood macrophage. The macrophage cells are not only the most efficient phagocytes of the body defense system but also have the ability to process the phagocytized antigen and present this antigen to the CD4 lymphocyte for an efficient and effective initiation of a primary immune response. Refer to Chapter 4.

Makler is the name of a counting chamber that is designed specifically for semen analysis (sperm counts).

Malignant refers to a life-threatening condition. Cancers are usually malignant, whereas a simple wart is benign or not life threatening.

Malignant erythrocytosis describes acute erythroleukemia (FAB M6, AEL) and demonstrates more than 50% erythroid dysplasia in the bone marrow. Megaloblastic normoblasts with diffuse blocks of cytoplasmic glycogen when stained with periodic acid-Schiff (PAS) stain will differentiate AEL from polycythemia. Differentiation from myelodysplastic syndrome can be done with monoclonal antibodies and flow cytometry. The old name for this disorder is Di Guglielmo's disease. Refer to Chapter 9.

Malignant histiocytosis is characterized by malignant (life-threatening) histiocyte proliferation, nuclear abnormalities, abundant cytoplasm, and infiltration of the body tissues. This interferes with the normal function of the body and results in organ failure. Refer to Chapter 4.

Malignant lymphocytosis includes acute lymphoblastic leukemia (ALL), chronic lymphocytic leukemia (CLL), and the leukemic phase of lymphoma. Refer to Chapter 5.

Managed care refers to health care costs that are dictated by third-party payers in the attempt to achieve quality health care in an efficient and least costly manner. Refer to Chapter 16.

Material safety data sheets (MSDS) must be available for each chemical used in the laboratory. The MSDS is provided by the manufacturer and provides instructions on storage, use, and emergency procedures.

Major histocompatibility complex (MHC I and II) constitutes a family of membrane proteins that are the antigens associated with self-recognition (MHC II) and organ rejection (MHC I). The MHC antigens are also referred to as histocompatible leukocyte antigens, HLA-I and -II. Refer to Chapter 5.

May-Hegglin anomaly is a rare inherited disorder characterized by the presence of Döhle bodies in the cytoplasm of the neutrophils, large poorly granulated thrombocytes, and thrombocytopenia. Refer to Chapter 3.

Mean ($\bar{x}$). Average value.

$$\bar{x} = \frac{\Sigma n \text{(sum of all the determinations)}}{n \text{ (the number of determinations)}}$$

Mean corpuscular hemoglobin (MCH) is the average hemoglobin per erythrocytic cell. The normal reference range is 26 to 32 picograms (pg). This calculation provides an indication of hemoglobin present but does not take into consideration the size of the cells. The MCHC includes cell size in the calculation and is more accurate and useful. Refer to Chapters 1 and 10 for the formulas and application.

Medullary hematopoiesis is the production of blood cells within the bone marrow. This is in contrast to blood cell production outside of the bone marrow as seen in lymphopoiesis, which is extramedullary hematopoiesis. Refer to Chapter 2.

Megakaryocytic leukemia (FAB M7) is a rare acute leukemia involving the early megakaryocytic cell. Refer to Chapter 11.

Megaloblastic describes a large nucleated erythroid cell with asynchronous maturation. The cytoplasm is more mature than is the nucleus. This is seen in vitamin B_{12} deficiency, because B_{12} is required for normal DNA synthesis. The resultant mature cell will be macrocytic and may have Howell-Jolly body inclusions, which are pieces of DNA. These inclusions will mark these cells for destruction by the phagocytic cells of the body. An erythrocyte can be macrocytic without having a megaloblastic nucleus, but a megaloblastic nucleated cell will always produce a macrocytic erythrocyte. Refer to Chapter 9.

Metamyelocyte is the last mononuclear stage in the granulocytic cell line. This cell is not capable of mitosis but continues to differentiate into the banded granulocyte and then the mature granulocyte. The nucleus is kidney shaped with a fairly granular cytoplasm. The granules present in the cytoplasm should be noted by preceding this name with an N for neutrophilic, an E for eosinophilic, or a B for basophilic. Refer to Chapter 3.

Methemoglobin (Hi) is formed by oxidation of the hemoglobin iron from the ferrous (Fe^{2+}) state to the ferric state (Fe^{3+}), which is not capable of transporting oxygen. A small amount of Hi is formed in the blood normally, but oxidative drugs can convert a significant amount that will result in hypoxia (decreased oxygen to the tissues). The glucose-6-phosphate dehydrogenase (G-6-PD) of the hexose monophosphate shunt is a major contributor in the reduction of methemoglobin to functional hemoglobin. Refer to Chapter 8.

Methylene blue stain is basic and stains the acid components of cells (e.g., DNA and RNA) dark blue. This stain is associated with the Wright-Giemsa stain and the reticulocyte stain.

Microcytic describes a small erythrocyte of less than 80 femtoliters (fl) in volume. This occurs in iron deficiency anemia and thalassemia, and when schistocytes (fragmented red blood cells) are present.

Microscope is an instrument to magnify very small objects in order to reveal the details of structure that are not visible with direct observation. The most common microscope is the compound light microscope used in the clinical laboratory; however, there are at least 15 different microscopes available for specific observations of small objects.

Microscopy refers to evaluation of a specimen under the microscope. Specific preparation is required for each specimen viewed. The correct size or number of objects must be considered. Too many, too few, too large, or too small objects are not suitable. Color enhancement through staining may also be required or helpful. The specimen preparation method is a written procedure in the laboratory manual. Urine and miscellaneous body fluids are the most common specimens to require microscopy for analysis. In hematology the most common specimen involving microscopy is the prepared blood smear.

Miller disk is used in the ocular of the microscope to facilitate the counting of reticulocytes on a prepared smear. Refer to Chapter 10.

Minerals are required for normal body function. The most commonly known of these are calcium (Ca^{2+}) and iron (Fe^{2+}). Others include magnesium (Mg^{2+}), Zinc (Zn^{2+}) and iodine. Calcium is a component of blood coagulation (clotting) as well as many other systems within the body. Several of the anticoagulants (e.g., EDTA, Na citrate, Na oxalate and Na fluoride) keep the blood from clotting by binding the calcium ions in the blood. Iron is necessary for hemoglobin synthesis in the erythrocyte. Lack of iron results in anemia. Overdoses of minerals may occur, due to storage in various organs of the body, and may be toxic. Tests to measure levels are performed in the clinical chemistry section of the laboratory.

Mission of the clinical laboratory is to: (1) provide test results that reflect the condition within the body (in vivo), not changes that took place once the blood was removed from the patient and placed into a glass tube (in vitro), and (2) correlate and validate all test information (puzzle pieces) available to provide the primary health care provider with a clear and accurate picture of the patient's state of health.

Monochrome stain, such as the reticulocyte stain, contains only one color to reveal only one component of interest. This is in contrast with a polychrome stain, which has more than one stain (color) in order to characterize more than one component.

Monoclonal refers to a multitude of cells derived from, and identical to, a single parent cell. This group of identical cells is called a clone. If this is a clone of B lymphocytes, they will all produce an identical antibody. This is in contrast with polyclonal, which refers to the proliferation of cells from several different parent cells.

Monoclonal antibody refers to one specific antibody directed against one antigen. This is not desirable in an immune response to a foreign substance (antigen) such as bacteria. One antibody is not sufficient to destroy the antigen. A healthy individual will produce many specific antibodies against several different antigens on the foreign substance, which increases the chances of elimination. Monoclonal antibody diseases are multiple myeloma and Waldenström's macroglobulinemia. Monoclonal antibodies are very useful tools of clinical testing and research. A single specific antibody can be produced to interact with a specific cell antigen (e.g., the CD4 protein on lymphocytes) in order to identify the substance of interest. Examples of methodology utilizing monoclonal antibodies are flow cytometry, latex agglutination, and enzyme linked immunoassay (EIA).

Monoclonal gammopathy of undetermined significance (MGUS) is a condition that mimics the initial onset of multiple myeloma (MM). A monoclonal antibody is produced in excess, suggesting a malignant disorder; however, the bone marrow has only slightly increased numbers of plasma cells. This condition is benign and will not progress any further unless it is misdiagnosed as a malignancy (e.g., MM) and chemotherapy is administered, which may alter the genetic material and induce a malignancy. On the other hand, if this presentation is an early MM, the sooner that the chemotherapy treatment is started the more successful it will be.

Monocyte is the peripheral blood macrophage and is an extremely important cell in the body's response to infection. The monocyte is a major phagocytic cell of the body that not only destroys the invading organism or substance but also processes the foreign antigen and relays information about the invader to other cells of the body. Due to this function, the monocyte is also called an antigen-presenting cell (APC). A third function of the monocyte is to store iron until needed by the body. The monocyte is discussed in Chapter 4.

Monocyte/macrophage system, also called the reticuloendothelial system (RES), includes the various macrophage cells throughout the body such as the bone marrow histiocytes; liver cells are Kupffer cells; the brain macrophages are microglial cells; osteoclasts are the phagocytic bone cells; Langerhans cells are the skin macrophages; and the monocyte is the peripheral blood macrophage. These cells are not only the most efficient phagocytic cells of the body defense but they also act as initiation agents, antigen-presenting cells (APCs), allowing an immune response to develop adequately. The macrophage stores body iron until it is needed. Refer to Chapter 4.

Monocytopenia is defined as a monocyte count of less than $0.2 \times 10^9/l$. This count is not easily established due to the low number of monocytes normally within the peripheral blood. Monocytopenia has been seen during and transiently after therapy with the drug prednisone and with hairy cell leukemia. Refer to Chapter 4.

Monolayer literally means one layer and, in hematology, refers to the evaluation area of a peripheral blood smear. The erythrocytes must be distributed evenly in a monolayer in order to evaluate the erythrocyte, leukocytes, and thrombocytes adequately. This good reading area is just inside the feather edge of a traditional blood smear. Refer to Chapter 6. See Figures 6–11 to 6–13.

Mononucleosis (infectious) is an acute self-limiting (days to weeks) infection of Epstein-Barr virus (EBV), a herpes virus. EBV is passed by exchange of saliva, which occurs during kissing; thus, the alternate name for this is the "kissing disease." It is most common in the 17 to 25-year-old age group. Infectious mononucleosis presents with a sore throat, lymphadenopathy (enlarged lymph nodes), and splenomegaly (enlarged spleen). The white blood cell count is usually elevated from 12 to $25 \times 10^9/l$ but can reach as high as $80 \times 10^9/l$ with 60 to 90% lymphocytes with over 20% reactive. The reactive lymphocyte (see Fig. 5–3) should not be mistaken for a monocyte. Abnormally elevated liver enzyme levels (aspartate aminotransferase [AST] and lactate dehydrogenase [LD]) are seen in most cases due to liver infection, and occasionally a normocytic, normochromic hemolytic anemia is seen. Cytomegalovirus (CMV) infection is similar to mononucleosis. The symptoms and blood picture are the same, with a negative result on a mononucleosis test. Large reactive lymphocytes will make up 90% of the peripheral blood leukocytes. The mode of transmission is multiple blood transfusions or exchange of saliva as seen with mononucleosis. A definitive diagnosis is made in the microbiology laboratory by isolating the CMV from blood or urine or by noting a rise in CMV antibody titer. The CMV isolation is done in the microbiology department or is sent to a reference laboratory. A titer is more useful if done several times over a period of days. The titer is significant only if a rise or a fall is seen. There are chronic cases of CMV causing chronic fatigue. Refer to Chapter 5.

Monopoiesis is the production of monocytes. This occurs in the bone marrow from the CFU-M, which differentiates into the promonocyte and then matures into the monocyte. Monocytes are the peripheral blood macrophages. Refer to Chapter 4.

Multiple myeloma (MM) is a monoclonal gammopathy, and the excessive antibody is usually IgG. The malignant cell in MM is the plasma cell, which becomes a myeloma cell. The production of monoclonal antibodies for research and clinical reagent use is done by fusing a myeloma cell with a lymphocyte sensitized to the antigen of interest. The resultant cell that produces mass quantities of the single antibody of interest is called a hybridoma cell. Refer to Chapter 5.

Mycosis fungoides is a chronic, malignant, lymphoreticular neoplasm of the skin. In late stages, the lymph nodes and body organs are involved, and large, painful ulcerating tumors develop. Refer to Chapter 5.

Myeloblasts are also called colony-forming unit–granulocyte (CFU-G, CFU-Eo, CFU-Ba) cells, which are the earliest definitive cells of the granulocytic cell line. In acute myelocytic or myeloblastic leukemia (AML, M1), the myeloblast has cytoplasmic azurophilic rod-like inclusions called Auer rods, which can be used to aid in cell identification. Refer to Chapter 3.

Myelocyte is an immature cell in the granulocytic cell line. The significant characteristic of this stage of granulocytic maturation is the development of specific (neutrophilic, eosinophilic, or basophilic) secondary granules in the cytoplasm. The secondary granules are the primary characteristic to differentiate the granulocytes. For this reason the myelocyte nomenclature should be preceded by an N or neutrophilic, or an E for eosinophilic, or a B for basophilic. This is the last stage to undergo division, and the nucleus is still round. Refer to Chapter 3.

Myelodysplastic syndrome (MDS) is seen in individuals older than 50 years of age and presents with anemia and bone marrow abnormalities that may affect all cell lines. Myelodysplasia has been divided into five categories by the French-American-British (FAB) hematology group, based on the bone marrow percentage of blasts, percentage of ringed sideroblasts, percentage of peripheral blood blasts, and number of peripheral blood monocytes. The categories are (1) refractory anemia (RA); (2) refractory anemia with ringed sideroblasts (RARS); (3) refractory anemia with excessive blasts (RAEB); refractory anemia with excessive blasts in transformation (RAEB-t); and (4) chronic myelomonocytic leukemia (CMML). Refer to Chapters 3 and 9.

Myelofibrosis is infiltration of the bone marrow with fibrous tissue. This results in the inability of the bone marrow to produce blood, thus producing anemia. Complete disruption of hematopoiesis is aplasia; decreased hematopoiesis is hypoplasia. A characteristic erythrocyte morphology seen due to the production of cells among invading fibers is the teardrop cell. Refer to Chapter 9.

Myeloid:erythroid (M:E) ratio is used to evaluate the bone marrow cellularity, which normally has three to four times as many myeloid cells as erythroid cells. The normal M:E ratio is 3:1 or 4:1. Refer to Chapter 2.

Myeloid growth factors are proteins that are produced and act on the bone marrow (myeloid) cells. These factors direct the hematopoietic stem cell to become a myeloid cell (e.g., the colony-forming unit–GEMM). Refer to Chapter 3.

Myeloid hypoplasia is the failure of the bone marrow to produce cells at an adequate level. Refer to Chapter 3.

Myeloid metaplasia is the transformation of cells, within a tissue in the adult, to form cells that are abnormal for the tissue in which they are present. An example of this is the extramedullary hematopoiesis in the spleen and liver to compensate for a failing bone marrow (e.g., in myelofibrosis). Immature blood cells are seen accompanied by a mild to moderate anemia. Refer to Chapters 3 and 9.

Myeloperoxidase (MPO) is a digestive enzyme found in the granules of the neutrophil and in a smaller amount in the monocyte granules. The MPO cytochemical stain can be used to differentiate a neutrophilic blast from a lymphocytic blast. Refer to Chapters 3 and 4.

Myeloproliferative disorders (MPDs) are abnormal and excessive production of myeloid (bone marrow) cells, such as chronic myelogenous leukemia (CML) and myelodysplasia (MDS).

Myocardial infarct (MI) is cardiac necrosis as a result of a blood clot blocking blood flow to a section of the heart. This would also qualify as a heart attack.

Natural killer lymphocyte (NK cell) is a cell whose function is to search throughout the body for cells that have become abnormal for any reason and destroy these cells. Included in the abnormal cells are viral infected cells and cancer cells. Refer to Chapter 5.

Necrotic tissue refers to dead tissue. Tissue necrosis occurs due to a lack of oxygen to the tissue, resulting in cell death.

Needle holders are required for routine venipuncture with the vacuum tube technique. This technique requires that the needle be attached to a plastic needle holder (sometimes called a jacket) in which the tubes are inserted. The needle holders, or jackets, have various sizes and require a needle with the same method of attachment. As seen in Figure 1–11, the needle holder may require a threaded needle or a bayonet-style needle that inserts and locks with a half turn. Some jack-

ets are disposable and are available with needle protectors that cover the needle when it is removed from the vein.

Needles of 20 or 21 gauge are appropriate for routine phlebotomy. The larger the gauge, the smaller is the diameter of the needle. If a larger gauge needle is used, there is a risk of hemolyzing the red blood cells as they are forced through a small bore. Using a smaller-gauge needle may limit the choice to veins with a greater diameter than the needle. The needle should be used with the slanted side (bevel) up (Fig. 1–10) and discarded immediately after the procedure into an appropriate sharps container. Never re-cap the needle or lay it down. Refer to Chapter 1.

Neimann-Pick disease is a lipid storage disease that is caused by a genetic lack of the sphingomyelinase enzyme necessary for lipid catabolism. The build-up of lipids in the cells of the body is detrimental and may be fatal. Refer to Chapter 3.

Neoplasm refers to growth of new or abnormal tissue. Neoplasms are also called tumors and can be benign or malignant.

Nephelometric immunoprecipitin assays are similar to the turbidimetric assays. The more antigen-antibody reaction that occurs, the more of the unknown protein is present; thus, more light scatter is required to indicate and quantitate the protein of interest.

Neutropenia is a decreased number of neutrophils in the blood. This can be caused by decreased production in the bone marrow as seen in leukemias, after bone marrow transplants, and as a result of radiation therapy. In these situations a granulocyte colony-stimulating factor (G-CSF) is available to enhance the production of neutrophils. Another reason for neutropenia is a bacterial infection in the initial phase when the peripheral blood neutrophils have migrated out of the blood to the site of infection and the bone marrow has not had time to release more, or the end of the infection when the bone marrow has exhausted all neutrophils available. This latter scenario paints a poor prognosis if the bacteria have outnumbered the defending neutrophils. This is undoubtedly a systemic sepsis, and the individual will probably succumb to the infection. Refer to Chapter 3.

Neutrophilia is a count of more than 60%, more than $6 \times 10^9/l$, neutrophils in the peripheral blood. Causes of neutrophilia include chronic myelogenous leukemia (CML) or a leukemoid reaction in response to a bacterial infection. The leukocyte alkaline phosphatase (LAP) score, also called the neutrophil alkaline phosphatase (NAP) test, is used to differentiate the leukemoid reaction from CML. Refer to Chapter 3.

Non-Hodgkin's lymphomas are a heterogeneous group of lymphomas characterized by a mixed population of cells that proliferate excessively in the lymph tissue. The only common feature of these lymphomas is the absence of the Reed-Sternberg cell, which is diagnostic for Hodgkin's lymphoma. Refer to Chapter 5.

Nonvital stains are used for fixed (dead or non-viable) cells prepared on a slide. Examples of nonvital stains utilized in hematology are the Wright-Giemsa stain, the stain for siderotic (iron) granules called Prussian blue stain, and the cytochemical stains. Vital stains are combined with blood while it is still viable (alive), and the slide is prepared after staining. Refer to Chapter 1.

Normochromic literally means normal color. The normal erythrocyte stained with Wright-Giemsa stain is red and has a slightly lighter center (normal central pallor) due to the bioconcave shape of the erythrocyte, which is thinner in the center. The erythrocyte indices, mean corpuscular hemoglobin (MCH), and mean corpuscular hemoglobin concentration (MCHC) indicate and correlate with the erythrocyte morphology. A normochromic erythrocyte population would have an MCH of 26 to 32 pg and a MCHC of 32 to 36%. Refer to Chapters 7 to 10.

Normocytic literally means normal size. The normal size of the erythrocyte is approximately the size of a small lymphocyte nucleus (6 to 8 μm). The erythrocyte indices, which would indicate and correlate with the erythrocyte size, are the mean corpuscular volume (MCV) and the red cell distribution width (RDW). The average erythrocyte volume (MCV) is 80 to 95 fl, and the population should be fairly homogeneous. The RDW is an indicator of the percentage of cells outside of the normal size range. In a normal blood specimen, 11.5 to 14.5% of the erythrocytes will fall out of the normal reference range for size. Variation in size of erythrocytes is generically termed anisocytosis, which can include microcytes and macrocytes as well as a variety of shapes that are generically termed poikilocytosis. Refer to Chapters 7 and 10.

Nuclear to cytoplasmic ratio (N:C) is one of the identification characteristics used to distinguish one cell from another and also estimate the maturity of a cell. Immature cells, such as blast cells, have a large nucleus that fills the cell, resulting in a high N:C ratio. This ratio decreases with maturity as the nucleus becomes smaller and the cytoplasm becomes more abundant. This transition occurs because early cells are primarily proliferating, whereas mature cells no longer divide and need cytoplasm, containing organelles, in order to carry out the cell's function, such as phagocytosis or production of proteins. There are exceptions, such as the small resting lymphocytes that have very little cytoplasm as mature cells.

Nucleated red blood cells (NRBC) are immature erythrocytes that still contain a nucleus, which is normally seen only in the bone marrow. The orthochromic normoblast stage of erythrocyte mat-

uration is the last nucleated stage, and upon expulsion of the nucleus a reticulocyte is formed, which becomes a mature erythrocyte. Refer to Chapter 7.

Nucleoli are areas of RNA found in the nucleus of immature or reactive cells. These areas are associated with cell division and proliferation. The nucleoli appear as light blue circular areas in the nucleus when stained with a methylene blue stain such as Wright-Giemsa stain. Nucleoli are not readily visible in many cells, and the light microscope's fine focus is required to see them.

Nutrients are required to allow a blood specimen to remain viable until testing or use, such as administration of a unit of blood. Most routine testing is done within a few hours of blood collection. There are enough nutrients in the blood to sustain the blood for the routine testing time period of less than 4 hours. After this time the blood may remain viable, but changes will begin to take place. Testing over a prolonged period of time, or storage of units of blood for up to 35 days for transfusion, requires additional nutrients to keep the cells viable. Glucose metabolism is a major source of energy. Glucose levels are measured as part of a routine chemistry profile. Accurate glucose levels depend on the diet prior to blood collection and the time the fluid portion of the blood remains in contact with the cells after blood collection. The cells will continue to metabolize the glucose at the rate of 5% per hour, resulting in a lower glucose value than is present in vivo. Heparin fluoride can be added to inhibit glycolysis by the erythrocytes. If bacteria are present in the specimen, they will utilize glucose also. The use of heparin fluoride will not affect bacterial glucose metabolism.

Objective lenses of the microscope range from a very low-power scanning objective to the oil immersion lens. The shorter scanning objective (4 to 5×) is used for the large, gross specimen; the longer low-power objective (10 to 15×) is used for the thinner and smaller specimen, such as peripheral blood smears, and for a clearer image of the gross specimen. Both the scan and low-power objectives can be focused with the coarse adjustment control. The high-dry objective (40 to 45×) is a little longer than the low-power objective and is brought into focus only with the fine adjustment control. If the coarse adjustment is used, the objective may be driven through the specimen, damaging the objective lens and destroying the specimen. The oil immersion objective (50 or 100×) requires a drop of oil on the specimen to alter the light rays passing through the specimen for better resolution of very small objects. Only the fine adjustment control can be used at this magnification. Refer to Chapter 1.

Occupational Safety and Health Administration (OSHA) mandates safety protocols of concern in any work environment. OSHA specifically requires safety devices, exits, safety manuals, and material safety data sheets (MSDS) to mention a few protocols. Refer to Chapter 1.

Oculars are lenses at the top of a compound light microscope. There will be one (monocular) or two (binocular) lenses that adjust to the width and focus of your eyes. It is important to always have both eyes open when doing microscope work (microscopy); even when looking through a monocular microscope, always keep the other eye open. Using a binocular microscope, the oculars must be adjusted to allow the individual to see a full field of vision with both eyes open. The object viewed is magnified 10× by the ocular lens. Refer to Chapter 1.

Oncogenes are genes associated with the production of tumors, often in association with cancer-causing viruses. These exist in the body as non-cancerous proto-oncogenes that are transformed into oncogenes by as yet unknown mechanisms.

Opsonins are substances, primarily proteins, that bind to foreign cells or particles and attract phagocytic cells to destroy the invading (opsonized) material.

Opsonization is the attachment of proteins to a cell or particle that will mark this cell or particle for phagocytosis and destruction. Often opsonization will result in particles sticking together or sticking to the PMN (immune adherence), which encourages phagocytosis, and a membrane enclosed phagocytic vacuole is formed around the opsonized cell or particle.

Optical clot detection is the methodology used by most automated coagulation instrumentation in the clinical laboratory. Light passes through the reaction well containing the patient's plasma, and the reagent and light passing through not absorbed by the specimen are detected on the opposite side of the reaction well. As the specimen begins to coagulate, more light is blocked due to the formation of the fibrin strands from the soluble fibrinogen. The time taken for a change of light detected is the coagulation time. Tests such as the prothrombin time (PT), partial thromboplastin time (PTT), thrombin time (TT), and fibrinogen, circulating anticoagulant test (mix), and factor assays can be performed with this instrument. Samples from many patients and for more than one test can be loaded onto the larger instruments at the same time, and the results will be printed to be validated and disseminated to the primary health care provider within a short time. Refer to Chapter 13.

Orthochromic normoblast is the last nucleated cell in the erythrocyte maturation sequence, which is normally found only in the bone marrow. This cell has a gray-blue cytoplasm that contains a significant amount of functional hemoglobin and a considerable amount of RNA, which is still synthesizing hemoglobin polypeptide chains for hemoglobin molecule construction. The nucleus is described as pyknotic and has no visible structure; once this is extruded, a reticulocyte is formed. Refer to Chapter 7.

Osmotic concentration refers to the cellular osmotic environment (diluent solution) that must remain isotonic, that is, maintain the same fluid and solute concentration as the body environment. The normal concentration of fluids and cells within the body is equivalent to a 0.85% NaCl solution. Any diluent used to suspend cells must be isotonic. Solutions with too much solute are hypertonic and will result in the shriveling of cells. Solutions that have too little solute are hypotonic, and the cells will take in fluid to equalize the osmotic concentrations, inside and out, resulting in swelling and lysis of the cell. These responses to the osmotic environment are characteristic of semipermeable membranes.

Osmotic fragility test is used to measure the ability of the erythrocytes in a specimen to withstand a range of osmotic concentrations without lysing. The normal healthy erythrocyte is able to take in a significant amount of water before it will lyse. A cell that is already spherocytic, as in hereditary spherocytosis, cannot take in much water before lysing and is therefore more osmotically fragile. Large flat erythrocytes, such as target cells, can take in more water than usual, demonstrating a decreased osmotic fragility. Refer to Chapters 7 and 10.

Osteoclasts are bone macrophage cells, which are also called antigen-presenting cells (APCs). The macrophage cells are not only the most phagocytic cells of the body defense but also have the ability to process and present antigen to the CD4 lymphocyte for an efficient and effective initiation of an immune response. In addition to the two functions stated earlier, the macrophages also store iron (Fe) for use within the body as needed.

Ouchterlony double immunodiffusion technique is used to compare the similarities and differences of various antigens and antibodies. A neutral (without antigen or antibody) agar gel medium in a Petri dish or on a glass slide has various wells cut into it. The known reagent antibody is placed into one well, and the unknown fresh, clear serum sample from the patient is added to another well. Several different preparations or samples are used in various wells to compare their antigen characteristics. The reaction chamber or slide is maintained at controlled temperatures and humidity for a specific time to allow the reactants to diffuse toward each other through the agar gel medium. If the antigens in the two wells are identical—demonstrate complete antigenic identity—a solid arc line of precipitation will be visible. If there is more than one antigenic determinant in the patient's sample and some are identical and some are not, a fused arc with a spur is visible, demonstrating partial identity. If the precipitation lines make an X, this indicates the lack of likeness, or non-identity. Refer to Chapters 5 and 6.

Outcome assessment is a measure of what was accomplished (the outcome) from a process or action. An example is how well a clinical laboratory technician student functions in the first position that he or she fills upon graduation. This would assess the outcome of the person's education and training. Refer to Chapter 16.

Oxygen saturation curve or oxygen dissociation curve is the amount of oxygen carried by the hemoglobin and is influenced by several factors, such as pH or 2,3-diphosphoglycerate (2,3-DPG or 2,3-BPG) levels, and the partial pressure of oxygen (PO_2). As these factors change, the ability to carry and release oxygen from the hemoglobin molecule changes the central sigmoid curve to a "shift to the left" or a "shift to the right." Refer to Chapter 8.

Oxyhemoglobin (HbO_2) is hemoglobin carrying oxygen to the tissues. The four heme groups contain iron (Fe^{2+}), and each binds one molecule of oxygen. When the erythrocyte reaches the tissue in need of the oxygen and releases the oxygen it is called deoxyhemoglobin. Refer to Chapter 8.

PF3 (platelet factor 3) is a phospholipid required as a surface for intrinsic pathway blood clotting (coagulation) to take place. Another source of phospholipid for coagulation is tissue factor III of the extrinsic coagulation pathway. Refer to Chapter 11.

PPL (platelet phospholipid), also called platelet factor 3 (PF3), is required as a surface for intrinsic pathway blood clotting (coagulation) to take place. Another source of phospholipid for coagulation is tissue factor III of the extrinsic coagulation pathway. Refer to Chapter 11.

Pallor literally means paleness. In hematology this refers to the center of the normal biconcave erythrocyte, which has a "central pallor" surrounded by the pink hemoglobin at the edges of the cell.

Palpate means to feel by lightly touching in order to determine the condition of parts beneath. The veins are palpated to determine an appropriate site for phlebotomy. By palpating the vein, the phlebotomist can determine the direction, depth, wall thickness, and stability of the vein. This information increases the chances of a successful venipuncture.

Panmyelosis is an increase or abnormality that affects all bone marrow (myeloid) cells.

Pappenheimer bodies are pale blue patches in the mature erythrocytes stained with Wright-Giemsa stain. When stained with Prussian blue iron stain, they appear as siderotic (iron) granules. Refer to Chapters 9 and 10.

Parasitic infections are the result of an organism living within a human, such as in malaria or a tapeworm infestation or infection. Parasitic infections result in an increased number of eosinophils in the peripheral blood. Refer to Chapters 3 and 9.

Paroxysmal cold hemoglobinuria (PCH) is a hemolytic anemia that occurs suddenly and transiently when the individual is exposed to cold temperatures, resulting in free hemoglobin in the urine. PCH is the result of a cold antibody that lyses the erythrocytes in the blood stream (intravascular hemolysis), thus releasing free hemoglobin, which is evident by red plasma, dark urine, and a decrease in the free hemoglobin carrier protein, haptoglobin. Refer to Chapter 9.

Paroxysmal nocturnal hemoglobinuria (PNH) is a sudden or transient anemia from lysis of the erythrocytes (hemolysis) during the night with a dark-colored urine in the early morning. The hemolysis is caused by the increased sensitivity of erythrocytes to the plasma protein complement that lyses erythrocytes. The occurrence at night is due to acidification of the urine during the long hours of sleep, which enhances the hemolysis. Tests to diagnose PNH are the acidified serum test and the sugar water (Ham's) test. Refer to Chapter 9.

Partial thromboplastin time (PTT) test measures the intrinsic coagulation pathway to initially detect factor deficiencies, as seen in hemophilia, and circulating anticoagulants, such as the antiphospholipid antibodies (APAs). The specimen required is a blue-top sodium citrate tube that is full for a 9:1 blood:anticoagulant ratio, which is fresh, clear, and well mixed. Refer to Chapters 12 and 13.

Pathogens are any disease-producing organisms or substances.

"Patient oriented" means the laboratory protocols and decisons are made with the patient's best interest as a priority. Refer to Chapter 16.

Pelger-Huët anomaly is an inherited or acquired defect in nuclear segmentation of the granulocytes that results in hyposegmented granulocytes. This anomaly must be differentiated from a leukemoid reaction (response to bacterial infection) in which there is an increased number of band (immature hyposegmented) neutrophils in the peripheral blood. Refer to Chapter 3.

Pericardial fluid is the lubricating fluid between the serous membranes surrounding the heart in the pericardial cavity. Approximately 10 to 50 ml is normal, and it is clear, sterile, and cell free. Refer to Chapter 14.

Peritoneal (ascitic) fluid bathes the abdominal membranes to allow visceral organ movement without friction pain. In healthy individuals, less than 100 ml of clear, straw-colored fluid lines the peritoneum. Ascites refers to the abnormal effusion (exudate or transudate fluid) and accumulation of serous fluid in the abdomen. Refer to Chapter 14.

Pernicious anemia (PA) is a macrocytic (large erythrocytes) and megaloblastic (abnormal nuclear maturation) anemia due to vitamin B_{12} deficiency. In most cases, this is an autoimmune disorder. Refer to Chapter 9.

Personal protective equipment (PPE) includes any items such as gloves, goggles, and laboratory coats that are worn to protect an individual from safety hazards.

Petechia is a minute red spot due to the escape of blood from the blood vessel. This is the result of poor platelet function or decreased vascular integrity (blood vessel strength). These are the indicators of a positive result on a tourniquet test for vascular integrity. Refer to Chapters 11 and 13.

pH refers to the hydrogen ion (H^+) concentration of a fluid. The pH of blood (approximately 7.4) is determined by many factors, which include respiration and metabolism. If an individual is not breathing properly, if the person's lungs are not functioning properly, or if the person is having kidney problems or is not metabolizing glucose properly, the blood pH may be altered. A normal blood pH is 7.36 to 7.41 for venous blood and 7.38 to 7.44 for arterial blood.

Phagocytic cells are cells that engulf (ingest) cells, particles, or debris and digest them. The most efficient phagocytic cells are the macrophages of the body, such as the monocytes and histiocytes. Neutrophilic granulocytes are also phagocytic, but they mostly ingest bacteria. Refer to Chapters 3 and 4.

Phlebotomy literally means the cutting or wounding of a vein with a sharp instrument. In practice, phlebotomy is the entry of a vein with a needle to obtain blood. The art of phlebotomy requires specific knowledge of the blood vessel anatomy, equipment used, specific test requirements, and proper patient identification and personal relations, including communication and ethics. The phlebotomist is the laboratory's major contact with the public via patients, who are the clients, requiring accurate, ethical, and personal treatment. The accuracy of the specimen drawn is critical. If the correct specimen is not drawn on the correct individual, the laboratory results are meaningless. Refer to Chapter 1.

Plasma is the liquid portion of whole blood made up of 90% water, with the remaining 10% nutrients, minerals, and proteins. Plasma makes up 45% of the whole blood and appears straw colored and hazy due to the high concentration of protein fibrinogen, which is the largest protein molecule.

Plasma cell leukemia (PCL) is a rare abnormal proliferation of malignant plasma cells in the bone marrow. This is the only disorder in which plasma cells would be seen in the peripheral blood. Refer to Chapter 5.

Plasma cells are the transformed B lymphocytes, which are the most efficient antibody producers of the body. Plasma cells make up about 5% of the bone marrow nucleated cell population and are not seen in the peripheral blood unless the rare plasma cell leukemia is present. The most common malignancy associated with abnormal plasma cell proliferation is multiple myeloma. Refer to Chapter 5.

Plasma volume is the amount of plasma in the entire body that is measured by radioactive dilution to aid in the diagnosis of polycythemia (excessive erythrocytes). This test, along with the erythrocyte cell mass test, equals the total blood volume.

Platelet factor (PF) assays are tests to measure the PF3 and PF4 available for proper platelet function. PF3 assays are done using a clotting time methodology, and the PF4 is measured by radioimmunoassay. Refer to Chapter 13.

Platelet index (MPV or mean platelet volume) is a calculated index to provide the average size of the platelets in a specimen. The normal reference range for MPV is approximately 7 to 10 fl. MPVs above 10 fl indicate a release of immature platelets in response to use of all the mature platelets due to clotting in the body, an anomaly, or a disorder. Refer to Chapters 11 and 13.

Platelet phospholipid (PPL), also called platelet factor 3 (PF3), is required as a surface for intrinsic pathway blood clotting (coagulation) to take place. Another source of phospholipid for coagulation is tissue factor III of the extrinsic coagulation pathway. Refer to Chapters 11 and 12.

Platelet-poor plasma (PPP) is plasma that does not contain platelets and is used for the coagulation tests such as the prothrombin time (PT) and the partial thromboplastin time (PTT). PPP is made by centrifuging a tube of whole blood (usually the blue-top tube containing sodium citrate) at 2500 g for 15 minutes, which will remove the erythrocytes, leukocytes, and platelets. Platelets are removed for these tests to eliminate them as a variable affecting the result. The platelet phospholipid needed for the PTT test is added in the reagent, and the PT reagent is tissue phospholipid in factor III. Refer to Chapter 13.

Platelet-rich plasma (PRP) is plasma containing the platelets for platelet function tests such as aggregation, adhesion, and factor assays. PRP is made by centrifuging a tube of whole blood (usually the lavender-top tube containing EDTA) at 50 g for 5 minutes, which will remove the erythrocytes and leukocytes while leaving the platelets suspended. Refer to Chapter 13.

Pleural (effusion) fluid is the lubricant fluid that bathes the lungs and allows expansion without membrane friction. In healthy individuals there is less than 15 ml of fluid between serous membranes of the lungs and the thoracic (chest) cavity. In response to an infection, malignancy, or body fluid shift, more than 1500 ml can be accumulated. Refer to Chapter 14.

Pluripotent stem cells (PSCs) make up a significant percentage (approximately 10%) of the umbilical cord blood cells of a newborn and less than 1% of the blood cells of an adult. The PSCs of the body are the earliest, undifferentiated progenitor cells from which all cells originate. When stimulated by hematopoietic factors, this cell becomes the hematopoietic stem cell (HSC), which is destined to become one of the blood cells of the body. Refer to Chapter 2.

Poikilocytosis describes the presence of abnormally shaped erythrocytes in a blood specimen. This general term is not as useful as a description of the specific abnormal shapes. The presence of poikilocytosis may be correlated with the RDW and MCV indices. Refer to Chapter 9.

Point of care testing (POCT) is testing being done at the patient's bedside, in doctor's offices, or in patients' homes (wherever the care is taking place). The laboratory practitioner must be prepared to work and communicate with other health care professionals in order to deliver the best health care. Refer to Chapter 16.

Polychromatophilic normoblast is an immature nucleated erythrocyte found in the bone marrow. Polychrome literally means many colors, due to the first visible synthesis of hemoglobin changing the cytoplasmic color from the blue of primarily RNA to a mixture of red hemoglobin and RNA producing a gray-blue color. Refer to Chapter 7.

Polychrome (Romanowsky) stain is a polychrome (many color) stain, such as Wright-Giemsa (see Fig. 1–22), used to examine blood specimen slides. This stain requires the cells to be fixed with methanol followed by a basic methylene blue stain and then counterstained with an acid eosin stain. By using more than one color stain, the various cell components will be visible for microscopic evaluation. Refer to Chapter 1.

Polyclonal response literally means many clones in the response resulting in the production of many antibodies in a normal immune response. Many antibodies are produced due to the development of many clones, which are identical cells all derived from one parent cell in response to this one foreign substance. Each clone produces an antibody to a different antigen on the foreign substance, so that many antibodies are produced in a normal infection. A polyclonal response to disease is necessary to eliminate the invading substance (e.g., bacteria) from the body. This is in contrast to a monoclonal response that involves only one clone of cells producing only one antibody. Refer to Chapter 5.

Polycythemia is an increase in red blood cell mass, elevated hematocrit test, and hemoglobin test values due to excessive production of erythrocytes (erythropoiesis). This proliferation of erythrocytes can be a benign response to a lack of oxygen or a malignant process that requires rigorous treatment. The hematocrit can reach 80% (reference is less than 54%), which is life threatening due to the inability of the heart to pump such viscous blood. If this increase in erythrocytes is due to polycythemia vera, which involves all of the bone marrow derived cells, the white blood cell count will be elevated and the thrombocyte count is often greater than 1000×10^9/l. Absolute benign polycythemia is the production of red blood cells in response to increased erythropoietin (EPO) levels due to a decreased supply of oxygen (hypoxia) from the lungs to the tissues. This occurs in smokers, in emphysema, and at high altitudes, all of which do not allow an adequate amount of oxygen to be transported from the lungs to the tissues. The body compensates by producing more cells in order to carry more oxygen. Refer to Chapter 9.

Porphyria is a hereditary inability to synthesize adequate heme for hemoglobin production. Tests to aid in the diagnosis of porphyria are elevated levels of alpha aminolevulinic acid (ALA) in a 24-hour urine, and an increase in free erythrocyte protoporphyrin (FEP). The urine of these individuals may appear dark. Refer to Chapters 8 and 9.

Posthemorrhagic anemia is anemia due to the loss of blood, which can be acute or chronic. An acute loss is loss of a large volume of blood over a short period of time. The characteristics are decreased blood volume (hypovolemia) and a low thrombocyte (platelet) count due to the activation and use of platelets. The platelet count will become elevated as the bone marrow responds, and there will be a neutrophilic leukocytosis with a slight left shift. The reticulocyte count will be normal due to the lack of time for the bone marrow to respond, and the erythrocytes will be normocytic and normochromic. Chronic posthemorrhagic anemia is a slow loss of blood with stress reticulocytes that are macrocytic and polychromatic (large and blue), an increased reticulocyte count, and possibly iron-deficient erythrocytes that are microcytic and hypochromic (small and pale) depending on the length of the anemia and the diet of the patient. Refer to Chapter 9.

Precision is demonstrated in the ability to duplicate results. Every test in the clinical laboratory must be performed more than once, and the same value must be attained each time in order to ensure the precision of the testing. If the value varies significantly each time that the test is performed, the values are meaningless for the patient's diagnosis or treatment.

Prednisone is a steroid drug that destroys lymphocytes (lymphocytotoxic) and thus inhibits the production of antibodies by the B lymphocytes. This is necessary in autoimmune disorders in which high levels of abnormal antibodies are produced, resulting in anemia, thrombocytopenia, or other life-threatening or painful outcomes. A complication of this therapy is the inability to produce normal healthy antibodies when needed to fight infection.

Primary immune response occurs after the first stimulation of the immune system with a foreign antigen. This antibody response takes several days after exposure to an antigen due to the need for a macrophage to phagocytize the antigen, process the antigen, and then pass this information on to the CD4 lymphocyte to initiate the primary immune response with the first production of antibodies specific for each specific antigen. Among the cells produced in a primary immune response are the T and B lymphocyte memory cells. The T and B memory cells remain in the body for years and have the ability to respond immediately to the antigen that it was produced against in the first antigen exposure. Upon a second exposure to the same antigen, the T and B memory cells will immediately respond and stimulate other cells to provide a rapid secondary immune response with a high titer of antibody produced. This is the mechanism for protection by a vaccination. Refer to Chapter 5.

Primary lymphoid organs are the thymus and bone marrow (bursa equivalent), which influence the lymphoblast to become a competent T or B cell. The T and B lymphocytes circulate within blood and the secondary lymphoid tissue, which include the spleen, lymph nodes, intestine-associated lymphoid tissue (Peyer's patches), and tonsils. The secondary lymphoid organs contain localized areas of T cells and B cells. The spleen also contains an abundance of macrophages. Refer to Chapter 5.

Proficiency testing (PT) is the term for outside agencies providing specimens with known values to be analyzed in the laboratory. Some agencies providing and evaluating PT are the state board of health and the College of American Pathologists (CAP). Refer to Chapters 1 and 16.

Progenitor cells are self-renewing cells for each cell line. The myeloid progenitor cell is committed to increasing the number of the cells in the myeloid hematopoietic cell line. The lymphoid progenitor cell is committed to increasing the cells in the lymphoid cell line. Refer to Chapter 2.

Prognosis is a prediction of the possible course and outcome of a disorder. Malignant (life-threatening) disorders such as cancer may have a poor prognosis. Benign (not life-threatening) disorders such as ovarian cysts have a good prognosis.

Proliferation is the division and multiplication of cells in order to produce more of the cells that are stimulated.

Promyelocyte is the granulocytic precursor cell between the myeloblast and the myelocyte characterized by its large size and prominent nonspecific (peroxidase) granules. Smaller peroxidase-positive granules are found in all granulocytes in addition to the specific neutrophilic, eosinophilic, or basophilic granules produced in the next stage of maturation. Excessive degranulation of promyelocytic granules, as seen in acute promyelocyte leukemia (FAB M3), can cause a disseminated intravascular coagulation (DIC) that can be life threatening. Refer to Chapter 3.

Pronormoblast is an early erythrocyte precursor cell in the bone marrow. Refer to Chapter 7.

Prothrombin time (PT) test evaluates the extrinsic coagulation pathway and monitors warfarin (Coumadin) oral anticoagulant therapy. The specimen of choice for this test is the sodium citrate (Na citrate, blue top) blood collection tube, which is full of fresh, clear blood that has been well mixed. It is important that the tube be full to ensure a 9:1 (blood:anticoagulant) ratio. Less blood in the tube results in excess anticoagulant, which will prolong the PT erroneously. The PT reference value is approximately 11 to 13 seconds as an observed result. The PT observed time is converted to an international normalized ratio (INR) before a report is given to the primary care provider. The INR is a calculation that includes the manufacturer's value for reagent activity. This allows a standardized method of evaluating PT results in terms of diagnosis and monitoring anticoagulant therapy. The INR reference range is less than 2.0. Refer to Chapter 13.

Proto-oncogene is a normal gene that, when altered, becomes an abnormal cancerous gene called an oncogene.

Prussian blue stain is a nonvital monochrome stain used to detect nonhemoglobin iron present in red blood cells and storage iron present in the histiocytes. Refer to Chapter 10.

Pure cutaneous histiocytosis is one of the original histiocytosis X proliferative histiocyte disorders. These diseases demonstrate a "foamy" cell in bone granulomas and are often found in young children who have a very short time of survival. Refer to Chapter 4.

Purpura is a purplish or red-brown discoloration in patches due to seepage of blood under the skin and into the tissues. It is common in the geriatric population. Refer to Chapter 11.

Pus is the visible accumulation of white blood cells as a result of chemotaxis and migration of leukocytes (PMN's) to the site of infection. This migration of leukocytes is initiated by chemotactants such as lipopolysaccharide (LPS) fragments of bacterial cell walls, various cytokines, and a variety of inflammatory proteins. Refer to Chapter 3.

Quality assurance (QA) is an all-encompassing term for addressing the accuracy, precision, and correlation of laboratory results as well as the overall application of quality to the personnel, environment, equipment, supplies, procedures, data presentation, data interpretation, and personal relations. QA is addressed and administered by the entire laboratory from the bench technician to the laboratory manager. Refer to Chapter 1.

Quality control (QC) testing, procedures, and calculations are done to determine if the values generated from known testing control material fall within acceptable limits and that the random patient values are accurate. The quality control calculations are used to assess the variation in values and the distribution of values within a laboratory. A Levey-Jennings quality control graph is used to plot and monitor laboratory QC results. Refer to Chapter 1.

Quality control calculations include the mean ($\bar{x}$) or average value within a population. The variance (s^2) and the standard deviation (SD or s) are the two most common measures of dispersion of results that provide more information than does the range of values. The coefficient of variation (CV) allows the comparison of variance and standard deviation with consideration of the mean. These calculations allow the laboratory to record on a graph the values pertinent to precise and accurate test results. If the values are rising, falling, or erratic, steps can be taken to correct the problem with the procedure, reagents, instruments, or individual performing the test before the laboratory produces erroneous results. These values are also information required to determine each laboratory's own reference ranges as well as when calculating the additional quality assurance values. The average value for a test at one hospital or clinical laboratory may be different from those at another. The values generated by one clinical laboratory facility are only relevant to the population serviced by that specific facility. Numbers mean nothing if there is no relevant point of reference. Refer to Chapter 1.

RDW is the red blood cell distribution width, which is an erythrocyte index providing the percentage of cells outside the normal size range (80 to 95 fl), or in other words, providing insight into the uniformity of the erythrocyte population. The RDW reference range is approximately 11.5 to 14.5%. The RDW provides additional information when used with the MCV, which is an average. If the erythrocytes range from small to large, the MCV will present a normal average cell volume. Refer to Chapters 9 and 10.

Radial immunodiffusion (RID) is an immunoassay (antigen-antibody reaction) using precipitation as the indicator of presence and quantity of the unknown patient antigen (or antibody) of interest. As the antigen diffuses in a circle from the central well of application through the medium, it becomes more dilute. At the point where the

concentration of antigen and the concentration of antibody in the gel are optimal (zone of equivalence, optimal concentrations), insoluble complexes form that are visible precipitation. The diameter of the precipitation ring is proportional to the amount of unknown antigen (or protein) of interest in the patient's serum. Refer to Chapter 6.

Radioimmunoassay (RIA) is an immunoassay (antigen-antibody reaction) using radioisotopes as an indicator of the presence and quantity of the patient's unknown antigen (or antibody) of interest. Refer to Chapter 6.

Random distribution refers to the distribution of cells and proteins undergoing testing in the laboratory and reflects a random, unbiased indication of the status within the patient's body (in vivo). The random distribution of the specimen collected from the patient is essential for precise and accurate test results. A liquid specimen must be well mixed; a cellular sample must be evenly distributed to ensure evaluation of the sample as a whole and not just one portion that is not representative or that is a reflection of poor specimen or patient preparation. Corrections must be made in procedures if a random distribution is not observed. Examples include adequately mixing a tube of blood before testing for a complete blood count; or counting all nine squares on the hemocytometer when a manual cell count is very low, as seen in body fluid counts, in order to get an accurate assessment of the cells present in the patient. Refer to Chapter 6.

Reactive lymphocyte refers to a normal healthy lymphocyte that is responding to a foreign antigen by proliferating and producing cytokines or antibodies, which is a benign cellular response. Reactive lymphocytes become large; the nucleus has an immature active appearance (euchromatin) and may have nucleoli; and the cytoplasm becomes more abundant and dark blue. The large immature nucleus is associated with cell division and proliferation. The dark blue cytoplasm indicates protein synthesis, and a clearing near the nucleus (Hof area or perinuclear halo) indicates an active Golgi apparatus preparing the proteins for secretion. Additional terms used to identify this cell are atypical lymphocyte, Turk cell, and Downey cell. The most common reasons for reactive lymphocytosis are viral infections. Refer to Chapter 5.

Reactive monocytosis ($>1.0 \times 10^9$/l monocytes) is a normal response of monocytes to infection and disease; however, this response may indicate either a good or poor prognosis (expected outcome). Monocytosis in the recovery phase of acute infection is a good sign (good prognosis). Monocytosis seen in association with tuberculosis indicates a poor prognosis for recovery. Refer to Chapter 4.

Reactive thrombocytosis is the normal response

to use of all circulating thrombocytes and increased production of thrombocyte growth factors by increased bone marrow release and production of thrombocytes to meet the body's need to stop bleeding. The bone marrow will release the larger, less mature thrombocytes if necessary. Causes of increased use of thrombocytes are hemorrhage, trauma, surgery, malignancy, chronic infections, chronic iron deficiency, and connective tissue disease (e.g., rheumatoid arthritis). Refer to Chapter 11.

Red cell distribution width (RDW) is an erythrocyte index providing the percentage of cells outside the normal size range (80 to 95 fl) or, in other words, providing insight into the uniformity of the erythrocyte population. The RDW reference range is approximately 11.5 to 14.5%. The RDW provides additional information when used with the MCV, which is an average. If the erythrocytes range from small to large, the MCV will present a normal average cell volume. Refer to Chapter 10.

Red cell mass is a radioisotope dilution test used to accurately determine the proportional mass of erythrocytes in the blood as suspended in the plasma. An aliquot of the patient's cells are tagged with radioisotope and placed back into the individual to be allowed to circulate, then an aliquot is redrawn and the amount of dilution of the radioisotope provides information regarding the total erythrocyte mass. This test and the plasma volume test provide total blood volume information. Refer to Chapter 10.

Red cell survival refers to a test to determine if the life span of the erythrocytes is shortened. This is not a common test and requires the collection of an aliquot of the patient's cells that are tagged with radioisotope and placed back into the individual to be monitored, via urine excretion of the radioisotope, for the tagged cell destruction. Refer to Chapter 10.

Red marrow is the active bone marrow engaged in the production of blood cells (hematopoiesis). Red marrow appears red in the bone and fills 90% of the bone marrow of the newborn baby's body, demonstrating active production of blood cells. Over time, the demand for hematopoiesis decreases, and the bone marrow of the long bones becomes white marrow (replaced with fat cells), which does not produce blood cells. The red marrow of the adult exists primarily in the large flat bones of the body, and at age 20 approximately 60% of the bone marrow is actively producing cells as red marrow. By age 65 approximately only 40% of the bone marrow is still actively producing blood cells.

Reference values are values for each test done in the laboratory. These values are established as the normal range for a specific population (e.g., adults, children) as performed within a specific laboratory to aid in the interpretation of a patient's value as being normal or abnormal. Refer to Chapters 1 and 16.

Relative anemia is an increase of fluid in the blood, not a decrease in erythrocytes; thus, this is not a true anemia. The increase in fluid in the blood stream may be due to pregnancy, intravenous fluid dilution, liver cirrhosis (damage from alcohol consumption), or nephritis (kidney inflammation). The reticulocyte count is normal (<1.5%), and the erythrocytes are normocytic, normochromic. Refer to Chapter 9.

Relative values are test values that erroneously appear abnormal or normal due to a change in the relationship to other components. In other words, the relative value has not changed in actual amount but appears to have increased or decreased due to a change in another component related to the original one. An example is a dehydrated patient who appears to have excess cells in his or her blood, when in fact the number of cells is normal but the fluid level has decreased, resulting in the concentration of the cells present. Once the fluid level is restored, the cell count will be normal. Compare this with an absolute test result that reflects the true test value. Another example is the percentage of lymphocytes relative to the other cells present in the specimen. If the number of neutrophils decreases, the number of lymphocytes will appear to increase relatively.

Reticulocyte count is an estimate of the number of reticulocytes (immature erythrocytes) in the peripheral blood, which is the best indicator of bone marrow function. The reference range for an observed reticulocyte count is 0.5 to 1.5% of the erythrocytes. If anemia is present, the bone marrow should respond by releasing reticulocytes that can carry oxygen although they are not quite mature. Other calculations for the reticulocyte count are the absolute count, the corrected reticulocyte count, and the reticulocyte production index (RPI). Refer to Chapters 11 and 13.

Reticuloendothelial system (RES) is the old name for the monocyte/macrophage system, which is made up of large phagocytic cells that are assigned different names depending on where they are located in the body. In the bone marrow they are histiocytes; liver cells are Kupffer cells; the brain macrophages are termed microglial cells; osteoclasts are called bone macrophage cells; Langerhans cells are skin macrophages; and the monocyte is the peripheral blood macrophage. The macrophage cells are not only the most efficient phagocytes of the body defense system but they also store iron and have the ability to process phagocytized antigen and present this antigen to the CD4 lymphocyte for an efficient and effective initiation of a primary immune response. Refer to Chapter 4.

Rheumatoid arthritis (RA) is an autoimmune disorder characterized by deposition of antigen-antibody complexes that stimulate chronic inflammation, degeneration, or metabolic derangement of the connective tissue structures, especially in the joints, resulting in pain, stiffness, limitation of movement, and joint disfiguration. The production of the antibody directed against connective tissue (rheumatoid factor [RF]) inhibits the production of normal proteins, may opsonize the erythrocytes for phagocytosis resulting in anemia, and interferes with normal body function such as coagulation. Latex agglutination tests are available to detect RF, and the erythrocyte sedimentation rate (ESR) will be elevated. Refer to Chapter 9.

Ringed sideroblasts are nucleated erythrocytes in the bone marrow with a ring of iron granules around the nucleus due to the inappropriate utilization of the iron that they contain for hemoglobin synthesis. This is associated with sideroblastic anemia and myelodysplastic syndrome (MDS). Refer to Chapters 7 and 9.

Sandhoff's disease is a lipid storage disease caused by a genetic lack of hexosaminidase A and B enzymes necessary for lipid catabolism. The build-up of lipids in the cells of the body interferes with body function and may be fatal. Refer to Chapter 4.

Scattergram is the name of the diagram produced from the characteristic light scatter of each cell as it passes through the automated cell counting instruments as part of the automated differential information. Refer to Chapter 6.

Sea-blue histiocytosis is a lipid storage disease that is caused by a genetic lack of a specific enzyme necessary for lipid catabolism. A specific enzyme deficiency in this case has not been found consistently, although low sphingomyelinase has been documented in some cases. The build-up of lipids in the cells of the body interferes with body function and may be fatal. Refer to Chapter 4.

Secondary immune response to foreign antigen involves the response of the T and B lymphocyte memory cells upon second exposure to the same antigen. The memory cells remain in the body for years, and they have the ability to respond immediately to a subsequent exposure to the antigen that it was produced against in the first antigen exposure (primary immune response). Upon a second exposure to the same antigen, the memory cells immediately respond and stimulate other cells to provide a rapid secondary immune response with a high titer of antibody produced. This is the mechanism for protection by a vaccine. Refer to Chapter 5.

Segmented eosinophil (Eo) is the mature cell derived from the colony-forming unit–eosinophil (CFU-Eo). The eosinophil is involved in hypersensitivity reactions and is seen in association with allergies, colds, and parasitic infections. The eosinophil is discussed in detail in Chapter 3.

Segmented neutrophilic granulocyte (seg), also called the polymorphonuclear (PMN or poly) cell, is the mature cell derived from the colony-forming unit–granulocyte (CFU-G) cell. This cell contains digestive granules in the cytoplasm and phagocytizes primarily bacteria. An increased neutrophil count and band cell count in response to a bacterial infection is called a leukemoid reaction. The seg makes up approximately 60% of the white blood cells peripheral blood in a normal, healthy individual. This cell is discussed in detail in Chapter 3.

Self-healing histiocytosis is one of the original histiocytosis X diseases, which are proliferative histiocyte disorders. This disease demonstrates a "foamy" cell in bone granulomas and is often found in young children. Refer to Chapter 4.

Seminal fluid, or semen, is a viscous fluid produced by the prostate, the testes, the epididymis, the seminal vesicles, and the bulbourethral gland. It is used to transport spermatozoa (sperm cells). The sperm present are counted and analyzed for motility, viability, and morphology. The fluid portion may be analyzed for viscosity, fructose value, acid phosphatase activity, citric acid levels, and zinc values. Refer to Chapters 14 and 15.

Serotonin is a hormone and neurotransmitter produced by many tissues (including platelets) that induces vasoconstriction (tightening of the blood vessels), stimulation of smooth muscle, and inhibition of gastric secretion. Refer to Chapter 11.

Serous fluids, such as pleural fluid, pericardial fluid, and peritoneal (ascites) fluid, exist between two thin mesothelium-lined membranes, which are referred to as serous membranes. If the serous fluid accumulates abnormally, it is called an effusion. The various mechanisms for accumulation of serous effusions include infections and tumors that produce exudative (high protein, cellular, secreted) effusions or cardiac failure that produces a transudative (thin, watery, cell free, shift of fluid) effusion. Refer to Chapter 14.

Serum is the liquid portion of clotted or coagulated blood. The color is pale yellow and clear due to the absence of coagulation proteins such as fibrinogen, which is converted to fibrin in the clot.

Serum ferritin is an iron-apoferritin complex that is a storage form of iron, and is the best indicator of the body's storage level. Refer to Chapters 8 and 10.

Serum iron is measured to contribute information concerning the body's iron level; however, the serum levels of iron vary depending on diet and other variables. Refer to Chapters 8 and 10.

Serum lactate dehydrogenase (LD or LDH) is

a group of isoenzymes found in various cells of the body and in the plasma. When cells are damaged, LDH is released. LDH can be measured to indicate which cells are damaged and how much damage has occurred. The isoenzymes are LD-1 through LD-5 (also called LDH_1 through LDH_5) and are found in cardiac (heart) cells, renal (kidney) cells, and erythrocytes. Excessive erythrocyte death releases LD; thus, an increase in LD is associated with hemolysis. The hemolysis-associated increase in LD may be considered part of the diagnosis in vitamin B_{12} and folate deficiencies. Refer to Chapter 9.

Serum transferrin is a protein that binds to and transports iron (Fe) to the bone marrow for use in new erythrocyte hemoglobin synthesis or to the bone marrow histiocytes for storage until needed. Free Fe would pass through the kidney and be lost for use in the body. A normal reference range for serum transferrin is approximately 240 to 480 mg/dl. Refer to Chapters 8 and 10.

Sézary syndrome is a T lymphocyte lymphoma that primarily involves the skin. Sézary syndrome is similar to mycosis fungoides and T cell lymphoma, both of which are found in older individuals and are usually discovered at the time of organ infiltration, when the person has a prognosis of several months. The Sézary cell is a large or small lymphocyte with folded or indented nuclei and prominent nucleoli. Refer to Chapter 5.

"Shift to the left" refers to an increase of immature, usually band, cells in the peripheral blood. This is seen most often in the neutrophil's response to a bacterial infection (leukemoid reaction) with the appearance of the band cells. Refer to Chapter 3.

Shilling urinary excretion test is a test to determine the ability of the stomach to absorb vitamin B_{12} for the diagnosis of vitamin B_{12} deficiency, which was previously called pernicious anemia (PA). This test is not often done and requires the individual to drink vitamin B_{12} tagged with radioisotope. Refer to Chapters 9 and 10.

Sickle cell hemoglobin trait and disease are genetic hemoglobin abnormalities (hemoglobinopathies) involving the production of hemoglobin S instead of hemoglobin A. Hemoglobinopathies are confirmed by hemoglobin electrophoresis. Refer to Chapters 8 to 10.

Sideroblastic anemia is a hypochromic, and often microcytic, anemia caused by the inability of the erythrocytes to utilize the iron for hemoglobin synthesis, resulting in ringed sideroblasts in the bone marrow, iron (siderotic) granules in the erythrocytes with iron stain, and Pappenheimer bodies with Wright-Giemsa stain. Refer to Chapter 9.

Sizes of the formed elements of the blood are important for data interpretation:

thrombocytes = 2–4 μm
erythrocytes = 6–8 μm
lymphocytes = 8–10 μm
basophils = 8–10 μm
neutrophils = 10–12 μm
eosinophils = 10–15 μm
monocytes = 10–15 μm

Specimen (plural specimens) is a small sample or aliquot of the whole organism (patient) for the purpose of identification and evaluation of the whole patient for prevention, diagnosis, and treatment of disease. Examples are urine, blood, and tissue fluids, and biopsies are used to determine the status of the individual from which the specimen was taken.

Spherocytic refers to erythrocytes that have lost their biconcave shape and become swollen and round, thus predisposing them to be destroyed (hemolysis). Hereditary spherocytosis results in intravascular hemolysis, and spherocytes can be a product of extravascular hemolysis. Spherocytes are uniformly dark red and round.

Standard deviation (SD or s) is a quality assurance calculation to measure the imprecision of analytical results. The calculation is the square root of the variance. Refer to Chapter 1.

$$SD = s = \sqrt{\frac{\Sigma(\bar{x} - x)^2}{n - 1}}$$
$$= \sqrt{\frac{\text{sum of (mean} - \text{the score})^2}{\text{number of determinations} - 1}}$$

Storage pool disease (gray platelet syndrome) or thrombocyte storage pool disease is a rare disease characterized by defective secondary aggregation due to the lack of granules and their contents. Refer to Chapter 11.

Storage pools of cells are located in the bone marrow, where a reserve of mature and less mature, but functional, cells is available when an additional demand is made on the body. Slightly immature cells will also be released into the peripheral blood stream if the need is great enough: This is called a "left shift." Refer to Chapters 2 and 3.

Sucrose hemolysis test is a test of erythrocyte sensitivity to lysis that is used to diagnose anemia, such as paroxysmal cold hemoglobinuria (PCH). Similar tests include the sugar water test and the acidified serum test (Ham's test). Refer to Chapters 9 and 10.

Sugar water test is a test of erythrocyte sensitivity to lysis used to diagnose anemia, such as paroxysmal cold hemoglobinuria (PCH). Similar tests include the sucrose hemolysis test and the acidified serum test (Ham's test). Refer to Chapters 9 and 10.

Sulfhemoglobin (HbS), or sulfmethemoglobin, is hemoglobin chemically modified (unable to transport oxygen) due to irreversible oxidation by certain drugs and chemicals such as sulfonamides. An individual with a significant amount of HbS will suffer from hypoxia and anemia. Refer to Chapters 8 and 9.

Synovial fluid is a small amount of fluid that is normally found in the joints as lubrication. This fluid may accumulate abnormally in the body during time of disease. The abnormal accumulation is the result of ultrafiltration of plasma across the synovial membrane and from secretion by synoviocytes. Synovial fluid is a viscous lubricant for the joints and has a unique composition. Normal synovial fluid is pale yellow or colorless and clear. Identification of crystals unique to this fluid will aid in diagnosis. Refer to Chapter 14.

Systemic refers to the entire body. A systemic infection is in the blood stream and involves the entire body compared with a local infection, which is confined to one area of the body.

T helper (CD4) lymphocyte is the key cell that orchestrates an immune response to foreign organisms or toxic substances (antigens), resulting in lymphocyte proliferation, cell-mediated immunity (production of cytokines and physical lysis of foreign cells), and humoral immunity (production of antibodies). This is the cell in which the human immunodeficiency virus (HIV) resides in order to produce the acquired immunodeficiency syndrome (AIDS). Refer to Chapter 5.

T lymphocyte is a mature cell developed from the lymphocyte stem cell (LSC) in the thymus gland. The T cell is responsible for the cell-mediated immunity (CMI) in an immune response. There are subsets of T cells with different functions. The T cell responsible for amplifying the immune response is called the CD4 cell due to the presence of the cluster differentiation marker no. 4 protein on the cell surface. The T cell responsible for suppressing and controlling the immune response as well as physically destroying abnormal cells is called the CD8 cell due to the presence of the CD8 protein marker on its cell membrane. The ratio of CD4:CD8 cells is normally 2:1. The T lymphocytic cell makes up approximately 80% of the peripheral blood lymphocytes. T memory cells remain in the body for years and have the ability to respond immediately to the same antigen. Refer to Chapter 5.

T memory cells are among the cells produced in response to antigenic stimulation of the immune system. The T memory cells remain in the body for years and have the ability to respond immediately to the antigen that it was produced against in the first antigen exposure (primary immune response; see Fig. 5–4). Upon a second exposure to the same antigen, the T memory cells will immediately respond and stimulate other cells to provide a rapid secondary immune response with high titer of antibody produced. Refer to Chapter 5.

Tay-Sachs is a lipid storage disease due to a genetic lack of hexosaminidase-A enzyme, which is necessary for lipid catabolism. Refer to Chapter 4.

Telangiectasia is a hereditary vascular lesion formed by dilation of a group of small blood vessels. Individuals with hereditary telangiectasia are subject to recurrent episodes of bleeding. The formation of telangiectasia demonstrates a loss of vascular integrity. Refer to Chapter 11.

Temperature is an important factor in laboratory testing as well as in body maintenance. The body temperature of 37° C is the temperature at which metabolism is quite rapid to meet the needs and demands of the body. When blood is drawn from the body, the metabolism of the cells will continue in the test tube. If the specimen will not be tested in a relatively short period of time, it should be refrigerated. The lower temperature (4° C) will slow down the metabolism and component degradation, which will keep the blood as close to the in vivo state as possible. A few special tests require the blood to be placed on ice immediately or kept warm (37° C) until testing. Most test protocols specify room temperature (25° C) for testing. If the test is done at an inappropriate temperature, the results will not be accurate. If blood is heated above 56° C, the cells will lyse and be destroyed. If blood is subjected to temperatures lower than 4° C, freezing and lysing of the cells may occur.

Terminology in the clinical laboratory is a language of its own. Here are some stems, prefixes, and suffixes used in medical terminology:

a = without	micro = small
blast = young, nucleated	myelo = marrow
cyte = cell	normo = normal
chromatic, chromic = color	oid = like
	osis = increase
dys = abnormal	penia = decrease
emia = blood	plasia = formation
hyper = more, increased	poiesis = cell production
hypo = less, decreased	poly = many
iso = equal to, same as	pro = before, previous
lympho = of the lymph	sidero/side/ferro = iron
macro = large	uria = urine
mega = large	

Thalassemia disease or trait is a hereditary decreased production of one of the globin chains needed to form the hemoglobin molecule, which results in anemia. The most severe form, α-thalassemia major, is more common in individuals of Mediterranean descent, (e.g., Italians) and demonstrates target cells, microcytic erythrocytes, and hypochromic erythrocytes. Testing for a normal iron level and an elevated hemoglobin A_2 on hemoglobin electrophoresis is recommended for the differential diagnosis. Refer to Chapters 8 to 10.

Thrombasthenia is a genetic absence of the

thrombasthenin contractile protein in thrombocytes (platelets) necessary for primary aggregation, resulting in abnormal clot retraction. Refer to Chapters 11 and 13.

Thrombin time (TT) test is a coagulation test that contributes to an evaluation of the common coagulation pathway of hemostasis. The production of thrombin (coagulation factor II) from the precursor prothrombin is measured. The specimen of choice is a full, well-mixed sodium citrate (blue-top tube) of blood containing clear, fresh plasma. Refer to Chapters 12 and 13.

Thrombocyte-aggregating agents stimulate the aggregation of platelets and are used as reagents for the testing of platelet aggregation. The most common aggregating agents are ADP, epinephrine, collagen, thrombin, ristocetin, and arachidonic acid. Substances such as heparin, alcohol, aspirin, radiographic contrast agents, and dextrans inhibit platelet aggregation and factor release. Refer to Chapter 13.

Thrombocyte function tests include the bleeding time test, the clot retraction, the platelet glass bead adhesion test, and aggregation studies. Drugs and substances such as heparin, alcohol, aspirin, radiographic contrast agents, and dextrans inhibit platelet aggregation and factor release. Refer to Chapters 11 and 13.

Thrombocyte storage pool disease (gray platelet disease) is a rare disease characterized by defective secondary aggregation of the thrombocytes due to the lack of granules and their contents. Refer to Chapter 11.

Thrombocytes (platelets) are cytoplasmic fragments of a cell in the bone marrow. These fragments are responsible for the initial arrest of bleeding by forming a plug at the site of the injured blood vessel. Mature thrombocytes are 2 to 4 μm in size, number 150 to 400 $\times$ 10^9/l, and demonstrate a gray-blue cytoplasm containing purple functional granules. Platelet factors (PF) are required for normal blood clotting. Refer to Chapter 11.

Thrombocythemia, also called essential thrombocythemia, is uncontrolled megakaryocyte and platelet production. Refer to Chapter 11.

Thrombocytopenia is a decrease in the number of thrombocytes (platelets) in the peripheral blood. This may be due to decreased production of thrombocytes or increased consumption of thrombocytes in clots being formed in the body, or it could be due to the thrombocytes being destroyed after being released from the bone marrow into the peripheral blood by autoimmune antibodies that mark them for destruction by the macrophages. Examples of disorders involving thrombocytopenia are thrombotic thrombocytopenic purpura (TTP), idiopathic thrombocytopenic purpura (ITP), disseminated intravascular coagulation (DIC), and decreased bone marrow

production. Thrombocytopenia is defined by a count of less than 100 $\times$ 10^9/l of blood. Refer to Chapter 11.

Thrombocytosis is the excessive production of thrombocytes as seen in a normal response to bleeding or as a result of a myeloproliferative disease. Refer to Chapter 11.

Thrombotic coagulopathy describes abnormal coagulation producing thrombi (blood clots). Refer to Chapter 11.

Thrombotic thrombocytopenic purpura (TTP) is a thrombocytopenia or decrease in platelets due to the formation of thrombi (blood clots). The erythrocytes are torn passing through the clots and form irregular erythrocyte pieces called schistocytes. Refer to Chapter 11.

Thrombus (pleural thrombi), also called a blood clot, is the result of blood coagulation. If thrombi form at a break in the blood vessel, they can be beneficial by stopping the loss of blood from the body. If thrombi form within the blood vessels and block the flow of blood to the body tissue, as seen in a stroke or heart attack, the tissue that is deprived of oxygen will necrose (die), which is life threatening. If a piece of the thrombus breaks off and travels to the lung, or other organs, where it blocks flow to the lung tissue (which is also life threatening), it is called a thromboembolism. Refer to Chapter 12.

Thromboxane A$_2$ is synthesized by platelets and functions to stimulate blood vessel vasoconstriction, platelet aggregation, and factor release. Refer to Chapter 11.

Thymus gland is a primary lymphoid organ that is located in the chest just above the heart where it produces competent T lymphocytes. Refer to Chapter 5.

Total iron-binding capacity (TIBC) test measures the transferrin that is not bound to iron (Fe) in order to determine the Fe level in the body. The opposite of this is the transferrin saturation test, which is the serum Fe divided by the TIBC. Refer to Chapters 8 to 10.

Total quality management (TQM) involves the administration of all of the quality assurance (QA) concepts, such as quality control (QC) and continuous quality improvement (CQI), which is usually the responsibility of the laboratory manager or an assigned quality management officer, as well as enforcing and monitoring the safety concepts. Refer to Chapters 1 and 16.

Tourniquet is a device, usually a band, tied around the area from which venous blood will be drawn or an intravenous line must be started, to stop the flow of blood. This action increases the prominence of the veins. Refer to Chapter 1.

Toxic granulation is prominent granulation visible in the cytoplasm of neutrophils in association with a neutrophil response to bacterial infection (leukemoid reaction). Also associated with toxic granulation are phagocytic vacuolation, cytoplasmic blue patches of RNA (Döhle bodies), and an increased number of slightly immature neutrophils (band cells), which is called a "shift to the left." Refer to Chapter 3.

Transferrin is a protein that binds and transports iron (Fe) to the bone marrow for use in new erythrocyte hemoglobin synthesis or to the bone marrow histiocytes for storage until needed. Free Fe would pass through the kidney and be lost for use in the body. A normal reference range for serum transferrin is approximately 240 to 480 mg/dl. Refer to Chapter 10.

Transferrin saturation (% Sat) is a test to evaluate the body's store of iron by dividing the serum iron level by the total iron-binding capacity (TIBC) of transferrin. Reference values are greater than or equal to 16%. Refer to Chapter 10.

Transudates are clear, colorless, and watery abnormal collections of fluid (effusions) in the body, due to decreased osmotic pressure and increased hydrostatic pressure. The specific gravity is less than 1.015, and the total protein is less than 3 g/dl. The leukocyte count is less than 100 × 10^9/l with more than 50% mononuclear. Fluid formation is a dynamic process, and the physician needs to know if the effusion is a transudate (shift in body fluid pressures) or an exudate, which is a much different secreted fluid caused by infection or cancer. Refer to Chapters 14 and 15.

Tumor necrosis factor (TNF) is a cytokine produced by lymphocytes and is detrimental to tumor cells. TNF also has other physiologic properties and is produced by other cells. Refer to Chapter 5.

Turbidimetric immunoprecipitin assay is a method of identifying and quantitating a protein of interest by use of the corresponding antigen or antibody. The greater the amount of antigen-antibody complexes, the more light is absorbed, which is related to the quantity. Nephelometric immunoprecipitin assays are similar. The more antigen-antibody reactions, the more of the unknown protein is present, and the more light scatter (instead of light absorption) will occur to indicate and quantitate the protein of interest.

Universal precautions (UP) are precautions that require treatment of all blood and body fluid specimens as if they are contaminated. Universal precautions specify the use of gloves, disposable or on-site laundered laboratory coats, appropriate sharp containers and biohazard bags, goggles and face guards, fresh (less than 1 week old) 10% bleach available for spills, and no contact with the mouth or mucous membranes.

Unopette is a trade name for small reservoirs of diluents and micropipettes used for manual counting and evaluation procedures, such as manual leukocyte, thrombocyte, and reticulocyte counts.

Uremia is an increase in urea in the blood due to renal (kidney) failure. The build-up of toxic substances normally excreted in the urine results in disorders such as hemolytic anemia or hemolytic uremic syndrome (HUS). Thromboxane A_2 is decreased.

Vacuolation of the cytoplasm of phagocytic cells signifies ingestion of foreign particles and is seen occasionally in lymphocytes due to exposure to EDTA anticoagulant, not phagocytosis. In association with the phagocytic vacuoles of neutrophils responding to a severe bacterial infection (leukemoid reaction) are toxic granulation (darker prominent cytoplasmic granules) and possibly Döhle bodies (blue cytoplasmic patches of RNA).

Vacuum venipuncture tubes are blood collection (phlebotomy) tubes used with a needle in a holder, which allows many different tubes to be filled with only one puncture of the vein. Table 1–1 presents the various phlebotomy tubes and their uses. Figure 1–12 represents the most commonly used blood collection vacuum tubes. The specific tube and amount of blood collected, the treatment of the blood in transit from the patient to the laboratory (well mixed and maintained at the proper temperature), and the identification of the blood tube are all essential to obtaining accurate test results. If the specimen is not correct, none of the subsequent testing is meaningful. Refer to Chapter 1.

Validity is the usefulness or meaningfulness of the results; in other words, "do the results make sense" or are they valid? Validity is a product of precision (duplication of results), accuracy (true value), correlation (comparison of more than one test procedure result for consistent information), and verification of the result leaving the laboratory to avoid clerical error or problems in getting valid information to the primary care provider. Refer to Chapters 1 and 16.

Variance (s^2) is a quality control (QC) calculation to express the amount of variation in results. The formula is the sum (Σ) of squared deviations around the mean, divided by n − 1. Refer to Chapter 1.

$$s^2 = \frac{\Sigma(\bar{x} - x)^2 \ (\text{mean} - \text{the score})}{n - 1 \ (\text{number of determinations} - 1)}$$

Vascular integrity is the normal blood vessel function of keeping the blood contained within the vessel. In order to maintain the blood within the vessels, an adequate number of circulating functional thrombocytes must be present and also an adequate level of collagen and hyaluronic acid, which holds the endothelial cells lining the blood vessels together. Vascular integrity is tested via the tourniquet test. Refer to Chapters 11 and 13.

Verification involves checking the clinical laboratory data for errors such as clerical error, lack of validation, and abnormal flags and correcting these errors before the final release of information to the primary care provider for diagnostic and treatment decisions. Refer to Chapters 1 and 16.

Viruses are infectious agents that are so small that they are not usually visible with a light microscope. The viruses are primarily made only of DNA or RNA and have no organelles for metabolism or replication. This inability to replicate on its own requires the virus to live inside a cell that has all of the organelles necessary for the viral replication. Examples of viruses associated with blood cells are the mononucleosis virus, which is the Epstein-Barr virus (EBV), the adult T-cell leukemia (ATL) virus, also called the human T-cell lymphotrophic virus-II (HTLV-II), and the acquired immunodeficiency syndrome (AIDS) virus, also called the human immunodeficiency virus (HIV) or the HTLV-I. All three of these viruses reside in lymphocytes. Refer to Chapter 5.

Vital stains are usually monochrome stains that are available to facilitate identification of specific cellular inclusions or contents. These stains are added to the blood while it is still viable. After the cells are stained, a slide is prepared. The reticulocyte stain is an example of a vital stain. Refer to Chapter 1.

Vitamins are substances required for normal body function and are usually obtained from food, such as vitamin K from green leafy vegetables for normal coagulation, vitamin B_{12} for normal DNA synthesis, and vitamin C for normal blood vessel (vascular) integrity. Tests to measure vitamin levels are performed in the clinical chemistry section of the laboratory. Refer to Chapters 10 and 13.

Vitamin B_{12} deficiency, also called pernicious anemia (PA), is often due to autoimmune production of antibodies to the intrinsic factor (IF) in the stomach necessary for the metabolism of vitamin B_{12}. The blood demonstrates macrocytic erythrocytes and hypersegmented neutrophils, with inappropriately immature (megaloblastic) nuclei in the erythroid cells in the bone marrow. Refer to Chapter 9.

Vitamin K deficiency and liver disease result in a decrease in the coagulation factors synthesized in the liver. The factors synthesized in the liver are factors II, VII, IX, and X. Of these, VII is the most sensitive to a lack of vitamin K. The oral anticoagulant administered to individuals with a clotting tendency, warfarin (e.g., Coumadin), inhibits clotting by competing with vitamin K in the liver. This vitamin K antagonist results in less of the vitamin K–dependent coagulation proteins being produced, reducing the risk of unnecessary clotting. Since factor VII is the most sensitive to this therapy and is part of the extrinsic coagulation pathway, the prothrombin time (PT) test, which tests the extrinsic pathway, is the test used to monitor warfarin therapy. Refer to Chapters 12 and 13.

Von Willebrand's disease is a genetic deficiency of von Willebrand's factor (vWF), which is necessary for normal platelet adhesion. This deficiency is diagnosed by a decreased platelet adhesion, prolonged bleeding time test, and decreased platelet aggregation in response to ristocetin. The vWF is associated with coagulation factor VIII. Individuals with this deficiency have a bleeding tendency that is not usually life threatening, although dental work and surgeries may cause excess bleeding. Refer to Chapter 12.

Waldenström's macroglobulinemia is the excessive and uncontrolled B cell/plasma cell proliferation and production of a single immunoglobulin M (IgM). This monoclonal gammopathy is most often seen in individuals older than 40 years of age who may demonstrate a normocytic, normochromic, hemolytic anemia, lymphocytosis, thrombocytopenia, or pancytopenia, an elevated erythrocyte sedimentation rate (ESR), and rouleaux phenomena. A lymphoma differs from a leukemia in terms of the primary site of neoplastic cells, e.g., in leukemia the neoplastic cells are primarily found in the bone marrow, while the lymphoma cells are primarily found in the lymph tissue. Refer to Chapter 5.

Warfarin is the generic name for the Coumadin oral anticoagulant. Warfarin inhibits the functional synthesis of vitamin K–dependent coagulation factors in the liver, and the result is a prolonged coagulation test result. Refer to Chapter 12.

Westgard multirule technique involves quality control (QC) criteria used to determine when a result is not considered within the acceptable limits. The small "s" represents a standard deviation from the mean. Refer to Chapter 1.

1. Reject when one observation falls outside of +3s.
2. Reject when two consecutive observations fall outside of +2s.
3. Reject when one control observation in a run is greater than +2s and another is less than −2s.
4. Reject when four consecutive control observations are greater than the mean +1s or are less than the mean −1s.
5. Reject when 10 consecutive control observations are on one side of the mean.

White marrow is primarily adipose or fat tissue in the bone that is no longer producing blood cells; however, under stress, it is capable of engaging in hematopoiesis. Refer to Chapter 2.

Whole blood (WB) is the blood as it exists in the body, which consists of free-moving erythrocytes, leukocytes, thrombocytes, and plasma. WB is the formed elements suspended randomly in the plasma. In order to obtain whole blood to analyze in the laboratory, an anticoagulant must be added to keep the blood from clotting. Refer to Chapter 1.

Wright-Giemsa stain is a nonvital (used on fixed cells) polychrome stain (stain of more than one color) used to stain the various cell components for microscopic examination. Refer to Chapter 1.

Yolk sac refers to the first site of blood cell formation in the early embryo. The yolk sac produces a very primitive nucleated erythroblast containing a primitive hemoglobin, called Gower 1 and 2. Refer to Chapter 2.

Index

Note: Page numbers in *italics* refer to illustrations.
Page numbers followed by the letter t refer to tables,
and those followed by d refer to definitions.

Abetalipoproteinemia, 189, 323d
Absolute anemia, 178
Absolute cell count, 10–11, *11*
Absolute lymphocytosis, 10
Absolute malignant polycythemia, 194
Absolute polycythemia, 11
  plasma volume in, 222
Absolute reticulocyte count, 211–212
Absolute value(s), 323d
Absorbed plasma (AP), 323d
  in coagulation testing, 272, *273*
Acanthocyte, *175, 208,* 323d
  in abetalipoproteinemia, 189
Accuracy, 323d–324d
  in cell counts, 10
ACD (anemia of chronic disease), 186–187, 326d
Acetylsalicylic acid, 327d
  platelet dysfunction from, 241
Acid, in seminal fluid, 293
Acid dye, in hematology stains, 26
Acid elution, 324d
  in erythrocyte testing, 215
  resistance to, 184
Acid phosphatase, in seminal fluid, 293
Acid-base balance, in oxygen transport, 154
Acid-fast stain, 324d
  of body fluids, 307
  of cerebrospinal fluid, 287
Acidified serum test, 324d, 339d
  in erythrocyte testing, 220–221
Acquired illness, 324d
  anemia of, 185–191. See also *Anemia.*
  hemorrhagic disorders of, 252–253, 255
  platelet dysfunction of, 241
Activated partial thromboplastin time (APTT) test, 268
Activin, in erythrocyte function, 148
Acute erythroleukemia (AEL), 195, 196t, 324d, 336d
  classification of, 64t
  cytochemistry in, 67t
Acute leukemia, 324d
  neutrophilia in, 63, 64
Acute lymphocytic leukemia (ALL), 324d
  classification of, 64t
  cytochemistry in, 67t
  lymphocytosis in, 98–101, *100, 101*
  neutrophilia in, 66
Acute megakaryocytic leukemia (AMegL), 324d, 350d
  classification of, 64t
  cytochemistry in, 67t
  thrombocytosis in, 236, 239
Acute monocytic leukemia (AMoL), classification of, 64t
  cytochemistry in, 67t
  monocytes in, 82, *82*
  neutrophilia in, 67

Acute myelogenous leukemia (AML), 325d
  classification of, 64t, 65
  cytochemistry in, 67t
  neutrophilia in, 63–66, *65, 66,* 67t
Acute myelomonocytic leukemia (AMML), 325d
  classification of, 64t
  cytochemistry in, 67t
  monocytosis in, 80, 81
  neutrophilia in, 66–67
  with eosinophilia, cytochemistry in, 67t
    monocytes in, 81
    neutrophilia in, 67
Acute posthemorrhagic anemia, 178–179
Acute promyelocytic leukemia (APL), 325d
  classification of, 64t
  cytochemistry in, 67t
  neutrophilia in, 66, *67*
ADCC (antibody-dependent cytotoxic cell), 96
Addison's disease, 222
Adenocarcinoma, *292*
Adenosine diphosphate (ADP), 230, 235, 323d
  in platelet aggregation studies, 268
Adenosine triphosphate (ATP), 230
Adhesion of thrombocyte(s), 232
  evaluation of, 267–268
ADP (adenosine diphosphate), 230, 235, 323d
  in platelet aggregation studies, 268
Adrenocortical hormone, in lymphocytopenia, 104
Adult T-cell leukemia (ATL), classification of, 64t
  cytochemistry in, 67t
  malignant lymphocytosis in, 100, *100*
AEL (acute erythroleukemia), 195, 196t, 324d, 336d
  classification of, 64t
  cytochemistry in, 67t
Aerobic culture, 325d
  of body fluids, 308
Agarose electrophoresis, 127, 342d
Aged serum (AS), 325d
  in coagulation testing, 272, *273*
Agglutination, in body fluid testing, 308
  in erythrocyte testing, 215–216
  in lymphocyte testing, 95
Agglutinin(s), cold, 332d
  in erythrocyte testing, 204
Aggregation, platelet, 233–235
  in coagulation, 250
  in manual platelet counting, 265
  testing of, 240, 268, *269*
Aggregometer instrument, 268
Aging. See *Elderly.*
Agnogenic, 325d
Agranulocytosis, *68,* 68–69, 69t
AHF (antihemophiliac factor), 247t
  deficiency of, 251

369

AIHA (autoimmune hemolytic anemia), 189, 327d
    diagnostic tests for, 218
ALA (aminolevulinic acid), 326d
    in erythrocyte testing, 219
    in hemoglobin synthesis, 160–162
    in porphyria, 185
Alcohol, bone marrow toxicity from, 180
    isopropyl, for phlebotomy, 18–19
Alcoholic liver disease, 188
Alder-Reilly anomaly, 70, *71*, 325d
Aldosteronism, 222
Alkali denaturation test, 184, 325d–326d
    in erythrocyte testing of, 215
Alkaline phosphatase score, 326d
    in chronic myelogenous leukemia, 64
    in leukemoid reaction, 62
    in microscopic leukocyte evaluation, 123, *123*
ALL. See *Acute lymphocytic leukemia (ALL)*.
Allergic reaction, 343d
    basophils in, 59, *59*
    delayed-type, 91
    eosinophils in, 58–59, 61–62
Alloimmune hemolytic anemia, 326d
    diagnostic tests for, 218
Alloimmune intravascular hemolysis, 188
Alpha-aminolevulinic acid (ALA), 326d
    in hemoglobin synthesis, 160–162
    in porphyria, 185
Alpha-thalassemia, 184
AMegL. See *Acute megakaryocytic leukemia (AMegL)*.
Amine, cerebrospinal, 287
Amino acid(s), in cerebrospinal fluid, 287
    in hemoglobins, 166, 168
Aminolevulinic acid (ALA), 326d
    in erythrocyte testing, 219
    in hemoglobin synthesis, 160–162
    in porphyria, 185
AML. See *Acute myelogenous leukemia (AML)*.
AMML. See *Acute myelomonocytic leukemia (AMML)*.
Amniocentesis, 294
Amniotic fluid analysis, 294–295
AMoL. See *Acute monocytic leukemia (AMoL)*.
Amyloidosis, 235, 236
Anaerobic culture, 326d
Analytic component, of clinical laboratory testing, 316
Anemia, 178–191, 326d
    absolute, 178
    aplastic, 180, 327d
    classification of, 192, 193
    definition of, 176
    erythrocyte metabolism in, 150
    etiology of, 178, *179*
    Fanconi's, 180, 337d
    folic acid deficiency, 187–188
    hemolytic, 188–191, 341d. See also *Hemolytic anemia*.
    hereditary spherocytic, 220
    hypoplastic, 180, 343d
    in elderly, 189, 335d
    in Hodgkin's lymphoma, 105
    in lead poisoning, 188, *188*
    in multiple myeloma, 103
    in Waldenström's macroglobulinemia, 102
    intravenous fluid dilution, 177
    iron deficiency, 185–186, *186*
    macrocytic, *179*, 188, *188*
    microcytic, *179*
    normocytic, *179*
    of abnormal production, 180–188

Anemia *(Continued)*
    in chronic disease, 186–187
    in folic acid deficiency, 187–188
    in glucose-6-phosphate dehydrogenase deficiency, 185
    in hemoglobinopathies, 180–185. See also *Hemoglobinopathy(ies)*.
    in iron deficiency, 185–186, *186*
    in lead poisoning, 188, *188*
    macrocytic, 188, *188*
    pernicious, 187, *187*
    sideroblastic, 186, 187t
    of chronic disease, 186–187, 326d
    of decreased production, 180
    of increased destruction, 188–191
    of pregnancy, 177, 326d
    pernicious. See *Pernicious anemia (PA)*.
    posthemorrhagic, 358d
        acute, 178–179
        chronic, 179–180, *180*
    refractory, 69, 69t
    relative, 177, 361d
    reticulocytes in, 147, 212
    sickle cell, 180–184, 363d
        screening tests for, 213
    sideroblastic, 186, 187t, 363d
Anisocytosis, 326d
    in chronic posthemorrhagic anemia, *180*
    in erythrocyte testing, 207
Anomaly(ies), 325d, 326d–327d
    genetic. See *Genetic anomaly(ies)*.
    neutrophil, 70, *70*, *71*
Anoxia, 327d
    in sickle cell disease, 181
Antibiotic(s), bone marrow toxicity from, 180
Antibiotic sensitivity test, 296
Antibody(ies), 95
    antiphospholipid, 327d, 348d
        hemorrhagic disorders and, 252
    monoclonal, 351d
Antibody-dependent cytotoxic cell (ADCC), 96
Anticoagulant(s), 249
    for synovial fluid analysis, 288
Antigen, 327d
Antigen presentation, monocytes in, 78, *79*
    T cells in, 90
Antigen-presenting cells (APCs), 323d, 327d
Antihemophiliac factor (AHF), 247t
    deficiency of, 251
Antiphospholipid antibody (APA), 327d, 348d
    hemorrhagic disorders and, 252
Antithrombin III, 255
    in coagulation pathway, 246, 247t, 249
    in thrombotic disorders, 254
    testing of, 274
AP (absorbed plasma), 323d
    in coagulation testing, 272, *273*
APA (antiphospholipid antibody), 327d, 348d
    hemorrhagic disorders and, 252
APCs (antigen-presenting cells), 323d, 327d
Aperture, 327d
    in erythrocyte testing, 201
    in leukocyte testing, 111, 112
APL. See *Acute promyelocytic leukemia (APL)*.
Aplasia, anemia in, 178
    neutropenia in, 68
    thrombocytopenia in, 236, 238
Aplastic anemia, 180, 327d
Apoptosis, 147

APTT (activated partial thromboplastin time) test, 268
Arachidonic acid, 327d
  in thrombocyte testing, 268
Arm, of microscope, *27*, 28
Arm band, identification, 17–18
Arneth count, 68, 327d
  for neutrophil segmentation, 123–124, *124*
Arterial blood gas analysis, 156
Arteriole, 231
Artery(ies), 231
Arthritis, rheumatoid, 362d
  autoimmune hemolytic anemia in, 189
  synovial fluid in, 290
  thrombocytosis in, 236, 239
AS (aged serum), 325d
  in coagulation testing, 272, *273*
Ascitic fluid, 292–293, 356d–357d
  testing of, 309
Aspartate aminotransferase (AST), 287
Aspiration, in cellular identification and evaluation, 43
  of amniotic fluid, 294
  of wound, 295–296
Aspirin, 327d
  platelet dysfunction from, 241
AST (aspartate aminotransferase), 287
Asthma, bronchial, eosinophils in, 61–62
Asynchronous maturation, 187
Atherosclerosis, fibrinolytic defects in, 254
Atherosclerotic plaque, 237, 327d
ATL (adult T-cell leukemia), classification of, 64t
  cytochemistry of, 67t
  malignant lymphocytosis in, 100, *100*
ATP (adenosine triphosphate), 230
Attitude, in clinical laboratory, 319
Auer rods, 65, *65*, 66
Auramine-rhodamine stain, 327d
  of cerebrospinal fluid, 287
Autoimmune hemolytic anemia (AIHA), 189, 327d
  diagnostic tests for, 218
Autoimmune intravascular hemolysis, 188–189
Automated complete blood count, 110–114, *113*, *114*
  in erythrocyte testing, 201–202
Automated reticulocyte count, 211
Average value, 13
Azurophilic granule(s), 88, 327d

B cell(s), 328d
  in cell-mediated immunity, 91t, *93*
  in hairy cell leukemia, 104
  in hematopoiesis, 42
  in Waldenström's macroglobulinemia, 102
  memory, 95, 328d
  origin of, 88, 89, *89*, 91t
  physiology and function of, *93*, *94*, 94–96
Bacteria, phagocytosis of, 60, *61*
Bacterial antigen detection test, 308
Bacterial infection, cerebrospinal fluid in, 286
  complete blood count in, 112
  leukemoid reaction in, 62
  leukocyte testing in, 127
  response to, 61, *62*
Bacterial meningitis, 286, *287*
Bacterial product(s), 328d
  phagocytosis of, 60
Band cell(s), 328d
  in acute posthemorrhagic anemia, 179

Band cell(s) *(Continued)*
  in bacterial infection, 61
  morphology of, *57*, 57–58
Base, of microscope, *27*, 28
Basic dye, for staining, 26
Basilic vein, in venipuncture, 18, *18*
Basket cell(s), in chronic lymphocytic leukemia, 101, *102*
  in complete blood count, 113
Basopenia, 72
Basophil(s), 328d
  decreased, 72
  in hematopoiesis, 41–42
  increased, 72
  information on, 72t
  origin, maturation, and morphology of, *59*, 59–60
  physiology and function of, 62
  reference value for, 110
  size of, 7, 363d
Basophilia, 72
Basophilic normoblast, 146, *146*, 149, 328d
Basophilic stippling, *182*
  in erythrocytes, *209*
  in lead poisoning, 188, *188*
Beer's law, 11, 328d
Bence Jones protein, 103
Benign, 328d
Benign polycythemia, 194
Benzene toxicity, 180
Bernard-Soulier syndrome, 240–241, 328d–329d
Beta-thalassemia, 184
BFU-E (burst forming unit-erythroid), 328d
  in erythrocyte maturation, 145–146
Bicarbonate, in oxygen transport, 154
Bilirubin, 329d
  from heme catabolism, 162
  in autoimmune hemolytic anemia, 189
  in erythrocyte testing, 218
Bioconcave shape, of erythrocyte(s), 150, *152*
Biopsy, in cellular identification and evaluation, 43
2,3-Biphosphoglycerate (2,3-BPG), 160, *161*
Blast cell(s), cytochemistry of, 66, 67t, 82, 83t
  in acute myelogenous leukemia, 66, *66*
  in leukemia, 63
  in myelodysplastic syndrome, 69, 69t
Bleeding time test, 23, 240, 329d
  in thrombocyte testing, 266, *267*
  in thrombotic thrombocytopenic purpura, 252
Blood, coagulation of, 244–257. See also *Coagulation.*
  collection of. See *Phlebotomy.*
  composition of, *6*, 6–7
Blood cell(s), in fetus, 54, *54*
  in hematopoiesis, 39–43, *40*
Blood gases, 329d
  in oxygen transport, 153–154
Blood islands, 36
Blood pH, in oxygen transport, 154
Blood pressure cuff, in tourniquet test, 260
Blood smear. See *Peripheral blood smear.*
Blood transfusion(s), for sickle cell disease, 181
  for sideroblastic anemia, 186
  for thalassemia, 185
Blood vessel(s), 231–232
  constriction of, in coagulation, 250
    protein regulators in, 233
  integrity of, 231–232, 366d
    loss of, *234*, 235–237, *237*, 251
    vitamins in, 16

Blood vessel(s) *(Continued)*
 lumen of, 232
 physiology and function of, 233–235, *234*
Blood volume, 329d
 in acute posthemorrhagic anemia, 178
 in erythrocyte testing, 223
Bloodborne pathogens, 29–30
Blood-brain barrier, 285
Body fluid(s), 279–310, *284,* 329d
 analysis of, 282–297
  amniotic fluid in, 294–295
  cerebrospinal fluid in, 284–288, *286, 287*
  serous fluids in, 291–294, *292, 294, 295*
  synovial fluid in, 288–290, *289, 290*
  urine in, 294
  wound aspirates in, 295–296
 characteristics of, 285
 testing of, 298–310
  cell counts in, 301–303, *302, 304*
  chemical analysis in, 306–307
  microbiologic and immunologic tests in, 307–309
  microscopy and cytology in, 303–306, *305–307*
  physical characteristics in, 300–301
 types of, 284, 285
Body substance isolation (BSI), 30, 329d
Body temperature, in homeostasis, 15–16
Body tube, of microscope, *27, 28*
Bone marrow, 329d
 hematopoiesis in, 36–39, *38,* 44, *45*
 in anemia, reticulocyte count and, 212
  smear of, *186*
 in blood cell proliferation, *55*
 in chronic myelogenous leukemia, 64, *65*
 in lymphopoiesis, 88, *89*
 in myeloid metaplasia, 67–68
 infiltration of, thrombocytopenia in, 236, 238
 macrophage cells in, 76
 microenvironment of, 36, *38,* 329d
 plasma cells in, 94
Boyden chamber, 329d
 in neutrophil function testing, 125–127
2,3-BPG (2,3-Biphosphoglycerate), 160, *161*
Brain, macrophage cells in, 76
Bronchial asthma, eosinophils in, 61–62
BSI (body substance isolation), 30, 329d
Buffy coat, 6, *6,* 329d
 for microscopic leukocyte evaluation, 123
Burkitt's lymphoma, 100–101, *101*
Bursa equivalent, 329d
 in lymphopoiesis, 88, *89*
Burst forming unit-erythroid (BFU-E), 328d
 in erythrocyte maturation, 145–146
Busulfan, for chronic myelogenous leukemia, 65

Ca. See *Calcium.*
Cabot rings, *182*
 in erythrocytes, *209*
CAE (chloroacetate esterase), in leukemia cytochemistry, 65, *65*
Calcium, in coagulation, 246, 247t
 in homeostasis, 17
Calcium pyrophosphate dihydrate (CPPD) crystal(s), 289
CAM (cell adhesion molecule), 330d
 in erythrocyte function, 147
 in hematopoiesis, 39

Cancer, 330d
 fibrinolytic defects in, 254
 hemorrhagic disorders in, 253, 255
 natural killer cells in, 96
CAP (College of American Pathologists), 31, 332d
Capillary(ies), 231
Carbon dioxide, partial pressure of, 154
 transport of, 152–153, *153*
Carbonic acid, in oxygen transport, 154
Carboxyhemoglobin, 154, 168, 330d
Cardiac disease, fibrinolytic defects in, 254
Catabolism, hemoglobin, 162, *164*
 lipid, ineffective, 82–83
CBC. See *Complete blood count (CBC).*
CD (cluster differentiation) marker(s), 90, 90t, 329d–330d, 331d
 in humoral immunity, 95
 to T suppressor cells ratio, 96, 97
Cell adhesion molecule (CAM), 330d
 in erythrocyte function, 147
 in hematopoiesis, 39
Cell agglutination test, 184
Cell count, body fluid, 301–303, *302, 304*
 complete blood. See *Complete blood count (CBC).*
 in cerebrospinal fluid testing, 286
 in synovial fluid testing, 288
 manual. See *Manual cell count(s).*
 relative and absolute, 10–11, *11*
Cell membrane, of erythrocyte, 150–152, *153*
Cell morphology, 43
Cell size and shape, 8–9
Cell volume, 7
Cell-Dyn 3000, in complete blood count, 111–112
Cell-mediated immunity (CMI), 90, 91t, *93*
Cellular identification and evaluation, 43–44
Cellular metabolism, 152
Cellular morphology, 44, *45*
Cellulose acetate hemoglobin electrophoresis, *166*
Center vein, in venipuncture, 18, *18*
Central nervous system (CNS), hypoxia in, 287
 inflammation of, 288
Centrifuge, in complete blood count, 200
Cephalic vein, in venipuncture, 18, *18*
Cerebral infarction, 287
Cerebrospinal fluid (CSF), 330d
 analysis of, 284–288, *286, 287*
 testing of, 309
Cerebrovascular disease, fibrinolytic defects in, 254
CFU-Baso (colony-forming unit–basophil), development of, 59
 in granulocyte origination, 54, *55*
 in hematopoiesis, 41
CFU-E (colony-forming unit–erythroid), 330d
 in erythrocyte maturation, 146
CFU-Eo (colony-forming unit–eosinophil), 332d
 in granulocyte origination, 54, *55*
 morphology of, 58
CFU-G (colony-forming unit–granulocyte), in acute myelogenous leukemia, 66, *66*
 origin, maturation and morphology of, 54–56, *55*
CFU-GEMM. See *Colony-forming unit–granulocyte, erythroid, monocyte, megakaryocyte (CFU-GEMM).*
CFU-GM (colony-forming unit–granulocyte monocyte), 332d
 in granulocyte origination, 54, *55*
 in hematopoiesis, 41
 origin and maturation of, 76

CFU-mega (colony-forming unit–megakaryocyte), 332d
 in thrombocyte maturation, 230
CFU-S (colony-forming unit–spleen), in erythrocyte maturation, 144–145
 in granulocyte maturation, 54, *55*
 in thrombocyte maturation, 230
CFU-x (colony-forming unit–x), 332d
CGD (chronic granulomatous disease), 69, 330d
 tests for, 125
CGL (chronic granulocytic leukemia). See *Chronic myelogenous leukemia (CML).*
CGP (circulating granulocyte pool), 60
Chédiak-Higashi anomaly, 70, *70*, 330d
Chelation therapy, for sideroblastic anemia, 186
Chemical analysis, in porphyria, 185
 of amniotic fluid, 294–295
 of body fluids, 306–307
 of cerebrospinal fluid, 285, 287
 of seminal fluid, 293
 of serous fluid, 291
 of synovial fluid, 289–290
Chemotaxis, 330d
 in granulocytic function, 60–61
 neutrophil response to, 125–127
Chemotherapy, bone marrow toxicity from, 180
 for acute promyelocytic leukemia, 66
 for chronic myelogenous leukemia, 65
 for polycythemia, 195
 lymphocytopenia from, 104
Chest, serous fluid in, 291
Chloramphenicol, bone marrow toxicity from, 180
Chloroacetate esterase (CAE), in leukemia cytochemistry, 65, *65*
Cholesterol, in synovial fluid, 288–289, *289*
 plaque from, 237
Choroid plexus cell(s), in cerebrospinal fluid, 286, *287*
Christmas factor, 247t
 deficiency of, 255
Chromatin, of monocyte, 76, *78*
Chromicity, 174, 178
 in erythrocyte testing, 207
Chromosomal abnormality(ies), amniocentesis in, 294
Chronic, 330d
Chronic disease, anemia of, 186–187, 326d
 serum ferritin in, 216
Chronic granulocytic leukemia. See *Chronic myelogenous leukemia (CML).*
Chronic granulomatous disease (CGD), 69, 330d
 tests for, 125
Chronic intravascular hemolytic anemia, 221
Chronic lymphocytic leukemia (CLL), 330d
 malignant lymphocytosis in, *101*, 101–102, *102*
Chronic myelogenous leukemia (CML), 330d
 leukemoid reaction vs., 62–63
 neutrophilia in, 62, 64–65, *65*
 thrombocytosis in, 236, 239
Chronic myelomonocytic leukemia (CMML), 330d–331d
 in myelodysplastic syndrome, 69, 69t
 monocytes in, 82
Chronic posthemorrhagic anemia, 179–180, *180*
Circulating anticoagulant test, 272, 331d
Circulating granulocyte pool (CGP), 60
Circulating inhibitor(s), 255, 331d
 in coagulation pathway, 246, 247t, 249
 in thrombotic disorders, 254
 testing of, 274
Circulating monocyte pool (CMP), 76
Circulatory system, 241–242, 331d. See also *Vasculature.*

Cirrhosis, of liver, pseudoanemia in, 177
 thrombocytopenia in, 236, 239
Citrate agar hemoglobin electrophoresis, *166*
Citric acid, in seminal fluid, 293
Cleansing, for phlebotomy, 19–20
Clerical error, 14
CLIA (Clinical Laboratory Improvement Act), 31, 331d
Clinical hematology, 4–33
 blood composition in, *6*, 6–7
 mathematics of, 8–14. See also *Mathematic(s).*
 microscope in, 23–29. See also *Microscopic evaluation.*
 phlebotomy in, 17–23. See also *Phlebotomy.*
 physiologic concepts of, 15–17, *16*
 practice of, 31–32
 quality assurance in, 30–31
 safety in, 29–30, *30*
 terminology in, 7–8
Clinical Laboratory Improvement Act (CLIA), 31, 331d
Clinical laboratory practice, 311–322
 correlation in, 316
 dissemination in, 318–319
 documentation in, 318
 mission of, 351d
 personnel in, *319*, 319–320, *320*
 validation in, 316–318
 verification in, 318
Clinical laboratory scientist (CLS), 319, *320*, 331d
Clinical laboratory technician (CLT), 319–320, 331d
Clinical pathways, 331d
CLL (chronic lymphocytic leukemia), 330d
 malignant lymphocytosis in, *101*, 101–102, *102*
Clot, 7, 331d
 composition of, 10
 detection of, 269–270, 355d
 formation of. See *Coagulation.*
Clot retraction, 240, 331d
 in coagulation, 250
 in thrombocyte testing, 266–267
Clotting time, 268
CLS (clinical laboratory scientist), 319, *320*, 331d
CLT (clinical laboratory technician), 319–320, 331d
Cluster differentiation (CD) marker(s), 90, 90t, 329d–330d, 331d
 in humoral immunity, 95
 to T suppressor cells ratio, 96, 97
CMI (cell-mediated immunity), T cells in, 90, 91t, *93*
CML. See *Chronic myelogenous leukemia (CML).*
CMML (chronic myelomonocytic leukemia), 330d–331d
 in myelodysplastic syndrome, 69, 69t
 monocytes in, 82
CMP (circulating monocyte pool), 76
CMV (cytomegalovirus) infection, 333d
 lymphocytosis in, 97–98
CNS (central nervous system), hypoxia in, 287
 inflammation of, 288
Coagulation, 7, 232–235, 244–257, 331d
 appropriate, 249–251
 disseminated intravascular. See *Disseminated intravascular coagulation (DIC).*
 in complete blood count, 112, 200
 in loss of vascular integrity, 237
 inappropriate, 251–255
 intravascular, 252–253
 pathways of, 246–249, *248*
 testing of, 268–273, *271*, *273*, 331d–332d
 vitamins in, 16–17
Coagulation factor(s), 246, 247t, 331d
 activation of, 233

Coagulation protein(s), 246, 247t
  deficiency of, 254, 255
  testing of, 274
Coagulopathy, dilutional, 253
  thrombotic, 251, 253–255, 365d
Coarse adjustment, of microscope, 27, 28
Cobalamin deficiency, 187, *187*
  neutropenia in, 68, *68*
  serum lactate dehydrogenase isoenzymes in, 221
  thrombocytopenia in, 236, 238
Coefficient of variation (CV), 14, 332d
Cold agglutinin(s), 332d
  in erythrocyte testing, 204
Collagen, 332d
  in coagulation, 246
  in thrombocyte testing, 268
  in vascular integrity, 232
College of American Pathologists (CAP), 31, 332d
Colony-forming unit–basophil (CFU-Baso), development
    of, 59
  in granulocyte origination, 54, *55*
  in hematopoiesis, 41
Colony-forming unit–eosinophil (CFU-Eo), 332d
  in granulocyte origination, 54, *55*
  morphology of, 58
Colony-forming unit–erythroid (CFU-E), 330d
  in erythrocyte maturation, 146
Colony-forming unit–granulocyte (CFU-G), in acute mye-
    logenous leukemia, 66, *66*
  origin, maturation and morphology of, 54–56, *55*
Colony-forming unit–granulocyte, erythroid, monocyte,
    megakaryocyte (CFU-GEMM), 332d
  in basophil origination, 59
  in erythrocyte maturation, 145
  in granulocyte origination, 54, *55*
  in hematopoiesis, 40–41
  in thrombocyte maturation, 230
  morphology of, 58
  origin and maturation of, 76
Colony-forming unit–granulocyte monocyte (CFU-GM),
    332d
  in granulocyte origination, 54, *55*
  in hematopoiesis, 41
  origin and maturation of, 76
Colony-forming unit–megakaryocyte (CFU-mega), 332d
  in thrombocyte maturation, 230
Colony-forming unit–spleen (CFU-S), in erythrocyte matu-
    ration, 144–145
  in granulocyte origination, 54, *55*
  in thrombocyte maturation, 230
Colony-forming unit–x (CFU-x), 332d
Colony-stimulating factor (CSF), 332d
  in erythrocyte function, 148
  in erythropoiesis, 144
Colony-stimulating factor–mega (CSF-mega), 230
Common coagulation pathway, 247–250, 332d–333d
Competitive immunoassay, 133–134, *134*
Complement, in immune response, 96
Complete blood count (CBC), 329d, 333d
  in erythrocyte testing, 200–205
    automated procedure for, 201–202
    correlation factors in, 204
    error in, 204–205
    indices for, 202–204, *203*
    laser light scattering technique for, 202
    light absorbance technique for, 202
    specimen collection for, 200
  in leukocyte testing, 110–114, *113*, *114*

Complete blood count (CBC) *(Continued)*
  in thrombocyte disorders, 237
  in thrombocyte testing, 261, *262*, *263*
Confidentiality, 21
Congestive heart failure, 177
Connective tissue disease, 236, 239
Constriction, in coagulation, 250
  protein regulators in, 233
Continuous quality improvement (CQI), 31, 333d
Copper sulfate, in erythrocyte testing, 206
Correlation, 316, 333d
  in erythrocyte testing, 204, 211–212
  in leukocyte testing, 118–119, 123
  in platelet testing, 264–265
  in validation, 317
Corticosteroid crystal(s), in synovial fluid, 289
Coulter scattergram, in complete blood count, *113*
Coumadin (warfarin), 333d, 367d
  coagulation pathway and, 247
  in protein C deficiency, 254
  in vitamin K deficiency, 252
  prothrombin time test monitoring of, 271
Counterimmunoelectrophoresis, in body fluid testing, 308
Covariance, 333d
CPPD (calcium pyrophosphate dihydrate) crystal(s), 289
CQI (continuous quality improvement), 31
Crenated erythrocyte(s), 15, *16*, 333d
Cryoprecipitate, in genetic factor deficiency, 251–252
Cryptococcus organism, in cerebrospinal fluid, 286, *287*
CSF (cerebrospinal fluid), 330d
  analysis of, 284–288, *286*, *287*
  testing of, 309
CSF (colony-stimulating factor), 332d
  in erythrocyte function, 148
  in erythropoiesis, 144
CSF-mega (colony-stimulating factor–mega), 230
CTCL (cutaneous T-cell lymphoma), 105, *106*
Cubital vein, in venipuncture, 18, *18*
Culture(s), of body fluid, 308
  of cerebrospinal fluid, 288
  of synovial fluid, 290
  of wound aspirates, 295–296
Cushing's syndrome, 222
CuSO$_4$. See *Copper sulfate.*
Cutaneous histiocytosis, 84, 359d
Cutaneous T-cell lymphoma (CTCL), 105, *106*
CV (coefficient of variation), 14, 332d
Cyanocobalamin deficiency, 68, *68*
Cyanosis, hemoglobin in, 155, 168
Cytocentrifugation slide differential, of body fluid,
    307
  of cerebrospinal fluid, 286
  of serous fluid, 291
  of synovial fluid, 288, 289
Cytocentrifuge, 305, *307*, 333d
Cytochemical stain, 333d
  in complete blood count, 112
  in erythrocyte testing, 212–213
  in leukemia, 63, 65, *65*
    to differentiate blast cells, 66, 67t, 82, 83t
  in microscopic leukocyte evaluation, 122, 122t
Cytokine(s), 333d
  in anemia, 180
  in blood cell proliferation, 54, *55*
  in cell-mediated immunity, 90, 91t, *93*
  in erythrocyte function, 149
  in granulocytic function, 60
  in thrombocyte maturation, 230

Cytokine(s) *(Continued)*
  response to, monocytes in, 78, *79*
  T cells and, 90
Cytologic examination, 333d
  of body fluids, 303–306, *305–307*
  of serous fluid, 291
Cytomegalovirus (CMV) infection, 333d
  lymphocytosis in, 97–98
Cytometry, flow. See *Flow cytometry.*
Cytoplasm, in cell maturation, 44–46
  in hairy cell leukemia, 104, *104*
  of band cell, 57, *57*
  of eosinophil, 59, *59*
  of lymphocyte, 88, *90*
  of metamyelocyte, 57, *57*
  of monocyte, 76, *78*
  of myeloblast, 54–55, *55*
  of myelocyte, 56–57, *57*
  of neutrophil, 58, *58*
    in May-Hegglin anomaly, 70, *70*
  of plasma cell, 94
  of promyelocyte, 55, *55*
  of reticulocyte, 147
  of thrombocyte, 230
Cytotoxic T (T_c cell), 90, 333d

Dacryocyte, *175, 208*
DAT (direct antiglobulin test), in autoimmune hemolytic
    anemia, 189
  in erythrocyte testing, 218–219
DDAVP (1-Desmino-8-D-arginine vasopressin), 333d–334d
  in genetic factor deficiencies, 252
D-dimer test, 249
  in coagulation testing, 269
  in fibrinolysis testing, 273–274
Deep vein thrombosis (DVT), 253–254, 255, 334d
Dehydration, plasma volume in, 222
Delayed-type hypersensitivity (DTH) reaction, 91
Delta check, 14, 334d
Delta-aminolevulinic acid (δ-ALA) synthetase levels, 219
Denatured hemoglobin, *209*
Denaturation, alkali, 184, 325d–326d
  in erythrocyte testing, 215
Deoxyhemoglobin, 154, 168, 334d
Deoxyribonucleic acid (DNA), of erythrocyte, *209*
  synthesis of, 16
1-Desmino-8-D-arginine vasopressin (DDAVP), 333d–334d
  in genetic factor deficiencies, 252
Diabetes, hemoglobin monitoring in, 168, 340d–341d
  vascular integrity in, 235, 236
Diamond-Blackfan syndrome, 180, 334d
Diapedesis, 60
DIC. See *Disseminated intravascular coagulation (DIC).*
Differentiation, 334d
  in hematopoiesis, 39–43, *40*
Digestion, in phagocytosis, 60, *61*
DiGuglielmo's disease, 195
Dilution method, for body fluid cell count, 301–302, *302*
  for leukocyte counts, 116–117, *117*
  for platelet count, 261, *263*
Dilutional coagulopathy, 253
2,3-Diphosphoglycerate (2,3-DPG), 160, *161*
Direct antiglobulin test (DAT), in autoimmune hemolytic
    anemia, 189
  in erythrocyte testing, 218–219
Discocyte, *175, 208*

Disseminated intravascular coagulation (DIC), 253, 255,
    334d
  in acute promyelocytic leukemia, 66
  thrombocytopenia in, 236, 238
  vascular integrity in, 235, 236
Disseminated thrombosis, 253
Dissemination, of information, 318–319
Dithionite, in sickle cell screening, 183, 213
DNA (deoxyribonucleic acid), of erythrocyte, *209*
  synthesis of, 16
Documentation, 318, 334d
Döhle body(ies), 61, *61, 62*, 334d
  in leukemoid reaction, 62–63
2,3-DPG (2,3-Diphosphoglycerate), 160, *161*
Drepanocyte, *175, 208*
  in sickle cell anemia, 181
Drug-induced immune response, thrombocytopenia in,
    236, 238–239
DTH (delayed-type hypersensitivity) reaction, 91
DVT (deep vein thrombosis), 253–254, 255, 334d
Dye, for staining, 26, 27t
Dyserythropoiesis, 334d
  anemia in, 178
Dysplasia, 334d

EBV (Epstein-Barr virus), 336d
  Burkitt's lymphoma in, 101
  in infectious mononucleosis, 97
Ecchymosis, 235, 251, 334d
Echinocyte, *175, 208*
  in abetalipoproteinemia, 189
EDTA. See *Ethylenediaminetetra-acetic acid (EDTA).*
EIA (enzyme immunoassay), 134–135, *135*, 336d
EID (electroimmunodiffusion), 131, 335d
Elderly, anemia in, 189, 335d, 338d
  hematopoiesis in, 38–39
  phlebotomy in, *21*, 21–22, 22t
Electroimmunodiffusion (EID), 131, 335d
Electrolyte solution, 335d
Electromechanical probe, 335d
  in coagulation testing, 270, *271*
Electronic impedance, 335d
  in complete blood count, 111
  in erythrocyte testing, 201
Electrophoresis, 335d–336d
  hemoglobin. See *Hemoglobin electrophoresis.*
  high-resolution agarose, 127, 342d
  in body fluid testing, 308
  in lymphocyte tests, 95–96
  in protein identification and quantitation, 127, *128*
Elliptocyte, *175, 208*
ELT (euglobin lysis test), 249
Elution, acid, in erythrocyte testing, 215
    resistance to, 184
Embden-Meyerhof pathway (EMP), 336d
  hemoglobin function in, 168
  in erythrocyte metabolism, 150, *151*
  in oxygen transport, 155
Embolization, in deep vein thrombosis, 254
Embryo, hemoglobin in, 166, *167*
EMP. See *Embden-Meyerhof pathway (EMP).*
Emphysema, polycythemia in, 194
Encephalopathy, cerebrospinal fluid in, 287
Endosmosis, 336d
Endothelium, damage to, 235, 236, 336d
  of lumen, 232

Enzyme(s), cerebrospinal, 287
  deficiency of, in porphyria, 185
  liver, in infectious mononucleosis, 97
Enzyme immunoassay (EIA), 134–135, *135*, 336d
Eosin stain, 26, 27t, 336d
Eosinopenia, 72
Eosinophil(s), decreased, 72
  development of, 54–58
  increased. See *Eosinophilia.*
  information on, 72t
  morphology of, 58–59, *59*
  physiology and function of, 61–62
  reference value for, 110
  segmented, 59, *59*, 362d
  size of, 7, 363d
Eosinophilia, 71
  AMML with, cytochemistry in, 67t
    monocytes in, 81
    neutrophilia in, 67
Eosinophilic granuloma, 83, 336d
Ependymal cell(s), in cerebrospinal fluid, 286, *287*
Epinephrine, 336d
  in thrombocyte testing, 268
Epitope, 336d
EPO. See *Erythropoietin (EPO).*
Epstein-Barr virus (EBV), 336d
  Burkitt's lymphoma in, 101
  in infectious mononucleosis, 97
Equipment, for phlebotomy, 18–20, *18–21*, 20t
Erythroblast(s), formation of, 142
  morphology of, 55–56, *56*
Erythrocyte(s), 6, *6*, 137–224. See also *Red blood cell* entries.
  basophilic stippling in, *182*, 188, *188*
  crenated, 15, *16*, 333d
  decrease in, abnormal, 178–191. See also *Anemia.*
    physiologic, 174–177, *175–177*
  function of, 152–156, *153*, *154*
  hemoglobin in, 158–171. See also *Hemoglobin.*
  Howell-Jolly bodies in, 181–183, *182*
  hypochromic. See *Hypochromic erythrocyte(s).*
  in bone marrow, 44
  in exudates, 291
  in hematopoiesis, 42
  in sickle cell disease, 181
  in synovial fluid, 288
  in Waldenström's macroglobulinemia, 102, *102*
  inclusions of, *182*
  increase in, abnormal, 194–196, 196t
    physiologic, 191–194
  indices of, 9, 12, 336d
  macrocytic, 174, 350d
    in chronic posthemorrhagic anemia, 180
    in liver disease, 188, *188*
  maturation of, 144–147, *145–147*
  metabolism of, 150, *151*
  microcytic. See *Microcyte(s).*
  morphology of, 147–150, *148*, 174, *175*
    abnormalities and, *208*
  nucleated 36, 354d
    in complete blood count, 113
    in pernicious anemia, 187
  normochromic. See *Normochromic erythrocyte(s).*
  normocytic. See *Normocyte(s).*
  origin of, 142–144, *143*, *144*
  physiology of, 150–152, *152–154*
  poikilocytic. See *Poikilocytosis.*
  relative and absolute count of, 10–11

Erythrocyte(s) *(Continued)*
  shape of, 10
    membrane abnormalities and, *176*
  sickling of, 181
  size of, 7, 10, 363d
  spherocytic, 174, *175*, *177*, 178, 189–191, 363d
    in thalassemia, 185
    morphology of, *208*
  testing of, 198–224
    acid elution test in, 215
    acidified serum test in, 220–221
    alkali denaturation test in, 215
    aminolevulinic acid levels in, 219
    bilirubin in, 218
    blood volume in, 223
    complete blood count in, 200–205, *203*. See also *Complete blood count (CBC).*
    direct antiglobulin test in, 218–219
    erythrocyte sedimentation rate in, *221*, 221–222
    erythropoietin levels in, 219
    folate concentrations in, 219
    free erythrocyte protoporphyrin in, 219
    free plasma in, 218
    glucose-6-phosphate dehydrogenase levels in, 219
    haptoglobin in, 216–218
    hemoglobin and hematocrit in, 206
    hemoglobin breakdown in, 216, *218*
    hemoglobin electrophoresis in, 213–215, *214*
    iron, 216, *217*
    lactate dehydrogenase isoenzymes in, 221
    lead levels in, 219
    microscopic, 206–213. See also *Microscopic evaluation.*
    osmotic fragility test in, *219*, 219–220
    plasma volume in, 222–223
    red blood cell mass in, 222
    red blood cell survival in, 222
    Shilling urinary excretion test in, 219
    sickle cell screening tests in, 213
    slide agglutination test in, 215–216
    sucrose hemolysis test in, 220–221
    sugar water test in, 220–221
    urine hemoglobin in, 218
    vitamin B$_{12}$ levels in, 219
    zinc protoporphyrin in, 219
Erythrocyte folate concentrations, 135
Erythrocyte sedimentation rate (ESR), in erythrocyte testing, *221*, 221–222
  in multiple myeloma, 103
  in Waldenström's macroglobulinemia, 102
Erythrocytosis, malignant, 195, 196t, 350d
Erythroleukemia, 195, 196t
  acute, 324d, 336d
    classification of, 64t
    cytochemistry in, 67t
Erythropoiesis, 142–144, *143*, *144*, 174
  in anemia, 176
    of decreased production, 180
    stress, 176
    in chronic posthemorrhagic anemia, 180, *180*
Erythropoietin (EPO), 336d
  in anemia, 176, 179–180, *180*
  in erythrocyte testing, 219
  in erythropoiesis, 143, 148, 174
  in hemoglobin synthesis, 160–162
  in polycythemia, 194
ESR (erythrocyte sedimentation rate), in erythrocyte testing, *221*, 221–222
  in multiple myeloma, 103

ESR (erythrocyte sedimentation rate) *(Continued)*
  in Waldenström's macroglobulinemia, 102
Essential thrombocythemia (ET), 236, 239, 336d
Esterase, in leukemia cytochemistry, 65, *65*
ET (essential thrombocythemia), 236, 239, 336d
Ethylenediaminetetra-acetic acid (EDTA), 334d–337d
  in erythrocyte testing, 200
  in leukocyte testing, 110, 111
  in microscopic leukocyte evaluation, 119
Etiology, 337d
Euchromatin, 337d
  in cell maturation, 44
Euglobin lysis test (ELT), 249
Examination, of cerebrospinal fluid, 285–288, *287*
  of pericardial fluid, 292, *292*
  of peritoneal fluid, 292, *292–293*
  of seminal fluid, 293, *294*
  of synovial fluid, 288–290, *289*, *290*
Extramedullary hematopoiesis, 36, 142, 337d
  in myeloid metaplasia, 68
Extravascular hemolysis, 337d
  anemia from, 189, *190*, 191
  in immune response, 96
  in spherocytosis, 191
  of hemoglobin, 162, *164*
Extrinsic coagulation pathway, 247, 250, 337d
Exudate, 291, 337d

FAB. See *French-American-British (FAB) classification.*
Fabry's disease, 83, 337d
FACS (fluorescence-activated cell sorter), 338d
  in leukocyte testing, 125, *126*
Factor substitution test, 272
Fanconi's anemia, 180, 337d
FDP (fibrinogen degradation products) test, 249
  in coagulation testing, 269
  in fibrinolysis testing, 273
Fe. See *Iron.*
Fecal-oral contamination, in hepatitis, 98
FEP. See *Free erythrocyte protoporphyrin (FEP).*
Ferric state, iron in, 163
Ferritin, 337d
  in anemia, 187
  in heme catabolism, 162
  in hemoglobin kinetics, 163–165, *164*
  serum, 216, 362d
Ferritin test, 185–186
Ferrous state, iron in, 163
Fetus, blood of, in maternal blood, 184
  production of, 54, *54*
  erythropoiesis in, 142
  hematopoiesis in, 36, *38*
  hemoglobin in, 166, *167*
FFP (fresh frozen plasma), 338d
  for disseminated intravascular coagulation,
    253
Fibrin, 337d
  in coagulation, 246, 248, 250
Fibrin split products (FSP) test, 249
  in coagulation testing, 269
  in fibrinolysis testing, 273
Fibrinogen, 6–7, 247t, 337d
  in coagulation, 246, 248, 250
  testing of, 249
Fibrinogen degradation products (FDP) test, 249
  in coagulation testing, 269
  in fibrinolysis testing, 273

Fibrinolysis, 244–257
  appropriate, 249–251
  defects in, 254, 255
  inappropriate, 251–255
  pathway of, 249, 250, 337d
  proteins of, 246–249, 247t, *248*
  systemic, 253, 255
  testing of, 273–274, *275*, 337d
Fibrin-stabilizing factor (FSF), 247t, 249
Fibrometer electromechanical coagulation instrument, *271*
Fine adjustment, of microscope, *27*, 28
Finger stick, in blood collection, 22, *23*
Fitzgerald factor, 246
Fletcher factor, 246
Flow cytometry, 337d–338d
  in aggregation studies, 268
  in cellular identification and evaluation, 44
  in complete blood count, 111
  in erythrocyte testing, 202
  in erythroleukemia, 195
  in leukemia, 63
  in leukocyte testing, 125, *126*
Fluorescence-activated cell sorter (FACS), 338d
  in leukocyte testing, 125, *126*
Fluorescent microscope, 29t
Folate, 338d
  deficiency of, anemia in, 187–188
    neutropenia in, 68
  identification and quantitation of, 135
  in erythrocyte testing, 219
  reference range for, 135
Forearm veins, in venipuncture, 18, *18*
Foreign immunogen, in humoral immunity, 95
Free erythrocyte protoporphyrin (FEP), 338d
  in anemia, 186–187
  in erythrocyte testing, 219
  in hemoglobin synthesis, 162
  in porphyria, 185
Free hemoglobin, in autoimmune hemolytic anemia, 189
Free plasma, 338d
  in autoimmune hemolytic anemia, 189
  in erythrocyte testing, 218
French-American-British (FAB) classification, of leukemia,
    64t, 337d
  cytochemical stains and, 122t
  erythrocytosis and, 196t
  lymphocytosis and, 99t
  monocytosis and, 81t
  thrombocytosis and, 240t
  of myelodysplastic syndrome, 69, 69t
  erythrocytes and, 186, 187t
Fresh frozen plasma (FFP), 338d
  for disseminated intravascular coagulation, 253
Fructose, in seminal vesicles, 293
FSF (fibrin-stabilizing factor), 247t, 249
FSP (fibrin split products) test, 249
  in coagulation testing, 269
  in fibrinolysis testing, 273
Functional assay, in protein C deficiency, 254, 255

Gammopathy, monoclonal, 102–103
  of undetermined significance, 103, 351d
Gaucher's disease, 83, 338d
Gaussian distribution, 13, *13*
Gene therapy, for sickle cell disease, 181
  for thalassemia, 185
Genetic abetalipoproteinemia, 189

Genetic alteration, 338d
Genetic anomaly(ies), 338d
  in leukemia, 63, 80
  in lymphocytopenia, 104
  neutropenia in, 68
  neutrophils in, 61
  of amino acid sequence, 168
  of thrombocytes, 236, 240–241
Genetic factor deficiency, 251–252, 255
Genetic predisposition, for lymphoma, 99
Geriatric. See *Elderly.*
Giemsa stain, 26, 27t. See also *Wright-Giemsa stain.*
Glanzmann's disease, 235, 240
Glass bead adhesion test, 240
  in thrombocyte testing, 267–268
Glass white blood cell pipette dilution method, for leukocyte count, 116, *116*
Glide stage, of microscope, *27*, 28
Globin, 160
  abnormal production of, 180–181
  decreased, 181
Gloves, 338d
  for body fluid testing, 301
  for manual platelet count, 264
  in clinical hematology, 29–30, *30*
  in phlebotomy, 18
Glucose, in cerebrospinal fluid, 287
  in synovial fluid, 288, 289
Glucose-6-phosphate dehydrogenase (G-6-PD), deficiency of, 185, 338–339d
  in erythrocyte testing, 219
  in oxygen transport, 155
Glutamine, cerebrospinal, 287
Glycolysis, in erythrocyte metabolism, 150, *151*
Glycoprotein(s), 246
  in platelet aggregation, 235
GM-CSF (granulocyte macrophage colony-stimulating factor), 144
Golgi apparatus, in cell maturation, 44
  of metamyelocyte, 57
  of plasma cell, 94
Gower 2, 166, 339d
G-6-PD (glucose-6-phosphate dehydrogenase), deficiency of, 185, 338d–339d
  in erythrocyte testing, 219
  in oxygen transport, 155
Gram stain, 339d
  of cerebrospinal fluid, 287
  of synovial fluid, 290
  of wound aspirates, 295
Granule(s), azurophilic, 88, 327d
  in acute promyelocytic leukemia, 66, *67*
  in bacterial infection, 61
  of basophil, 59, *59*
    in hypersensitivity reactions, 62
  of eosinophil, 58–59, *59*
  of myeloblast, 55
  of myelocyte, 56, *57*
  of neutrophil, 58, *58*
  of promyelocyte, 56, *56*
  of thrombocytes, 230, *233*
  siderotic, *209*
Granulocyte(s), 50, 52–73
  basic information on, *51*
  in abnormal neutrophil function, 69–70
  in basophilia, 72
  in eosinopenia, 72
  in eosinophilia, 71–72

Granulocyte(s) *(Continued)*
  in hematopoiesis, 42
  in neutropenia, *68*, 68–69, 69t
  in neutrophil anomalies, 70, *70*, *71*
  in neutrophilia, 62–68, 64t, *65–67*, 67t. See also *Neutrophilia.*
  information on, 72t
  lupus erythematosus cell in, 70–72, *71*
  origin, maturation, and morphology of, 54–60, *55–57*
    basophils in, *59*, 59–60
    eosinophils in, 58–59, *59*
    neutrophils in, 58, *58*
  physiology and function of, 60–62, *61*, *62*
Granulocyte macrophage colony-stimulating factor (GM-CSF), 144
Granulocytic leukemia, chronic. See *Chronic myelogenous leukemia (CML).*
Granuloma, eosinophilic, 83, 336d
Granulomatous disease, 69, 330d
  tests for, 125
Granulopoiesis, 54, *54*, 55, 339d
Gray platelet syndrome, 241, 339d, 363d, 365d
Growth factor(s), 339d
  in hematopoiesis, 39–41
  myeloid, 353d

HA (hydroxyapatite) crystal(s), 289
Haemophilus influenzae, 307
Hageman factor, 247t
Hairy cell leukemia (HCL), 104, *104*, 339d
  monocytopenia in, 82
Ham's test, 324d, 339d
  in erythrocyte testing, 220–221
Hand-Schüller-Christian syndrome, 83, 339d
Haptoglobin, 162, 339d–340d
  in autoimmune hemolytic anemia, 189
  in erythrocyte testing, 216–218
Hashimoto-Pritzker syndrome, 83, 340d
HAV (hepatitis A virus) infection, 98, 339d
Hay fever, eosinophils in, 61–62
Hb. see *Hemoglobin.*
HbCO. See *Carboxyhemoglobin.*
HbO$_2$. See *Oxyhemoglobin.*
HBV (hepatitis B virus) infection, 98, 339d
HCL (hairy cell leukemia), 104, *104*, 339d
  monocytopenia in, 82
HCO$_3^-$. See *Bicarbonate.*
H$_2$CO$_3$. See *Carbonic acid.*
HCV (hepatitis C virus) infection, 98, 339d
HDL (high-density lipoprotein), in plaque development, 237
HDN (hemolytic disease of newborn), 341d
  diagnostic tests for, 218
  erythrocyte testing in, 215
Health care provider, 319, 340d
Heart, pericardial fluid and, 292
Heart attack, serum lactate dehydrogenase isoenzymes in, 221
Heinz body(ies), 154–155, *182*, *209*, 341d
  stains of, 212
Helmet cell(s), *175*, *208*
Hematocrit, 340d
  determination of, 12
  in anemia, 180
  in complete blood count, 110
  in erythrocyte testing, 206
  in polycythemia, 191

Hematology, 4–33, 340d
  blood composition in, *6*, 6–7
  mathematics of, 8–14. See also *Mathematic(s).*
  microscope in, 23–29. See also *Microscopic evaluation.*
  phlebotomy in, 17–23. See also *Phlebotomy.*
  physiologic concepts of, 15–17, *16*
  practice of, 31–32
  quality assurance in, 30–31
  safety in, 29–30, *30*
  terminology in, 7–8
Hematology clinical laboratory scientist, 319–320
Hematoma, 250–251, 340d
Hematopoiesis, 34–48, 340d
  blood cell proliferation and differentiation in, 39–43, *40*
  cell structure and maturation in, 44–47, *45*, *46*
  cellular identification and evaluation in, 43–44
  extramedullary, 36, 142, 337d
    in myeloid metaplasia, 68
  fetal, 36, *38*
  granulopoiesis and, 54, *55*
  in bone marrow, 44, *45*
  medullary, 142, 350d
  monopoiesis and, 76, *77*
  pediatric and adult, 36–39, *38*
  scheme of, 39, *40*
Hematopoietic stem cell (HSC), 40, 340d
  in erythrocyte maturation, 144–145
  in granulocyte maturation, 54, *55*
  in lymphocyte maturation, 88, *89*
  in monocyte maturation, 76
  in thrombocyte maturation, 230
Heme groups, 160
Heme synthesis, 160–162, *163*
  interference with, 181
    lead poisoning in, 188
Hemochromatosis, 340d
  in sideroblastic anemia, 186
Hemocytoblast, 36
Hemocytometer method, of body fluid cell count, 301, *302*, 302–303, *304*
  of manual leukocyte count, 115, *115*, 117–118, *118*
  of manual platelet count, 261–264, *264*
Hemoglobin, 158–171, 174, 178, 340d
  catabolism of, 162, *164*
  classification and function of, 165–170, *166*, *167*
  decrease in, 178–191. See also *Anemia.*
  denaturated, *209*
  determination of, 11–12, *13*
  in complete blood count, 110
  in erythrocyte testing, 206, 216, *218*
  in oxygen transport, 152–153
  in polycythemia, 191
  iron kinetics and, 163–165, *164*
  structure, synthesis, and breakdown of, 160–163, *161–163*
  urine, 338d
    in erythrocyte testing, 218
Hemoglobin A, 166, *167*, 170, 183, 340d
Hemoglobin A_2, 166, *167*, 170, 341d
Hemoglobin A_{1c} monitoring of diabetic diet, 168, 340d–341d
Hemoglobin C, *182*, 183, 341d
  in erythrocytes, *209*
Hemoglobin D disease, 183
Hemoglobin electrophoresis, 166, *166*, 168–169, 341d
  in erythrocyte testing, 213–215, *214*
  in sickle cell disease, 181, 183, 213–215, *214*
  in thalassemia, 184

Hemoglobin F, 183, 341d
Hemoglobinopathy(ies), 180–185, 341d
  hemoglobin disease in, 183
  hemolytic disease of newborn in, 183–184
  porphyria in, 185
  sickle cell anemia in, 180–183, *181*
  thalassemia in, 184–185, *185*
Hemoglobin-oxygen dissociation curve, 154, *154*
Hemoglobinuria, 218
  paroxysmal cold, 189, 356d
    diagnostic tests for, 218
  paroxysmal nocturnal, 188–189
    diagnostic tests for, 220–221
    fibrinolytic defects in, 254
Hemolysis, 162, *164*, 341d
  complete blood count in, 112
  extravascular. See *Extravascular hemolysis.*
  free plasma or urine hemoglobin in, 218
  in erythrocyte testing, 204, 220–221
  in phagocytosis, 78
  in sickle cell disease, 181
  intravascular. See *Intravascular hemolysis.*
  serum lactate dehydrogenase isoenzymes in, 221
Hemolytic anemia, 178, 188–191, 341d
  alloimmune, 326d
    diagnostic tests for, 218
  autoimmune, 189, 327d
    diagnostic tests for, 218
  chronic intravascular, 221
  in infectious mononucleosis, 97
  in Waldenström's macroglobulinemia, 102
  red blood cell survival in, 222
Hemolytic disease of newborn (HDN), 183–184, 341d
  diagnostic tests for, 218
  erythrocyte testing in, 215
Hemolytic transfusion reaction (HTR), 218
Hemophilia, 251, 255
  factor VIII in, 246
Hemorrhage, 251–253, 255, 341d
  obstetric, 253, 255
  thrombocytosis in, 236, 239
Hemosiderin, 162, 341d
Hemosiderinuria, 218
  diagnostic tests for, 220–221
Hemostasis, 225–277, 341d–342d
  coagulation in, 244–257. See also *Coagulation.*
  testing of, 258–277
    coagulation in, 268–273, *271*, *273*
    fibrinolysis in, 273–274, *275*
    flow chart of, *275*
    thrombocytes in, 261–268. See also *Thrombocyte(s).*
    vasculature in, 260
  thrombocytes in, 228–243. See also *Thrombocyte(s).*
Heparin, 342d
  antithrombin III and, 249
  coagulation pathway and, 247
  for disseminated intravascular coagulation, 253
  in acute promyelocytic leukemia, 66
  in basophil, 59, *59*
  in synovial fluid testing, 288
  partial thromboplastin time monitoring of, 271
  platelet dysfunction from, 241
Hepatic. See also *Liver.*
Hepatic hematopoiesis, 142
Hepatitis, 339d, 342d
  lymphocytosis in, 98
  serum ferritin in, 216
Hepatitis A virus (HAV) infection, 98, 339d

Hepatitis B virus (HBV) infection, 98, 339d
Hepatitis C virus (HCV) infection, 98, 339d
Hereditary spherocytic anemia, 220
Hereditary telangiectasia, 235, 236
Hereditary thrombocyte disorders, 236, 240–241
Heterochromatin, 342d
  in cell maturation, 44
  of neutrophils, 58, *58*
Hexose monophosphate shunt (HMPS), 342d
  hemoglobin function in, 168
  in erythrocyte metabolism, 150, *151*
  in oxygen transport, 155
Hi. See *Methemoglobin.*
HI (humoral immunity), 343d
  B cells in, *93*, *94*, 94
High blood pressure, from polycythemia, 191
High dry objective, 28
High-density lipoprotein (HDL), in plaque development, 237
High-molecular-weight kininogen (HMWK), 246, 247t
High-resolution agarose electrophoresis, 127, 342d
Histamine, in basophil, 59, *59*
Histamine-neutralizing substance, in eosinophil, 58–59
Histiocyte(s), 76, 77, *78*, 342d
  in erythrocyte testing, 212
Histiocytosis, 83–84
  malignant, 350d
  pure cutaneous, 359d
  self-healing, 362d
Histiocytosis X, 83, 342d
Histogram, 342d
  in complete blood count, for erythrocyte testing, *203*, 203–204
    for leukocyte testing, 112, *113*
  in platelet count, 261, *262*
HMPS (hexose monophosphate shunt), 342d
  hemoglobin function in, 168
  in erythrocyte metabolism, 150, *151*
  in oxygen transport, 155
HMWK (high-molecular-weight kininogen), 246, 247t
Hodgkin's lymphoma, 104, *105*, 342d
Homeostasis, 15–17, *16*, 342d
Hormones, 342d–343d. See also *Erythropoietin (EPO).*
Howell-Jolly body(ies), *209*
  in erythroleukemia, 195
  in sickle cell anemia, 181–183, *182*
HSC. See *Hematopoietic stem cell (HSC).*
HTLV-II (human T-cell lymphotropic virus-II), 104
HTR (hemolytic transfusion reaction), 218
Human parvovirus, bone marrow toxicity from, 180
Human T-cell lymphotropic virus-II (HTLV-II), 104
Humoral immunity (HI), *93*, *94*, 94, 343d
Hyaluronic acid, in vascular integrity, 232
Hybridoma cell, 103
Hydrogen ion concentration. See *pH.*
Hydrogen peroxide, 343d
  from phagocytosis, 60
Hydrostatic pressure, serous effusions and, 291
Hydroxyapatite (HA) crystal(s), 289
Hypercoagulability, 249
Hypergammaglobulinemia, 343d
  leukocytes in, 102
  platelet dysfunction in, 241
Hypergranulation, in acute promyelocytic leukemia, 66, *67*
Hyperplasia, in bone marrow, 64, *65*
Hypersegmented cell, 58
Hypersegmented neutrophil, 343d
  in pernicious anemia, 187, *187*

Hypersensitivity reaction, 343d
  basophils in, 59, *59*
  delayed-type, 91
  eosinophils in, 58–59, 61–62
Hypertonic solution, 343d
  cells in, 15, *16*
Hypochromic erythrocyte(s), 174, *177*, 178, 343d
  in chronic posthemorrhagic anemia, 180
  in iron deficiency anemia, 186, *186*
  in sideroblastic anemia, 186
  in thalassemia, *184*, 184–185
Hypoplasia, myeloid, 353d
  neutropenia in, 68
Hypoplastic anemia, 180, 343d
Hyposegmented cell, 58
Hyposegmented neutrophil, 343d
  in Pelger-Huët anomaly, 70, *71*
Hypotonic solution, 343d
  cells in, 15, *16*
Hypovolemia, in anemia, 178
Hypoxia, 343d
  central nervous system, 287
  in anemia, 176
  in erythropoiesis, 174

¹²¹I. See *Radioactive albumin.*
Icterus, 343d
Identification, patient, 17–18
Identification marker(s), lymphocyte, 90, 90t
Idiopathic thrombocytopenic purpura (ITP), 236, 238, 343d
IEP (immunoelectrophoresis), 344d
  in protein identification and quantitation, 127–129, *129*
IFN (interferon), 91t, 345d
  in erythropoiesis, 180
  monocytes and, 79
Ig. See *Immunoglobulin(s).*
ILs. See *Interleukins (ILs).*
Immune adherence, 60
Immune destruction, thrombocytopenia in, 236, 238
Immune response, in pregnancy, 183
  primary, 92, *94*, 359d
  secondary, 92, *94*, 362d
Immunity, cell-mediated, 90, 91t, *93*
  humoral, *93*, *94*, 94, 343d
Immunoassay, 343d
  competitive, 133–134, *134*
  enzyme, 134–135, *135*, 336d
  in protein C deficiency, 254, 255
  noncompetitive, 133
  of body fluids, 307–309
  of cerebrospinal fluid, 285, 287–288
  of lymphocytes, 95
  of synovial fluid, 290
Immunodiffusion, 343d
  in lymphocyte tests, 95
  Ouchterlony double, 131–133, *132*, 355d–356d
  radial, 129–131, *130*, 360d
Immunoelectrophoresis (IEP), 127–129, *129*, 344d
Immunogen, 344d
  foreign, in humoral immunity, 95
  presentation of, monocytes in, 78, *79*
Immunoglobulin(s), 95, 344d
  cerebrospinal, 287
  in cell-mediated immunity, 90, 91t, *93*

Immunoglobulin(s) *(Continued)*
  in parasitic and hypersensitivity reactions, 62
  in Waldenström's macroglobulinemia, 102
Immunoprecipitin tests, 133, 344d, 353d, 366d
Immunotherapy, 96
In vitro, 345d
Inclusion(s), erythrocyte, 207, *209*
India ink stain, 344d
  of cerebrospinal fluid, 287
Indices, 9, 12, 344d–345d
  in erythrocyte testing, 202
Infant, hematopoiesis in, 36
  newborn. See *Newborn.*
  phlebotomy in, 22, *22*, *23*
Infarction, cerebral, 287
  in sickle cell disease, 181
  myocardial, 221, 353d
Infection, bacterial. See *Bacterial infection.*
  monocytosis in, 80
  neutropenia in, 68
  of meninges, 285
  parasitic, 356d
    eosinophils in, 61–62
    of erythrocytes, *182*, *209*
    serum ferritin in, 216
    thrombocytosis in, 236, 239
  viral. See *Viral infection.*
Infectious lymphocytosis, 97, 345d
Infectious mononucleosis, 345d, 352d
  lymphocytosis in, 97
Inflammation, 345d
  central nervous system (CNS), 288
  serum ferritin in, 216
  serum lactate dehydrogenase isoenzymes in,
    221
Initiating event, 345d
  in leukemia, 63, 80
  in lymphoma, 99
Instrument(s), for complete blood count, 111–
  112
Interferon (IFN), 91t, 345d
  in erythropoiesis, 180
  monocytes and, 79
Interleukins (ILs), 345d
  in erythrocyte function, 148, 149
  in erythropoiesis, 144
  in hematopoiesis, 40
  in lymphopoiesis, 50
  response to, monocytes in, 78, *79*
Intestine-associated lymphoid tissue, 88
Intravascular coagulation, 252–253
Intravascular hemolysis, 162, *164*, 345d
  anemia from, 188–189, *190*
    diagnostic tests for, 221
  in immune response, 96
  in spherocytosis, 191
Intravenous (IV) fluid dilution anemia, 177
Intrinsic coagulation pathway, 246–247, *248*, 250,
  345d
Iodine, in homeostasis, 17
Iris diaphragm, of microscope, *27*, 28
Iron, 345d–346d
  deficiency of, anemia in, 185–186, *186*, 346d
    thrombocytosis in, 236, 239
  in heme catabolism, 162
  in hemoglobin, 160
  in thalassemia, 184
  serum, 216, 362d

Iron stain, 26, 27t, 346d
  in erythrocyte testing, 212, 216, *217*
  in sideroblastic anemia, 186
Irradiation, lymphocytopenia from, 104
Isopropyl alcohol, 186
  for phlebotomy, 18–19
ITP (idiopathic thrombocytopenic purpura), 236, 238,
  343d
IV (intravenous) fluid dilution anemia, 177

Joint(s), fluids of, 288–290, *289*, *290*
Joint Commission on the Accreditation of Healthcare Or-
  ganizations (JCAHO), 30

K (killer) cell(s), 96, 346d
Kaposi's sarcoma, 235, 236
Karyotyping, of amniotic fluid, 295
Kidney(s), disorders of, hemorrhage in, 253, 255
    in polycythemia, 194
    pseudoanemia in, 177
  in erythropoietin production, 143
  in urine production, 294
Killer (K) cell(s), 96, 346d
Kininogen, high-molecular-weight, 246, 247t
Kliehauer-Betke method, 184
Kupffer cell(s), 76, 346d

LA (lupus anticoagulants), 327d, 348d
  hemorrhagic disorders and, 252
Labile factor, 247t, 248
Laboratory information systems (LIS), 318, 346d
Laboratory practitioner, 319–320
Lactate, cerebrospinal, 287
  synovial, 289–290
Lactic dehydrogenase (LD), 346d
  cerebrospinal, 287
  in erythrocyte testing, 221
  serum, 362d–363d
LAK (lymphokine-activated killer) cell(s), 96
Lancet, in phlebotomy, 22, *22*
Langerhans cell(s), 76, 346d
Langerhans cell histiocytosis, 83, 346d
LAP. See *Leukocyte alkaline phosphatase (LAP) score.*
Laser light scattering, 346d–347d
  in erythrocyte testing, 202
  in leukocyte testing, 111–112
Late reticulocyte, 147
Latex agglutination test, 347d
  of cerebrospinal fluid, 287
Lazy leukocyte syndrome, 69, 347d
  testing for, 127
LD (lactic dehydrogenase), 346d
  cerebrospinal, 287
  in erythrocyte testing, 221
  serum, 362d–363d
LDL (low-density lipoprotein), in plaque development,
  237
LE (lupus erythematosus), 70–72, *71*
  autoimmune hemolytic anemia in, 189
  synovial fluid in, 290
  testing of, 124–125, *125*

Lead, in erythrocyte testing, 219
  poisoning from, 188, *188*, 347d
Lecithin/sphingomyelin (L/S) ratio, in amniotic fluid, 295
Lee-White clotting time test, 272, 347d
Left shift, 58, 347d, 363d
  in acute posthemorrhagic anemia, 179
  in bacterial infection, 61
  neutrophils in, 58
Leptocyte, *175, 208*
Letterer-Siwe disease, 83, 347d
Leukemia, 324d, 347d
  acute lymphocytic. See *Acute lymphocytic leukemia (ALL).*
  acute megakaryocytic. See *Acute megakaryocytic leukemia (AMegL).*
  acute monoblastic, 64t
  acute monocytic. See *Acute monocytic leukemia (AMoL).*
  acute myelogenous. See *Acute myelogenous leukemia (AML).*
  acute myelomonocytic. See *Acute myelomonocytic leukemia (AMML).*
  acute promyelocytic. See *Acute promyelocytic leukemia (APL).*
  adult T-cell, classification of, 64t
    cytochemistry of, 67t
    malignant lymphocytosis in, 100, *100*
  chronic granulocytic. See *Chronic myelogenous leukemia (CML).*
  chronic lymphocytic, 330d
    malignant lymphocytosis in, *101*, 101–102, *102*
  chronic myelogenous. See *Chronic myelogenous leukemia (CML).*
  chronic myelomonocytic, 330d–331d
    in myelodysplastic syndrome, 69, 69t
    monocytes in, 82
  development of, 80–81
  hairy cell, 104, *104*, 339d
    monocytopenia in, 82
  lymphoid, 64t
  lymphosarcoma, 101–102
  neutrophilia in, 63, 64
  plasma cell, 103, 357d
Leukemic phase of lymphoma, 98, 347d
Leukemoid reaction, 58, 347d
  neutrophilia in, 62–63
Leukocyte(s), 6, *6*, 49–136, 347d–348d
  granulocytes in, 52–73. See also *Granulocyte(s).*
  in body defense, 50–51
  in exudates, 291
  in Hodgkin's lymphoma, 105
  in synovial fluid, 288
  in transudates, 291
  information in, *51*
  lymphocytes and plasma cells in, 86–107. See also *Lymphocyte(s); Plasma cell(s).*
  monocytes in, 74–85. See also *Monocyte(s).*
  shape of, 10
  size of, 10
  testing of, 108–136
    counts in, 110–119. See also *Leukocyte count.*
    flow cytometry in, 125, *126*
    lupus erythematosus preparation in, 124–125, *125*
    microscopic, 119–124. See also *Microscopic evaluation.*
    protein identification and quantitation in, 127–135. See also *Protein identification and quantitation.*
    vitamin identification and quantitation in, 135–136
    white blood cell function tests in, 125–127
Leukocyte alkaline phosphatase (LAP) score, 326d, 346d, 347d

Leukocyte alkaline phosphatase (LAP) score *(Continued)*
  in chronic myelogenous leukemia, 64
  in leukemoid reaction, 62
  in microscopic leukocyte evaluation, 123, *123*
Leukocyte count, 9, 110–119
  complete blood count in, 110–114, *113, 114*
  correlation factors in, 118–119
  error in, 119
  glass white blood cell pipette dilution method in, 116, *116*
  hemocytometer method in, 115, *115*, 117–118, *118*
  unopette dilution method in, 116–117, *117*
Leukocytosis, neutrophilic, 179
Leukopoiesis, 348d
Levey-Jennings Quality Control graph, 13, *14*, 348d
Light absorbance, 348d
  in erythrocyte testing, 202
  in leukocyte testing, 112
Light microscope, 27, *27*, 29t
  in reticulocyte counting, 210
Lipemia, 348d
  complete blood count in, 112
  in erythrocyte testing, 204
Lipid catabolism, ineffective, 82–83
Lipid plaque, 237
Lipid storage disease, 83, 348d
Lipopolysaccharide (LPS), 348d
  in granulocytic function, 60
LIS (laboratory information systems), 318, 346d
Liver, 348d
  bilirubin detoxification in, 218
  cirrhosis of, pseudoanemia in, 177
    thrombocytopenia in, 236, 239
  disease of, hemorrhagic disorders in, 252, 255
    macrocytic anemia in, 188
    target cells in, 181
  hematopoiesis in, 36, 142
  in erythropoietin production, 143
  in infectious mononucleosis, 97
  injury to, 221
  inflammation of. See *Hepatitis.*
  macrophage cells in, 76
Low-density lipoprotein (LDL), in plaque development, 237
Low-power objective, 27, 28
LPS (lipopolysaccharide), 348d
  in granulocytic function, 60
L/S (lecithin/sphingomyelin) ratio, in amniotic fluid, 295
LSC (lymphoid stem cell), 349d
  in hematopoiesis, 41
  in lymphopoiesis, 88, *89*
LSL (lymphosarcoma leukemia), 101–102
Lumbar puncture, in cerebrospinal fluid collection, 285, *286*
Lumen, endothelial surface of, 232
Lupus anticoagulants (LA), 327d, 348d
  hemorrhagic disorders and, 252
Lupus erythematosus (LE), 70–72, *71*
  autoimmune hemolytic anemia in, 189
  synovial fluid in, 290
  testing of, 124–125, *125*
Lymph flow obstruction, 291
Lymph node(s), hematopoietic activity in, 142
  lymphocytes in, 88
Lymphatic reabsorption, 291
Lymphoblastic leukemia, acute. See *Acute lymphocytic leukemia (ALL).*
Lymphocyte(s), 50, 86–107, 348d–349d

Lymphocyte(s) *(Continued)*
  decreased, 104, *104*
  in cerebrospinal fluid, 288
  in malignant lymphomas, 104–106, *105*, 105t, *106*
  in pericardial fluid, 292
  in peritoneal fluid, 293
  in pleural fluid, 291, *292*
  increased, 97–103. See also *Lymphocytosis.*
  information on, *51*
  origin, maturation, and morphology of, 88–90, *89,*
    90, 91t
  physiology and function of, 90–96
    B cells in, *93, 94,* 94–96
    killer cells in, 96
    natural killer cells in, 96
    T cells in, 90–94, 91t, *93, 94*
  reactive, 88, *90,* 360d
  reference value for, 97
  relative count of, 10
  size of, 7, 363d
Lymphocytic leukemia, acute. See *Acute lymphocytic leuke-*
  mia (ALL).
  chronic, 330d
    malignant lymphocytosis in, *101,* 101–102
Lymphocytopenia, 104, *104,* 349d
Lymphocytosis, 97–103, 349d
  absolute, 10
  infectious, 97, 345d
  malignant, 98–103, 350d. See also *Malignant lympho-*
    cytosis.
  reactive, 97–98
  relative, 10
  T cells in, 90
Lymphoid growth factor(s), 41
Lymphoid leukemia, 64t
Lymphoid organs, 88, 359d
Lymphoid proliferation, 253, 255
Lymphoid stem cell (LSC), 349d
  in hematopoiesis, 41
  in lymphopoiesis, 88, *89*
Lymphokine-activated killer (LAK) cell(s), 96
Lymphoma, 98, 349d
  Burkitt's, 100–101, *101*
  cutaneous T-cell, 105, *106*
  genetic predisposition for, 99
  Hodgkin's, 104, *105,* 342d
  leukemic phase of, 98, 347d
  malignant, 104–106, *105,* 105t, *106*
  monocytosis in, 80
  non-Hodgkin's, 105, 105t, 353d–354d
  viral infection in, 99
Lymphopoiesis, 50, 349d
Lymphosarcoma leukemia (LSL), 101–102
Lysosome, in phagocytosis, 60, *61*

Macrocyte(s), 174, 350d
  in chronic posthemorrhagic anemia, 180
  in liver disease, 188, *188*
Macrocytic anemia, *179,* 188, *188*
Macroglobulinemia, Waldenström's, 102, 367d
Macrophage(s), 50. See also *Monocyte(s).*
  in autoimmune hemolytic anemia, 189
  in immune response, 96
  in pericardial fluid, 292
  in peritoneal fluid, 292

Macrophage(s) *(Continued)*
  in pleural fluid, 291, *292*
  in synovial fluid, 289
Magnesium, in homeostasis, 17
Magnification, calculation of, 29, 29t
Major histocompatibility complex (MHC), 88, 350d
Malaria, in erythrocytes, *209*
Malignancy, 350d
  complete blood count in, 112
  peritoneal fluid in, 292
  pleural fluid in, 291–292, *292*
  serum ferritin in, 216
  thrombocytosis in, 236, 239
  vascular, 235, 236
Malignant erythrocytosis, 195, 196t, 350d
Malignant histiocytosis, 84, 350d
Malignant leukemic cell(s), 64
Malignant lymphocytosis, 98–103, 350d
  in acute lymphoblastic leukemia, 100–101, *101*
  in acute lymphocytic leukemia, 98–100, *100*
  in adult T-cell leukemia, 100, *100*
  in chronic lymphocytic leukemia, *101,* 101–102
  in monoclonal gammopathy of undetermined signifi-
    cance, 103
  in multiple myeloma, 102–103, *103*
  in plasma cell leukemia, 103
  in Waldenström's macroglobulinemia, 102
Malignant lymphoma, 104–106, *105,* 105t, *106*
Malignant monocytosis, 80
Malignant polycythemia, 194
Managed care, 32, 350d
Manual cell count(s), 8–10
  of leukocytes, 114–119. See also *Leukocyte count.*
  of platelets, 261–268. See also *Platelet count.*
  of sperm, 301–302, *302*
MAPSS (multiangle polarized scatter separation),
  112
Marginal granulocyte pool (MGP), 60
Margination monocyte pool (MMP), 76
Massive transfusion, 253, 255
  thrombocytopenia in, 236, 239
Mast cell, 59–60
Material safety data sheets (MSDS), 30, 350d
Mathematic(s), 8–14
  erythrocyte and thrombocyte indices in, 12
  hematocrit determinations in, 12
  hemoglobin determinations in, 11–12, *13*
  manual cell counts in, 9–10
  quality control calculations in, *13,* 13–14, *14*
  relative and absolute cell counts in, 10–11, *11*
  size and shape calculations in, 8–9
May-Hegglin anomaly, 70, *70,* 350d
MCH (mean corpuscular hemoglobin), 9, 174, 178, 349d,
  350d
  in erythrocyte testing, 202
  units used for, 13
MCHC (mean corpuscular hemoglobin concentration), 9,
  174, 178, 349d
  in erythrocyte testing, 203, *203*
  units used for, 13
MCV (mean corpuscular volume), 9, 349d
  in erythrocyte testing, 202, 203, *203*
  units used for, 13
MDS (myelodysplastic syndrome), 352d
  neutropenia in, 68–69, 69t
  sideroblastic anemia in, 186, 187t
M:E (myeloid:erythroid) ratio, 44, 353d
Mean, 13, 350d

Mean corpuscular hemoglobin (MCH), 9, 174, 178, 349d, 350d
  in erythrocyte testing, 202
  units used for, 13
Mean corpuscular hemoglobin concentration (MCHC), 9, 174, 178, 349d
  in erythrocyte testing, 203, *203*
  units used for, 13
Mean corpuscular volume (MCV), 9, 349d
  in erythrocyte testing, 202, 203, *203*, 204
  units used for, 13
Mean platelet volume (MPV), 9, 349d–350d, 357d
Mechanical trauma, intravascular hemolysis in, 188
Medial cephalic vein, 18, *18*
Medial cubital vein, 18, *18*
Medullary granulopoiesis, 54, *54*, 55
Medullary hematopoiesis, 142, 350d
Mega-CSF (colony-stimulating factor–mega), 230
Megakaryoblast, in hematopoiesis, 42
Megakaryoblastic leukemia, acute. See *Acute megakaryocytic leukemia (AMegL)*.
Megakaryocyte, 230, *232*
  in hematopoiesis, 42
Megakaryocyte colony-stimulating factor–mega (mega-CSF), 230
Megakaryocytic leukemia, acute. See *Acute megakaryocytic leukemia (AMegL)*.
Megaloblastic nucleus, 350d
  in pernicious anemia, 187
Membrane, of erythrocyte, 150–152, *153*
Meninges, 285
Meningitis, 286, *287*
Mesothelial cell(s), in pericardial fluid, 292
  in peritoneal fluid, 292
  in pleural fluid, 291, *292*
Metabolic disorder(s), cerebrospinal fluid in, 287
Metabolism, erythrocyte, 150, *151*
Metamyelocyte, 57, *57*, 350d
  eosinophilic, 59
Metaplasia, myeloid, 353d
  neutrophilia in, 67–68
Metarubricyte, 146–147, *147*, 149
Methemoglobin, 155, 168, 350d–351d
Methemoglobin reductase pathway, 168
  in erythrocyte metabolism, *151*
  in oxygen transport, 155
Methylene blue stain, 26, 27t, 351d
Mg^{2+}. See *Magnesium*.
MGP (marginal granulocyte pool), 60
MGUS (monoclonal gammopathy of undetermined significance), 103, 351d
MHC (major histocompatibility complex), 88, 350d
MI (myocardial infarction), 353d
  serum lactate dehydrogenase isoenzymes in, 221
Microbiologic testing, of body fluids, 307–309
  of cerebrospinal fluid, 285, 287–288
  of serous fluid, 291
  of synovial fluid, 288, 290
  of wound aspirates, 295
Microcyte(s), 174, 351d
  in iron deficiency anemia, 186, *186*
  in sideroblastic anemia, 186
  in thalassemia, *184*, 184–185
Microcytic anemia, *179*
Microenvironment, bone marrow, 36, *38*, 329d
Microglial cell(s), 76
Micromegakaryocyte, 113

Microscopic evaluation, 23–29, 351d
  blood smear preparation in, 24–26, *25*
  cell size in, 7–8
  in manual platelet count, 265–266
  magnification in, 29, 29t
  microscope in, 27–29
  of body fluids, 303–306, *305–307*
  of cerebrospinal fluid, 285–286
  of erythrocytes, 206–213
    cytochemical stain in, 212–213
    Heinz body stains in, 212
    iron stain in, 212
    peripheral blood smear in, 206–212, *207–210*. See also *Peripheral blood smear*.
  of leukocytes, 119–124
    Arneth count for neutrophil segmentation in, 123–124, *124*
    buffy coat preparation for, 123
    correlation factors in, 123
    cytochemical stains in, 122, 122t
    error in, 123
    leukocyte alkaline phosphatase score in, 123, *123*
    leukocyte differential and peripheral blood smear procedure in, 119–122, *120*, *121*
  of pericardial fluid, 292
  of peritoneal fluid, 292
  of seminal fluid, 293
  of serous fluid, 291
  of synovial fluid, 288–289
  staining and, 26, *27*, 27t
Microthrombus, in disseminated intravascular coagulation, 253
  vascular integrity in, 235, 236
Miller disk procedure, *210*, 210–211, 351d
Mineral(s), 351d
  in homeostasis, 16–17
Mission of clinical laboratory, 351d
Mitochondria, hemoglobin synthesis in, 160–162, *163*
MM (multiple myeloma), 102–103, *103*, 352d
MMP (margination monocyte pool), 76
Monochrome stain, 26, 27t, 351d
  in erythrocyte testing, 212
Monoclonal, 351d
Monoclonal antibody, 351d
Monoclonal gammopathy, 102–103
  of undetermined significance, 103, 351d
Monoclonal response, 93
Monocyte(s), 50, 74–85, 351d. See also *Macrophage(s)*.
  decreased, 82–84, 83t
  in diseases and malignancies, 84
  in pericardial fluid, 292
  in peritoneal fluid, 292
  in pleural fluid, 291
  in synovial fluid, 289
  increased, 80–82, 81t, *82*, 83t
  information on, 80
  origin, maturation, and morphology of, 76–77, *77*, *78*
  physiology and function of, 77–80, *79*
  reference value for, 110
  size of, 7, 363d
Monocytic leukemia, acute. See *Acute monocytic leukemia (AMoL)*.
Monocytopenia, 82–84, 352d
Monocytosis, 80–82, 81t, *82*, 83t
  reactive, 360d
Monolayer, 352d
  peripheral blood smear in, 174, *177*, 178

Mononuclear cell(s), in cerebrospinal fluid, 286
  in hairy cell leukemia, 104
Mononucleosis, infectious, 345d, 352d
  lymphocytosis in, 97
Monopoiesis, 76, *77*, 352d
Monosodium urate (MSU) crystal(s), 288, *289*
Motility, of seminal fluid, 293
  of sperm, 304
Mouth cell(s), *175, 208*
MPD (myeloproliferative disorder), 353d
  fibrinolytic defects in, 254
  platelet dysfunction in, 241
  thrombocytosis in, 236, 239
MPO (myeloperoxidase), 353d
  in leukemia cytochemistry, 65, *65*
  in myeloblast, 55
  in myelocyte, 56
  in promyelocyte, 56
MPV (mean platelet volume), 9, 349d–350d, 357d
MSDS (material safety data sheets), 30, 350d
MSU (monosodium urate) crystal(s), 288, *289*
Multiangle polarized scatter separation (MAPSS), 112
Multiple myeloma (MM), 102–103, *103*, 352d
Multiple sclerosis, cerebrospinal fluid in, 287
Muscle injury, serum lactate dehydrogenase isoenzymes
    in, 221
Mycobacterium tuberculosis, 307
Mycosis fungoides, 105, *106*, 352d
Myeloblast(s), 352d
  in acute myelogenous leukemia, 65, *65*
  origin, maturation and morphology of, 54–56, *55,
    56*
Myelocyte(s), basophilic, 59
  eosinophilic, 58
  morphology of, 56–57, *57*
Myelodysplastic syndrome (MDS), 352d
  erythroleukemia in, 195, 196t
  neutropenia in, 68–69, 69t
  sideroblastic anemia in, 186, 187t
Myelofibrosis, 352d–353d
  neutrophilia in, 67–68
Myelogenous leukemia, acute. See *Acute myelogenous leuke-
    mia (AML)*.
  chronic. See *Chronic myelogenous leukemia (CML)*.
Myeloid cell(s), 51
Myeloid growth factor(s), 353d
  in hematopoiesis, 40, 41
Myeloid hypoplasia, 353d
  neutropenia in, 68
Myeloid metaplasia, 353d
  neutrophilia in, 67–68
Myeloid proliferation, hemorrhagic disorders in, 253,
    255
Myeloid:erythroid (M:E) ratio, 44, 353d
Myeloma, multiple, 102–103, *103*, 352d
Myelomonocytic leukemia, acute. See *Acute myelomonocytic
    leukemia (AMML)*.
  chronic, 330d–331d
  in myelodysplastic syndrome, 69, 69t
  monocytes in, 82
Myeloperoxidase (MPO), 353d
  in leukemia cytochemistry, 65, *65*
  in myeloblast, 55
  in myelocyte, 56
  in promyelocyte, 56
Myelopoiesis, 54, *54, 55*
Myeloproliferative disorder (MPD), 353d
  fibrinolytic defects in, 254

Myeloproliferative disorder (MPD) *(Continued)*
  platelet dysfunction in, 241
  thrombocytosis in, 236, 239
Myocardial infarction (MI), 221, 353d

NAP (neutrophil alkaline phosphatase) score, 326d, 346d,
    347d
  in leukemoid reaction, 62
  in microscopic leukocyte evaluation, 123, *123*
Natural killer (NK) cell(s), 96, 353d
NBT (nitroblue tetrazolium reduction test), 125
N:C. See *Nuclear to cytoplasmic (N:C) ratio*.
Neck, of microscope, *27*, 28
Necrosis, 353d
  in protein C deficiency, 254
Needle(s), *19*, 19–20, 353d
Needle holder(s), 20, *20*, 353d
Neimann-Pick disease, 353d
Neisseria meningitidis, 307
Neonate. See *Newborn*.
Neoplasm(s), 353d
  in multiple myeloma, 103
  peritoneal fluid in, 292
  pleural fluid in, 291–292, *292*
Nephelometric immunoprecipitin assay, 133, 353d
Nephritis, pseudoanemia in, 177
Neubauer Hemocytometer Counting Chamber, *115, 302*
Neutropenia, *68*, 68–69, 69t, 353d
Neutrophil(s), abnormal function of, 69–70
  anomalies of, *70, 70, 71*
  decreased, *68*, 68–69, 69t
  development of, 54–58, *55–57*
  hypersegmented, 343d
  hyposegmented, 343d
  in cerebrospinal fluid, 286
  in exudates, 291
  in fetus, 54, *54*
  in pericardial fluid, 292
  in peritoneal fluid, 292
  in pleural fluid, 291
  in synovial fluid, 289
  increased, 62–68, 64t, *65–67*, 67t. See also *Neutrophilia*.
  information on, 72t
  morphology of, 58, *58*
  phagocytosis of, 60
  physiology and function of, 60–61, *61, 62*
  segmented. See *Segmented neutrophil(s)*.
  size of, 7, 363d
  testing of, 125–127
Neutrophil alkaline phosphatase (NAP) score, 326d, 346d,
    347d
  in leukemoid reaction, 62
  in microscopic leukocyte evaluation, 123, *123*
Neutrophil count, reference value for, 110
Neutrophilia, 62–68, 353d
  in acute leukemias, 63–64, 64t
    myelogenous, 64t, *65*, 65–66, *66*, 67t
    myelomonocytic, 64t, 66–67
    promyelocytic, 66, *67*
  in chronic myelogenous leukemia, 64–65, *65*
  in leukemoid reaction, 62–63
  in myelofibrosis and myeloid metaplasia, 67–68
Neutrophilic granule(s), 187
Neutrophilic leukocytosis, 179
Newborn, blood cell production in, 54, *54*
  hematopoiesis in, 36

Newborn *(Continued)*
  hemolytic disease of, 183–184, 341d
    diagnostic tests for, 218
    erythrocyte testing in, 215
    phlebotomy in, 22, *22, 23*
Niemann-Pick disease, 83
Nitroblue tetrazolium reduction test (NBT), 125
NK (natural killer) cell(s), 96, 353d
Nocturnal hemoglobinuria, paroxysmal, 188–189
    diagnostic tests for, 220–221
    fibrinolytic defects in, 254
Noncompetitive immunoassay, 133
Non-Hodgkin's lymphoma, 105, 105t, 353d–354d
Nonvital stain, 26, 27t, 354d
Normoblast(s), basophilic, 146, *146*, 149, 328d
  orthochromic, 146–147, *147*, 149, 355d
  polychromatophilic, 146, *147*, 149, 358d
Normochromic erythrocyte(s), 174, *177*, 178, 207, 354d
  in anemia, acute posthemorrhagic, 179
    chronic posthemorrhagic, 180
    of chronic disease, 187
    of decreased production, 180
    sickle cell, 181, 183
  in glucose-6-phosphate dehydrogenase deficiency, 185
  in Hodgkin's lymphoma, 105
  in infectious mononucleosis, 97
  in multiple myeloma, 103
  in sideroblastic anemia, 186
  in Waldenström's macroglobulinemia, 102
Normocyte(s), 174, *175*, 207, *208*, 354d
  in anemia, acute posthemorrhagic, 179
    chronic posthemorrhagic, 179–180
    of chronic disease, 187
    of decreased production, 180
    sickle cell, 181, 183
  in glucose-6-phosphate dehydrogenase deficiency, 185
  in Hodgkin's lymphoma, 105
  in infectious mononucleosis, 97
  in multiple myeloma, 103
  in Waldenström's macroglobulinemia, 102
Normocytic anemia, *179*
NRBC (nucleated red blood cells), 36, 354d
  in complete blood count, 113
  in pernicious anemia, 187
Nuclear remnant(s), in erythrocytes, *209*
Nuclear to cytoplasmic (N:C) ratio, 354d
  of band cell, 57, *57*
  of metamyelocyte, *57*
  of myeloblast, 54
  of myelocyte, *57*
  of neutrophil, 58, *58*
  of promyelocyte, 55, *55*
Nucleated red blood cells (NRBC), 36, 354d
  in complete blood count, 113
  in pernicious anemia, 187
Nucleoli, 44, 354d
  loss of, 46
Nucleus, in cell maturation, 44, 46
  of band cell, 57, *57*
  of eosinophil, 59, *59*
  of lymphocyte, 88, *90*
  of megaloblast, 350d
    in pernicious anemia, 187
  of metamyelocyte, 57, *57*
  of monocyte, 76, *78*
  of myeloblast, 54, *55*

Nucleus *(Continued)*
  of myelocyte, *57*
  of neutrophil, 58, *58*
  of plasma cell, 94
  of promyelocyte, 55, *55*
  of thrombocyte, 230, *232*
Null cell(s), 96
Nurse, 319
Nutrient(s), 354d
  in homeostasis, 16

Objective lens, 27, *27*, 354d
Obstetric hemorrhage, 253, 255
Occupational Safety and Health Administration (OSHA), 30, 354d–355d
Ocular lens, 27, *27*, 355d
Oil immersion objective, 28
Oncogene(s), 99, 355d
Opaque solution, in sickle cell screening tests, 213
Opsonin(s), 355d
  in autoimmune hemolytic anemia, 189
  in phagocytosis, 60
Opsonization, 355d
Optical clot detection, 269–270, 355d
Orientation, in clinical laboratory, 319
Orthochromic normoblast, 146–147, *147*, 149, 355d
OSHA (Occupational Safety and Health Administration), 30, 354d–355d
Osmotic concentration, 355d
  in homeostasis, 15, *16*
Osmotic fragility test, 355d
  in erythrocyte testing, *219*, 219–220
Osmotic pressure, serous effusions and, 291
Osteoclast, 76, 355d
Ouchterlony double immunodiffusion technique, 131–133, *132*, 355d–356d
Outcome assessment, 356d
Oxygen, partial pressure of, 154
Oxygen dissociation curve, 156, 356d
  of hemoglobin, 154, *154*, 160, *162*
Oxygen saturation curve, 156, 356d
  of hemoglobin, 154, *154*, 160, *162*
Oxygen transport, erythrocytes in, 152–156, *153, 154*
Oxyhemoglobin, 154, 168, 356d
Oxyhemoglobin dissociation curve, 156

PA. See *Pernicious anemia (PA)*.
Pallor, 356d
Palpation, 356d
  in phlebotomy, 18, 19
Pancytopenia, 104
Panmyelosis, 67, 356d
Pappenheimer body(ies), *182*, 356d
  in erythrocytes, *209*, 212
  in sideroblastic anemia, 186
Parasitic infection, 356d
  eosinophils in, 61–62
  of erythrocytes, *182, 209*
Parkinson's disease, 287
Paroxysmal cold hemoglobinuria (PCH), 189, 356d
  diagnostic tests for, 218
Paroxysmal nocturnal hemoglobinuria (PNH), 188–189
  diagnostic tests for, 220–221
  fibrinolytic defects in, 254

Partial pressure, of carbon dioxide, 154
  of oxygen, 154
Partial thromboplastin time (PTT) test, 247, 356d
  in coagulation testing, 271–272
  in hemophilia A, 251
Parvovirus, 180
PAS (periodic acid-Schiff) stain, in erythrocyte testing, 212–213
Pathogen, 29–30, 356d
Patient oriented, 320, 356d
Patient preparation, for phlebotomy, 17–18, *18*
PCH (paroxysmal cold hemoglobinuria), 189, 356d
  diagnostic tests for, 218
PCL (plasma cell leukemia), 103, 357d
PCO. See *Partial pressure, of carbon dioxide.*
Pelger-Huët anomaly, 70, *71*, 356d
Percent saturation, of iron, 185, 186
  of transferrin, 216, 366d
Pericardial fluid, 292, *292*, 356d
  testing of, 309
Periodic acid-Schiff (PAS) stain, 212–213
Peripheral blood lymphocyte, 89. See also *Lymphocyte(s).*
Peripheral blood monocyte, 76. See also *Monocyte(s).*
Peripheral blood pool, 44, *45*
Peripheral blood smear, in complete blood count, 112
  in microscopic erythrocyte evaluation, 206–212
    morphology and inclusions in, 207, *208*, *209*
    reticulocyte count in, 207–212. See also *Reticulocyte count.*
    stress reticulocytes in, 207, *207*
  in sideroblastic anemia, 186
  in thrombocyte disorders, 237–238
  polychrome stained, 174, *177*, 178
  preparation for, 24–26, *25*
Peritoneal fluid, 292–293, 356d–357d
  testing of, 309
Pernicious anemia (PA), 187, *187*, 357d, 367d
  neutropenia in, 68, *68*
  serum lactate dehydrogenase isoenzymes in, 221
  thrombocytopenia in, 236, 238
Peroxidase, in bacterial infection, 61
  in leukemia cytochemistry, 65, *65*
Personal protective equipment (PPE), 30, 357d
  for body fluid testing, 301
  for manual platelet count, 264
  for phlebotomy, 18
Personnel, *319*, 319–320, *320*
Petechiae, 232, 235, 251, 357d
  in tourniquet test, 260
Peyer's patches, lymphocytes in, 88
PF (platelet factor) assay, 268, 357d
pH, 357d
  in homeostasis, 15
  in oxygen transport, 154
  of spermatozoa, 293
Phagocytic cell(s), 357d
Phagocytosis, granulocytic function in, 60, *61*
  monocytes in, 78, *79*
Pharmacist, 319
Phase contrast microscope, 29t
Phlebotomy, 17–23, 357d
  completion of, 20–21
  equipment for, 18–20, *18–21*, 20t
  for polycythemia, 195
  in elderly patients, *21*, 21–22, 22t
  in newborns and infants, 22, *22*, *23*
  patient preparation for, 17–18, *18*

Phospholipid, platelet, 356d, 357d
  in coagulation, 246, 247, 248
Phosphotidylglycerol level, in amniotic fluid, 295
Physical examination, of cerebrospinal fluid, 285
  of seminal fluid, 293
  of serous fluid, 291
  of synovial fluid, 288
Physician, 319
Physiologic polycythemia, 222
PL (prolymphocytic leukemia), 101–102
Plaque, atherosclerotic, 237, 327d
Plasma, *6*, 6–7, 357d
  absorbed, 323d
    in coagulation testing, 272, *273*
  free, 338d
  fresh frozen, 338d
    for disseminated intravascular coagulation, 253
  ultrafiltration of, 288
Plasma cell(s), 50, 86–107, 357d. See also *Lymphocyte(s).*
  in multiple myeloma, 103
  in Waldenström's macroglobulinemia, 102
  origin, maturation, and morphology of, 88–90, *89*, *90*, 91t
  physiology and function of, *94*, 94–96
Plasma cell leukemia (PCL), 103, 357d
Plasma thromboplastin, 247t
Plasma volume, 357d
  in erythrocyte testing, 222–223
Plasma–synovial fluid glucose difference, 289
Plasminogen, 247t
  in fibrinolytic pathway, 249
Platelet(s). See also *Thrombocyte(s).*
  adhesion of, 267–268
  in hematopoiesis, 42
  in May-Hegglin anomaly, 70, *70*
  size and shape of, 10
Platelet aggregation, 233–235
  in coagulation, 250
  in manual platelet counting, 265
  testing of, 240, 268, *269*
Platelet count, 261–268
  correlation factors in, 264–265
  hemocytometer method of, 261–264, *264*
  in acute posthemorrhagic anemia, 178–179
  in complete blood count, 110
  microscopic evaluation in, 265–266
  safety precautions for, 264
  unopette dilution method of, 261, *263*
Platelet factor(s), 233, 356d
  in coagulation, 250
  in platelet aggregation, 235
Platelet factor (PF) assay, 268, 357d
Platelet index, 9, 357d
Platelet phospholipid (PPL), 356d, 357d
  in coagulation, 246, 247, 248
Platelet-poor plasma (PPP), 267, 357d
Platelet-produced protein regulator, 232
Platelet-rich plasma (PRP), 267, 268, 357d
Pleomorphism, in peritoneal fluid, 293
  in pleural fluid, 291–292
Pleural fluid, 291–292, *292*, 357d–358d
  testing of, 309
Pluripotent stem cell (PSC), 39, 358d
  in erythrocyte origination, 144
  in granulocyte origination, 54, *55*
  in lymphocyte origination, 88, *89*
  in monocyte origination, 76
  in thrombocyte origination, 230

PMN (polymorphonuclear cell), 58, 58
PNH (paroxysmal nocturnal hemoglobinuria), 188–189
  diagnostic tests for, 220–221
  fibrinolytic defects in, 254
PO. See *Partial pressure, of oxygen.*
POCT (point of care testing), 32, 313, 358d
Poikilocytosis, 358d
  in chronic posthemorrhagic anemia, 180
  in erythrocyte testing, 207
  in sickle cell anemia, 181
  in thalassemia, 185
Point of care testing (POCT), 32, 313, 358d
Poisoning, lead, 188, 188
Polarized microscope, 29t
Polychromasia, in chronic posthemorrhagic anemia, 179, 180
  in thalassemia, 184, 184
Polychromatic cell(s), 211
Polychromatophilic normoblast, 146, 147, 149, 358d
Polychrome stain, 26, 26, 27t, 358d
  of peripheral blood smear, 174, 177, 178
Polyclonal response, 93, 358d
Polycythemia, 191–194, 358d
  absolute, 11, 194
  diagnosis and treatment of, 194–195
  plasma volume in, 222
  red blood cell mass in, 222
  relative, 10–11
  thrombocytosis in, 236, 239
Polymorphonuclear cell (PMN), 58, 58. See also *Segmented neutrophil(s).*
Polypeptide chain, of hemoglobin, 160
Porphyria, 180, 185, 358d
Postanalytic phase, of clinical laboratory testing, 316
Posthemorrhagic anemia, 358d
  acute, 178–179
  chronic, 179–180, 180
Postsurgery, thrombocytosis in, 236, 239
PPE (personal protective equipment), 30, 357d
  for body fluid testing, 301
  for manual platelet count, 264
  for phlebotomy, 18
PPL (platelet phospholipid), 356d, 357d
  in coagulation, 246, 247, 248
PPP (platelet-poor plasma), 267, 357d
Preanalytic component, of clinical laboratory testing, 316
Pre-B cell, 89
Precipitation, in Ouchterlony double immunodiffusion, 131, 132
  in radial immunodiffusion, 130, 130–131
Precision, 358d
  in cell counts, 10
Prednisone, 358d–359d
  monocytopenia after, 82
Pregnancy, anemia of, 177, 326d
  fibrinolytic defects in, 254
  hemoglobinopathies and, 183–184
Prekallikrein, 246, 247t
Prenatal erythropoiesis, 142
Primary immune response, 93, 94, 95, 359d
Primary lymphoid organs, 88, 359d
Proficiency testing (PT), 31, 359d
Progenitor cell, 359d
  in hematopoiesis, 40–41
Prognosis, 359d
Progranulocyte, 56, 56, 58
Proliferation, 359d
  blood cell, cytokines in, 54, 55

Proliferation *(Continued)*
  in hematopoiesis, 39–43, 40
  lymphoid, 253, 255
  myeloid, 253, 255
Prolymphocytic leukemia (PL), 101–102
Promegakaryocyte, 230
Promonocyte, 76
Promyelocyte(s), 359d
  basophils and, 59
  eosinophils and, 58
  in acute myelogenous leukemia, 66, 66
  in acute promyelocytic leukemia, 66, 67
  morphology of, 56, 56
Promyelocytic leukemia, acute. See *Acute promyelocytic leukemia (APL).*
Pronormoblast, 146, 146, 149, 359d
Prorubricyte, 146, 146, 149
Prostate function, seminal fluid in, 293–294
Protamine sulfate test, 272
Protein(s), Bence Jones, 103
  coagulation, 246, 247t
    deficiency of, 254, 255
    testing of, 274
  fibrinogen, 6–7
  in cerebrospinal fluid, 287
  in erythrocyte regulation, 149
  in synovial fluid, 289
Protein identification and quantitation, 127–135
  electroimmunodiffusion in, 131
  electrophoresis in, 127, 128
  enzyme immunoassay in, 134–135, 135
  immunoelectrophoresis in, 127–129, 129
  immunoprecipitin tests in, 133
  Ouchterlony double immunodiffusion technique in, 131–133, 132
  radial immunodiffusion in, 129–131, 130
  radioimmunoassay in, 133–134, 134
Prothrombin, 247t
Prothrombin consumption test, 272
Prothrombin time (PT) test, 247, 359d
  in coagulation testing, 268, 270–271
  in warfarin therapy, 252
Proto-oncogene, 99, 359d
Protoporphyrin, of hemoglobin, 160–162, 161
  of zinc, 219
PRP (platelet-rich plasma), 267, 268, 357d
Prussian blue stain, 26, 27t, 346d, 359d
  in erythrocyte testing, 212
  in sideroblastic anemia, 186
PSC. See *Pluripotent stem cell (PSC).*
Pseudoanemia, 177
PT (proficiency testing), 31, 359d
PT (prothrombin time) test, 247, 359d
  in coagulation testing, 268, 270–271
  in warfarin therapy, 252
PTT (partial thromboplastin time) test, 247, 356d
  in coagulation testing, 271–272
  in hemophilia A, 251
Pure cutaneous histiocytosis, 84, 359d
Purpura, 235, 251, 359d
  idiopathic thrombocytopenic, 236, 238, 343d
  thrombotic thrombocytopenic, 236, 238, 252, 365d
Pus, 359d
  formation of, 61
Pyknotic cell, 113, 114

Quality assurance (QA), 14, 316, 359d–360d
  in clinical hematology, 30–31
Quality control (QC), 360d
  calculation of, *13*, 13–14, *14*

RA (refractory anemia), 69, 69t
RA (rheumatoid arthritis), 362d
  autoimmune hemolytic anemia in, 189
  synovial fluid in, 290
  thrombocytosis in, 236, 239
Radial immunodiffusion (RID), 360d
  in protein identification and quantitation, 129–131, *130*
Radioactive albumin, in plasma volume test, 222
Radioimmunoassay (RIA), 360d
  in body fluid testing, 308
  in platelet factor testing, 268
  in protein identification and quantitation, 133–134, *134*
Random distribution, 360d
  in cell counts, 10
Rapoport-Luebering pathway, in erythrocyte metabolism, *151*
rbc fragment, *175, 208*
RDW (red blood cell distribution width), 9, 360d, 361d
  in erythrocyte testing, 202, 203, *203*
RE (reticuloendothelial) cell(s), in autoimmune hemolytic anemia, 189
Reactive lymphocyte, 88, *90*, 360d
Reactive lymphocytosis, 97–98
Reactive monocytosis, 80, 360d
Reactive thrombocytosis, 236, 239, 360d–361d
Red blood cell(s). See *Erythrocyte(s)*.
Red blood cell count, 9, 201
  in complete blood count, 110
Red blood cell distribution width (RDW), 9, 360d, 361d
  in erythrocyte testing, 202, 203, *203*
Red blood cell mass, 222, 361d
Red blood cell survival, 222, 361d
Red marrow, 142, *144*, 361d
  hematopoiesis in, 36, 37
Reed-Sternberg cell, 104–105, *105*
Reference value(s), 361d
  for erythrocyte testing, 201
  for folate, 135
  for leukocyte testing, 110
  for lymphocytes, 97
  for serum ferritin, 216
  for serum iron, 216
  for vitamin B$_{12}$, 135
Refractory anemia (RA), 69, 69t
Relative anemia, 177, 361d
Relative cell count, 10–11, *11*
Relative lymphocytosis, 10
Relative polycythemia, 10–11
  plasma volume in, 222
Relative values, 361d
Renal disorder(s). See also *Kidney(s)*.
  hemorrhage in, 253, 255
  in polycythemia, 194
  pseudoanemia in, 177
RES (reticuloendothelial system), 74–85, 351d–352d, 361d. See also *Monocyte(s)*.
Resistance to acid elution, 184
Reticulocyte(s), 147, *148*, 149
  in pseudoanemia, 177
  stress, 147, *147*
  in erythrocyte testing, 207, *207*

Reticulocyte count, 207–212, 361d
  automated, 211
  correlation factors in, 211–212
  error in, 211
  in anemia, chronic posthemorrhagic, 179
    of chronic disease, 186
    of decreased production, 180
  light microscope method of, 210
  Miller disk procedure for, *210*, 210–211
  stains for, *207*, 207–210, *210*
Reticulocyte production index (RPI), 211–212
Reticuloendothelial (RE) cell(s), in autoimmune hemolytic anemia, 189
Reticuloendothelial system (RES), 74–85, 351d–352d, 361d. See also *Monocyte(s)*.
Revolving nosepiece, 27, *27*
Rh immune globulin (RHIg), 184
Rh negative, 183
Rh positive, 183
RhD, testing for, 215
Rheumatoid arthritis (RA), 362d
  autoimmune hemolytic anemia in, 189
  synovial fluid in, 290
  thrombocytosis in, 236, 239
RHIg (Rh immune globulin), 184
RIA (radioimmunoassay), 360d
  in body fluid testing, 308
  in platelet factor testing, 268
  in protein identification and quantitation, 133–134, *134*
Ribonucleic acid (RNA), in erythrocyte(s), *209*
Ribosome(s), hemoglobin synthesis in, 160–162, *163*
RID (radial immunodiffusion), 360d
  in protein identification and quantitation, 129–131, *130*
Right shift, in vitamin B$_{12}$ deficiency, 68, *68*
  neutrophils in, 58
Rigid cell(s), in sickle cell disease, 181
Ringed sideroblast, 362d
Ristocetin, in thrombocyte testing, 268
RNA (ribonucleic acid), in erythrocytes, *209*
Romanowsky stain, 26, *26*, 358d
  of peripheral blood smear, 174, *177*, 178
Rouleau phenomenon, in erythrocyte testing, 204
  in Waldenström's macroglobulinemia, 102, *102*, 103
RPI (reticulocyte production index), 211–212
Rubricyte, 146, *147*, 149

s^2. See *Variance*.
Safety, 29–30, *30*
  in body fluid testing, 301
  in manual platelet count, 264
  in phlebotomy, 18
Sandhoff's disease, 83, 362d
Sandwich technique, 133
Sarcoma, Kaposi's, 235, 236
Satellitism, 236, 237
  in manual platelet counting, 265
  in thrombocyte testing, 261
SBB (Sudan Black B), in leukemia cytochemistry, 65, *65*
Scanning electron microscope, 29t
Scanning objective, 27
Scattergram, 362d
  in erythrocyte testing, *203*, 204
  in leukocyte testing, 112, *113*
SCF (stem cell factor), in erythropoiesis, 143–144
  in hematopoiesis, 39–40
Schistocyte(s), *175, 177, 208*
  in thalassemia, 185
  in thrombocyte testing, 261

Schistocyte(s) *(Continued)*
   in thrombocytopenia, 238, *238*
   in thrombotic thrombocytopenic purpura, 252
Schistocytosis, 191
Screening, for sickle cell anemia, 183
Scurvy, vascular integrity in, 235, 236
SD (standard deviation), 14, 363d
Sea-blue histiocytosis, 83, 362d
Secondary immune response, 93, *94*, 95, 362d
Segmented basophil, 41–42
Segmented eosinophil, 59, *59*, 362d
Segmented neutrophil(s), 58, *58*, 362d
   Arneth count for, 123–124, *124*
   in chronic myelogenous leukemia, 64
   in granulocytic function, 60
   in meningitis, *287*
   in Pelger-Huët anomaly, 70, *71*
   in pernicious anemia, 187, *187*
   in phagocytosis, 60, *61*
   in vitamin B_{12} deficiency, 68, *68*
Seizure disorder(s), 287
Self-healing histiocytosis, 84, 362d
Seminal fluid, 293–294, *294*, 362d
   microscopic and cytologic evaluation of, 303–305, *305, 306*
   testing of, 309
Sensitivity test, antibiotic, 296
Serotonin, 235, 362d
Serous fluid, 362d
   analysis of, 291–294, *292, 294, 295*
   testing of, 309
Serum, 250, 362d
   aged, 325d
     in coagulation testing, 272, *273*
Serum ferritin, 216, 362d
Serum iron, 216, 362d
Serum lactate dehydrogenase, 362d–363d
Serum transferrin, 216, 363d
Sézary syndrome, 105, *106*, 363d
SF (synovial fluid), 364d
   analysis of, 288–290, *289, 290*
   testing of, 309
SHb. see *Sulfhemoglobin.*
Shift to left, 58, 347d, 363d
   in acute posthemorrhagic anemia, 179
   in bacterial infection, 61
   neutrophils in, 58
Shift to right, in vitamin B_{12} deficiency, 68, *68*
   neutrophils in, 58
Shilling urinary excretion test, 135–136, 363d
   in erythrocyte testing, 219
Sickle cell disease, 180–183, *181*, 363d
   screening tests for, 213
Sickled cell, *175, 180, 181*
Sideroblast(s), 362d
   in erythroleukemia, 195
Sideroblastic anemia, 186, 187t, 363d
Siderocyte, 212
Siderotic granule(s), *209*
Size, cell, 363d
   measurement of, 8–9
Skin, macrophage cells in, 76
   necrosis of, 353d
     in protein C deficiency, 254
   puncture of, in blood collection, 22, *23*
Slide, of body fluids, 307
   of cerebrospinal fluid, 286
   of seminal fluid, 305

Slide *(Continued)*
   of serous fluid, 291
   of synovial fluid, 288, 289
Slide agglutination test, in erythrocyte testing, 215–216
Smoker, polycythemia in, 194
Smudge cell(s), in chronic lymphocytic leukemia, 101, *102*
   in complete blood count, 113
Sodium citrate, in erythrocyte testing, 200
   in leukocyte testing, 110
Sodium heparin. See *Heparin.*
Sodium-potassium pump, in erythrocyte physiology, 150
Solid phase technique, 133
Solutes, in plasma, 6–7
Specimen, 363d
   for body fluid testing, 300
   for complete blood count, 200
   for leukocyte testing, 110
   for protein testing, 127
   for seminal fluid testing, 293
Sperm cell(s), 293–294, *294, 295*
   microscopic and cytologic evaluation of, 303–305, *305, 306*
Sperm count, 293
   dilution method for, 301–302, *302*
   reference values for, 303
Spherocyte(s), 174, *175, 177*, 178, 189–191, 363d
   in thalassemia, 185
   morphology of, *208*
Spherocytic anemia, hereditary, 220
Spinal column, spinal fluid in, 285
Spleen, hematopoietic activity in, 142
   lymphocytes in, 88
Splenectomy, for autoimmune hemolytic anemia, 189
   for spherocytosis, 191
   thrombocyte distribution after, 236, 239–240
Splenomegaly, in hairy cell leukemia, 104
   plasma volume in, 222
   thrombocytopenia in, 236, 239
Stab cell(s), 328d
   in acute posthemorrhagic anemia, 179
   in bacterial infection, 61
   morphology of, *57*, 57–58
Stable factor, 247t
Stage, of microscope, *27*, 28
Stain(s), acid-fast, 324d
   of body fluids, 307
     of cerebrospinal fluid, 287
   auramine-rhodamine, 327d
     of cerebrospinal fluid, 287
   cytochemical. See *Cytochemical stain.*
   Giemsa, 26, 27t. See also *Wright-Giemsa stain.*
   Gram. See *Gram stain.*
   hematology, 26, *26*, 27t
   in complete blood count, 112
   in erythrocyte testing, 212–213
   in hairy cell leukemia, 104
   in microscopic leukocyte evaluation, 119
   in sideroblastic anemia, 186
   india ink, 344d
     of cerebrospinal fluid, 287
   iron, 26, 27t, 346d
     in erythrocyte testing, 212, 216, *217*
     in sideroblastic anemia, 186
   methylene blue, 26, 27t, 351d
   monochrome, 26, 27t, 351d
     in erythrocyte testing, 212
   nonvital, 26, 27t, 354d
   of body fluids, 305–309

Stain(s) *(Continued)*
  of cerebrospinal fluid, 287
  of pericardial fluid, 292
  of peripheral blood smear, 174, *177*, 178
  of peritoneal fluid, 292
  of pleural fluid, 291
  of seminal fluid, 305
  of synovial fluid, 290
  of wound aspirates, 295
  periodic acid-Schiff, 212–213
  polychrome, 26, *26*, 27t, 358d
    of peripheral blood smear, 174, *177*, 178
  prussian blue, 26, 27t, 346d, 359d
    in erythrocyte testing, 212
    in sideroblastic anemia, 186
  Romanowsky, 26, *26*, 358d
    of peripheral blood smear, 174, *177*, 178
  tartrate-resistant acid phosphatase, 104
  vital, 26, 27t, 367d
    in iron deficiency anemia, 186
  Wright-Giemsa. See *Wright-Giemsa stain.*
Standard(s), in quality assurance, 31
Standard deviation (SD), 14, 363d
Staphylococcus aureus, 307
Starvation, plasma volume in, 222
Stem cell(s), hematopoietic. See *Hematopoietic stem cell (HSC).*
  lymphoid, 349d
    in hematopoiesis, 41
    in lymphopoiesis, 88, *89*
  pluripotent. See *Pluripotent stem cell (PSC).*
  transplantation of, in thalassemia, 185
Stem cell factor (SCF), in erythropoiesis, 143–144
  in hematopoiesis, 39–40
Stem cell pool, bone marrow, 44, *45*
Stomatocyte, *175, 208*
Storage pool, 363d
  bone marrow, 44, *45*
Storage pool disease, 241, 339d, 363d, 365d
Streptococcus pneumonia, 307
Streptokinase, in fibrinolytic pathway, 249
Stress erythropoiesis, 176
  in chronic posthemorrhagic anemia, 180, *180*
Stress reticulocyte(s), 147, *147*
  in erythrocyte testing, 207, *207*
Stuart-Prower factor, 247t, 248
Subarachnoid hemorrhage, 285
Subarachnoid space, 285
Substage condenser, of microscope, *27, 28*
Sucrose hemolysis test, 363d
  in erythrocyte testing, 220–221
Sudan Black B (SBB), in leukemia cytochemistry, 65, *65*
Sugar water test, 363d
  in erythrocyte testing, 220–221
Sulfhemoglobin, 154, 168, 363d–364d
Surgery, thrombocytosis after, 236, 239
Synovial fluid (SF), 364d
  analysis of, 288–290, *289, 290*
  testing of, 309
Synoviocyte, 289, *290*
Synthesis, hemoglobin, 160–163, *161–163*, 168–169
Systemic, 364d
Systemic fibrinolysis, 253, 255

T cell(s), 364d
  helper, 90, 90t, 329d–330d, 364d
    in humoral immunity, 95

T cell(s) *(Continued)*
    to T suppressor cells ratio, 96, 97
  in hematopoiesis, 42
  memory, 91, 364d
  origin of, 88–89, *89*, 91t
  physiology and function of, 90–94, 91t, *93, 94*
  suppressor, 90, 330d
    ratio of T helper to, 96, 97
Target cell(s), *175, 208*
  in hemoglobinopathies, 181, *181*
  in liver disease, 188, *188*
  in sickle cell anemia, 181
  in thalassemia, 184
Tart cell, 71
Tartrate-resistant acid phosphatase (TRAP) stain, 104
Tay-Sachs disease, 83, 364d
T_c (cytotoxic T) cell, 90, 333d
T-cell leukemia, classification of, 64t
  cytochemistry of, 67t
  malignant lymphocytosis in, 100, *100*
T-cell lymphoma, 105, *106*
Teardrop cell, *175, 208*
Technicon scattergram, in complete blood count, *113*
Telangiectasia, 364d
  vascular integrity in, 235, 236
Temperature, 364d
  in complete blood count, 112, 200
  in homeostasis, 15–16
Terminology, 7–8, 364d
T_h (T helper) cell(s), in humoral immunity, 95
  to T suppressor cells ratio, 96, 97
Thalassemia, 180, 184–185, *185*, 364d
Therapeutic phlebotomy, for polycythemia, 195
Thoracentesis, 291
Thoracic cavity, serous fluid in, 291
Thrombasthenia, 235, 240, 364d–365d
Thrombin, in coagulation, 246, 250
  in thrombocyte activation, 233
  in thrombocyte testing, 268
Thrombin time (TT) test, 249, 365d
  in coagulation testing, 268
Thrombocyte(s), 6, *6*, 228–243, 365d
  abnormal distribution of, 236, 239–240
  abnormal function of, 240–241
  adhesion of, 232
    evaluation of, 267–268
  aggregation of, 233–235
    in coagulation, 250
    in manual platelet counting, 265
    testing of, 240, 268, *269*
  general information on, 242
  hereditary disorders of, 236, 240–241
  in thrombocytopenia, 237–239, *238*
  in thrombocytosis, *239*, 239–240
  in vascular integrity, 231–232
  loss of, *234*, 235–237, *237*
  indices of, 12
  origin, maturation, and morphology of, 230–232, *231–233*
  physiology and function of, 233–235, *234*
  size of, 7, 363d
  storage pool disease of, 241, 339d, 363d, 365d
  testing of, 261–268, 365d
    aggregation studies in, 268
    bleeding time test in, 266, *267*
    clot retraction in, 266–267
    complete blood count in, 261, *262, 263*
    glass bead retention test in, 267–268

Thrombocyte(s) *(Continued)*
　　manual platelet count in, 261–268. See also *Platelet count.*
　　platelet factor assays in, 268
　　platelet-poor plasma in, 267
　　platelet-rich plasma in, 267
Thrombocyte count, 9
　　in acute posthemorrhagic anemia, 178–179
　　in thrombocyte disorders, 237
Thrombocyte index, 9
Thrombocyte-aggregating agent(s), 365d
Thrombocythemia, 365d
　　essential, 236, 239, 336d
Thrombocytopenia, 236, 237–239, *238,* 365d
　　coagulation in, 252
Thrombocytosis, 236, *239,* 239–240, 365d
　　reactive, 236, 239, 360d–361d
Thromboplastin, plasma, 247t
　　tissue, 246, 247, 247t
Thromboplastin generation time test, 272
Thrombopoietin-like factor (TPO), 230
Thrombosis, deep vein, 253–254, 255, 334d
　　disseminated, 253
Thrombotic coagulopathy, 251, 253–255, 365d
Thrombotic thrombocytopenic purpura (TTP), 236, 238, 252, 365d
Thromboxane A$_2$, 233, 365d
Thrombus, 331d, 365d. See also *Clot.*
Thymus gland, 365d
　　in lymphopoiesis, 88, *89*
TIBC (total iron-binding capacity), 216, 365d
　　in anemia, 185–186
Tissue mast cell, basophil and, 59–60
Tissue plasminogen activator (tPA), 249
Tissue thromboplastin, 246, 247, 247t
TNF (tumor necrosis factor), 366d
　　in erythrocyte function, 149
Tonsils, lymphocytes in, 88
Total cell count, in cerebrospinal fluid, 286
　　in synovial fluid, 288
　　of white blood cells, 110
Total iron-binding capacity (TIBC), 216, 365d
　　in anemia, 185–186
Total quality management (TQM), 31, 365d
Tourniquet, 365d
　　for phlebotomy, 19, *19*
　　vascular integrity and, 232
Tourniquet test, 260
Toxic granulation, 61, *62,* 365d–366d
Toxicity, bone marrow, 180
Toxin(s), hemorrhagic disorders and, 253, 255
　　phagocytosis of, 60, *61*
tPA (tissue plasminogen activator), 249
TPO (thrombopoietin-like factor), 230
TQM (total quality management), 31, 365d
Transferrin, 366d
　　in heme catabolism, 162
　　in hemoglobin kinetics, 163–165
　　in iron transport, 185
　　serum, 216, 363d
Transferrin saturation, 366d
　　in erythrocyte testing, 216
Transfusion(s), for sickle cell disease, 181
　　for sideroblastic anemia, 186
　　for thalassemia, 185
　　massive, thrombocytopenia in, 236, 239
Transfusion-acquired hepatitis, 98
Transmission electron microscope, 29t

Transplantation, of stem cells, 185
Transudate, 291, 366d
TRAP (tartrate-resistant acid phosphatase) stain, 104
Trauma, intravascular hemolysis in, 188
　　thrombocytosis in, 236, 239
True polycythemia, 222
T$_s$ (T suppressor) cell(s), 90
　　ratio of T helper to, 96, 97
TT (thrombin time) test, 249, 365d
　　in coagulation testing, 268
TTP (thrombotic thrombocytopenic purpura), 236, 238, 252, 365d
Tube, for phlebotomy, 20, 20t, *21*
Tuberculosis, monocytosis in, 80
Tumor(s), in polycythemia, 194
　　peritoneal fluid in, 292
　　pleural fluid in, 291–292, *292*
　　vascular, 235, 236
Tumor necrosis factor (TNF), 366d
　　in erythrocyte function, 149
Turbidimetric immunoprecipitin assay, 133, 366d
Turbidity, of body fluids, 300
　　of synovial fluid, 288

Ultrafiltration, of plasma, 288
Universal precautions (UP), 30, 366d
Unopette, 366d
Unopette dilution method, for body fluid cell count, 301–302, *302*
　　for manual leukocyte counts, 116–117, *117*
　　for manual platelet count, 261, *263*
UP (universal precautions), 30, 366d
Uremia, 366d
　　platelet dysfunction in, 241
Uric acid, in synovial fluid, 288, 289
Urinalysis, in porphyria, 185
Urinary excretion test, 135–136, 363d
　　in erythrocyte testing, 219
Urine, 294
　　excretion of protoporphyrin in, 185
　　free hemoglobin in, in autoimmune hemolytic anemia, 189
Urine hemoglobin, 338d
　　in erythrocyte testing, 218
Uterus, amniotic fluid in, 294–295

Vacuolation, 366d
Vacuole, in phagocytosis, 60, *61*
　　of monocyte, 76, *78*
Vacuum tube, 366d
　　for phlebotomy, 20, 20t, *21*
Validation, 316–318
Variance, 14, 366d
Variation, coefficient of, 14, 332d
Vascular disorder(s), fibrinolytic defects in, 254
Vascular integrity, 231–232, 366d
　　loss of, *234,* 235–237, *237,* 251
　　vitamins in, 16
Vascular malignancy, vascular integrity in, 235, 236
Vascular testing and evaluation, 260
Vasculature, 231–232
　　physiology and function of, 233–235, *234*
Vasoconstriction, *234,* 235
Vein(s), 231

Venipuncture sites, 18, *18*
Venipuncture tube, 366d
  for phlebotomy, 20, 20t, *21*
Venous blood gas analysis, 156
Venule(s), 231
Verification, 318, 366d–367d
Viability, of sperm cells, 293
Viral hepatitis, 216
Viral infection, 367d
  autoimmune hemolytic anemia in, 189
  bone marrow toxicity from, 180
  cerebrospinal fluid in, 286
  complete blood count in, 112
  in leukemia, 63, 79
  in lymphoma, 99
  lymphocytes in, 88, 91t
  natural killer cells in, 96
Viral meningitis, 286
Viscosity, of body fluids, 300–301
  of cerebrospinal fluid, 285
  of seminal fluid, 293
  of synovial fluid, 288
Vital stain, 26, 27t, 367d
  in iron deficiency anemia, 186
Vitamin(s), 367d
  identification and quantitation of, 135–136
  in homeostasis, 16–17
Vitamin B$_{12}$, deficiency of, 367d
    anemia in, 187, *187*
    neutropenia in, 68, *68*
    serum lactate dehydrogenase isoenzymes in, 221
    thrombocytopenia in, 236, 238
  identification and quantitation of, 135
  in erythrocyte testing, 219
  in homeostasis, 16
  normal reference range for, 135
Vitamin C, deficiency of, 235, 236
  in homeostasis, 16
Vitamin K, deficiency of, 367d
    hemorrhagic disorders in, 252, 255
  in homeostasis, 16–17
Volume, of body fluids, 300
von Willebrand factor (vWF), 233, 246
von Willebrand's disease, 240, 367d
vWF (von Willebrand factor), 233, 246

Waldenström's macroglobulinemia, 102, 367d
Warfarin (Coumadin), 333d, 367d
  coagulation pathway and, 247
  in protein C deficiency, 254
  in vitamin K deficiency, 252
  prothrombin time test monitoring of, 271
WB (whole blood), 6, *6*, 39, 367d–368d
  composition of, 10

Westergren method, for erythrocyte sedimentation rate, *221*, 222
Westgard multirule technique, 13, 367d
Wet preparation, of seminal fluid, 303–305
  of synovial fluid, 288–289
White blood cell(s). See also *Leukocyte(s)*.
  in erythrocyte evaluation, 207
  in fetus, 54, *54*
  in leukocyte testing, 125–127
  May-Hegglin anomaly in, 70, *70*
  production of, 50
White blood cell count, in chronic myelogenous leukemia, 64
  in infectious mononucleosis, 97
  in leukemia, 63
  total, 110
White clots, 252
White marrow, 142, 367d
  hematopoiesis in, 36
Whole blood (WB), 6, *6*, 39, 367d–368d
  composition of, 10
Winged needle apparatus, in phlebotomy, *21*, 21–22
Wintrobe method, for erythrocyte sedimentation rate, *221*, 222
The Working Formulation of Non-Hodgkin's Lymphoma for Clinical Use, 105, 105t
Wound aspirate analysis, 295–296
Wright-Giemsa stain, 26, *26*, 27t, 368d
  in erythrocyte testing, 207, *207*
  in microscopic leukocyte evaluation, 119
  of body fluids, 305
  of pericardial fluid, 292
  of peripheral blood smear, 174, *177*, 178, 186
  of peritoneal fluid, 292
  of pleural fluid, 291
  of seminal fluid, 305

Xanthochromic cerebrospinal fluid, 285

Yellow marrow, 142
Yolk sac, 368d
  hematopoiesis in, 36, *38*

Zinc, in erythrocyte testing, 219
  in homeostasis, 17
  in seminal fluid, 293–294